Elements of Paediatric Physiotherapy

Illustrator: Robert Britton

For Churchill Livingstone

Publisher: Mary Law
Project Development Editor: Mairi McCubbin
Copy Editor: Eleanor Flood
Production Controller: Mark Sanderson
Sales Promotion Executive: Hilary Brown

Elements of Paediatric Physiotherapy

Edited by

Pamela M. Eckersley BA MCSP

CHURCHILL LIVINGSTONE
EDINBURGH LONDON MADRID MELBOURNE NEW YORK AND TOKYO 1993

CHURCHILL LIVINGSTONE
Medical Division of Longman Group UK Limited

Distributed in the United States of America by Churchill
Livingstone Inc., 650 Avenue of the Americas, New York,
N.Y. 10011, and by associated companies, branches and
representatives throughout the world.

First published 1993

ISBN 0 443 03894 5

British Library Cataloguing in Publication Data
A catalogue record for this book is available from the
British Library.

Library of Congress Cataloging in Publication Data
Elements of paediatric physiotherapy/edited by Pamela
   M. Eckersley.
      p. cm.
   Includes index.
   1. Physical therapy for children. I. Eckersley,
Pamela M. (Pamela Margaret)
   [DNLM: 1. Physical Therapy — in infancy &
childhood. WS 366 E38]
RJ53.P5E44   1992
618.92′0062 — dc20
DNLM/DLC
for Library of Congress   91–47869

Produced by Longman Singapore Publishers Pte Ltd
Printed in Singapore

The
publisher's
policy is to use
**paper manufactured
from sustainable forests**

Preface

Working with children and parents adds a new perspective to standard physiotherapy practice. Children are not just small adults. The therapist needs an understanding of both child development and the experiences of childhood, as well as a knowledge of the nature of children's diseases and disabilities and of relevant physiotherapeutic intervention.

The physiotherapist entering paediatrics needs a grounding in all areas of clinical practice. He or she must also understand the roles of co-workers and the importance of working in partnership with parents, and be aware of relevant child-care legislation. Most of all, he or she needs to see the child first, and the child with problems second.

This book aims to provide both the theoretical and the practical information needed by the pacdiatric physiotherapist in any setting. It is intended primarily for three groups:

* student physiotherapists and physiotherapists who are beginning a paediatric placement
* physiotherapists who have entered the specialism of paediatrics
* physiotherapy teachers and course tutors.

It is also hoped that teachers, nurses, parents and other colleagues will find the book a helpful introduction to the field.

Approaches to therapy intervention are presented separately from the problems and disorders of childhood. This is to encourage development of treatment strategies related to the particular needs and skills of the child, rather than to the condition the child is experiencing.

The book is divided into five sections:

SECTION 1: THE PHYSIOTHERAPIST IN PAEDIATRICS details the history of the specialism and explores the roles and responsibilities of clinical practice.

SECTION 2: CHILD DEVELOPMENT first provides a genetic and embryological background, then covers the motor, cognitive and social development of the child. Practices in child health relating to promotion of general health, early identification through screening and routine developmental assessments, and the prevention of disease and disability are then discussed.

SECTION 3: PROBLEMS AND DISORDERS IN CHILDHOOD covers those conditions, diseases and disabilities that the paediatric physiotherapist meets. Respiratory, cardiac, neurological, neuromuscular and orthopaedic conditions are included. There are also chapters on sensory disorders and on learning and behavioural problems. The subject of non-accidental injury and child abuse is introduced.

SECTION 4: PHYSIOTHERAPY IN PRACTICE looks at the systems and methods of therapy available to the clinician. It begins with an outline of common assessment procedures, and goes on to describe a broad range of treatment approaches, physical activities and philosophies of management. Individual learning programmes, activities of daily living and the use of aids and appliances are included, ending with a chapter on Planning for Progress.

SECTION 5: ALLIES IN THE PROVISION OF SERVICES explores the concept of the paediatric physiotherapist as a member of a team and highlights the importance of working towards a common objective. The perspective of the parent is emphasised throughout this section, which ends by examining current child-related health, education and social service legislation.

An APPENDIX lists Voluntary and Statutory Resources.

GLOSSARIES of Physiotherapy Terms, and of Syndromes and Genetic Disorders are also included.

Finally, I would like to thank each of the contributors to this multi-author book. They come from a wide range of clinical and professional backgrounds, and are all experienced in their particular fields. In editing, I have aimed at a common style of presentation throughout so that the reader can move easily from one section to another, and hope that the individual perspective of each contributor has been retained. I hope also that the book will encourage physiotherapists to explore the field of paediatrics and to develop their own experience and understanding of working with children.

September 1993   Pamela M. Eckersley

Editor's note

For ease of reading, the term 'he' has been used throughout to refer to children. This should not be taken to imply that all patients are male, nor conversely that all physiotherapists are female.

Contributors

Pamela M. Eckersley BA MCSP

Director, Special Education Resource Information Service
(SERIS), Manchester City Council Education Committee,
Manchester, UK; Former Paediatric Superintendent
Physiotherapist, South Manchester Health Authority,
Manchester, UK

13   *Thermal injuries*
16   *Section on 'The clumsy child'*
18   *Treatment systems*
19   *Sections on 'Exercise and activity' and 'Hydrotherapy'*
22   *Planning for progress*
25   *Legal aspects in paediatric physiotherapy*

Geoff Bardsley BEng PhD

Senior Rehabilitation Engineer, Tayside Rehabilitation
Engineering Services, Dundee Limb Fitting Centre,
Dundee, UK

21   *Section on 'Seating'*

Veronica M. Bastow MSc MCSP

Senior Paediatric Physiotherapist, Queen Elizabeth
Hospital, King's Lynn, Norfolk, UK

7   *Respiratory conditions and cardiothoracic disorders*
17   *Section on 'Respiratory function'*
19   *Section on 'Respiratory therapy'*

Roger Bates
Teacher's Certificate

Director, Northern ACE Centre (Aids to Communication
in Education), Oldham, UK

20   *Section on 'Computer technology'*

Stuart M. Bedford BA MCSP

Former Superintendent Paediatric Physiotherapist, North
Staffordshire Health Authority, UK

4   *The developing child*
8   *Section on 'Cerebral palsy and spina bifida'*

Elma J. Bell MCSP

Private Practice. Former Head Physiotherapist and
Coordinator of Therapy Services, The Scottish Council of
Spastics (Eastern Region), Edinburgh, UK

10   *Section on 'Posture and deformity'*
19   *Section on 'Hydrotherapy'*
19   *Section on 'Vibration therapy'*

Mary Pamela Clegg DipPhys MCSP SRP

Superintendent 1, Paediatric Physiotherapy Services,
Leicestershire, UK; Course Director, Birmingham
Polytechnic, Birmingham, UK

9   *Developmental delay*
17   *Section on 'Development'*

W. J. K. Cumming BSc MD FRCPI FRCP

Consultant Neurologist and Honorary Lecturer in
Medicine and Cell and Structural Biology, University
Hospitals of South Manchester, Manchester, UK

11   *Neuromuscular Disorders*

Dian Donnai MBBS FRCP DCH DObstRCOG

Consultant Clinical Geneticist, Regional Genetics Service,
St Mary's Hospital, Manchester, UK

3   *Section on 'Genetics'*

Peggy Freeman MBE
Diploma for Teachers of Handicapped Children

Founder and Vice-President, National Deafblind and
Rubella Association

14   *Sensory disorders*

Margaret I. Griffiths MD FRCP

Former Consultant Paediatrician (West Midlands), UK;
Honorary Research Fellow, University of Birmingham,
UK; Member Emeritus, American Academy of Cerebral
Palsy and Developmental Medicine

5   Practices in child health
13   Section on 'Accidental injury and child abuse'

Ann M. D. Grimley

District Physiotherapist, Preston Health Authority, Preston, Lancashire, UK; Former Paediatric Superintendent Physiotherapist, Royal Manchester Children's Hospital, Pendlebury, Manchester, UK

1   A historical perspective
2   Roles and responsibilities
24   Team workers

Gay Hall DipCOT SROT

Head Occupational Therapist, Paediatric and Mental Handicap Services, Preston District Health Authority, Preston, UK

20   Section on 'Dressing and toileting'

Patricia Hartley PhD BA(Hons) BA(Gen) CertEd CertCounselling AFBPsS CPsychol

Reader in Health Studies, Centre for Health Studies, University College Salford, Manchester, UK

23   Parents and children

Margaret Jones GradDipPhys MCSP SRP

Former Superintendent Paediatric Physiotherapist, Burnley General Hospital, Lancashire, UK

17   Section on 'Gait'
19   Section on 'Serial splinting and strapping'
21   Section on 'Orthoses, footwear and bracing'

Lauren Kerzin-Storrar BA MSc

Genetic Associate, Regional Genetic Service, St Mary's Hospital, Manchester, UK

3   Section on 'Genetics'

Linda M. King MSc GradDipPhys MCSP CertEd DipTP FETC ONC

Senior Lecturer in Physiotherapy, University College Salford, UK

17   Section on 'Tone'
18   Treatment systems

Jeanne E. Lamond MCSP

Former Superintendent Physiotherapist — Mental Handicap, Lancaster Health Authority, UK

10   Section on 'Behaviour, self-help and reality'

T. G. Marshall MB ChB MRCP

Consultant Paediatrician, Royal Hospital for Sick Children, Edinburgh, UK

13   Section on 'Infection in babies and children'

Ian McKinlay BSc(Hons) MB ChB DCH FRCP (Lond.)

Senior Lecturer in Community Child Health, University of Manchester, Royal Manchester Children's Hospital, Manchester, UK

8   Section on 'The epilepsies'

Kathleen Newton BLing DipCST MCST

Senior Lecturer in Speech Pathology and Therapy, Department of Psychology and Speech Pathology, Manchester Polytechnic, Manchester, UK

20   Section on 'Feeding'

Annette Parker MCSP

Superintendent Physiotherapist, King's College Hospital, London, UK

6   Neonatal problems and the neonatal unit

Patricia M. Pott GradDipPhys MCSP

Senior 1 Physiotherapist, Community Paediatrics, Lancasterian School, Manchester, UK

20   Section on 'Feeding'

James E. Robb BSc(Hons) FRCS

Consultant Orthopaedic Surgeon, Princess Margaret Rose Hospital, Edinburgh, UK

12   Orthopaedic aspects of childhood disorders

Sue Steel MEd (Special Education)

Deputy Head Teacher, Lancasterian School, Manchester, UK

16   Section on 'Behavioural barriers to learning'
19   Section on 'Individual learning programmes'

Peter Wigmore BSc PhD

Lecturer, Department of Biomedical Sciences, Marischal College, University of Aberdeen, UK

3   Section on 'Embryology'

James Edmond Wraith MB ChB MRCP

Consultant Paediatrician, Willink Biochemical Genetics Unit, Royal Manchester Children's Hospital, Manchester, UK

15   Inborn errors of metabolism

Contents

The history and growth of the Chartered Society of Physiotherapy are outlined in Chapter 1, along with the development of a philosophy and body of knowledge specific to the paediatric field. Chapter 2 explores the roles and responsibilities of clinical practice and the professional and personal skills of the paediatric physiotherapist.

SECTION 1
The physiotherapist in paediatrics

1

A historical perspective

A. M. D. Grimley

INTRODUCTION

Physiotherapists in the field of paediatric practice are members of a health care team concerned with children from birth through to adulthood. They practise at all three levels of health care:

- primary
- secondary
- tertiary

within the medical, educational, social and community fields of child care.

Primary health care services are at the frontline of all health services to all people (HMSO 1986). They comprise the Family Practitioner Services and Community Health Services provided outside a hospital by family doctors, dentists, retail pharmacists, opticians, community nurses, midwives, health visitors and members of the professions allied to medicine and speech therapy.

Secondary health care is provided by a doctor or other health professional to whom the primary health care worker has referred the patient. Referrals may be for investigations, treatment or direct care. In the UK referrals are most often by general practitioners to NHS hospital consultants.

Tertiary health care is usually provided by specialised health care workers at the request of a secondary health care professional (Fig. 1.1).

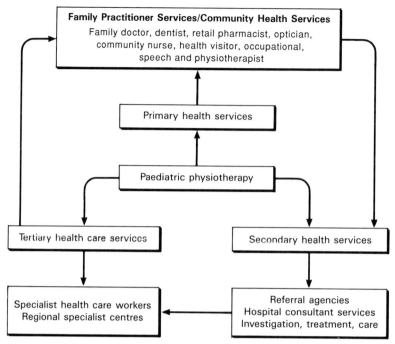

Fig. 1.1 Health care services.

Paediatric physiotherapists working in each of these sectors have a professional responsibility to meet both individual and statutory needs of children within the parameters of professional practice. The scope of that professional practice is determined in the United Kingdom by the Chartered Society of Physiotherapy (CSP).

This chapter outlines the history and growth of the Chartered Society of Physiotherapy and the development of a philosophy and body of knowledge specific to work in the field of paediatrics.

A HISTORY OF THE PHYSIOTHERAPY PROFESSION

The Chartered Society of Physiotherapy (CSP) is the educational, professional and trade union organisation for Britain's chartered physiotherapists (CSP 1990). It is also the professional body that defines the core curriculum for initial training, scope of practice and ethical standards. The CSP validates postbasic training, and itself organises various workshops and courses. It also provides a director of education to coordinate

and support postgraduate education and research activities. Assistance is given to individual members, to clinical interest groups and to colleges of further and higher education in course planning and validation.

Historical background

In 1894 the Society of Trained Masseuses was founded by four nurses: Lucy Marianne Robinson, Rosalind Paget, Elizabeth Anne Manley and Margaret Dora Palmer. All were trained in massage and 'medical rubbing'. They aimed to make massage a reputable profession within the framework of medicine and stipulated the need for good professional habits and training. Regular examinations were held to maintain high standards and rules of conduct were published and circulated to medical professionals and their organisations.

In 1900 membership reached 250 and the parent society acquired the legal and public status of a professional organisation and became the Incorporated Society of Trained Masseuses.

This parent society amalgamated in 1920 with

the Manchester Institute of Massage and Remedial Gymnastics to become the Chartered Society of Massage and Medical Gymnastics. By 1930 the Society had its own journal, teachers' certificates and examinations in massage, medical gymnastics, light and electrotherapy.

New qualifying exams were continually being introduced and, in 1942, the Society adopted its present name, The Chartered Society of Physiotherapy.

The Faculty of Physiotherapists and the Physiotherapy Association Ltd amalgamated with the CSP in 1968 and 1970, respectively, and the Society of Remedial Gymnasts merged with the CSP in 1985. Current membership of the CSP stands at 24 500 (March 1991).

THE DEVELOPMENT OF PAEDIATRIC PHYSIOTHERAPY

In the archives of the Royal Manchester Children's Hospital (RMCH) Louis Borchardt (RMCH 1857) stated that objectives of medicine with children were not only cure but prevention of disease and its processes. He also advocated:

'diet and infantile gymnastics to promote digestion, strengthen muscles, assist development, quicken the circulation, deepen respiration and to enliven the spirit' (RMCH 1862).

In the same archives (RMCH 1891) there are requests for qualified nurses accustomed to the treatment and nursing of children. Skilled nurses in the dispensary were said to be invaluable, particularly in the application of splints and surgical appliances.

Early twentieth century developments

The early part of the twentieth century saw a growing interest in the use of electrotherapy and remedial exercise. Massage, breathing and remedial exercises, splinting and applications of artificial sunlight were the modalities in main use with children at that time.

In 1914 massage, Swedish drill and gymnastics were reported to play an important part in the treatment of certain diseases of children, and in 1921 the same hospital archives state that:

'effective treatment of a diseased condition of childhood implies not only the saving of life in some cases, the immediate relief of suffering in others, the prevention of deformity and crippling in yet others but it also gives the firm assurance of a proportionate diminution in the amount of sickness and disability among the adults of the future' (RMCH 1914–1921).

Rickets, bronchiectasis, whooping cough, skin diseases, fractures, deformities (congenital and acquired), poliomyelitis, osteomyelitis and tuberculosis (of the chest, spine and joints) were amongst the conditions treated by CSP members in hospitals, clinics and dispensaries throughout the country up to the middle of this century. Treatments were ordered by the doctor (usually an orthopaedic surgeon or public health clinic doctor) and were mainly massage, splinting, stretching, exercising and postural drainage for children with chronic respiratory disorders.

Up to the Second World War, and until the widespread use of antibiotics and improvements in nutrition and social conditions, physiotherapists worked mainly for medical, orthopaedic and skin specialists (CSP 1990).

Modern developments

With the advances of modern medicine, surgery, obstetric and special care, the therapist of the late 1950s and early 1960s began to be faced with increasing numbers of neurologically damaged and surviving sick or frail children, including those with cerebral palsy, postmeningitis, haemophilia, spina bifida, hydrocephalus, cystic fibrosis and oncological, metabolic, neuromuscular and genetically determined diseases. The importance of using physiotherapeutic skills, knowledge and attitudes for assessment, problem-solving and management of children with minimal or perceptuomotor difficulties and severe learning difficulties became increasingly recognised.

There has been gradual acceptance by paediatricians, neurologists, psychologists and teachers of the need to include the paediatric physiotherapist in the child development and assessment centre care teams (Barton & Grimley 1977). Similarly, paediatric physiotherapists are now numbered amongst essential members of most clinical specialist child care teams in hospital and community.

The Association of Paediatric Chartered Physiotherapists (APCP)

In 1973 a group of chartered physiotherapists working in the Midlands invited all UK colleagues to come together for peer support and to advance the profession in paediatric practice. They formed the Association of Paediatric Chartered Physiotherapists (APCP), a clinical interest group of the CSP.

They believed that basic professional education, training and general experience provides a firm foundation upon which to acquire postgraduate specialist clinical knowledge, abilities in problem identification and resolution, and team membership skills.

The APCP's objectives were, and are, to:

1 Improve the training, education and professional status of its members.
2 Promote and advance a curriculum for the obtaining of post-registration qualifications.

In 1984 the first CSP-validated post-qualification course, 'An Introduction to Paediatric Physiotherapy', was held in Salford, Greater Manchester. This formed the basis, in 1991, for the Certificate in Paediatric Physiotherapy (Advanced) at Birmingham Polytechnic.

National APCP Conferences are now held throughout the UK each year. A quarterly journal and many regional and local workshops, courses and education activities have contributed to meeting the objectives of the association. In 1990 APCP published guidelines for good practice as a basis for acceptable practice from which further measurable standards may be developed (Dunn et al 1990). The APCP maintains a register of chartered physiotherapists engaged in the practice of physical therapy in paediatrics, with 1700 members registered in December 1990. In addition, associate membership is welcomed by professionals working in the field of paediatrics, and includes occupational therapists, speech therapists and doctors.

THE PHILOSOPHY OF PAEDIATRIC PHYSIOTHERAPY

The principles, ethical parameters and objectives of the CSP founders remain constant, although the scope, practice and method of service delivery of chartered physiotherapists in paediatrics may have changed and developed over the years. The paediatric physiotherapist is involved in the management of children with physical and learning difficulties; the acutely and chronically ill child; those with severe learning difficulties; and children sustaining injury or with joint and soft tissue problems. This involvement may extend from birth to school leaving age. Working closely with the family, the physiotherapist aims to encourage the child to the best of his ability in order to lead the fullest life possible (Dunn et al 1990).

The APCP recognises that the work of therapists with children is not confined to the traditional image of 'hands on' activities with hospitalised sick children nor those in special educational or care establishments. Members have examined their extended role and realise they have to accommodate to the constantly changing statutes, clinical needs and roles demanded of them by the law, children themselves, their families and other agents of the child centred multiprofessional team (see Chapter 2). It is stated (APCP 1990) that practitioners need:

• a sound base of core skills
• an appreciation of the needs of both parent and child
• an ability to establish empathetic relationships
• to be professional
• to communicate effectively
• to work harmoniously with other professionals
• to continue to learn and to develop their skills.

Skills and knowledge

To work successfully with children, families, educationalists, medical and nursing colleagues, or social and voluntary care workers, paediatric physiotherapists have themselves specified that they require not only a knowledge of normal child development, specific clinical knowledge and skills but also enhanced interpersonal skills as communicators, educators, skill sharers and counsellors.

The skills and knowledge needed by therapists are summarised in the following statements:

1 Specialist skills must be built onto a firm foundation.
2 Learning is a continuous process, therefore knowledge and skills must be regularly updated.
3 Knowledge of normal child development is necessary so that deviations can be recognised.
4 Knowledge of pathologies plus the theories, philosophies and treatment modalities available to manage childhood disorders.
5 A variety of handling skills must be acquired and refined.
6 Knowledge of specialist equipment is essential.
7 Statutory obligations must be understood.
8 Counselling skills should be acquired.
9 Confidentiality is paramount. (Dunn et al 1990)

Working with parents

Paediatric physical therapists are members of multiprofessional teams aiming to meet the personal, clinical and statutory needs of a child. This team will include parents and the child itself whenever possible to identify and to meet the needs and choices of each individual child.

Physiotherapists also need to be aware of social, environmental and cultural variables which influence family structure, dynamics and motivation. They will need to recognise and empathise with parents who choose alternative patterns of clinical therapies that may not coincide with the therapist's own skills or chosen mode of treatment. This can give an opportunity for each physiotherapist to examine their own practice, its strengths, weaknesses, and to identify gaps in service delivery.

Joint service planning

In the UK, Health and Local Authority joint service planning underpins the development and facilitation by the various professionals of services for children. This planning should include physiotherapy as well as parental or consumer representation. The bringing of direct medical care close to individual people includes preventative medicine, professional cooperation and participation of the patients in diagnostic and decision-making activities concerning their care and the health care in their community.

Objective (iv) of the APCP states that the Association aims to improve communications and understanding between various authorities, e.g. hospital and local and other authorities responsible for paediatric physiotherapy. Health Care is best provided when family doctors, community nurses, practice nurses and therapists work together as members of a local health care team (Dunn et al 1990).

Conclusion

Physiotherapists should remember that constant evaluation of practice is essential and that research is needed to extend knowledge and skills. This takes place within a framework of:

1 The parameters of professional practice identified by the Chartered Society of Physiotherapy.
2 Statutory legal instruments, such as the 1981 Education Act and the 1990 Children Act (see Chapter 25 Legal Aspects).
3 The rights of the child.

The paediatric physiotherapist has a professional duty to meet established standards of practice and to continually update knowledge and skills. In this way competency in practice is ensured and allied to the continued development of paediatrics as a specialism within physiotherapy.

REFERENCES

Barton M, Grimley A M D 1977 Setting up an assessment unit. APCP/CSP, London

Chartered Society of Physiotherapy 1990a Physiotherapy taking care of you and your family: Promotional literature. CSP, London

Chartered Society of Physiotherapy 1990b The history of the Chartered Society of Physiotherapy: Promotional literature. CSP, London

Dunn C L, Williams V, Young C S 1990 Paediatric physiotherapy — guidelines to good practice. APCP/CSP, London

HMSO 1986 Primary health care. HMSO, London

Royal Manchester Children's Hospital 1857, 1862, 1891, 1914, 1921 Annual reports. RMCH, Manchester

FURTHER READING

Court Report 1986 Report of the Committee on Child Health Services: Fit for the future. HMSO, London

NHS Act 1977 HMSO London

United Nations 1971 Declaration of general and special rights of the mentally handicapped. Department of Social Affairs, New York

World Health Organization 1986 Charter for health promotion. WHO, Geneva

2

Roles and responsibilities

A. M. D. Grimley

INTRODUCTION

Physiotherapy is defined as

a systematic method of assessing musculoskeletal, cardiovascular, respiratory and neurological disorders of function, including pain and those of psychosomatic origin and of dealing with or preventing those problems by natural methods based essentially on movement, manual therapy and physical agencies' (Trent Regional Health Authority 1989).

ROLE OF THE PAEDIATRIC PHYSIOTHERAPIST

The physiotherapist in paediatric practice applies physiotherapy skills and knowledge to the assessment, design, delivery and evaluation of physiotherapeutic treatments in the management of neonates, babies, children and adolescents with a range of problems. Such clients may have acute or chronic conditions of sickness, disability or handicap. They may have physical, mental, developmental, learning or emotional disorders with concomitant clinical, educational, family and social problems and needs.

Paediatric physiotherapists work in hospital wards and departments; clinics; health centres; child assessment and support units; nurseries; preschool, special and mainstream school premises and in the child's home. They work closely with family members and with members of the health care, social and education teams.

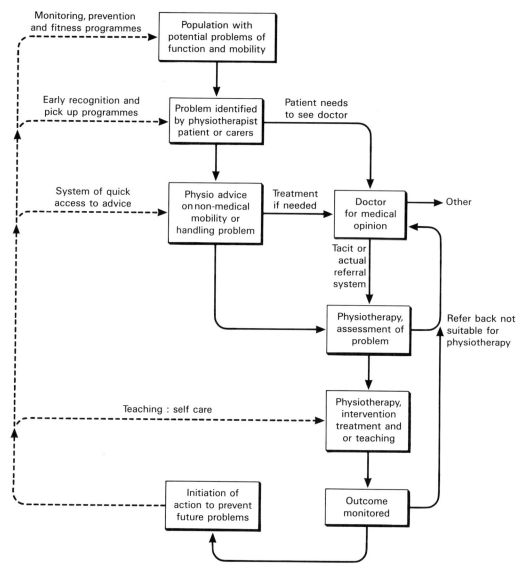

Fig. 2.1 A workload model for physiotherapy. (Reproduced by kind permission of Mrs J I Williams, District Physiotherapist, Doncaster Health Authority, from Williams 1985 Caseload, casemix, workload and costing. Doncaster Health Authority, Workshop Report I.)

To fulfil this sharing role they need skills as a physiotherapist, facilitator, motivator, communicator, educator, listener and counsellor, as well as being a flexible health care and support worker.

A physiotherapist is expected to do the following:

1. Demonstrate a knowledge of, and ability

to apply, an investigative approach to academic and clinical subjects.

2. Assess the physical, psychosocial and environmental state of the patient from a physiotherapeutic point of view.

3. Synthesise knowledge and assessment of the patient to identify treatment objectives.

4. Plan a therapeutic programme for each patient to achieve treatment objectives while

recognising the involvement and priorities of the other members of the health-care team.

5. Evaluate the effectiveness of the assessment and therapeutic programmes according to the patient's progress and potential for recovery.

6. Teach and advise patients, relatives, medical practitioners and other members of the health-care team on the physiotherapeutic management and prevention of disorders.

Clinical role

Many aspects of the clinical role of a paediatric physiotherapist are no different from those of all chartered physiotherapists except that therapy is often delivered to the child through another person, such as a parent. Referrals are generally from general practitioners, hospital or community consultants, medical officers or members of the health-care teams.

Assessment

Physiotherapy assessments determine the aims and objectives of treatment with the referrer, the child's key worker, other team members, parents and the child, whenever possible (see Chapter 17 Common Assessment Procedures). Assessment records should include a database, observations (general and local), physical test procedures, a problem list, the diagnosis, treatments, short- and long-term goals, progress notes and reviews (Dunn et al 1990).

Treatment

The therapist will choose a mode of treatment and design a method of physical management to meet the agreed aims, but the treatment may be delivered by:

- the therapist
- other members of the care team
- parents, who will be taught by the therapist (see Chapter 18 Treatment Systems and Chapter 19 Treatment Methods).

Aids and equipment

Assessment for fitting and adjusting aids to mobility and development and physiotherapy health-care equipment should include instructing all concerned in their use (see Chapter 21 Aids and Appliances). This is to ensure that everyone complies with the safety and maintenance checks and with the Health and Safety Notices. The family, carers and equipment users must be able to understand written instructions and progress reports. Translations or diagrammatic written information must be provided if required for clarity and compliance.

Recording systems

Clinical and managerial activity records and outcomes are kept by the therapist for clinical and service review and to evaluate the standards and results of physiotherapeutic treatment activities with referred babies and children. Confidentiality and storage of record regulations must be adhered to at all times (see Chapter 22 Planning for Progress).

Monitoring and discharge

Physiotherapists must regularly review outcomes and, after consultation with others concerned, reset goals and sometimes change methods of treatment or management. In this way new goals that take account of the changing clinical, educational and daily needs of a child can be met. Therapists may make the decision to discharge the child and family from active physiotherapy services. Children are often placed on an inactive physiotherapy register with the option for re-referral by the family or a professional.

Advisory, liaison and counselling role

Advisory role

To establish a coordinated service for a child, the physiotherapist will need to attend a number of advisory meetings (see Chapter 24 Team Workers). These meetings will range from case conferences to curriculum design and classroom management or planning sessions. Therapists also need to attend clinic and ward consultations and participate in clinical audit and service planning meetings. Therapists often advise on:

- furniture design, purchase and use
- classroom or ward organisation
- recreational or occupational activity.

Liaison

Liaison skills are needed when making contact with other agencies in the statutory, health, private or voluntary fields. The therapist may also need to liaise between the family and another team member, or may use another team member as their liaison link.

At all times there is a need for therapists to work positively towards promotion and maintenance of good relationships in the physiotherapy department and amongst other disciplines.

Counselling

Counselling the child, family members or carers is an important aspect of the role of a therapist. The therapist may be likened to the 'professional wise person' by the family. The act of 'hands on' therapy will often lead to parents asking questions and to a gradual sharing of their anxieties and aspirations. They frequently seek clarification of information received from a variety of sources, such as the popular press, other parents or clinical reviews. Professional rules of practice govern clinical disclosures so the therapist must be in possession of all the information given to the family by the doctor.

Educational role

The induction and in-service training of professional staff is an important task for the experienced paediatric physiotherapist. Many physiotherapists have been attracted to the clinical field of paediatrics by the teaching and demonstrations of senior clinical therapists. Junior physiotherapy staff will spend time in the paediatric specialty team for observational and supervised clinical practice placements.

Senior physiotherapists need to monitor and assist evaluation of therapeutic management and treatment programmes carried out by junior staff,

support workers and others such as family, education staff, nurses, carers or the child. Senior physiotherapists also participate in the undergraduate training programmes of students from many health and education disciplines in order to widen their knowledge of physiotherapy and the aims, objectives and methodologies used to meet individual children's needs. This training may also involve health promotion and the prevention of lifting and load-handling injuries.

Within all departments, the encouragement of involvement in journal clubs, case presentation, and for all staff to initiate or to become involved in research projects is important for efficiency and job satisfaction.

Teaching the child, family, care staff and all personnel involved in therapy tasks is important for comprehensive management of the child. Skills can be developed through demonstration, written information and discussion. Evaluation is a joint process with the family. When language, cultural, communication or learning difficulties are present the services of a liaison worker must be employed.

Managerial role

Chartered physiotherapists are responsible for themselves professionally and accountable not only for their actions but also for the use of equipment, time and skill.

Accountability includes the keeping of clinical records, managerial records on staffing and resources, the submission of statistics and the maintenance of policies and procedures. Such records are used for planning and accounting purposes.

Prioritisation and planning

A senior therapist will need to prioritise the daily demands made on the service and upon each therapist (Butson 1989). They should ensure that case- and workloads, and utilisation of skills, are shared fairly amongst physiotherapy staff. Information systems with line management staff will need to be well-established if they are to respond to varying clinical and administrative demands.

Table 2.1 Caseload

Type of Caseload	Definition
Total	All that is contained within the job description and implied within the professional role
Potential	A defined population which is directly monitored, from which the current caseload is derived and for which the physiotherapist is responsible
Current	Those patients who have been assessed, have entered an episode of physiotherapy care and are not yet discharged
Daily	Patients from current caseload dealt with on one day

Therapists should advise the managing physiotherapist on the shortfalls, problems, possibilities and recent developments of the clinical specialty service. This will include assisting in the planning process in the health district or area and in job determination and personnel specifications for selection and recruitment processes.

Professional development

Each staff member needs to set and monitor standards of patient care through professional audit and to identify job satisfaction and training needs both for themselves and for other staff through individual performance reviews and appraisal. It is important to undertake self-examination through such reviews and, by identifying skills, personal development needs and achievements, job satisfaction and personal effectiveness can be enhanced.

Health and safety

It is part of the duty of all staff to ensure compliance with health district and area policies and procedures regarding health and safety at work, infection control, control of substances hazardous to health, accident, emergency, fire, smoking, alcohol, load and patient handling and moving, data protection, confidentiality, etc (see Chapter 25 Legal Aspects).

RESPONSIBILITIES OF THE PAEDIATRIC PHYSIOTHERAPIST

Professional and personal responsibilities are determined by the various roles of the paediatric therapist. They include maintaining high professional standards in record keeping, health and safety issues, confidentiality, and in direct service delivery (Bromley et al 1987). Therapists should aim to meet the individual and statutory needs of the child and their family within the parameters of professional practice.

Physiotherapists in the field of paediatric practice apply postgraduate training, skills and knowledge in the medical, educational and community spheres of family life. Involvement with children and with families may be directed towards child development, physical treatment, therapeutic management, disability prevention, independence training and health promotion.

Personal responsibility

Physiotherapists are responsible for accommodating themselves to the constantly changing needs and roles demanded of them by the varying circumstances of a child, family or other team members. They need to ensure that their professional skills include originality, good communication and interpersonal skills, combined with flexibility of mind and work practices. The personal responsibility of a paediatric physiotherapist is to ensure professional, physical and mental competency for the tasks, and that the nature and purpose of the job are understood.

Through study, skills training and regular personal update, the physiotherapist must develop an understanding and knowledge not only of the theories, philosophies and sciences involved in the management of most disorders but also of situations commonly encountered within paediatric practice.

Clinical responsibility

Clinical knowledge should include the major stages and influences on child development (see Chapter 4 The Developing Child), relevant information on epidemiology and genetics (see Chapter 3 Genetics), the psychology and sociology of sickness, handicap and dying (see Chapter 23 Parents and Children), the causation, pathology and processes of major systems disorders in children and their possible sequelae,

and the major handicapping conditions of childhood (see Section 3 Problems and Disorders in Childhood).

Professional knowledge and skills will be

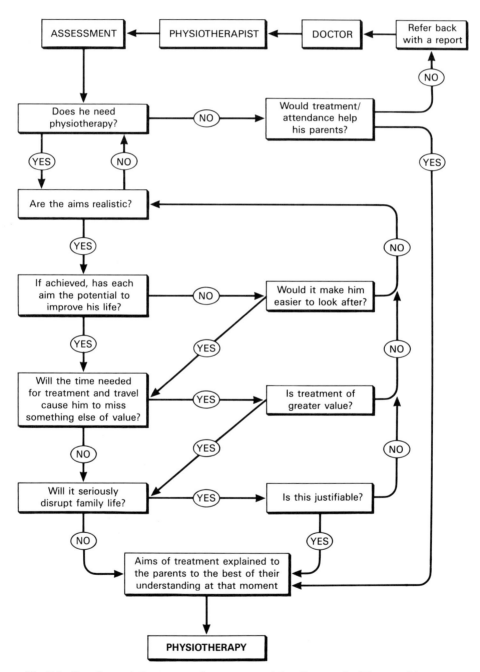

Fig. 2.2 Questions relating to outpatient treatment (after Scrutton D, Gilbertson M. 1975 Physiotherapy in Paediatric Practice, by permission of Butterworths, London).

needed to choose, apply and develop appropriate methods of record keeping, assessment, problem identification, realistic goal-setting, treatment design, delivery and management, case weighting and outcome measuring and evaluation of physiotherapeutic inputs (see Section 4 Physiotherapy in Practice).

There should be clear explanations of assessment (in an appropriate language or visual form) of therapeutic management aims and methods for others involved with the child. Shared case records are often useful to multidisciplinary team members. Named 'key workers' and professionals (and even parents) may change throughout the life of a child. A good, clear, concise and easily understood record is essential for good communication between the team members and the families they serve.

Professional responsibility

It is the therapist's responsibility to learn the various statutory and voluntary provisions and supporting services, the available resources and access to these and the formal and informal links between the agencies (see Appendix A Voluntary and Statutory Resources). The therapist is also responsible for ensuring compliance at all times with statutory, legal, professional, managerial and local policies and procedures. They must have a working knowledge of the professional code of practice and need to find out local procedures and policies for whichever site or service where they work. They will also need a working knowledge of legal issues relating to children (see Chapter 25 Legal Aspects).

Many paediatric physiotherapists work in a number of community settings and a proportion of work-time each day is spent travelling between local clinics, schools and home settings. It is important to balance the most effective use of physiotherapy time with the benefits gained by seeing children in their own setting, where treatment can be coordinated on a day-to-day basis with those people who are in regular contact with the child.

Time management may often be dictated to the therapist by school, ward or domiciliary circumstances and time will need to be allocated to case reviews, clinical hospital appointments and interdisciplinary planning meetings, as well as to report writing, compiling and analysing statistics, service and clinical audit and review.

SUMMARY

The role of the physiotherapist in paediatrics can be summarised as one of sharing: with the child, the parents, carers, doctors, nurses, educationalists and other health, welfare and social workers (see Chapter 24 Team Workers). This sharing is the result of joint assessment, problem identification, goal-setting and fulfilment and the evaluation of inputs and outcomes for the betterment of the child and its family.

The paediatric physiotherapist is responsible for fulfilling this role by using physiotherapeutic and interpersonal skills to identify problems, define a realistic baseline for therapies and management, gain recognition and understanding of the child in their family, social, hospital ward and/or classroom setting, and to facilitate (often through skill-sharing) remediation, amelioration, acceptance and sometimes circumvention of intractable difficulties in an individual child.

The job calls for tact, empathy, sensitivity, flexibility, curiosity, clear thinking, creativity, patience, practicality, generosity, and skill-sharing between physiotherapists. It is a demanding, responsible, but most rewarding role.

REFERENCES

Association of Paediatric Chartered Physiotherapists 1987 Task list compiled during APCP study weekend, May 1987, Cheadle

Bromley I, Hunter A, Sutcliffe B 1987 Physiotherapy services. A basis for development of standards. King's Fund Centre, London

Butson J 1989 Caseload priorities for a paediatric PT service. Therapy Weekly

Dunn C, Williams V, Young C 1990 Paediatric physiotherapy guidelines for good practice. Association of Paediatric Chartered Physiotherapists/CSP, London, ch 2, p 18

Trent Regional Health Authority 1989 Physiotherapy. An examination of demand and supply issues. Trent RHA Manpower Planning Advisory Group, para 1.2.11

This section outlines the major stages of child development. Chapter 3 first describes the development of the human baby from conception to birth, including the causes and detection of abnormal development. The factors contributing to congenital anomalies and disease are then covered in greater detail.

Chapter 4, on child development, details the progression of gross and fine motor skills and introduces the development of cognition, play, hearing, vision and perception.

Chapter 5 discusses the practices in child health that relate to promotion of general health, early identification through screening and routine development assessments, and the prevention of disease and disability.

SECTION 2
Child development

3

Genetics and embryology

D. Donnai   L. Kerzin-Storrar
P. Wigmore

INTRODUCTION

The process of development of the human embryo from a fertilised egg to the birth of an infant is complex and follows numerous well-defined stages. The physical appearance and biochemical makeup of the infant is determined by the genetic code contained within each cell.

In this chapter the processes of prenatal development are described and the various factors that may lead to the birth of a developmentally disabled child are discussed.

GENETICS
D. Donnai   L. Kerzin-Storrar

INTRODUCTION

Genetic disorders account for a significant number of the conditions causing neonatal mortality and morbidity and for many admissions to paediatric wards. The impact of a diagnosis of a genetic disorder often extends beyond the nuclear family. The clinical speciality of genetics aims, by investigation and counselling, to help families understand and come to terms with the problems of the disorder and the genetic implications.

A normal person has 46 chromosomes in each cell, 23 derived from each parent. These consist of 22 pairs of autosomes (the chromosomes common to men and women, numbered 1 to 22) and one pair of sex chromosomes (XX in a female, XY in a male). Each chromosome contains a large number of genes. Genes, like chromosomes, come in pairs and are made up of deoxyribonucleic acid (DNA). Each gamete (egg cell or sperm cell) contains only one of each pair of the parental chromosomes. When an egg containing 23 chromosomes is fertilised by a sperm containing 23 chromosomes, the fertilised egg contains 46 chromosomes (Fig. 3.1). As the embryo develops, the same set of 46 chromosomes is then copied into each new cell.

CATEGORIES OF GENETIC DISORDERS

The mechanisms by which genetic factors contribute to the aetiology of congenital anomalies and disease fall into three main groups of disorder:

- chromosomal
- single gene
- multifactorial.

In this section of the chapter we will describe and illustrate these mechanisms and then discuss the organisation of genetic services and the genetic counselling process.

Chromosomal disorders

The exact amount and correct balance of chromosome material is essential for the normal formation and function of a baby. A normal female pattern is called 46,XX and a normal male 46,XY (Fig. 3.2). Extra or missing chromosomal material may result in major problems with physical and mental development. Chromosomal abnormalities can be detected in children by microscopic analysis of the chromosome pattern of cultured blood cells or skin fibroblasts. Common groups of abnormalities include:

- trisomies (extra chromosome present)
- deletions and duplications (when part of a chromosome is missing or duplicated)
- translocations (where chromosomal material is rearranged)
- mosaics (where only some cells have an abnormal chromosome pattern).

Trisomy 21

Trisomy 21 is the most common chromosome pattern found in children with Down's syndrome. It occurs because either the egg or the sperm contains two (instead of the normal one) number 21 chromosomes. This occurs because of a process called non-disjunction. There is an increased risk of trisomy 21 in a baby as the mother's age increases, but in fact most trisomy 21 children are born to younger women, even though the risk is low, because so many more young women are having babies. The risk of recurrence of trisomy 21-type Down's syndrome is low, in the order of 1%, but prenatal diagnosis may be offered for reassurance.

Other common chromosome disorders. The other common trisomies are trisomy 13 (Patau syndrome) and trisomy 18 (Edwards

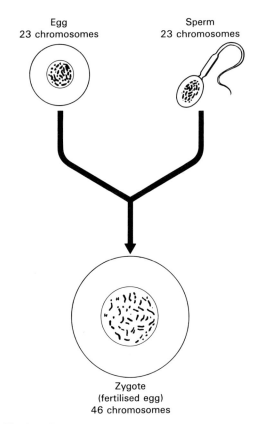

Fig. 3.1 Fertilisation.

Egg
23 chromosomes

Sperm
23 chromosomes

Zygote
(fertilised egg)
46 chromosomes

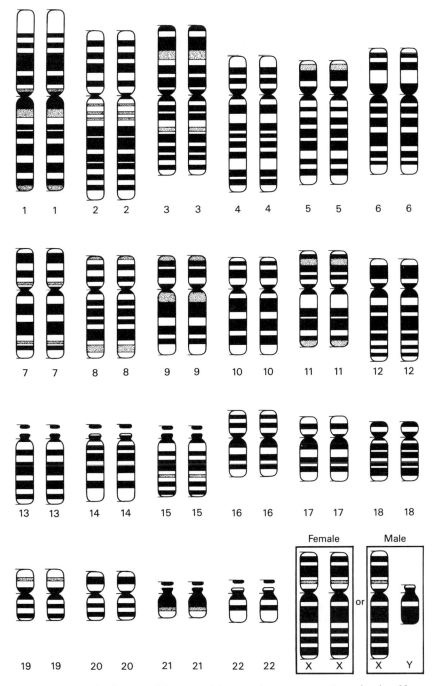

Fig. 3.2 Schematic diagram of the normal human chromosome pattern showing 22 pairs of autosomes and one pair of sex chromosomes.

syndrome). These are almost always lethal in infancy and are associated with severe multiple congenital anomalies.

Variation in the number of sex chromosomes usually gives rise to milder physical and intellectual problems.

Turner syndrome. This condition affects girls and arises when a fertilised egg has only one X chromosome (45,X). These girls have normal intellectual development, are short and need hormone replacement at puberty because their ovaries are not fully formed.

Klinefelter syndrome. This condition affects boys and arises when the fertilised egg contains an extra X chromosome (47,XXY). These boys are usually intellectually within the normal range, although a few may require special education. Like Turner syndrome, the individuals are infertile and require hormone replacement therapy at puberty.

Deletion and duplication

Sometimes only part of a chromosome is missing or duplicated. There are many hundreds of such conditions and only some are common enough to have been named. For example, when a particular part of chromosome 5 is missing, the condition is known as cri-du-chat syndrome (46,XX 5p–) (see Glossary List of Syndromes). It is often difficult to obtain information on the problems or prognosis associated with duplications or deletions because they are so rare. The regional genetic service may be helpful as an information resource. Many of the deletions and duplications happen as spontaneous isolated events but some can be due to inherited translocations.

Translocations

A person who has the correct number of chromosomes, but these are rearranged, is called a balanced translocation carrier. A common translocation is where a chromosome 14 and a chromosome 21 are joined together. Individuals who carry such a translocation are at risk of having a child with translocation Down's syndrome. This chromosome pattern accounts for approximately 5% of all children born with Down's syndrome.

Sometimes a translocation is more complex, involving parts of two or more chromosomes and resulting in duplications and deletions of chromosome material in offspring.

It is important to identify translocations because a carrier is at risk of having recurrent miscarriages and physically and mentally handicapped children.

Mosaicism

This refers to a situation where the chromosome abnormality exists in only a proportion of the body cells. Mosaicism arises when the fertilised egg contains the normal chromosome number (46) but where a subsequent faulty cell division gives rise to a cell with an abnormal chromosome number. The resulting baby has a mixture of cells with normal and abnormal chromosome numbers. The clinical syndrome may be milder than if all the cells carried the abnormality. For example, girls with mosaic Turner syndrome (45,X/46,XX) may be taller than girls with 45,X in each cell (see Glossary List of Syndromes).

Single gene disorders

Alterations (mutations) in single genes can give rise to malformations or diseases of all body systems. There are over 4000 known single gene disorders. For many years analysis of the pedigree patterns of certain conditions have made it clear that they are due to the effects of faulty genes (Fig. 3.3). However, it is now possible, in many conditions, to detect the actual fault in the chemical makeup (DNA) with 'gene probes'. For some conditions the chemical product for which the gene is responsible can be measured and deficiencies identified.

Single gene disorders can be inherited in families in three main ways:

- autosomal dominant
- autosomal recessive
- X-linked recessive.

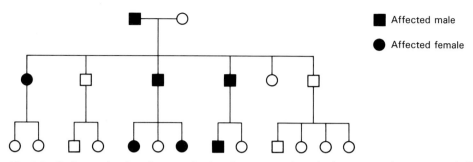

Fig. 3.3 Pedigree showing disease affecting three generations, both sexes, and on average half of the offspring of affected individuals, suggesting autosomal dominant inheritance.

Autosomal dominant disorders

These are disorders determined by genes on any one of the autosomal chromosomes. A dominant disorder is due to just one of a pair of genes being faulty. The term 'dominant' means that the mutated gene is stronger than its normal partner.

An individual carrying an abnormal dominant gene manifests signs of the condition and each of their children will have a 50% (1 in 2) risk of also being affected (Fig. 3.4). Some dominant conditions, such as achondroplasia (a type of short-limb dwarfism) affect all gene carriers in a very similar fashion, so there is no doubt as to which members of a family are affected and which are not. However, many dominant disorders, for example, myotonic dystrophy (a disorder of muscle weakness and spasm), are very variable in their clinical expression. Deciding who in the family carries the gene can be difficult and requires detailed examination and a range of investigations.

Examples of autosomal dominant disorders include:

- tuberous sclerosis
- neurofibromatosis
- type 1 osteogenesis imperfecta
- Huntington's chorea
- myotonic dystrophy
- retinitis pigmentosa (dominant type)
- achondroplasia
- Marfan syndrome
  (see Glossary List of Terms and Syndromes).

Autosomal recessive disorders

These disorders are also determined by genes on the autosomal chromosomes. In this case both genes in the pair are faulty. An individual with a recessive disorder has inherited one faulty gene from each parent. The parents (carriers) will have only one faulty gene in the pair and will be unaffected because the abnormal gene is the weaker (recessive) one of the pair. If a couple both carry the same faulty gene there is a 25% (1 in 4) chance of each child having the disease (Fig. 3.5). Recessive disorders are more common in the children of consanguineous (cousin) parents. However, most couples do not discover they are both carriers of a recessive gene until they have had an affected child. Some recessive disorders are common in particular ethnic groups and carrier tests can be performed for members of these groups. Examples include sickle-cell anaemia in individuals of African black extraction and Tay–Sachs' disease in the Ashkenazi Jewish population.

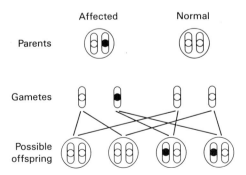

Fig. 3.4 Autosomal dominant inheritance.

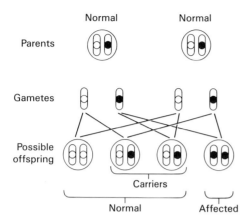

Fig. 3.5 Autosomal recessive inheritance.

The siblings of an individual with a recessive disorder such as cystic fibrosis (CF) often ask if they themselves could have an affected child. Their chance of being a carrier is 2 in 3, but for them to have an affected child their partner must also carry the gene. Because about 1 in 20 of the Caucasian population carry the CF gene, a population-based screening programme could help to reduce the incidence of CF. DNA techniques have now made this possible.

Examples of autosomal recessive disorders include:

- cystic fibrosis (see Chapter 7 Respiratory Conditions and Cardiothoracic Disorders)
- sickle-cell anaemia
- infantile spinal muscular atrophy (Werdnig–Hoffmann disease) (see Chapter 11 Neuromuscular Disorders)
- Tay–Sachs' disease (see Chapter 15 Inborn Errors of Metabolism)
- deafness (many forms)
- Phenylketonuria (see Chapter 15 Inborn Errors of Metabolism)
- Friedreich's ataxia

(see Glossary List of Syndromes).

X-linked recessive disorders

These are disorders determined by recessive genes on the X chromosome. If a male (XY) inherits the faulty gene he will be affected because he has only one set of X chromosome genes. However, a female (XX) who inherits the recess-ive gene is only a carrier — she has two sets of X chromosome genes. Because of a genetic mechanism (lyonisation) which controls the action of X chromosome genes in cells, some female carriers show mild signs of the disorder, which can aid in carrier detection. If a woman is a carrier, her sons will have a 50% (1 in 2) risk of being affected and her daughters a 50% (1 in 2) risk of being carriers (Fig. 3.6).

Molecular genetic techniques ('genetic engineering') have enabled the identification of the exact chromosomal location of many of the genes for genetic diseases on a specific chromosome. Research has been particularly fruitful for the X-linked disorders because geneticists knew that these genes must lie somewhere on the X chromosome. This has enabled the abnormal genes to be tracked in many families for accurate carrier and prenatal tests. This technology has greatly improved the situation for many Duchenne muscular dystrophy (DMD) families where, in the past, women have not had a clear idea of their carrier status. In Figure 3.7 gene probes have shown that the sister of a boy with DMD inherited from her mother the opposite X chromosome to her affected brother, and she is therefore almost certainly not a carrier.

Examples of X-linked recessive disorders are:

- Duchenne muscular dystrophy (DMD)
- Becker muscular dystrophy (BMD)
- haemophilia A and B
- hypogammaglobulinaemia (X-linked)

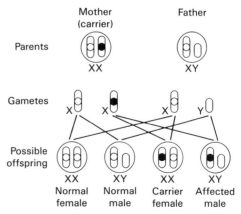

Fig. 3.6 X-linked recessive inheritance.

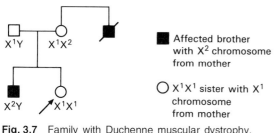

Fig. 3.7 Family with Duchenne muscular dystrophy. Using a gene probe it has been possible to distinguish between the X chromosomes in the consultand's mother, and to show that she has not inherited the same X chromosome from her mother as her affected brother, giving her a very low risk of being a carrier.

- Hunter syndrome (mucopolysaccharidosis type II)
- X-linked mental retardation (including fragile X)
  (see Glossary).

It has long been known that there is an excess of boys amongst the mentally retarded population and that in some families mental retardation is inherited in an X-linked recessive pattern. In some of these families a chromosomal marker has been identified, described as fragile X because down the microscope the lower part of the X chromosome appears to be loosely attached. The finding of this marker has helped with the detection of carrier females in these families. However, it is hoped that gene probes will soon allow more accurate testing. This condition is important in numerical terms because it may account for as many retarded individuals as Down's syndrome.

Multifactorial disorders

In addition to chromosomal and single gene disorders, where the genetic aspects are clear, there are a large number of conditions where genetic factors play a part but where they are less well understood and probably interact with environmental factors.

Many of the common single structural anomalies, including heart disease, cleft lip and palate, and neural tube defects, fall into this group. Although the mechanism underlying so-called multifactorial conditions is far from clear, it is known that some families have a 'predisposition'. Unlike the single gene disorders where a personal risk can be given based on the pedigree and knowledge of mendelian genetics, in multifactorial conditions risks must be based on empirical risk figures (risks derived from studies that look at how many families with the condition have more than one affected member). In general, the risk of recurrence after one affected child is in the region of 3–5%; the risk goes up if there are additional affected family members. For some conditions, whilst the genetic component cannot be altered, if the environmental component is identified there is the prospect of true prevention. Recent work suggests that periconception vitamin supplementation in mothers who have had one child with neural tube defect lowers the risk of recurrence.

Examples of multifactorial conditions are:

- neural tube defects (see Chapter 8 Disorders of the Central Nervous System)
- congenital heart defects (see Chapter 7 Respiratory Conditions and Cardiothoracic Disorders)
- cleft lip and plate
- epilepsy (some types) (see Chapter 8 Disorders of the Central Nervous System)
- congenital dislocation of the hip (see Chapter 12 Orthopaedic Aspects of Childhood Disorders)
- asthma and eczema
- diabetes (juvenile onset).

GENETIC COUNSELLING AND CLINICAL GENETIC SERVICES

Most regions have a centralised clinical genetics service run by consultant clinical geneticists in liaison with genetic laboratories. Referrals for genetic counselling are usually made by other specialists and general practitioners, although they may occasionally come from other health professionals, and very occasionally from the families themselves.

When parents discover that their child has a disorder that is genetically determined, the psychological sequelae are often compounded by feelings of guilt, anger, fear and concern for other family members. Genetic counselling aims to:

- establish a precise diagnosis where possible

- assess the risk of recurrence for individual family members
- communicate to the family the implications of the diagnosis and the genetic risks.
- discuss, where appropriate, reproductive options including prenatal diagnosis, and help families choose for themselves the most appropriate options
- provide support to help family members cope with the implications of the genetic diagnosis and risks.

Clearly this cannot be done by one person or in a single outpatient appointment. Genetic counselling is normally done by a team of doctors and counselling staff (genetic associates and nurses) combining home visits, clinic appointments and long-term follow-up, where appropriate, by genetic family registers.

The ability to diagnose and assess risk in genetic conditions is improving at a rapid pace, due largely to advances in molecular genetic techniques. However, it is the responsibility of medical genetic counsellors to ensure that these advances are applied to clinical practice so that families receive both accurate information and sensitive counselling to help them make their own personal decisions in the face of genetic risk.

EMBRYOLOGY
P. Wigmore

INTRODUCTION

The development of the human baby is one of nature's most remarkable achievements. The maternal and paternal chromosomes combine to provide a blueprint for the development of the adult so that from a single cell many millions of cells descend, each differentiated into the different tissues and organs. During this period the embryo must produce not only its own tissues but also the placenta, in itself a specialised organ, for the uptake of nutrients from the mother. Finally the fetus must prepare itself for the rapid changes in its environment that birth brings about. In the vast majority of instances the mechanisms of development proceed smoothly and a perfectly formed full-term infant is born.

However, as in any complex biological system, faults may develop and it is now realised that the developing child is susceptible to a variety of harmful influences. The following sections give a brief account of some of the major events during development while further sections describe some of the causes and detection of abnormal development.

AN OVERVIEW OF DEVELOPMENT FROM CONCEPTION TO BIRTH

Conception and the first week of development

During the normal menstrual cycle an unfertilised ovum is released from one of the ovaries and fertilisation must normally occur between 12 and 24 hours, or the ovum will be lost during the next menstrual bleeding.

Within 30 hours the fertilised egg divides into two cells and cell division continues rapidly until a ball of cells, the morula, is produced. This soon becomes hollow, the innermost cells will form the embryo while the outer cells will form the placenta. After 4–5 days the developing embryo and placenta attaches to the wall of the uterus and becomes implanted.

THE SECOND AND THIRD WEEKS

The placenta develops rapidly during the second and third weeks and invades the surrounding uterine tissue until the outer layer of placental cells is in contact with the maternal blood. The developing embryo consists of a flat disc, two cells thick. One layer of cells is called the ectoderm, the other the endoderm (see Fig. 3.8). Ectodermal cells migrate to form a third cell layer, the mesoderm, lying between the ectoderm and endoderm. All the tissues of the body will be derived from these three layers:

- the ectoderm will produce skin and nervous tissue
- the mesoderm will produce muscles, bone, cartilage, connective tissue and blood
- the endoderm will produce the digestive tract and its associated structures.

A

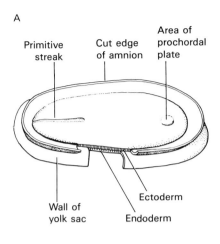

Primitive streak — Cut edge of amnion — Area of prochordal plate

Wall of yolk sac — Ectoderm — Endoderm

B

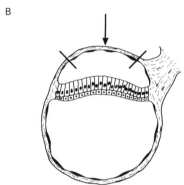

Fig. 3.8 (A) Schematic view of the germ disc at the end of the second week of development. (B) Dorsal view of amniotic cavity showing position of germ disc. (After Sadler 1985 by permission of Williams & Wilkins.)

THE FOURTH TO THE EIGHTH WEEK

Many of the organ systems, including eye, ear, nervous, respiratory, digestive and urogenital systems will be laid down during the fourth to the eighth week, together with the early stages of limb development. For this reason this time is particularly critical for the developing embryo and is the age when most congenital defects arise. During this period the embryo will grow from 5 mm to 30 mm in length and folding at the ends and sides of the embryo change it from a flat plate of tissue into a more recognisable embryonic shape. This folding closes the anterior abdominal wall and allows the formation of the digestive tract from the endodermal layer of cells.

Nervous tissue

One of the first systems to start to develop is the central nervous system. The formation of the brain and the spinal cord starts as a strip of ectodermal cells running the length of the embryo. The edges of this strip rise up to form the neural folds with a groove running between them. The neural folds continue to grow until they meet in the midline above the neural groove to form the neural tube. Fusion between the folds begins in the future neck region and then extends forward and backwards along the length of the embryo. The result is the neural tube, initially open at both ends but fully closed by day 27 of development (see Fig. 3.9). The parts of the neural tube in the head will expand to form the brain while the remainder will form the spinal

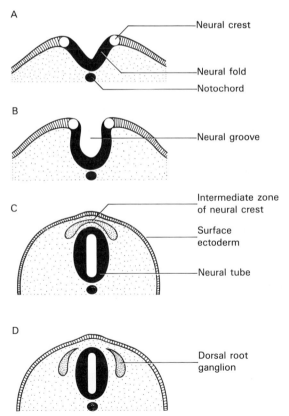

Fig. 3.9 Schematic drawing of a number of transverse sections through successively older embryos, showing the formation of the neural folds, neural groove and neural tube. (After Sadler 1985 by permission of Williams & Wilkins.)

cord. The development of the nervous system continues and new nerve cells are added until the end of the first year after birth. At the time of closure of the neural tube, cells detach from the tips of the neural folds and migrate into the embryo. These cells, called neural crest cells, will form the neuronal cell bodies in the dorsal root ganglia and ganglia of the autonomic nervous system.

Tissues derived from the mesoderm

As the neural tube is forming the mesoderm breaks up into square blocks of tissue, the somites, which lie on either side of the neural tube. Cells from the somites will contribute to many tissues in adjacent regions of the embryo. For example, parts of each somite will produce bone cells for the vertebrae surrounding the spinal cord. Cells will migrate out from other parts of the somite to produce the dermis of the skin and, still further, cells will provide the muscles. Small areas within the mesenchyme (a connective tissue derived from the mesoderm) within the head ossify and form the flat plates of bone of the skull. These areas of bone expand but remain separated from one another by narrow seams called sutures. Where several bones meet the suture is particularly wide and is called a fontanelle, the largest of which is the anterior fontanelle found above the baby's forehead. Continued growth of the skull bones in the first few years after birth closes these sutures.

Heart

The heart starts as a straight tube from which develops the four-chambered adult heart with its separated pulmonary and aortic circulations. This is achieved by folding the heart tube into a 'U' shape and by dilation of those parts destined to become the atria and ventricles. Division of these dilated regions into left and right atria and ventricles is achieved by the growth of shelves of tissue (septa) across the centre of the tube. As this is taking place, valves develop as flattened outgrowths of tissue between each atrium and ventricle and at the bases of the pulmonary and aortic arteries. These two great arteries are them-

selves derived from a single vessel, which is divided into two by the growth of a septum across its lumen. The formation of these septa within the heart occurs between 27 and 45 days of gestation and is one of the most critical aspects of its development.

One further complication is that the route taken by blood flowing through the heart in the unborn child is different from that in the post-natal infant. The reason for this is quite simple. The unborn child receives its oxygen through the placenta, from the maternal blood. Its lungs, though formed, do not serve any function until immediately after birth. The prenatal circulation therefore largely bypasses the lungs by passing blood from the right atrium directly into the left atrium and by further diverting the blood from the pulmonary circulation by a shunt, the ductus arteriosus, between the pulmonary artery and the aorta. At birth these two bypasses must close so that deoxygenated blood is directed through the lungs.

Development of the limbs

The limb buds appear at 5 weeks as flat paddle-like outgrowths. The limb bud elongates under the influence of cells near its tip and at 6 weeks the hand is visible as a flat plate of tissue. From about this time cartilage cells are found in the centre of the limb; these will form the early skeleton. The digits are visible as ridges within the hands and feet. For the digits to separate, the cells between them must die, a process that is normally complete by 8 weeks (see Fig. 3.10). Failure of this cell death will result in fusion between the digits.

After the cartilage skeleton has formed it is replaced by bone cells, which will produce the mineral matrix of normal bone. Bone cells are initially found in the centre and at each end of the long bones at sites called the centres of ossification. The expansion of the centres of ossification reduces the cartilage to a plate at each end of the bone, the epiphyseal plate, whose growth enables the bone to continue to elongate. The epiphyseal plate itself only becomes ossified in the late teens. Occasionally a child is born with a limb that appears to have been amputated. This

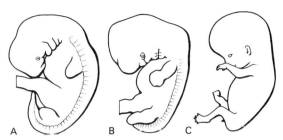

Fig. 3.10 Schematic drawings of human embryos to demonstrate the development of the limb buds. (A) At 5 weeks. (B) At 6 weeks. (C) At 8 weeks. Note that the hindlimb buds are somewhat behind in comparison with the forelimbs. (After Sadler 1985 by permission of Williams & Wilkins.)

is probably due to a localised region of vascular insufficiency after the limb has formed.

Respiratory system

At about 4 weeks of age, when the embryo is only 3 mm long, a pouch develops from the anterior side of that part of the foregut destined to become the oesophagus. This pouch, called the respiratory diverticulum, grows downwards into the thorax and subsequently loses its connection with the oesophagus. The tip of the respiratory diverticulum divides into the left and right lung buds. Each lung bud then grows and divides repeatedly to form the branching pattern of the bronchi. This pattern of growth will continue throughout prenatal life and into postnatal life. Smooth muscle, cartilage and blood vessels differentiate around the developing lung bud from the surrounding mesoderm. After birth, gas exchange will take place at the tips of the bronchi where they are expanded into thin walled sacs, the alveoli. These develop from about 7 months and are essential for the functioning of the lung. A few weeks before birth, specialised cells in the lung produce a phospholipid material that will lower the surface tension of the thin layer of fluid within the alveoli when the lung becomes filled with air immediately after birth. Without this surfactant the alveoli would tend to collapse and respiratory movements would be impaired. Before birth the lungs are filled with amniotic fluid, which is rapidly absorbed into the blood vessels at birth, allowing the lung to fill with air.

The third to the ninth month

From the third to the ninth month the organ systems mature and grow and the fetus will put on 50% of its weight (see Fig. 3.11). Few malformations arise during this period but in some cases the fetus can fail to thrive and grow as it should and is consequently born significantly lighter in weight than normal. External changes include the face taking on a more human appearance as the eyes move to a more anterior location. Subcutaneous fat is deposited in the final few months which gives the baby its rounded shape.

Birth

A full-term pregnancy lasts approximately 266 days from conception to birth (280 days from the last menstrual bleeding) and the baby should weigh between 3000 and 3500 g and have a crown to heel length of about 50 cm.

Small-for-dates babies

Babies born at full-term but who are significantly smaller than usual are called small-for-dates. It is usual to make a distinction between small-for-dates babies, who are small for their age, and premature babies who are the correct size for their age but who are born before full-term. The cause of small-for-dates babies is often uncertain but it is probably due to placental dysfunction,

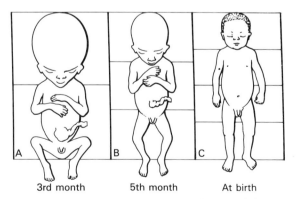

3rd month   5th month   At birth

Fig. 3.11 Schematic drawing showing the size of the head in relation to the rest of the body at various stages of development. (After Sadler 1985 by permission of Williams & Wilkins.)

which leads to undernutrition of the developing fetus, or to heavy smoking by the mother. Small-for-dates babies are born lighter in weight with an absence of subcutaneous fat and consequently have a more wrinkled appearance.

Premature babies

Premature babies normally survive if they are at least 28 weeks old but they suffer from a lack of surfactant in their lungs, which affects the efficiency of gas exchange.

CAUSES OF CONGENITAL DEFECTS

Congenital defects are defined as abnormalities present in the child at birth. The combined incidence of all types of defects is between 3 and 4% of live births, although some may not be discovered until some time after birth. A great deal of effort has been expended in trying to identify the causes of different defects but the vast majority (80%) are still of unknown origin. The known causes of congenital defects are called teratogenic factors and it is usual to differentiate between those with a hereditary basis and those due to an environmental factor. However, even these two classes may interact and be difficult to separate.

Critical time periods

The time at which the teratogenic factor acts on developing embryo or fetus will determine the type and severity of the defects produced. Teratogenic factors acting very early in development (before 3 weeks) may kill the embryo or cause defects that are repairable during later development. For this reason, congenital defects rarely arise during this stage; most arise during the second and third months of gestation, when the major organ systems are being laid down. Most organs have a critical period early in their development when cell division is very rapid and the particular processes involved in forming the organ must take place. Teratogenic factors acting on organs during this period will lead to permanent defects, while the same factors acting

later in development may only retard growth. Some organs, notably the brain, have particularly long critical periods and are susceptible to permanent damage throughout intrauterine life.

Hereditary teratogenic factors

Genetic teratogenic factors can vary from the inheritance of a single abnormal gene to alterations in the structure and number of whole chromosomes. Congenital defects due to a single mutated gene are relatively rare; examples are: achondroplasia, a condition where abnormal ossification of the long bones leads to dwarfism, and polydactylism (the development of additional digits).

The most common type of chromosomal abnormality is for there to be an extra chromosome. Certain chromosomes appear to be particularly susceptible to this, causing a condition known as trisomy. Down's syndrome is caused by trisomy of chromosome 21. Its incidence increases with maternal age from 1 in 2000 in mothers under 25 to 1 in 100 in mothers over 40. The symptoms of Down's syndrome include mental retardation and heart defects. Other chromosomal abnormalities can involve an additional sex chromosome (either X or Y) leading to a variety of syndromes whose symptoms may include infertility and mental retardation.

Some environmental agents, notably radiation and some drugs, can cause breaks in chromosomes. The effects of this will depend upon which chromosomes are involved (see pages 19–25 for a more in-depth discussion of genetics).

Environmental teratogenic factors

These are factors from outside the developing conceptus that have a deleterious effect on its development. Most will pass from the mother to the fetus because the placenta, although providing a barrier between maternal and fetal tissues, can readily be crossed by many drugs and infectious agents.

Viral factors

Rubella, the german measles virus, has long been

recognised as an environmental teratogen. Its effect on development depends upon the age of the fetus. Infection at 6 weeks produces cataracts in the eyes while infection at 9 weeks can cause deafness. Defects in the development of the heart can occur if infection occurs between 6 and 9 weeks. Another virus causing congenital defects is cytomegalovirus which, like rubella, can cross the placenta from an often asymptomatic but infected mother to cause blindness and a failure of the brain to grow (microcephaly).

Drugs

Many drugs have been shown to cause congenital defects, the most well known being thalidomide, an antinausea and sleeping pill prescribed during the late 1950s and early 1960s. This drug caused partial or total absence of the limbs and heart and digestive tract defects. Other drugs suspected of causing congenital defects include drugs used to treat epilepsy, antipsychotic and anti-anxiety agents together with some hormones.

Ingested substances

Substances not taken for medical reasons which disrupt development are mercury, alcohol and radiation. Even when doses of these substances have no long-term effect on the mother, the fetus may be affected showing its greater susceptibility to outside influences.

DEFECTS IN PARTICULAR SYSTEMS

Congenital defects of the heart

Congenital abnormalities of the heart and its associated great vessels are among the most common defects seen in new-born babies, occurring in 8 out of every 1000 live births. One form of defect is a failure of the changes that should occur at birth. This happens more frequently in premature babies where the ductus arteriosus fails to close, leading to a persistent bypass of the pulmonary circulation.

Structural defects arising during development can take the form of a failure to completely separate the right and left sides of the heart due to incomplete septal growth. These so-called hole-in-the-heart defects can occur between the atria, ventricles or great vessels, and again lead to a bypass of the pulmonary circulation. Other defects take the form of a narrowing or mispositioning of the aorta, pulmonary artery, or the valves of the heart. It should be noted that in many cases a heart can suffer from several of these anomalies (see Chapter 7 Respiratory Conditions and Cardiothoracic Disorders).

Symptoms

The symptoms of congenital heart defects are variable but include heart failure and cyanosis, a bluish appearance of the skin and lips due to insufficient oxygenation of the blood. Symptoms may be present immediately after birth or over the following weeks and months, often accompanied by a general failure to thrive.

Small defects may close spontaneously or remain undetected until the individual is examined in later life, while larger defects will require surgery.

Cause

In most cases the cause of congenital heart defects is unknown but it is associated with Down's syndrome children and may occur if the mother has been infected with rubella.

Congenital defects of the nervous system

These are most commonly due to a failure of the neural tube and its surrounding tissues to close, either in a localised region or along its whole length. Defects of this kind have an incidence of 2 in 1000 live births. Complete failure of the neural tube to close in the region of the brain is called anencephaly and is always fatal to the new born child.

Spina bifida

Spina bifida is the term used to describe a range of defects of different severity associated with the spinal cord. Spina bifida children often survive, their degree of disability depending on the extent of the defect. In its least severe form spina bifida is a failure of the dorsal side of a single vertebra to form. This will be covered by skin (often with a small tuft of hair at the site) and will not be associated with neurological symptoms. If several vertebrae are affected, the meningeal membranes covering the spinal cord may bulge outwards, resulting in a large swelling. Neurological symptoms are usually present, particularly in parts of the spinal cord found within the swelling. In its most severe form spina bifida is a failure of the neural tube to close. This results in the exposure of the undeveloped neural plate to the surface, and has severe neurological symptoms. Twenty per cent of neural tube defects are skin-covered and approximately one-third of infants with open lesions survive but with severe handicap (see Chapter 8 Disorders of the Central Nervous System).

Hydrocephalus

Hydrocephalus is a condition where the normal outflow of cerebrospinal fluid from the ventricles of the brain is blocked. This leads to an excessive accumulation of fluid within the ventricles, causing a build-up of pressure and an enlargement of the brain and cranium. This may be fatal if untreated but recent advances in prenatal surgery have enabled treatment by the release of fluid pressure before birth.

Causes

The causes of congenital defects of the nervous system are largely unknown. Spina bifida shows geographic and seasonal variations, which may indicate an environmental cause, while radiation and infection by the protozoan *Toxoplasma* have also been shown to cause defects. The central nervous system may also be damaged at birth due to internal bleeding and lack of oxygen, which can lead to cerebral palsy.

DETECTION OF FETAL ABNORMALITIES
Amniocentesis

Structural defects in the fetus can be detected by taking a sample of amniotic fluid (amniocentesis) or by visualisation of the fetus by ultrasound. Amniocentesis involves removal of 10–20 ml of amniotic fluid by passing a needle through the mother's abdominal wall, normally at between 16 and 20 weeks' gestation. This fluid contains cells that have detached from the fetus and these may be cultured in the laboratory. Analysis of the number and staining pattern of the chromosomes of these cells can reveal the sex of the fetus and some genetic abnormalities. Women over the age of 35 are routinely screened in this way to see if they are carrying a Down's syndrome fetus, which will be characterised by an additional chromosome.

Recent techniques of recombinant DNA technology have enabled the detection of markers for several other genetic diseases, including Duchenne muscular dystrophy and Huntington's chorea, thus allowing identification of fetuses liable to suffer from these hereditary diseases.

The amniotic fluid can also be screened for the presence of metabolites that may indicate that the fetus is developing abnormally. For example, an open neural tube acts like an open wound, allowing proteins from the fetus to leak into the surrounding fluid. One of these, alphafetoprotein, is easily detected and elevated levels are taken to indicate a neural tube defect of this type.

Ultrasound

Ultrasound imaging techniques use high frequency (2–5 MHz) sound waves which are reflected by the interface between adjacent tissues to visualise both the internal and external features of the fetus.

Ultrasound is used routinely to check the fetal measurements and the position of the placenta. It can also detect many structural defects in the fetus, including heart defects, anencephaly, spina bifida, hydrocephalus, cranial anomalies, limb abnormalities, tumours, and general intrauterine growth retardation.

FURTHER READING

Burn J 1988 Clinical genetics, a review. Journal of the
  Royal College of Physicians of London 22: 212–225
Davies K E, Read A P 1988 Molecular basis of inherited
  disease. IRL Press, Oxford
Emery A E H, Pullen I (eds) 1984 Psychological aspects of
genetic counselling. Academic Press, London
Harper P S 1988 Practical genetic counselling, 3rd edn.
  John Wright and Sons, Bristol
Sadler T W 1985 Longman's medical embryology, 5th
  edn. Williams & Wilkins, Baltimore

4

The developing child

S. Bedford

INTRODUCTION

In the first few years of life, rapid changes occur in development. From being totally dependent, with reflex-controlled movements, the newborn baby is transformed over 5 years into a comparatively independent child who is ready for school. The child changes in many ways: in personality, the way he communicates, how he perceives and thinks about his world, and his movement ability becomes complex and graceful. Although motor development is of primary importance to paediatric physiotherapists, knowledge of other aspects of development is valuable, because it provides an understanding of the total child. Therefore an introduction to the development of cognition, play, hearing, vision and perception is included in this chapter.

Sensory and motor development

Sensory and motor development are interdependent. Sensations not only provide input from the environment stimulating movement; they also create an awareness of our bodies, and feedback on the variety of movements that take place. Early postures and movements are in total patterns of flexion or extension and, together with the stereotyped reflexes of the neonate, they provide a foundation for voluntary movement. It is only as these movements become integrated that the child acquires the skills and abilities to perform differentiated movements that combine flexion and extension. Movements also become more selective, as the infant learns to isolate movement to specific parts of his body, e.g. at 8 months, if he tries to poke an object, the infant uses all his extended fingers, but by 9 months he can poke with his extended index finger only, the other fingers remain flexed.

From his earliest days the infant experiences new positions and movements. Righting reactions (see p. 42), which help to orientate his head and body upright in space, and to keep his head and trunk in alignment, start to evolve when the child starts to achieve positions such as sitting and standing, equilibrium or balance reactions will develop in these positions and these, together with protective extensions of the arms and legs, will eventually save the child from falling.

Most children follow a fairly predictable sequence of development but there is a wide variation in the age at which children reach milestones. Some stand and walk without crawling, and generally these are the early walkers. Others who do not crawl are often bottom shufflers, and

have a tendency to walk late. These children usually have some degree of low tone, and a dislike of prone lying. Bottom shuffling in normal children is usually familial.

GROSS MOTOR DEVELOPMENT

A dynamic posture is an essential framework for gross motor activities. This requires a normal postural reflex mechanism with normal postural tone, which provides stability, yet simultaneously has enough flexibility to allow for postural change. Reflexes are functional and adaptive to the environment throughout the life cycle. Mature reflexes provide an assistive framework for voluntary movement and exploration in the environment (Campbell 1984).

Tonic reflexes (see Table 4.1)

In the very early stages of development the changes in the distribution of postural tone are influenced in part by the tonic reflexes. Later they become integrated with other postural

Table 4.1 Reflex development, 0–5 years

Category	Reflex	Appears at	Integrated by
Neonatal	Moro	Birth	6 months
	Galant	Birth	2 months
	Crossed extensor	Birth	1–2 months
	Flexor withdrawal	Birth	1–2 months
	Extensor thrust	Birth	1–2 months
	Reflex walking	Birth	6 months
	Palmar grasp	Birth	6 months
	Plantar grasp	Birth	9 months
Postural	Tonic labyrinthine	Birth	6 months
	ATNR	2 months	4 months
	STNR	4–6 months	10 months
	Positive supporting	Birth	2 months
Righting and protective	Neck	Birth	4–6 months
	Labyrinthine	2 months	Lifelong
	Optical		Lifelong
	Body on body }	7–12 months	Lifelong
	Body on head }		5 years
	Protective extension — forwards	6–9 months	Lifelong
	— sideways	8 months	Lifelong
	— backwards	10 months	Lifelong
	Landau	3–6 months	1–2 yrs
	Equilibrium — prone	6 months	Lifelong
	— supine and sitting	7–8 months	Lifelong
	— all-fours	9–12 months	Lifelong
	— standing	12–21 months	Lifelong

mechanisms and are then under cortical control. They may persist and dominate the movements of children with cerebral palsy, and can sometimes be seen as tendencies to patterns of movement in children and adults under stress.

Tonic labyrinthine reflex

The tonic labyrinthine reflex operates when the head is horizontal. The sensory organ is in the internal ear and is stimulated by gravity. When the child's head is horizontal and the face is downwards, for example, when he is lying prone, there is an increase of postural tone in all flexor muscle groups. This is very apparent in the neonate, who is much more flexed in prone lying than in other positions. When the child is lying supine, or when the head is tilted backwards, there is a generalised increase in extensor tone. However, as the neonate has a tendency to be flexed in all non-weight-bearing positions, this increase in extensor tone may manifest only as a decrease in flexor tone. This reflex is fully integrated by the age of 6 months.

Asymmetrical tonic neck reflex

The asymmetrical tonic neck reflex (ATNR) is produced by rotation of the head, the stimulus originating in the proprioceptors of the neck. The reaction is more immediate with active than passive rotation. It is usually seen when the child is extended, as in supine lying. With the head rotated to one side, most commonly to the right, the right arm would extend and the left arm flex. The infant tends to gaze at the outstretched hand for a long time. The ATNR occurs in the second and third months; it is not obligatory in the normal infant, and starts to be integrated in the fourth month. The infant may continue to look in the direction of the extended arm, even when the ATNR is no longer active.

Symmetrical tonic neck reflex

The symmetrical tonic neck reflex emerges at 4–6 months and is integrated by 10 months. It is thought that it helps the infant to get into early crawling positions on all fours. The reflex can be demonstrated by supporting an infant in ventral suspension across the knees. If the head is passively or actively flexed, the arms will bend and the legs extend; however, if the head is extended, the arms extend and the legs flex.

Positive supporting reaction

The positive supporting reaction reflex, which is important for neonatal standing, is present at birth and is integrated by 2 months. This reaction operates when the infant is supported vertically, and there is pressure on the ball of the foot and stretching of the intrinsic muscles of the foot. The response is co-contraction of the leg muscles so that the leg becomes a rigid column, with a marked increase in extensor tone. The infant also has slightly flexed hips and knees. When integrated and under cortical control, this reaction will eventually play a major role in voluntary standing.

The neonate

The neonate's movements are determined by reflexes. In most positions his body is flexed, except for his neck (Fig. 4.1); but periodically he totally extends, for instance, when he stretches, or if he is startled. He also extends when he is held upright with his feet on a supporting surface.

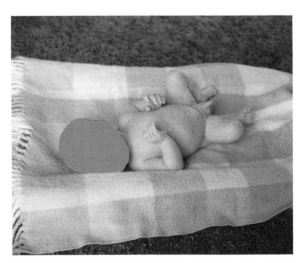

Fig. 4.1 Neonate aged 14 days. Note flexed position of limbs.

Neonatal reflexes can be most successfully observed when the neonate is comfortable, happy and alert (see Table 4.1).

Rooting reflex

If the corner of the mouth or cheek is touched, a neonate will turn his face towards the stimulus. The rooting reflex orientates the baby's mouth to his mother's nipple. However, if the baby has been fed recently, the rooting reflex may be difficult to elicit. When suckling, the mouth seals around the nipple and the baby uses negative pressure, together with a milking action by the tongue, to take in milk.

Moro reflex

The Moro reflex occurs when the baby's head suddenly falls backwards. The arms immediately abduct, with extended elbows, wrists and fingers. When the head regains its normal position, the arms flex. This reflex disappears about the age of 6 months and seems to be associated with the infant attaining head control.

Galant reflex, or lateral incurvation of the trunk

The galant reflex can be elicited by pricking or briskly stroking the paravertebral area of the back about 3 cm from the spine, from the bottom rib to the iliac crest. In response, the trunk flexes sideways towards the stimulus. This reflex is usually integrated by 2 months, but remains if the trunk is unstable.

Crossed extension reflex

The crossed extension reflex is demonstrated with the infant supine. One leg is held in extension and the sole of that foot is stimulated. The contralateral leg first flexes, then extends, adducts and inwardly rotates. The crossed extension reflex augments the positive supporting reaction, which was described with the tonic reflexes (see p. 36).

Flexor withdrawal reflex

When the sole of the foot of an extended leg is stimulated, the leg quickly flexes.

Extensor thrust

If pressure is put on the sole of a flexed leg that leg extends.

The crossed extension, flexor withdrawal and extensor thrust remain for 1–2 months before integration.

Reflex walking

Reflex walking can be seen when an infant is supported vertically. With the feet on the ground the legs will extend, and the infant will start to take steps if their weight is gently moved forward. This reflex will continue for about the first 6 weeks of life.

Placing reaction of the foot

The placing reaction of the foot can be elicited when the infant is held vertically and the dorsum of the foot is gently brushed against the lower edge of a table. The infant will lift the leg upwards and step onto the table. A similar response in the arm does not develop before the age of about 3 months.

Plantar grasp

Plantar grasp occurs in the foot when pressure is put on the ball of the foot and the toes flex. This reflex remains until the infant is 9 months old; up to this age the toes will curl when standing.

Grasp reflex

The grasp reflex of the hand can be demonstrated when a finger is inserted into the palm of the hand, followed by traction to the fingers. The result is strong, total flexion of the infant's arm and fingers.

The main changes in the first 6 months

During the first 6 months of life there is a gradual diminution of reflex activity. As reflexes become integrated and under cortical control, voluntary movement, with its potential for variety and choice, begins. There is also a change in the distribution of tone, from flexor muscle groups to extensor. In supine lying, the early asymmetry of head position, as well as the asymmetry produced by ATNRs in the second and third months, will disappear by the fourth month. The symmetrical infant should have acquired the ability to bring his hands together in the midline. Most 6-month-old infants will have developed head and trunk control; and will be able to sit on the floor supported with their hands. The infant will roll with his legs flexed, but without trunk rotation. When held, he may stand and possibly bounce, to the delight of his parents. His recently acquired eye–hand coordination will allow him to reach for and grasp objects.

A number of factors may influence development in the first 6 months, and these will now be considered (see also Table 4.2).

The development of extensor tone

Maturation or 'the importance of simply growing older' (Kagan 1973) plays its part in aspects of development. It is interesting to note that children from cultures that do not encourage playing on the floor, or creeping and crawling, eventually achieve the same milestones as Western children. It should be noted that creeping and crawling are used with opposite meanings in Britain and America. British usage is given in this chapter, where crawling refers to the 'on all fours' position.

A number of factors encourage the development of extensor tone and postural stability. If infants are carried upright, particularly if the holding hand is giving sufficient, but not too much, support, this will assist them to develop head and trunk control. Weight-bearing in a supported standing position promotes the development of extensor tone, and prone lying also has an important influence in the development of early standing (see Table 4.2).

Developments in prone lying

In prone lying the neonate can turn his head to one side. In this position the neonate is very flexed; the arms are under the body with hands

Table 4.2 Development 0–12 months

Age	Skill
2 months	Lifts head in prone
4 months	Lifts head in prone, weight on forearms Brings hands to midline Head kept in line with trunk when pulled to sitting
5 months	Lifts head in supine Lifts bottom in supine — 'bridges' Rolls to side Pushes up on straight arms in prone Reaches with one arm in prone
6 months	Sits with hands in front for support Rolls supine to prone Takes both feet to mouth Helps pull self to sitting
7 months	Pivots and pushes self backwards in prone
8 months	Creeps forwards on forearms Sits unsupported with straight back Can reach in sitting Can get into lying
8–10 months	Crawls on all fours Pulls to standing
10–12 months	Gets down from standing Walks with both or one hand held
12 months	Some children walk independently

fisted, and thumbs inside the palms. Gradually the arms will be able to move sideways and forwards away from the body. Yet by 3 months, when lying prone, the arms will still be partly flexed, with the elbows held behind the shoulders and the infant will be unable to reach forwards. The legs will also slowly become less flexed.

At 2 months, the infant starts to lift his head, although initially somewhat asymmetrically. Head-lifting is probably encouraged by the labyrinthine righting reaction which, together with the optical righting reaction, orientate the head in space.

By 4 months the infant will be lifting his head much higher, with his back quite extended. His arms will be further forward and he will now be able to bear weight on his forearms with his hands open. This is the so-called 'puppy position'.

At 5–6 months old, when lying prone, the infant can reach forward towards objects on the floor with two hands. He will also be able to take weight on one forearm while reaching with the other arm (Fig. 4.2). Another achievement is to push up on straight arms, with a very extended back (Fig. 4.3), which in many children will also result in extended and abducted legs.

By this stage the infant will have achieved a good degree of extensor tone. This ability to support himself on straight arms will occur at the same time as he is able to reach out to be picked up, either when lying supine, or sitting in a high-chair. The straight arms of the normal infant at 6 months will also give him the ability to support himself while sitting on the floor.

In Western culture, the infant's development in prone lying can be considered as the most usual way of laying the foundation for standing, and his development in supine lying as a preparation towards sitting. Head and trunk raising in prone lying is an extensor activity, preparing for extension against gravity and standing. The flexion associated with head raising in supine, together with being helped to sit up from supine, help towards learning to sit.

Developments in supine lying

The neonate lying supine is flexed, except for his head, which tends to be turned to one side, usually to the right. Most of the time his arms are flexed near to his body, with his hands clenched, often with the thumb inside the palm.

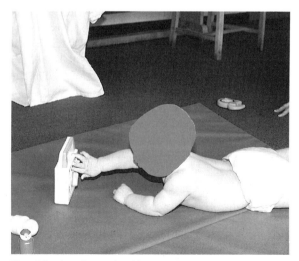

Fig. 4.2 Age 5 months. He can take weight on one forearm whilst reaching with the other.

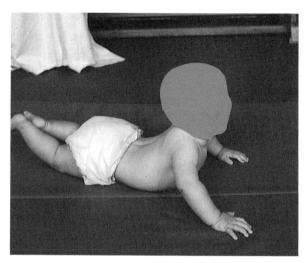

Fig. 4.3 5 months. He can push up on straight arms.

Occasionally he may totally extend, as when he stretches or is startled. The neonate does not usually show an ATNR (see p. 37) and, although some infants start to show one at 1 month old, ATNRs are most obvious when the baby is 2 months old. They are not obligatory in normal infants.

During the first and second months the infant's arms and legs will gradually become less flexed. By the age of 2 months the thumbs should be outside his palm, although in prone lying they may still be inside on exertion. At 4 months old the infant's posture will be more symmetrical, his head will face forwards, and he will not show ATNRs; he will be able to bring his hands together in midline and to take them to his mouth. When pulled up to sitting, he should be able to keep his head in line with his trunk.

At 5 months old, and lying supine, the infant will start to lift his head from the supporting surface. Also, with his knees bent and his feet flat on the floor, he may raise his bottom off the ground to make a 'bridge'. He will now be able to roll over to one side (Fig. 4.4) and, by 6 months, roll from supine to prone, like a log without trunk rotation. Sometimes he may hold his hands together while he rolls.

By 6 months the infant may lift both feet up towards his mouth, or reach for his feet and play with them. He will also reach out to be picked up, or to be taken out of a chair and, if ignored,

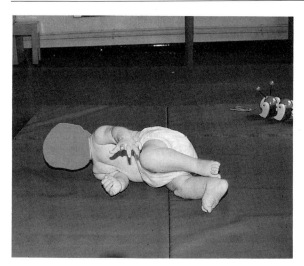

Fig. 4.4 5 months. He is now able to roll over to his side.

may cry as he reaches out to communicate his needs.

Head and trunk control

Initially, head and trunk control develop together. For example, when the infant is carried upright with a decreasing amount of support, his head and trunk have to compensate and gradually attain more postural stability. This also requires the infant to be able to adjust or balance his body and to cope with gravity as his position changes. The infant gradually learns to control his balance in changing circumstances and this will continue for a number of years. In prone lying an infant starts raising his head by 2 months, and succeeds in lifting it quite well by 3 months. At about 4 months old, when held upright, a baby should be able to maintain his head position when tilted to 45° in all directions.

Head control when pulled from supine to sitting. This is useful not only for checking the infant's head control, but for observing a general response. To test this response the infant's wrists may be grasped or the infant encouraged to grasp the tester's thumbs, with the wrists supported in extension. The infant's arms are kept straight as he is pulled to sitting. The responses at various ages are as follows. When the neonate is pulled to sitting his head lags and his shoulders, elbows,

wrists and fingers all flex strongly. This is called the traction reflex:

- 2 months: the head will lift a little
- 3 months: the head will be kept in line with the body
- 5 months: the infant will start to assist by bringing his head forward
- 6 months: he will help to pull himself to sitting, and he may extend and abduct his legs as he comes up.

Reflex to voluntary standing

When held upright, the neonate stands reflexively using the positive supporting reaction (Fig. 4.5). From 2–6 months the infant goes through a stage when he may be unable to take weight on his legs. Some children, when held upright, may even bend their legs up in the air. This is known as physiological abasia. There is also a stage during which, if attempts are made to walk a child, he is unlikely to take steps and will drag his feet.

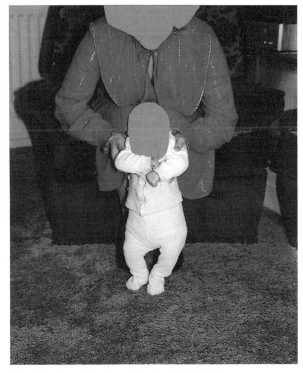

Fig. 4.5 6 weeks. Neonate stands reflexively.

This is the stage of physiological astasia. By 6 months, infants, when held, start taking weight voluntarily and by 9 months they will be pulling themselves to standing (Fig. 4.6).

Development in sitting

At 4 months the child is unable to sit on the floor without support (Fig. 4.7). As he sits, his legs will most likely be in a ring position, with knees and hips flexed and feet together.

Some infants will still need a little help at 5 months, whilst others may be sitting independently, using their hands for support. Children at this age usually have rounded backs when they sit on the floor, some may throw themselves backwards, possibly because they are still unable to keep their hips flexed, and extend their backs simultaneously. Occasionally a child may sit very steadily at 5 months, even without hand support. Usually these early sitters have good extensor tone, with straight extended knees and abducted hips, which provides a wide and firm base.

Most children should be able to sit with hand support by 6 months, and by 8 months sit unsupported for at least a short time.

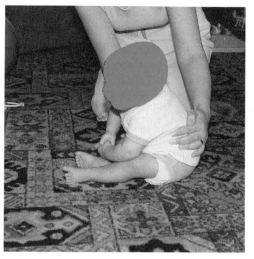

Fig. 4.7 4 months. He cannot sit on the floor without support.

Reactions in the first year

A number of reactions will only be evident by the end of the first year, but many of them start to appear at 6 months (see Table 4.1, p. 36).

Righting reactions

These orientate the head and body in space, and maintain alignment of the body parts. The righting reactions are not obligatory.

Neck righting reaction. This is present in the neonate and is integrated at 4–6 months. When the infant turns his head so that the chin points to the shoulder, the body will immediately come into line with the head.

Labyrinthine righting and optical righting reactions. Both these reactions are concerned with orientating the head in space. Unless we wish otherwise, the head is kept vertical, providing a consistent base from which we perceive the world. Labyrinthine righting reactions may be more useful in the early months when vision is limited, and they are similarly useful later in life if visual problems occur. These reactions operate when an infant is held upright and he keeps his head vertical, even when his body is moved. At 2.5 months the infant can hold his head upright while being carried, and by 4 months he can maintain the vertical when tilted to 45°. They

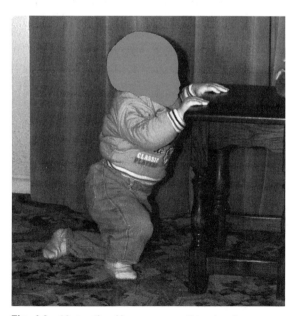

Fig. 4.6 10 months. He can now pull to standing.

also operate when the child lifts his head in prone and in supine.

Both reactions remain for life; however, many individuals are unable to right their heads unless their eyes are open and optical righting can be used.

Body on head, and body on body righting reactions. These reactions are stimulated when feedback from tactile receptors enables the individual to align himself according to distribution of body weight. If there is pressure on the soles of the feet, the whole body will be induced to stand upright. Tactile information that pressure on the buttocks in sitting is unequal will automatically result in correction of the weight distribution, and will assist in upright sitting.

In lying if the head is turned to the side or tilted out of alignment with the trunk, this information is received through touch and pressure. The body on head righting reaction will facilitate a return to the correct alignment. Similarly, when the trunk is rotated the body on body righting reaction facilitates subsequent derotation.

This reaction can be observed in children before the age of about 5 years. When they are sitting up from lying supine they still need to use rotation to first roll into prone, or to their sides.

Protective extension of the arms. As the child's weight moves outside his base, so that he is about to fall, the arm(s) automatically extend for protection.

Protective extension forward. At 6 months the infant will usually be able to protect himself from falling forwards by taking weight on his arms. This ability may be used as a test and is known as the downward parachute of the arms. The infant is held vertically in the air, supported by holding both sides of his chest. He is then tilted fairly quickly towards the ground, and the arms and fingers extend forward and abduct. At 6 months, only one-third of children show a full response, but most children will do so by 9 months. This protective reaction is not dependent on the use of vision.

Protective extension sideways. At 8 months infants will protect themselves with abduction of their arms sideways.

Protective extension backwards. At 10 months the infant will save himself on his elbows as he goes

backwards; by 12 months he will use extended arms.

Downward parachute of the legs. From about the fourth month, if a vertically held child is brought down rapidly towards the floor, his legs will extend and abduct and his toes splay.

The Landau reaction. The child is held horizontally, face downwards, with one hand under the lower thorax and the other on top. From 4 months old the head and back will extend, with the legs at first partially extended, and later fully extended. However, if the head is passively flexed, the whole body flexes. This reaction is strong at 1 year of age, but between 1 and 2 years it will integrate.

Equilibrium reactions. Equilibrium reactions in any position begin to develop once that position has been attained. They will first be present:

- in prone at 6 months
- in supine and sitting between 7 and 8 months
- in on all fours position between 9 and 12 months
- in standing between 12 and 21 months.

Reactions will continue to improve and become more skilful for many years as the child achieves increasingly difficult motor abilities. For example, he may stand and balance well, but when he starts to throw a ball in this position he will at first find balancing difficult, and will have to do more motor learning before he can achieve this satisfactorily. If equilibrium reactions are not adequate to prevent falling, the child will save himself by using protective reactions or propping of arms or legs.

Development between the ages of 6 and 12 months (see Table 4.2, p. 39)

Developments in prone lying

At 5–6 months old, an infant lying prone should be reaching out for objects with one hand, while taking his weight on the opposite forearm, and by 7 months his weight should be supported on his hand. Also at 7 months, while lying prone, infants may pivot round or push backwards, before they eventually start creeping forwards. When infants first creep, the forearms will do the work, but gradually their legs become involved and make reciprocal movements. While they are learning to creep, they may be trying to achieve a crawling or all fours position, facilitated by the symmetrical tonic neck reflex.

Sitting

By 8 months infants should be sitting with a straight back, without hand support. At last they can use both their hands to play with objects that are within reach (Fig. 4.8). By 8 months infants no longer roll with flexed legs like a log, but use trunk rotation assisted by the body on body righting reaction. This recently acquired trunk rotation will make possible a new range of activities. The infant can now reach across to the other side of his body to touch or pick up objects. He can also develop the ability to go from sitting on the floor, to either prone lying or to a crawling position; and eventually he will use rotation to get back from the floor to sitting again. There are at least two ways of going down to the floor. Some infants put both hands down to the floor on one side of their bodies, and then either roll over to prone or to all fours. From sitting, others

go straight forward over their flexed legs, into a crawling position.

Crawling

Early crawling is slow as the infant moves one limb at a time in a contralateral pattern. Eventually the arm and leg of opposite sides will be used together. Variations in crawling may develop. Some infants may periodically bring one foot through and put the sole on the ground; others may 'bear walk' with hands and toes on the ground, and with fairly straight arms and legs. Crawling may continue even after the child has started to walk.

Pull to stand

Between 8 and 10 months, when they are crawling on all fours, infants may grab their parents' legs or the seat of a chair, and pull themselves up to standing. They can stand holding a support for quite a long time, and they very quickly learn to hold with only one hand. It may be another 2 months before they learn how to get down from standing but their very short legs and well-covered bottoms make bumping down backwards a regular procedure, which most do not appear to find too unpleasant.

Walking

Between 10 and 12 months most children will be able to walk, when either one or both hands are held by an adult. Some may also walk sideways supporting themselves on furniture, while a few will be walking independently.

Development between 12 and 18 months

Walking and running

The normal age range for starting to walk is 10–15 months, with the average being around 13 months (Fig. 4.9). Occasionally, children may not walk before they are 2 years old. Some health authorities investigate children who are not walking at 18 months, to try to make sure there are no causating disorders. When children first walk, they walk with their legs wide apart and with their

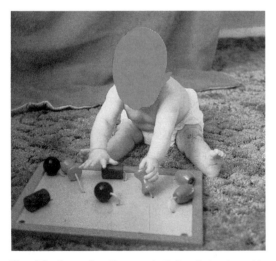

Fig. 4.8 8 months. Can use both hands to play with objects within reach.

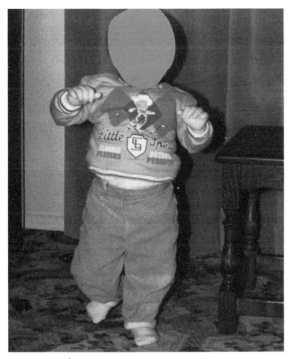

Fig. 4.9 $10\frac{3}{4}$ months. Starts to walk. Note the position of the arms in abduction.

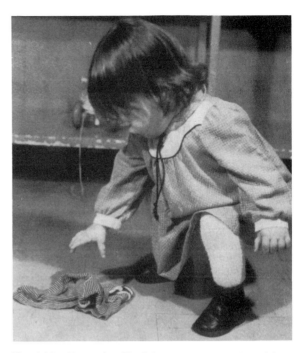

Fig. 4.10   18 months. The infant can now squat to pick objects up. (Reproduced by permission of Churchill Livingstone from Gassier J 1984 A guide to the psycho-motor development of the child.)

knees and hips slightly flexed, and usually their arms are abducted at or above shoulder level.

At 18 months a child may be walking with his arms down by his sides and his feet probably turned out. His base will become narrower as his balance improves. At 18 months he can push a toy truck as he walks; and is also able to run carefully.

Independent rise to standing

By 15 months many children stand up by themselves from the floor. They first roll into prone, then they push themselves backwards with their hands until they are squatting on hands and feet, and finally they heave themselves up to standing. When standing, with no support to hold on to by which they can lower themselves, they either sit down with a bump, or fall forward onto their hands.

At 18 months the child will be able to squat to pick up objects and play as he remains squatting (Fig. 4.10).

Stairs

Children of 15 months who are given the opportunity, may creep up stairs, and some may come down slowly, backwards.

Kneeling

At approximately 15 months the child begins to kneel up whilst holding on to a support, and by 18 months he should be able to high kneel without a support.

Sitting

Children of this age, wanting to sit on an adult chair, first climb forwards onto the chair and then turn round to sit down. However, if they wish to sit on a small chair they will probably walk backwards towards it, and then sit down.

Development at the age of 2 years

By 2 years of age the child should be running

confidently, avoiding obstacles, starting and stopping at will. If he has a tricycle, he will be able to sit on it, although as he moves around on it his feet remain on the ground because he is still unable to keep them on the pedals.

Specific motor skill development

There is a wide range in the age at which various motor skills develop in different children, and it is important to observe how children perform these skills. A number of examples are given below (Table 4.3).

Table 4.3 Gross motor skills, 12 months–5 years

Age	Skill
13 months	Walks
15 months	Independent rise to stand Comes down stairs backwards Creeps up stairs Kneels up holding on
18 months	Kneels up without support Squats to play
18–30 months	Goes upstairs — holding on — both feet on each step
2–2½ years	Jumps off floor, both feet together
2½–3 years	Alternate feet up and down stairs
3 years	Jumps off bottom step Stands momentarily on one leg
4 years	Stands on one leg 3–5 seconds
5 years	Jumps over knee-high cord feet together

Climbing stairs

At 13 months infants are able to creep up stairs, and by 15 months slowly come down backwards. The variability in age of attainment for climbing stairs holding a support is illustrated by the Bayley Motor Scales, with a range of 12–23 months for this activity. Children go up and down stairs without holding on, putting both feet on each step, somewhere between 18 and 30 months; and between 30 and 36 months they manage with alternate feet on each step. In each mode, they go up stairs about a month earlier than they come down.

Jumping

Children can jump off the floor with two feet between 2 and 2.5 years, and by 3 years they should be able to jump off a bottom step. When 5 years old, most children can jump over a knee-high cord, with their feet together. It is important to observe whether the child can jump both with feet together and bend his knees on landing.

Standing on one leg

Children should be able to stand on one leg for a short time at 3 years of age, and by 4 years they can usually manage this for 3–5 seconds.

Throwing and catching a ball
(Table 4.4)

When standing up, children should be able to throw a ball overhand without falling when they are between 2 and 2.5 years old. By 3.5 years they may throw it overhand a distance of 2 m (Fig. 4.11). Throwing a ball underhand should be possible for a child of 2.5–3 years. Catching is a more difficult skill than throwing, as much depends on the thrower and the size of the ball. The thrower should aim for the ball to go towards the chest of the child, and a medium sized, non-slippery ball is easier than a tennis ball. By 5 years children should be able to catch either a ball of about 2.5 cm diameter or a beanbag, at a distance of about 2 m. Also at 5 years, they should bounce a tennis ball with one hand and catch it with two hands for about half the trials. By 6–7 years they should be able to bounce and catch a tennis ball with one hand, using either hand, and succeed for at least half the trials (Cohen & Gross 1979). It is important to observe whether the child catches the ball clear of his body, or whether his body is used to help.

FINE MOTOR DEVELOPMENT

Fine motor development is closely associated with gross motor development (Table 4.5). Good head and trunk control, together with a good posture, shoulder stability and normal arm movements, are all useful for fine motor activities.

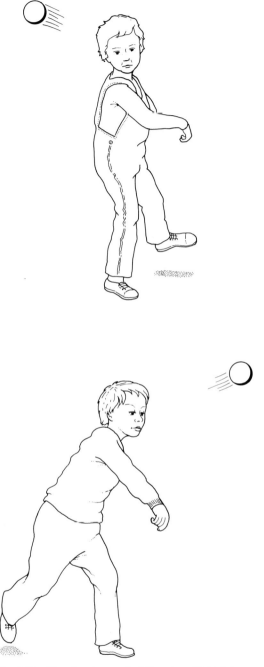

Fig. 4.11 The development of throwing. Note the progression to rotation of the body and stepping forward with weight on the opposite foot to the throwing arc.

Table 4.4 Development of projection skills

Age	Skill
9–10 months	Throws object to ground
18 months–$2\frac{1}{2}$ years	Throws ball without falling over
$2\frac{1}{2}$–3 years	Throws underhand
$3\frac{1}{2}$ years	Throws overhand 2 metres
5 years	Body rotates when throws 2-handed catch from bounce
6 years	1-handed catch from bounce
8 years	2-handed catch in air
9 years	1-handed catch in air
10 years	Moves to intercept ball

fingers and hand are essential. Fine motor development occurs in a predictable sequence of events, which allows the following generalisations to be made:

1. Early reflexes and basic voluntary movements, which are in total patterns, provide a foundation for more skilled movements.
2. Development progresses from the proximal parts of the arm to the distal.
3. Pronation of the forearm is achieved before supination.
4. Grasp is learned before release.

Early reflexes and reactions

Grasp reactions

The neonate does not show a true grasp reflex, but a 'tonic reaction of the fingers' (Bobath 1969). If a finger is inserted into the hand and traction applied, the whole arm and the fingers strongly flex.

By the fourth month, an instinctual grasp reaction occurs when a gentle stimulus touches the radial or ulnar side of the hand, and results in the hand automatically turning towards that stimulus. At 6–7 months, the stimulus touching the ulnar side of the hand will cause the hand to pronate, while one to the radial side will cause supination. Each is followed by the infant automatically trying to grasp the object. At this stage

Vision is also helpful but not essential for the learning of manipulatory skills; but grasp and release, and good sensorimotor control of the

Table 4.5 Development of hand use

Age	Skill
1 month	Hand clenches on contact, thumb idle Drops object immediately
2 months	Grasp in pronation
2–3 months	Retains rattle briefly Looks at hands
3 months	Holds rattle actively
4 months	Reaches with two hands
5–6 months	Releases object by throwing or dropping
6 months	Grasps cube with palmar grasp Visually directed reach
7 months	Grasps object in half supination Extends wrist with grasp
8 months	Releases with pressure on a surface Passes object from one hand to other Inferior scissor grip
9 months	Releases object into large container
10–11 months	Grasp integrated with vision
12 months	Fine pincer grasp Precision release into small container
12–18 months	Grasps pencil in fisted hand and scribbles
18 months	Builds tower of three bricks
18 months–3 years	Pencil held in pronated hand
$2\frac{1}{2}$ years	Builds tower of six to eight bricks Lines bricks into a train
3 years	Imitates bridge of three bricks Cuts with scissors
4 years	Threads small beads
$4\frac{1}{2}$–6 years	Holds pencil in dynamic tripod

of grasping the hand orientates towards the stimulus, even when the object or stimulus cannot be seen. Integration of the instinctual grasp reaction with vision occurs at 10–11 months.

Avoidance reaction

Up to the age of 6 months an avoidance reaction may occur when an infant grasps an object, so

that if the finger tips touch the object the fingers may open involuntarily, dropping the object.

Learning about hands

Infants suck their fists and fingers, which provides some awareness of their hands, but in the second and third months they also spend a lot of time looking at their hands. When ATNRs occur, their vision will be focused on their outstretched hand, which may provide a foundation towards achieving eye–hand coordination. At 4 months old they will look at both hands together.

The hand as an instrument of investigation

The hand is not only a tool for manipulating objects, but is also an instrument of investigation, with the help of which the immediate environment is explored. Infants in their first year of life pick up objects, shake and bang them, or transfer them from hand to hand; they also take them to their mouths. However, it is mainly in the second year that they deliberately investigate objects with their hands by feeling, squeezing and turning objects over and over while looking at them. During this exploration they learn about texture, shape, size, weight, consistency and temperature.

Reaching

In both supine and sitting positions the 4-month-old infant tries to reach out with two hands. Shoulder movements are used mainly, with the backs of the hands approaching the object in a circuitous manner, but because of his partly flexed arms the distance he can reach is very limited. He is able to stretch further at 5 months, but sometimes under-reaches, and later he may for a time tend to over-reach; but by 6 months he is starting to develop eye–hand coordination.

Eye–hand coordination

At 5 months a child may reach for an object. Sometimes his reach is accurate but at other times it is not, and when he misses the target he tries again. This is called visually initiated reaching, as the child initially looks at the object that motivates him; this also gives him an indication of the direction of the object, but at this stage his reaching is not yet visually monitored. At 6 months, when he reaches for an object but his aim is inaccurate he can correct the movement, as he is now receiving visual feedback. His reaching is now visually directed (Bower 1974). At 6 months of age he can look at the object and his hand at the same time, he can monitor his movement, and has started to develop eye–hand coordination. When the infant is 12 months old, once he has visually located the object, he should be able to reach for it without having to visually monitor his reach (Cohen & Gross 1979).

All these early volitional movements will be performed with pronated forearms until the child is 12 months old, when he becomes able to supinate his forearms voluntarily.

Voluntary grasp

The ability to grasp an object must in part depend on the size and shape of the object. A small object like a pea may not be picked up before 7 months, and then very clumsily, but a larger cube is grasped earlier.

A 3-month-old infant will grasp a small cube only when the cube actually touches the hand, but at 4 months the infant will be able to locate and grasp the cube if it is close to his hand. In both the above instances, when the cube is grasped a total flexor pattern occurs in the hand and the arm.

Ulnar palmar grasp. At 5 months a cube is grasped with all the flexed fingers and adducted thumb pressing the cube against the ulnar side of the palm, using *ulnar palmar grasp*.

Radial palmar grasp. At 6 and 7 months the child will probably use a *radial palmar grasp*. The object is now held on the radial side of the palm with flexed fingers, and at 6 months an adducted thumb, which may be opposed by the seventh month. At 7 months he will also be starting to extend his wrist when he grips.

Radial digital grasp. At 8 months old the child should be using his finger tips and opposed thumb only, with a space between the object and

his palm, when picking up a cube. This is a *radial digital grasp*.

Scissors grip. By 8 months a small object such as a pea can be grasped between the thumb and the side of the partly flexed finger, a *scissors grip*.

Inferior pincer grip. A 9-month-old infant can extend his index finger, while keeping his other fingers bent; this allows a new range of activities to be undertaken. He will be able to point with the index finger, which will help with communication, and also to poke objects with one finger, a movement that will prepare for a pincer grip. Small objects will now be grasped with the pads of his index finger and thumb in an *inferior pincer grip*.

Fine pincer grip. A *fine pincer grip* should be perfected by an infant of 12 months old, when he should be able to pick up small objects using only the tips of his index finger and thumb. When using these more skilled forms of hand grasp (prehension), children of this age often mirror the movement with the other hand.

Release of an object

A child finds it more difficult to voluntarily release an object than to grasp it. At 5–6 months he drops objects reflexively, but will only be able to let an object go voluntarily if it is also held by his mouth or his other hand; which allows him to transfer objects from one hand to the other. By 7 months he may learn to release an object when he presses it against a surface. At 9 months he will be able to freely release an object into a large container. He will be 12 months old before he can precisely release an object into a small container.

Use of a pencil

At 12–18 months old, a child will grasp a crayon or pencil with a fisted hand and will scribble using large movements of the whole arm (Fig. 4.12A). Between 18 months and 3 years children often use a pronated hold, with the hand facing downwards and the pencil in the palm of the hand. The index finger rests on the upper surface of the pencil, the thumb on one side and the remaining fingers on the other (Fig. 4.12B).

Dynamic tripod grip. During this period some children might experiment with a more mature grip, with the pencil resting between the thumb and first finger, supported by the radial side of the middle finger. This is the start of the tripod grip. Between the ages of 4.5 and 6 years, the child will learn small intricate movements of the interphalangeal joints; this grip is now called the *dynamic tripod grip* (Rosenbloom & Horton 1971) (Fig. 4.12C). Using these movements of the fingers the child should be able to form individual letters and shoulder movement, aided

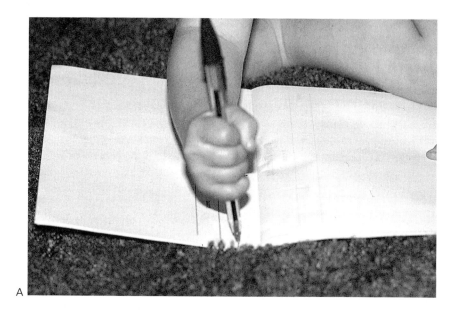

A

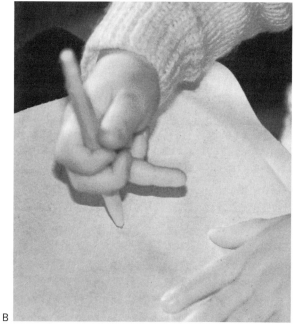

B

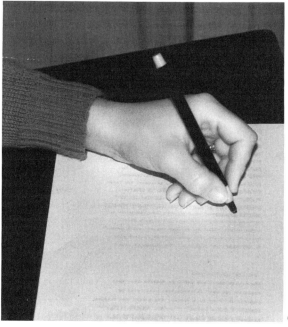

C

Fig. 4.12 Development of a mature pencil grip. (A) 20 months. (B) 2/4 years. (C) Mature grip.

by wrist and elbow movements, will be used to direct the flow of writing or drawing across the page.

Manipulatory skills

The following is a list of approximate ages for copying geometrical shapes. When copying these shapes, a variety of reasons may cause differences in performance between children. There may be differences in sensorimotor ability, learning ability, spatial and/or perceptual ability; some may have more experience of handling and recognising the shapes by touch; others may use pencils more often, or have a lot of experience of handling similar shaped tools, e.g. chopsticks (Ziviani 1987).

Copying geometric shapes. According to Alston & Taylor (1987), the ages at which the child should be able to copy the various geometric shapes are as follows:

- 2 years: vertical line
- 2.5 years: horizontal line
- 3 years: circle
- 4 years: cross
- 5 years: square
- 5.5 years: triangle
- 7 years: diamond.

Building with small cubes. Sheridan (1975) has produced a similar comparison for a child's ability to build with small cubes (Fig. 4.13):

- 15 months: builds a tower of two cubes after a demonstration
- 18 months: builds a tower of three cubes
- 2 years: builds a tower of six cubes
- 3 years: builds a tower of nine cubes
- 3.5 years: builds a bridge with three cubes.

HEARING

Babies appear to have normal hearing, although like other young children they can hear higher frequencies than adults. If a sound is made to one side, the young infant's eyes turn towards the sound.

Simple hearing tests at 3 months can consist of tinkling a spoon in a cup, or gently ringing a bell, with the object out of sight, about

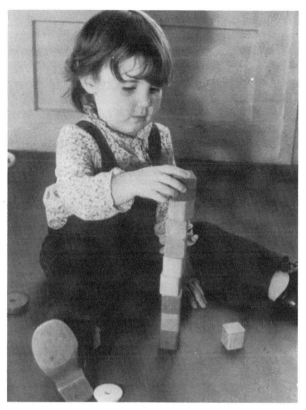

Fig. 4.13 3 years. The child can build a tower of eight to nine cubes. (Reproduced by permission of Churchill Livingstone from Gassier J 1984 A guide to the psycho-motor development of the child.)

15–30 cm away, and with a noise duration of 3–5 seconds.

Even from their earliest days, babies have a preference for human voice sounds to other sounds. Recent research has shown that babies a few days old will bodily move in synchrony with human speech sounds, and no other sounds (Condon & Sander 1974). By 4 months babies can recognise one parent from the other by their voice.

Some indication of children's hearing ability may be obtained from listening to the sounds that they make. Babies start babbling at about 1 month and deaf babies also babble at that age (see Chapter 14 Sensory Disorders: the deaf and blind child). But at 6 months the quality of babbling changes; normal babies start to imitate sounds that they hear, but the babbling from deaf babies tends to fade. From 8 months infants use

Table 4.6 Development of auditory skills and communication

Age	Skill
1 month	Babbles
2 months	Localises source of sound
3–4 months	Turns head to sound Interested in voice
5–6 months	Sensitive to intonation and music Imitates sound
6–9 months	Listens attentively
8 months	Strings syllables together, i.e. 'da-da-da'
9–12 months	Reaches for sound without sight
15 months	2–6 single word utterances
18 months	Uses 20 recognisable words
2 years	Joins in nursery rhymes
3 years	Uses plurals and pronouns Asks what, who, where
4–5 years	Acts out stories
5 years	Fluent speech

strings of syllables such as 'da-da-da', practising sounds they are trying to imitate. Children also use intonation with their jargon, the prelanguage vocalisations that they use indicating they can hear and listen to the intonation of adults. Lieberman (1967) has shown that infants also listen to pitch. Children between 10 and 13 months were observed and it was noted that changes in the pitch of their babbling occurred depending upon which parent they were with; when with the mother the babbling was higher pitched than when they were with their father (Table 4.6).

Between 12 and 18 months, children are alert when they can hear very quiet sounds that could be meaningful, but if the sounds are repeated without an interesting result they soon get bored.

After 18 months, his own spontaneous listening behaviour, and his standard of verbal communication, are good indicators of his hearing ability.

DEVELOPMENT OF COMMUNICATION

Communication consists of language and non-verbal communication. We listen to the words, the intonation, the voice quality of the speaker, and we are also influenced by his facial expression, his bodily posture, gestures and any eye contact he makes.

Language has a number of uses:

1. Objects and events are represented symbolically by words in verbal or printed forms.
2. Language helps us to communicate our thoughts to others.
3. With language we talk to ourselves overtly or covertly, reflecting on what we are doing or thinking.

To use language successfully, the communicants must have a shared understanding of the meaning, grammar, and how their culture uses words (Table 4.6).

Non-verbal communication

Non-verbal communication is most important in infancy before the ability to speak has been developed. Wolff (1969) has described three different types of crying for discomfort such as hunger, pain and anger. Many mothers understand why their infant is crying and can therefore respond appropriately to different types of cry. Infants will also communicate their feelings and wishes through body movements, facial expression and vocalisation.

Learning to communicate

An infant needs to realise that his behaviour can produce an effect on other people's actions before he is able to communicate in a purposeful, intentional way. Rogers (1985) gives the following example of how intentionality might arise:

'An infant of 6 months may reach unsuccessfully for an object, and his mother gives it to him. But by 9 months he will look at his mother and then reach and point, to indicate his need for her help. Now he is intentionally communicating his needs.'

To communicate successfully, babies have also to learn to take turns; to give attention and then act (Bruner 1979). Babies are not very good at giving attention, as they are constantly distracted by novel stimuli. They need to learn to attend to their mother's face while she talks to them.

Learning to use language

As with other forms of development, there are wide variations in the age at which children use language. To learn language infants need hearing and to have reached an appropriate level of cognitive development. Infants do not learn language from television (Clark & Clark 1977), which suggests that speech needs to be directed personally to them. Before learning language, babies in the sensorimotor stage will have interacted with and experienced their environment. Kessen & Nelson (1979) believe babies are most interested in making 'a functional analysis of the world of what is moveable, eatable, and touchable'. As a result of their interaction, babies construct mental concepts about how they perceive, feel and think about their world. Piaget says that children, before they have language, think without the use of words, much as we might think about human faces, or music without words.

Receptive language

Children usually understand a number of words by 12 months. These will usually be words that they have frequently heard in specific situations, such as 'bye, bye', 'hello' or 'pat-a-cake'. This is the start of receptive language. At this stage children do not appreciate that words represent objects and other concepts. Between 8 and 18 months they will learn that objects still exist even when they cannot be perceived (see cognitive development, p. 56). When the child has acquired this concept of object permanence (see p. 56), his receptive language ability will further develop. He will now be able to use symbols such as words to represent objects and other concepts that he has previously formed.

Verbal comprehension

The child will soon have understood short sentences such as 'fetch your shoe' and, by 3 to 3.5 years, he will verbally comprehend instructions with more than one concept, e.g. 'put dolly in the bath and wash her face'.

Expressive language

Infants babble and practise imitating sounds in their first year. By 15 months most children will be able to use expressive language for two to six single words, but they overextend their use of words, for example, cows, horses and dogs may all be called 'dogs', and all men 'dadda'. An 18-month-old child may use up to 20 recognisable words, understanding many more.

Children may use up to 50 different words singly before they start putting two words together. Two-word utterances usually consist of essential words only, which has led to their being called telegraphic speech. Children will soon add prepositions such as 'in' and 'on', followed by 's' to make nouns plural, and afterwards the articles 'a' and 'the'. There has been much debate on how children learn syntax or the rules of grammar, and Snow & Ferguson (1977) suggest a major influence is the way mothers talk to their children. Most mothers use what has been called 'baby talk register' or 'motherese'. They adjust their speech to their child's level of understanding, and talk slowly with an exaggerated intonation, in concrete terms about the 'here and now'. Mothers use short, simple, grammatically correct sentences that they repeat with slight variations, e.g. 'Pick up the red one. No, the red one. That's right, pick the red one up.' Young children often take the incentive in interaction, the mother following their lead.

By the time they are 3 years old, children have a large vocabulary, use plurals, pronouns, and ask 'what', 'who' and 'where' questions, although it may be another year before they use questions that ask 'how', 'when' and 'why'. Although speech is usually fluent by the time children are 5 years old, investigators have recently found that children of this age may still misunderstand some words, for instance 'more' and 'less' (Donaldson 1978), and 'ask' and 'tell' seem to cause difficulty for some children (Chomsky 1969).

VISION

The eyes of neonates are different in shape to those of adults, and the lens is fixed in focus at 20 cm, which is about the distance of the mother's face from the baby when she nurses him. Neonates are attracted to dim light, but turn away from bright light; they quickly learn to use the pupillary reflex to regulate the amount of light entering the eye. Neonates use only monocular vision, but binocular vision starts at 2 months and by 4 months infants are using binocular vision well. Neonates also move their eyes randomly, uncoordinated with their head movements, but by 1 month they move their eyes and head together, and at 6 months they can move their eyes independently. Infants seem able to discriminate colours at about 3 weeks, and by 3 months they prefer red and orange to other colours.

Accommodation

The lens needs to adjust rapidly when objects are seen at different distances. When the infant is 2 months old, this accommodation will have developed to the extent that he can vary his focus for distances between 18 cm and 162 cm. By 4 months of age his level of accommodation will be equal to that of an adult.

Acuity

The acuity of neonates is poor, but it greatly improves over the first six months of life (Table 4.7). By 6 months of age infants can probably track objects as well as an adult, and scan between three or more targets.

PERCEPTION

Bower (1974) has defined perception as 'the

process by which we gain immediate awareness of what is happening outside ourselves'. Perception is concerned with how we interpret sensations which reach the brain from our sense organs. Attention and memory are both essential components of this process.

Figure 4.14 is a simple model of how it is thought perception may occur. Input from the sensory organ 'A' is transformed into neural impulses, which go to the brain. Units of sensory information are individually briefly stored in 'B'. Perception is selective, so relevant impulses are filtered out from those which are not required. The remaining impulses are then differentiated into figure and ground. These interpreted units may be too small to form a recognisable pattern, so they are passed into short-term memory 'C', which is a temporary holding reservoir of limited capacity, where the perceptual units are briefly held and collected together, until they form a recognisable pattern. This information is then passed to the long-term memory 'D', which as a reservoir of past experience gives feedback to 'B' and 'C', to provide interpretation at those levels.

Perceptual concepts

Visual perception has been analysed into a number of concepts, which include the following:

Figure–ground discrimination

This is the most fundamental organisation in perception, where the percept is differentiated into

Table 4.7 Visual Acuity

Age	Distance (cm)	Acuity
1 month	25	Black stripe 0.3 cm wide
6 weeks	22–30	Follows small dangling object
3 months	182	Recognises family
6 months	600	Recognises people
	300	Tracks rolling ball 5 cm diameter
	25	Black stripe 0.04 cm wide

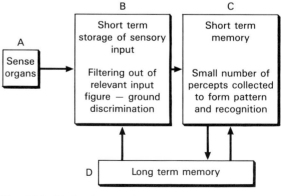

Fig. 4.14 Mode of perception.

objects that stand out and have shape or form — the figure — and a background or ground, which tends to be formless.

Appreciation of depth and distance

How do we know that the tiny car we can see is a good distance away, and not a toy car a few yards away? Bower (1966) has demonstrated that babies 6 weeks old are aware of depth and distance. When objects are a different distance away, if the head is moved sideways, say to the left, the near objects appear to move away to the right more quickly than the distant ones.

This motion parallax appears to be the major factor used by young babies in judging depth and distance. Sloboda (1985) points out that this phenomenon is obvious when you look out of the side window of a railway carriage, and the near objects flash by, while distant ones look almost stationary. Other optical factors and experience are probably also involved when babies get older.

Size and shape constancy

With experience we tend to see objects as being of constant size and shape, whatever the distance they are away, or the perspective in which we see them. For instance, we perceive a coin lying on the table as being circular, although it is probably an elipse that we actually see.

Closure

With closure there is a tendency to see incomplete objects as being complete, e.g. the spaces in a dotted line may be filled in so that an outline drawing is seen as complete (Table 4.8).

Perception in infancy

Ingenious experiments have recently shown that neonates have some perceptual abilities, including the appreciation of depth and distance. But they do not seem able to appreciate shape, form or orientation (Sloboda 1985). A model of a human face does not interest the neonate any more than a jumbled set of facial features. They start to have a conception of shape and form at

Table 4.8   Development of visual skills

Age	Visual skill
1 month	Eyes and head move together
2–4 months	Stares at hands Follows object 180° side to side Fascinated by bright colours and light Uses binocular vision
5–6 months	Associates touch and vision Uses eyes to explore Uses eyes independently of head
9–12 months	Watches moving objects
12–18 months	Form constancy develops
4 years	Visual concept of part–whole relationships

about 3 months, probably due to maturation of the visual perceptual area of the cerebral cortex.

However, a wide range of visual experience is essential for the development of normal perceptual abilities. Sloboda questions whether confining babies to cots and cribs provides them with the wealth of visual experience that would be of optimal benefit to them. He contrasts their experience with that of infants in cultures who are constantly carried around by their mothers.

As visual experience accumulates, memory and interpretation increase their role in perception; by 3 months a baby will discriminate between a pattern of a human face and other patterns, and will smile at it. By 5–6 months the child is likely to reserve his smiling for his mother or other care givers. At 8 months he may perceive the mood his mother is in, by looking at her face. With experience, he gradually becomes able to discriminate increasingly fine detail about the human face.

This increasing skill in perceiving patterns appears to be dependent on the child having the opportunity to gain experience in perceiving relevant material. More than one sensory modality is used, and the child will use both looking and feeling at the same time.

The perception of pattern is essential when the child begins to learn to read and write. He must now become aware that symbols not only have a shape, but also a left–right and an upper–lower orientation.

COGNITIVE DEVELOPMENT

Cognition refers to the activities of thinking, conceiving and reasoning. There are many theories of cognitive development, but those of Piaget have attracted most attention. Piaget investigated how children think, and considered that their thinking was very different to that of adults. He believed that children need to interact dynamically with their environment to develop their intellect. At first they interact physically, but later they interact with the action of the mind, i.e. perception and cognition.

Children use their past experience to link together previously practised movements and to construct ways of achieving objectives, e.g. how to reach for a biscuit, take it to the mouth and eat it. Piaget calls the mental plan of any activity a *schema*. The child's understanding of the object will be in terms of his interaction with it; what he did and how the object reacted. If he successfully repeats his reaching and eating technique with other objects, he will perceive these objects to have common attributes, and will form a concept of 'things he can grasp and eat'.

In time, with increased understanding, this generalised concept will be broken down into more rigorously defined concepts, each concept containing objects with common attributes, and differing from other concepts in specific ways, e.g. biscuits and puddings may become concepts. Once the child has the use of language, it will be easier to construct a range of concepts.

Piaget believes children have an invariant inborn capacity to develop in stages, with each stage building on the previous one. However, all children do not progress through the stages at the same rate, or achieve the same ultimate grade of cognition (Table 4.9).

Sensorimotor stage, 0–2 years

The infant's world is one of action and perception, and he will think in images until he develops language. The infant practises motor skills with much repetition, learning to use his body and to cope effectively with the environment. He acquires prelinguistic skills (see communication, p. 52), as well as achieving the

Table 4.9 Development of cognitive skills

Age	Skill
4 months	Brings object in hand to mouth
7 months	Pats a mirror
8 months	Removes cover from favourite toy
9 months	Explores objects in hand with interest
10 months	Waves goodbye Removes small toy from under cup
12 months	Puts comb to hair Looks for object out of sight Recognises 'No'
18 months	Points to distant interesting objects Obeys simple instructions Points to body parts
2 years	Refers to self by name Actively curious with no sense of danger Make-believe play
$2\frac{1}{2}$ years	Understands up, down, sideways, 200+ words
3 years	Matches colours, mainly red and yellow
4 years	Appreciates past, present, future Counts to 20
5 years	Acts out stories
6 years	Begins to understand rules and negotiation

concepts of 'object permanence' and instrumentation'. He will also learn to behave meaningfully with intent, termed 'intentionality' (see communication, p. 52).

Object permanence or object concept

Until the age of 1 year infants are not aware that objects exist when they are out of sight. This concept of object permanence is gradually attained between the age of 8 and 18 months. At 6 months, when an object is put under a container or cloth the infant loses interest, even though he sees it being hidden. This will occur even when the infant wants the object more than the article that covers it. Between the ages of 8 and 12 months the infant will immediately look under the cover and find the object. If, after a number of repetitions, the object is hidden under a different cover while the child is watching, he will still look for it under the first cover, where it was placed the first time. Between 12 and 18 months, he should look immediately under the correct cover, but not until 18–24 months is he likely to attain the final stage. One method of testing object concept uses three cloths. The child is shown an object lying in the open palm of an adult's hand. The adult makes a fist to conceal the object. The adult then places the fist in turn under each of the cloths and leaves the object under one of them. The child is then asked to find the object. By systematically looking under each cloth the child should be able to find the object.

Once the child has achieved an understanding that objects exist even when they cannot be seen, he will begin to develop an awareness that they can be represented by symbols.

Instrumentation

At about 8 months an infant can obtain an object which is out of reach by using another object or instrument, e.g. a piece of string to pull a toy. By 15 months, if a desired object is out of reach and a stick is available, he might realise that he can use the stick to get the object.

Pre-operational stage, 2–7 years

The term operation means a higher form of thinking, in which reversals can occur, e.g. a child will appreciate that a sausage-shaped roll of plasticine, when rolled out flat, can be returned to its original form. In the pre-operational stage children are unable to reverse mental thought in this way. For example, if they are shown the same amount of water in two identical containers, A and B (Fig. 4.15), they will agree that there is the same amount of water in each; however, if they then see the water from B being poured into the taller, narrower container C, and if A and C are then compared and the child asked which has the most water, a child at this stage will invariably say C. This is because he relies on his perception, but can only take one dimension into consideration.

Children of this age are egocentric, in that they find it difficult to take another person's point of view. They may think an appropriate present for

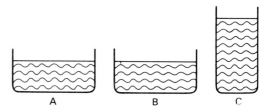

Fig. 4.15 Pre-operational stage 2–7 years: only one dimension taken into consideration in perception of quantity. A child would judge (A) and (B) to contain similar amounts of fluid, but that (C) contains more than (A).

their mother is something they would like themselves. This is also a time of pretending, and role play (see play, p. 59), although occasionally the child may not be able to differentiate between fantasy and reality.

Concrete operational stage, 7–11 years

Children at this stage are no longer egocentric, although they are still tied to the 'here and now'. The child is able to work things out mentally and can accept that some actions are reversible, and therefore understands the concept of conservation. He can use concrete thought to do arithmetic calculations with objects that are present, but has difficulty with algebra, which requires abstract thought. Nine-year-olds are still unable to do abstract verbal propositions, e.g. 'Helen is taller than Mary, Mary is taller than Jane, who is tallest of the three?'

Formal operational stage, 11–15 years

At this stage children can think abstractly, and no longer have to rely on concrete situations. They can reason about the hypothetical and, in solving a problem, can apply their reasoning in a practical way so as to consider all the possible factors that could lead to its solution. The child has now developed a logical, sequential process of thought in which internal language is used to analyse the many general concepts that have been acquired. Appropriate answers are deduced from the various hypotheses the child poses to itself.

Not all children in Britain reach this stage, and in some societies even the adults do not develop this form of thinking. Some societies use alternative methods and think in a holistic rather than a logical manner.

PLAY

By definition, play has no goals other than enjoyment, yet it can have a major influence on a child's development of motor, perceptual, communicational and social skills.

Most play is of a social nature. In the first year this is usually with cooperative, predictable parents or older siblings. In their second year of life, most children who play with peers do so in parallel, each playing independently but spending much of their time watching each other. By 2 years of age they manage to play cooperatively for up to a quarter of their time together, with disruptions as toys are snatched away or other disputes arise. As Garvey (1977) points out, 2-year-olds have a lot to learn about how to cope with 'other volatile equally inept playmates'. By 3 years of age they are more prepared to share their toys.

Piaget has pointed out that different types of play develop with increasing cognitive competence, and the following is his classification of play:

Sensorimotor stage, 0–2 years

Before the age of 2 years, play mainly consists of sensorimotor activities or practice play. By frequent repetition the child learns to control his movements, gain eye–hand coordination, and learn about his environment.

0–4 months

The infant is looking and listening. Simple hanging toys and mobiles are useful, but should look good from the baby's viewpoint, not the adult's. Mother and child often spend a lot of time looking at each other and when the infant starts babbling they take turns to make noises.

4–8 months

From 4 months the infant will hold toys with two hands and will soon reach for toys (Fig. 4.16). At 5–6 months if he finds reaching in prone difficult, a thin roll of carpet under his chest may help. He can now pick cubes up and pass them from hand to hand. He likes to play games like 'pat-a-cake' and 'this little piggy'. The infant also likes playing with his parents' face, and comes to learn that mother is a separate person from himself.

8–12 months

The infant will tend to grasp an object and take it to his mouth, then grasp another and take that to his mouth at the same time. He will also wave and bang objects, and learn that objects exist even when he cannot see them (see cognitive development, p. 56). He should also learn to pull a mobile toy towards himself with a piece of string. Anticipation and turn-taking games with his parents are good for developing the pre-linguistic skills of giving attention, and learning to look at the adult's face to determine whose turn it is next (Bruner 1979). Many parents will start to play a little more robustly with their children at this age.

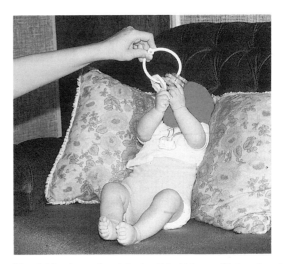

Fig. 4.16 4 months. Infant will hold toys with two hands.

15 months

Children now inspect and investigate objects when they first pick them up. They also learn to associate objects that are conventionally used together, such as a cup and saucer, and they will brush their own hair. They will start building with bricks, and scribbling with a crayon.

18–24 months

They are now starting pretend games, such as giving dolly a drink. They also like sand and water play and outdoor activities.

Representational or symbolic stage, 2–6 years

New forms of play evolve as the child becomes aware that objects can be represented by words, pictures or another object, for example, a dish may become the steering wheel of a car. He may also pretend to play 'house', 'hospitals', 'shops', and take the role of 'mother', 'baby', 'shopkeeper' and 'nurse', at first with his older siblings and later with his peers. Mead (1984) believes role play may help children to see other people's point of view. He will also enjoy stories from picture books.

Games with formal rules stage, 6 years plus

Children start to play formal games with their peers, and learn the rules of these games. This helps them to appreciate the use of rules, and they begin to understand that rules can be changed by negotiation, to suit circumstances.

CONCLUSION

An important role of the physiotherapist when working with children is to encourage and guide the development of movement and the child's exploration of the environment. This can only take place when the stepping stones of gross and fine motor skills are understood and combined with cognitive and communication skills to set up a holistic approach to therapy. All children learn naturally and willingly through play, which has a value for physical, intellectual, social and emotional development (Burns 1986).

ACKNOWLEDGEMENTS

I wish to acknowledge Dr and Mrs Bobath, Jenny Bryce and Judy Murray for much information acquired during lectures at the Bobath Centre, on Gross and Fine Sensori-Motor Development, and Play.

REFERENCES

Alston J, Taylor J 1987 Handwriting, theory, research and practice. Croom Helm, London
Bobath K 1969 The motor deficit in patients with cerebral palsy. Clinics in Developmental Medicine No 23. Heinemann Medical, London
Bower T G R 1966 The visual world of infants. Scientific American 215: 80–92
Bower T G R 1974 The perceptual world of the child. Fontana, London
Bruner J 1979 From communication to language — a psychological perspective. In: Lee V (ed) Language development. Croom Helm, London
Burns R B 1986 Child development. A text for the caring professions. Croom Helm, London
Campbell S K 1984 Paediatric neurologic physical therapy. Churchill Livingstone, Edinburgh
Chomsky C 1969 The acquisition of syntax in children from five to ten. Massachusetts Institute of Technology Press, Cambridge, Massachusetts
Clark H H, Clark E V 1977 Psychology and language. Harcourt Brace, Jovanovich, New York
Cohen M A, Gross P J 1979 The developmental resource Vol. 1. Grune and Stratton, New York
Condon W S, Sander L W 1974 Neonate movement is synchronized with adult speech: interactional participation and language acquisition. Science 1(11): 99–101
Donaldson M 1978 Children's minds. Fontana, London
Garvey C 1977 Play. Fontana, London
Kagan J 1973 New Society, 14 June 1973: 610–612

Kessen W, Nelson K 1979 In: Pulaski M A S Your baby's mind and how it grows. Piaget's theory for parents. Cassell, London

Lieberman P 1967 Intonation, perception, and language. Massachusetts Institute of Technology Press, Cambridge, Massachusetts

Rogers D 1985 Language development. In: Branthwaite A, Rogers D (eds) Children growing up. Open University Press, Milton Keynes

Mead G N 1984 Mind, self and society. University of Chicago Press, quoted in: Open University 1984 Social Psychology Unit 4. Section 5: symbolic interactionism: 102–113

Rosenbloom L, Horton M E (1971) The maturation of fine motor skill in young children. Developmental Medicine and Child Neurology 13: 3–8

Sheridan M D 1975 The developmental progress of infants and young children. Her Majesty's Stationery Office, London

Sloboda J 1985 Perception and knowledge. In: Branthwaite A, Rogers D (eds) Children growing up. Open University Press, Milton Keynes

Snow C E, Ferguson C A 1977 Talking to children: language input and acquisition. Cambridge University Press, London

Wolff P H 1969 The natural history of crying and other vocalisations in early infancy. In: Foss B M (ed) Determinants of infant behaviour, vol 4. Methuen, London

Ziviani J 1987 Pencil grasp and manipulation. In: Alston J, Taylor J (eds) Handwriting, theory, research and practice. Croom Helm, London

5

Practices in child health

M. I. Griffiths

INTRODUCTION

Child health is a major concern of all members of the health professions involved in any way with the care of children.

Although physiotherapists are largely concerned with the effects of disease and disability, the thrust of their work is directed to enabling each person to experience the greatest amount of physical (and mental and emotional) fulfilment within their capacity. In the case of children who are developing and learning at great speed, this approach to aiding the whole person is particularly important and is one basis of the provisions for child health.

The aim of the Child Health Service must be to encourage the optimal physical, emotional and mental development of all children. To achieve this aim the following practical objectives need to be addressed:

1. to promote good general health
2. to detect and identify as early as possible potential chronic, lethal or disabling conditions by screening procedures
3. to provide treatment and management for acute and chronic disease and disability
4. to prevent causes of disease or disability later in childhood.

Child Health Services are administered by District Health Authorities through community and hospital sectors that respectively offer primary or specialist care. Children have need of the services of both sectors and their health and development are greatly enhanced when close working relationships are fostered.

Physiotherapists may work in either or both sectors and are in a good position to effect liaison and to ensure cooperation with consistency of treatment.

PROMOTION OF GENERAL HEALTH

Environmental factors

Factors such as:

- the physical environment of the home
- type of accommodation
- heating
- washing facilities
- cooking facilities
- the child's need for clothing, food, play, sleep

have a significant effect upon all aspects of health and development. These factors are equally, if not more, important in the life of a disabled child, but many are not readily available for some patients who may be part of a family suffering some form of deprivation. Although a health authority is not responsible for ensuring that these social needs are met, health professionals have every right, and indeed duty, to urge their partners and colleagues in administrative posts in other professions to assist in the health care of a family by remedying some of their disadvantages.

Care for family health

The physical, mental and emotional health of parents and children interact. A father who is unemployed, bored, frustrated and perhaps ill-tempered, or a mother who is tired, depressed, ill or inadequate, are unable to give their children the care and support they need. The care of babies and young children demands physical and emotional energy during the early months, which are crucial in a child's growth and development. Pregnancy brings additional strains and the mother's general health at this time is most important in giving her baby a good start in life.

Antenatal care is available in the community and in hospital and should be coordinated to ensure the health of mother and child. Mothers are encouraged to report to their family doctor or local clinic as soon as they suspect that they are pregnant. Once registered, the pregnancy will be monitored regularly until the baby is delivered. Mothers will receive advice on their own health, on preparation for labour and breast feeding, and on child rearing practices; they will be carefully screened for any conditions that may affect their health or that of the baby. The intention of good antenatal care is to support the growth and development of the fetus in utero, and to lead towards a safe delivery.

This is the start of health education. After the birth of the baby the midwife is responsible for follow-up advice until the tenth day, when the health visitor takes over. Increasing emphasis (Hall 1989) is now being placed on the important role of parents in all aspects of their children's lives, and the health visitor is a person who can support, encourage and advise them in this important task before the children are of school age.

Growth and development

Surveillance is particularly important during the first 2 years of life when the child is growing very rapidly, both physically and mentally. Research has shown the importance of weight gain as an indicator of health (World Health Organization 1986). Regular weighing and charting of gains not only monitors the child's physical progress but gives an opportunity for discussion on feeding, sleep and other points of behaviour and development (Fig. 5.1). This type of surveillance is then carried on through the school health service. This can become a shared opportunity for parents and professionals. All aspects of growth and development can be considered together so that parents can take part in observation and training of their children, can come to understand problems of diet, learning play and behaviour, and enthusiastically promote procedures such as weighing, measuring, clinical examination and even immunisation.

Name _____
      Birth date _____ Reg. No. _____

Girls 9—18
Standing height (cm)

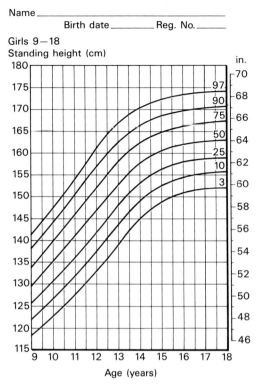

Fig. 5.1 Centile chart: Girls' Growth Assessment Chart. University of London Institute of Child Health (reproduced by permission of Castlemead Publications, Herts, England).

EARLY DETECTION AND IDENTIFICATION

Screening procedures

Screening procedures are used to detect conditions in the mother or baby that may be:

- amenable to treatment to prevent any adverse clinical effects
- responsive to control and improvement where basic disease cannot be prevented
- unchangeable or likely to be progressive.

There are certain principles to be observed in the setting-up and administration of any screening tests:

- There must be a definite objective. It is necessary to know what is being sought.
- Tests must be simple, safe to administer and easy to read.

- Some form of action should be possible if the test is positive.
- The population to be screened must be defined.
- Tests should be specific. They should identify only the abnormality that is being sought. There should be no false positives.
- Tests should be sensitive. No cases should be missed. There should be no false negatives.

In all children screening starts before they are born and continues into early childhood. Some tests are applied to all children and others only to a selected group who are known to be at risk. This chapter is only concerned with the nature and objectives of the tests; descriptions of treatments of the conditions identified will be found in other chapters.

Prenatal screening

Routine surveillance of mothers during pregnancy is carried out for the benefit of mother and baby. In most instances this can be undertaken in the health centre or doctor's surgery with referral to the local or a specialist hospital where necessary. Routine antenatal care includes:

- Health education — advice to the mother on diet (especially with regard to tobacco and alcohol), exercise (including exercises in the last trimester with a view to labour), sleep and working habits.
- Clinical examination, including the condition of breasts, height of the uterus, position of the fetus and blood pressure.
- Taking samples of blood and urine for routine tests (Table 5.1A).

Other more complex investigations (Table 5.1B) must be carried out in hospital, and are described in detail by Kingston (1989). These test the baby in utero and are offered to special groups of mothers when there is an increased risk of some handicapping condition. These investigations need thorough explanation and discussion with parents before they are undertaken, so that they may understand the implications for the baby and their family. In many cases termination of

Table 5.1(A) Prenatal screening

Population (pregnant women)	Specimen	Condition sought	Test		Action to be taken
			Nature	Timing	
All	Urine	Phenylketonuria	Phenestix or ferric chloride, if positive blood test as for newborns	Routine	Low phenylalanine diet
All	Urine	Glycosuria (diabetes)	Routine for glucose in urine, if positive glucose estimation in blood	Throughout	Blood analysis, if positive, diet and insulin
All	Urine	Albuminuria (toxaemia)	Qualitative and quantitative	Throughout	Blood pressure estimation, renal and liver function tests, rest and diet
All	Blood	Rhesus incompatibility	Blood groups and antibodies	Once, with retest if Rh negative	Exchange transfusion possibly in utero
All	Blood	Congenital syphilis	When required	Once	Antibiotics
All	Blood	Rubella embryopathy	Rubella antibody	Once only if high at outset, repeat if necessary	Abortion offered
All	Blood	Neural tube defects	Alphafetoprotein	14–16 weeks	Amniocentesis
Selected at-risk groups on request	Blood	AIDS	HIV antibodies	Repeated at least once	Abortion offered

pregnancy may be offered, and, although this may not be acceptable to all parents, they may wish to proceed with the investigation in the hope of reassurance that the fetus is normal.

Ultrasonography. This is available to all patients and, if carried out at 8–12 weeks, will confirm the pregnancy and afford a fairly accurate assessment of gestation period. Thereafter, fetal growth can be monitored and at 16–18 weeks a more accurate picture of fetal parts can be gained, and congenital abnormalities in various organs detected (Fig. 5.2).

Amniocentesis. This technique is carried out at 16–18 weeks of pregnancy. A small amount (16–18 ml) of amniotic fluid, which also contains fetal amniotic cells, is removed by a needle (with trochar) and syringe via the mother's abdomen under vision on the ultrasound screen. Anaesthetic is unnecessary (Giles & Nye 1987). The procedure is not without risk (< 1% above spontaneous abortion rate) and, as none of the conditions that can be detected are amenable to

treatment, the test is limited to those pregnancies thought to be at risk of producing a handicapped child. Biochemical tests may be carried out directly and results are available within a few days. When chromosome analysis is needed the fetal amniotic cells must be cultured and the result is not available until approximately 3 weeks later. If the test is positive, termination of pregnancy is the only solution that can be offered. Careful counselling and discussion with parents is necessary, as even if termination is requested it is a traumatic procedure, for the mother especially, as the results are only returned some weeks after the amniocentesis, when the fetus is already making its presence felt. Indications for amniocentesis are given by Giles & Nye (1987) and are noted in Table 5.1B.

Chorionic villus sampling. This is a technique that can be used much earlier in pregnancy (8–11 weeks) than amniocentesis and carries only a slight additional risk (2%) of spontaneous abortion (Leschot et al 1987). It is carried out by the

Table 5.1(B) Prenatal screening (contd)

Population (pregnant women)	Technique	Condition sought	Nature of test	Timing (weeks)	Action to be taken
All	Scanning	Growth, gestation period	Ultrasound	8–12	Monitoring growth, estimating gestation period
All	Scanning	Congenital defects of skull, limbs, heart and kidneys	Ultrasound	17–20	For observation unless gross when abortion might be offered
Alphafetoprotein in serum, previous infant affected	Amniocentesis	Neural tube defects	Alphafetoprotein estimation confirmed ultrasound	16–18	Termination
Previous history of sex-linked conditions	Chorionic villus analysis* or amniocentesis	Sex	Identification of sex chromosomes	8–12 16–18	Abortion of males
Older mothers on request or previous history	As above	Chromosome abnormalities	Analysis of chromosomes	As above	Carry on or termination
Previous sibling or family history	As above	Increasing numbers of inborn errors of metabolism and other enzyme deficiencies, including Hunter's, Hurler's syndromes, Tay–Sachs' disease, etc	Appropriate biochemical tests*	As above	Termination
As above and in races from around the Mediterranean, Africans and West Indians or universal	As above	Haemoglobinopathy	Haemoglobin electrophoresis	As above	Early warning system or termination

* These tests and techniques are not available at all centres

transcervical route. Chromosomes are studied by direct typing and so the result comes through more quickly and termination, if necessary, can be carried out earlier in pregnancy than following amniocentesis. The method is slightly less accurate but if there is any doubt of the result there is plenty of time for an amniocentesis to be carried out. More recent use of this technique has enabled the detection of many biochemical disorders (Kingston 1989).

Postnatal screening

Screening procedures in the immediate neonatal period and during the first 2 years of life can lead to the detection of some clinical or biochemical disorders which, without adequate treatment, may cause death or serious disability. Learning difficulties of various kinds may require more prolonged observation. All screening procedures need to be undertaken in the context of a supportive framework of a team of professionals so that the parents, whilst receiving encouragement and guidance, may feel that they are key participants.

Clinical methods. A full physical examination is always undertaken at birth. This includes measurement of weight, height and skull circumference, check for hip dislocation (MacFarlane 1980) and, in boys, testicular descent. A neonatal neurological examination is also carried out by medical staff.

This procedure is repeated at the age of 6 weeks by a family doctor or paediatrician. Any

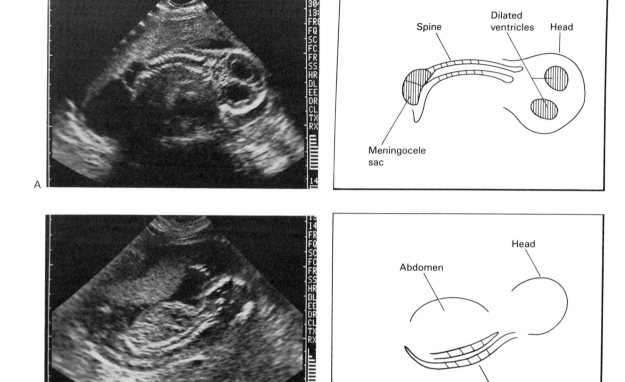

Fig. 5.2 Ultrasound scan at 18–20 weeks. (A) Longitudinal (coronal) view showing spina bifida with hydrocephalus and meningocele. (B) Normally developing spine: longitudinal view. Plates and drawings supplied by Dr Lesley Arkell and photography by A Coote, Wordsley Hospital, Dudley Health Authority.

abnormalities detected are then followed up as necessary.

Biochemical methods. Biochemical disorders are due to some form of gene abnormality that is present at conception. The fetus usually develops normally up to the time of birth because the mother undertakes all metabolism on its behalf. After birth the baby is independent and has to cope biochemically for itself, and many conditions only manifest themselves as the child grows up, by which time treatment may be ineffectual as irreversible damage may have taken place. Blood specimens are taken by heel prick at 2–5 days of age and repeated where necessary. Several spots of blood are collected on a special filter paper and allowed to dry before it is sent off to the laboratory. All the screening tests that are commonly used have been so devised that one-

eighth-inch circles of impregnated filter paper contain sufficient material for any of the appropriate tests (Naylor 1985) (Table 5.2).

In some cases the biochemical disorder can be directly treated and the child enabled to develop normally provided that treatment is started as soon as possible after birth (e.g. phenylketonuria, hypothyroidism — see Chapter 15 Inborn Errors of Metabolism); in others the symptoms of the disorder can be treated, the tests serving as an 'early warning' system (e.g. cystic fibrosis — see Chapter 7 Respiratory Conditions and Cardio-thoracic Disorders — and the haemo-globinopathies) so that suitable symptomatic treatment can be given early to prevent the more serious consequences and complications of the disorder. In some conditions only palliative help can be given and the downhill progress over a

Table 5.2 Postnatal screening: biochemical tests

Condition sought	Clinical effect	Incidence	Population to be tested	Retest (weeks)	Test		Action to be taken
					Specimen	Nature of test	
Phenylketonuria	Mental handicap	1/10 000	All neonates	4–6	Heel prick, dried blood on filter paper	Bacterial inhibition or fluorimetry	Phenylalanine-free diet
Homocystinuria	Lens dislocation, thrombo-emboli, mental handicap, osteoporosis	1/200 000	All neonates, only 50% detection	4–6	As above	Bacterial inhibition	50% respond to pyridoxine
Galactosaemia	Cataract, liver disease, mental handicap	1/50 000	All neonates	4–6	As above	Bacterial inhibition	Diet free from lactose and galactose
Maple syrup urine disease	Death, only 5–10% survive (with mental handicap)	1/225 000	Not universal in neonates		Dried urine on filter paper	Test for leucine	Medical emergency followed by leucine-free diet
Congenital hypothyroidism	Cretinism, mental handicap	1/4000	All neonates		Dried blood on filter paper	Radioimmuno-assay for TSH	Treatment with synthetic thyroid hormone
Haemoglobino-pathy, thalassaemia, sickle cell anaemia	High morbidity and mortality unless treated: splenic sequestration crises, infections, severe anaemia	Some races more prone than others, 1/1000 total newborns (see Table 5.1B)	Neonates, universal or selective		Dried blood on filter paper	Electrophoresis of haemolysate	Surveillance and prompt treatment of crises
Cystic fibrosis	Meconium ileus, chest infections	1/2000	Neonates, not yet in universal use		Dried blood on filter paper (also meconium or faeces)	Immunoreactive trypsin	Very early treatment with antibiotics, inhalation, etc
Duchenne muscular dystrophy	Progressive muscular dystrophy	1/4400 males	Considerable discussion re: ethics (see Table 5.1B)		Dried blood on filter paper	For creatine kinase	No treatment available but families benefit by genetic counselling

long or short period is inexorable (e.g. Duchenne muscular dystrophy — see Chapter 11 Neuro-muscular Disorders). The value of early detection in these children is that the parents can be warned of the risk before another child is conceived.

Electronic scanning. During the neonatal period physiotherapists are becoming more and more involved in the management of babies in special care baby units who are thought to be at risk of neurodevelopmental problems. The prognosis for individual children who need intensive care and suffer from cerebral damage is still unclear, and it is not usually possible to differentiate in the nursery which babies are likely to recover completely and which will turn out to be disabled. Active research is being carried out in a number of neonatal units using ultrasound, CAT (computer assisted tomography) scanning and MRI (magnetic resonance imaging) to locate areas of haemorrhage, tissue damage or cysts and to chart their progress. Eventually it may be possible to give a much more accurate prediction of the likely outcome, although prospects of reversing the harmful process seem remote.

Developmental screening

This is now an important universal function of child health services, and all mothers are urged to see that they and their children take part. At the start of their lives all babies have a neurological check, preferably by a paediatrician, before leaving the nursery for home, and a full neurological examination is part of the 6 week check by a doctor who has had paediatric training. Thereafter all children should be screened frequently during the first 2 years of life and at increasing intervals during the preschool period.

Although health authorities follow DHSS guidelines in the administration of tests, there are considerable local differences in practice. Certain basic criteria need to be observed:

1. There is an objective — to identify any significant delay in development so that the child may be referred for comprehensive assessment and a suitable individual programme of support.

2. It is possible to select those tests that are simple and easy to administer and record, and to carry out whenever the child is seen.

3. There should be sufficient trained personnel experienced in child development working together.

4. There should be easy access to facilities (if necessary home visits should be arranged).

5. The whole population of children under five should be involved.

6. These tests cannot be as sensitive and specific as biochemical tests, which are designed to detect only a single easily identifiable gene disorder.

Developmental tests identify varied clinical effects of a multitude of different conditions. However, the tests should be sensitive in detecting delay and specific in eliminating those children whose development is normal. Abnormal results at these ages are not necessarily predictive, but the detection of any abnormality should engender careful follow-up.

With these points in mind, schemes for surveillance can be made sufficiently flexible to be carried out wherever and whenever a child is encountered, without too much disruption of family life.

It has been suggested that personnel who are highly experienced in child development do not need specific scales to decide whether a child's performance lies within normal limits (Hall 1989). However, to meet the demands of a large, often mobile, population adequately, the use of appropriate scales by field workers will probably need to continue. Most of these scales assume that they will be carried out as part of a team service, usually by health visitors with the support of paediatrically trained general practitioners and community health doctors. These scales need to be simple, to require little in the way of equipment and to be speedy to carry out. Examples are given on page 69.

Those who carry out the tests need to be professionals who have ready access to families in the course of their duties, most commonly health visitors, family doctors or community clinical medical officers. It is essential that these individuals should have a good knowledge of paediatrics, particularly child development, and be acquainted with the approach to test scales used in their locality. Physiotherapists may need to undertake some form of developmental screening to get an idea of a child's stage of development at the commencement of treatment, either using the scale practised by others in the authority or a scale better known to them by experience. Levitt (1984) has produced a table for physiotherapists' use as a 'screening assessment'. In it she selects several items in four parameters at various ages, which are markers for average development at that age. She points out that although it is essential to discuss any problems with colleagues in other disciplines, it is important that physiotherapists should have some knowledge of normal development in parameters other than movement.

Box 5.1 Developmental scales

• Record cards compiled by Curtis-Jenkins (1977) give simple tests at various ages for use by general practitioners, health visitors and others, which can be completed in 15 min. These tests can be carried out at home, and it is essential that all children are seen. Specialist support services must be available, and there must be clear responsibility for provision of day-to-day care in the community. Curtis-Jenkins found that the benefit of such a programme improved the quality of overall paediatric care in the practice, particularly with the involvement of, and reassurance to, mothers.
• Simple developmental schedules for health visitor testing at home during their routine visits are provided in the Dundee Development Screening Programme. These are combined with more structured examinations by a medical officer, the two sets forming a sensitive network to ensure the fullest possible surveillance (Drillien & Drummond 1983).
• A pocket textbook was produced by MacFarlane (1980) for use by clinical medical officers and junior paediatricians. It contains a short, quick developmental screening chart.
• The Birmingham Chart, devised by Wood (1970), and slightly amended in Fig. 5.3, is used by doctors working in child health in the community and by health visitors. It is readily administered at any time, anywhere and requires little in the way of test material. There is an item in each parameter for each month, but because children vary considerably in the way they attain various skills, they may succeed in some actions beyond their chronological age whilst failing in earlier ones; the use of the scale is described in the Notes to Fig. 5.3. Although this is not a finite test of ability, profiles give a good idea of a child's attainment in individual fields and a quotient gives an idea of overall competence. These scores can then be followed in subsequent tests to give an idea of rate of progress that Drillien (1977) considers gives a better idea of potential than status at one period only.

Screening for vision and hearing

Screening is carried out concurrently with the clinical and developmental screening procedures described (Hall 1989).

Vision. Careful examination of the eyes is always included in the neonatal examination. Observation of eye movements, visual attention and use of the eye/hand items in developmental scales should give warning of possible visual problems (Hall 1989). Cover tests for squint should be carried out by experienced observers from 7–9 months onwards.

Hearing. Distraction tests can be carried out from 7–9 months and thereafter, if speech and language development progesses normally, no further testing is necessary until a sweep test is administered at entry to school.

Developmental assessment

Delays identified by developmental screening indicate fuller investigation. Developmental assessment may then be considered, using some of the more formal testing schemes such as the Griffiths, the Denver or Bayley scales, all described by Francis-Williams (1977). However, the results of such an assessment, whilst offering a more definite score, do not usually define the nature of the impairments that a child suffers and it is then necessary to consider a comprehensive assessment programme, of which the developmental assessment is part. The principles of comprehensive assessment entail:

• that it is a continuing process
• that it is undertaken by a team, each member of which has a particular expertise and skill to offer
• that it evaluates strengths and weaknesses in all fields of attainment
• that it leads to the promulgation of a programme of action adapted to the needs of each individual child.

Such an assessment cannot be undertaken by a single professional at one session, and the facilities needed for these specialist services are usually provided at child development centres or paediatric assessment units associated with children's or general hospitals (see Chapter 17 Common Assessment Procedures). As nursery activities are usually found to be essential, nursery units attached to primary schools or local clinics may be used. The physiotherapist is usually a core member of the assessment team, and an important contributor to the treatment programme in a variety of conditions (Moore 1973, Drillien 1977, Griffiths 1985).

Date Month		Motor	Social	Hearing and Speech	Eye and Hand	Month
	1	Head erect for few seconds	Quieted when picked up	Startled by sounds	Notices bright objects close to	1
	2	Head up when prone (chin clear)	Smiles	Listens to ball or rattle	Follows ring up, down and sideways	2
	3	Kicks well	Alert. Follows person with eyes	Searches for sound with eyes	Glances from one object to another	3
	4	Lifts head and chest prone	Returns examiner's smile	Laughs	Clasps and retains cube	4
	5	Holds head erect with no lag	Frolics when played with	Turns head to sound	Pulls paper away from face	5
	6	Rises on to wrists	Turns head to person talking	Babbles or coos to music	Takes cube from table	6
	7	Rolls from front to back	Friendly with strangers	Makes four different sounds	Looks for fallen object	7
	8	Tries to crawl vigorously	Shows toy	Shouts for attention	Passes toy from hand to hand	8
	9	Turns around on floor	Helps to hold spoon	Says 'Mama' or 'Dada'	Manipulates two objects at once	9
	10	Stands when held up	Rings bell in imitation	Listens to watch, responds to talking	Clicks two bricks together	10
	11	Pulls up to stand	Finger feeds	Understands 'No'	Pincer grip	11
	12	Walks or side-steps round furniture	Plays 'Pat-a-cake'	Three words with meaning	Points with index finger	12
	13	Stands alone	Waves 'Bye Bye'	Looks at picture	Picks up small object	13
	14	Walks alone	Uses spoon	Knows own name	Makes mark with pencil	14
	15	Climbs upstairs	Shows shoes	Four to five clear words. Points to familiar toy	Places one object upon another	15
	16	Pushes pram, toy horse etc.	Curious	Knows 'give', 'show', 'get'	Scribbles freely	16
	17	Climbs onto chair	Manages cup well	Babbled conversation	Watches from window	17
	18	Picks up toys without falling	Takes off socks and shoes	Enjoys pictures in books	Constructive play with toys	18
	19	Climbs stairs up and down	Knows one part of body	6–20 words	Tower of three bricks	19
	20	Jumps	Imitates activities	Echoes words	Removes wrapper from sweet	20
	21	Runs	Puts on garment	Two-word sentences	Circular scribble	21
	22	Walks up stairs	Tries to tell experiences	Listens to stories	Tower of five or more bricks	22
	23	Seats himself at table	Knows two parts of body	Demands by pointing	Copies perpendicular stroke	23
	24	Walks up and down stairs	Knows and names four parts of body	Names four toys	Copies horizontal stroke	24

Notes

1 Test items in each parameter, placing √s or Xs in adjacent right-hand columns, and starting at child's chronological age.
2 Carry on until three Xs consecutively are marked. If necessary, go back and check earlier items.
3 Add √s in each column.
4 Compare number of √s with chronological age in months. Marked divergence in column suggests a specific problem in an area of delay which should be checked.
5 A tape-slide set 'Developmental Screening' 81/24, explaining the use of the chart, is obtainable from Graves Medical Audiovisual Library, Chelmsford.

Fig. 5.3 Developmental screening: The Birmingham chart (published by permission of Graves Medical Audiovisual Library).

TREATMENT AND MANAGEMENT

Neither promotion of health nor early identification of health-threatening conditions can give total protection against childhood disease or disability, and therefore a network providing for management and treatment must be set up for acute and chronic conditions. This provision rests upon the two sectors of the health service, community/primary care and hospital/specialist care. Successful management of disease and disability is contingent upon close co-operation between the two. Acute conditions will first be encountered in the family practice and may or may not need referral to hospital. Chronic conditions often require hospital facilities for investigation and some monitoring, although day-to-day management will fall upon the community. The specialist, hospital aspects of these conditions are considered in other chapters.

Community aspects

The contribution of the community/primary health services in the promotion of health and in screening has been outlined, and forms a large part of the work undertaken in child health. Their responsibility for treatment and management of acute and chronic disease and disability is equally important.

Diagnosis and treatment of acute conditions

The child's general practitioner is normally the first person to be consulted, except possibly in large urban areas where some families may not be registered with a doctor and the local casualty department is more readily accessible. The child may be seen at home or at a health centre and, where diagnosis is simple and treatment straightforward, will stay within the community. Where diagnosis is in doubt, or treatment complicated, referral to hospital may be necessary. Acute conditions are largely infections, accidents and surgical emergencies.

Infections. The pattern of acute infections is changing year by year (see Chapter 13 Infection and Trauma).

1. With the gradual elimination of those specific fevers that can be prevented by immunisation, for example, diphtheria, poliomyelitis, tetanus, measles, whooping cough, rubella and mumps, chickenpox is the only common specific fever still uncontrollable.

2. Meningococcal meningitis is endemic and therefore presents as a mini-epidemic in unexpected localities, engendering a great deal of parental anxiety; early diagnosis and effective treatment with antibiotics mean that most children recover completely, but fulminating cases associated with septicaemia may be fatal, or late diagnosis and delayed treatment may lead to neurological sequelae.

3. AIDS is at present a rare condition in children, but it is important that physiotherapists should have some knowledge of its characteristics and modes of transmission, as infected children who may be symptomless or who may present with neurological problems may become their patients. It is important that these children should attend school and be able to mix with their peers, so education of those professionals who will come into contact with them is essential. Tandy & Bax (1987) discuss the role of the community health services in a practical and informative review.

4. The most common acute episodes are due to non-specific viral infections, which cause respiratory and gastrointestinal symptoms; these do not respond to antibiotics but usually clear up with expectant treatment.

5. Renal infections may pose problems of diagnosis and, in upper respiratory infections, ear infections may be an important complication.

6. Any high fever may, in susceptible children, cause febrile convulsions that may recur with other episodes of high temperature until the age of 4–5 years. In a few children, epilepsy may develop.

Treatment and management of chronic disease and disability

Whereas acute conditions are relatively transient and can usually be dealt with on medical grounds alone, chronic conditions require teamwork between health, education and social services departments. There are a number of categories of chronic disease and disability:

1. Conditions in which diet or medication can counteract the effects. Many will have been identified by screening techniques, and all will have been seen in hospital where diagnosis has been confirmed and specific treatment commenced (e.g. phenylalanine-free diet in phenylketonuria; synthetic thyroid hormone in hypothyroidism; diet and insulin in diabetes). These children will live ordinary lives and attend ordinary schools, and their treatment will be monitored in the community by the primary health care team, with occasional review at hospital or referral if control seems to be inadequate.

2. Conditions in which treatment of symptoms will enable the child to live an almost normal life, e.g. asthma, cystic fibrosis, epilepsy and some forms of cancer.

3. Orthopaedic conditions corrected by surgery.

4. Neurodevelopmental conditions for which there is no specific treatment but in which appropriate management, including therapy, education, training and support of the family, will enable the child to be as active and healthy as possible and to attain his potential.

All members of the community team have a role in supporting these children, at home and at school. Their cooperation can ensure that such children can get the best out of themselves despite their difficulties.

Personnel

The differences in administrative procedures between health authorities has already been stressed. In deciding which personnel within the community should undertake specific tasks there is additional variation within each local service. So that, in defining the role of various professionals, it will be noted that several may be equipped to undertake similar functions.

Consultant paediatrician with special interest in the community

This post is a new development within paediatrics and in some areas may still be designated as consultant community paediatrician or senior clinical medical officer. The consultant is usually based at the hospital child development centre, heading the local assessment team and being responsible for the clinical aspects of the care of handicapped children and child abuse. These aspects will involve one- to two-thirds of time for work in the community. The remaining period will include sharing in the day-to-day hospital paediatric and neonatal care in wards and outpatients.

Family doctors

The core of provision of health care in the home rests upon family doctors (GPs), who are independent practitioners and lead the primary care team. Nowadays most are grouped into partnerships, with several doctors working from a health centre. The doctor(s) heads a team of ancillaries, receptionists, secretaries, practice nurse (who is based at the centre and carries out all kinds of nursing duties), health visitor(s) and community nurse(s). A practice manager undertakes the day-to-day administration.

The GP is a family doctor who has responsibility for patients of all ages. Some GPs have a special interest and extensive experience in child health and may be consulted by their colleagues on such problems. So that within the life of a child the GP's responsibility may include:

1. Antenatal supervision of the mother, including the possible obstetric care of the mother in a GP maternity unit.

2. Surveillance of the baby's growth and development, partially delegated to the health visitor and carried out in a developmental clinic within the practice premises.

3. Clinical care of acute and chronic childhood disease including total care of many childhood illnesses that can be treated at home; referral to hospital of those children who need further investigation, skilled nursing or specialist treatment procedures such as surgery or intensive care; follow-up treatment on discharge from hospital, particularly of children with chronic conditions.

4. Organisation and supervision of immunisation procedures.

5.   Some GPs may act as school doctors when requested by the local health authority.

Clinical medical officers

In contrast to GPs, who are self-employed, clinical medical officers are employed by the health authority. Their responsibilities may be entirely in the field of child health or, if the authority so decides, they may be expected to undertake other duties in the field of community health. There is no question that in the field of child health, particularly when that is their only duty, the work they carry out is essential and can be defined as:

- Working with and supervising health visitors in the general care and surveillance of infants and young children.
- Either undertaking, or acting as adviser to health visitors in, developmental screening.
- Undertaking routine clinical examinations of children, in the clinic or at home, as specified by the procedures of the health authority by whom they are employed.
- Acting as a nominated school doctor in ordinary schools, taking referrals from head teachers, parents or the school nurse, and following-up children with special educational needs.
- As a result of clinical judgement in these circumstances, prescribing medication or referring children for specialist advice, in cooperation with the family doctor.
- Advising on, and taking part in, immunisation sessions and any special occurrences within the school that need medical advice.

It will be noted that there are similarities and overlap between the duties and responsibilities of GPs and clinical medical officers. Their professional relationship is under discussion at the present time, and it is hoped that their complementary roles will be evolved to the benefit of the child patients.

Health visitors

Health visitors, who are nurses with additional training in community work, are normally attached to GPs and work closely with them. Like GPs, their responsibility is with the whole family, although their main concern is with the young and the old and with families who have social problems or disabled members. Their role can be summed up as:

- Prenatal, getting to know mother and any domestic problems she may have.
- Advice and help to mothers on care of a new baby after the midwife has ceased her visits, usually on the tenth day.
- Continuing surveillance of growth and development of the infant and the preschool child.
- Advice to the mother on infant feeding, sleep, play activities, immunisation, home safety and any other problems that may occur in the normal course of development.
- Developmental screening in localities where it is the practice for health visitors to do so.
- Referral to GP or clinic doctor when in doubt or when further advice is needed.
- Health visitors may arrange for children to receive help from playgroups, toy libraries, or such systems of home education as Portage (Cameron 1982) where it seems that the child needs additional stimulation from the environment.

School nurses

These nurses are based in schools, maybe more than one, depending on its size. Their duties include:

- simple testing of vision and hearing
- advice and help for children with special educational needs
- a source of counselling and confidential discussion with adolescents
- taking part in immunisation sessions
- supporting the head teacher and class teachers in health problems and acting as a link between the medical and educational services.

Other professional staff

Occupational therapists, physiotherapists and speech therapists all have an important role in community care. Some are based at GP health centres, others at community clinics run by the health authority. Social workers employed by the local authority social services, and psychologists employed by the education authority, should also have close links with medical practices.

PREVENTION OF DISEASE AND DISABILITY

We have considered how to prevent disease or disability affected by conditions in the home environment, in the mother or baby during pregnancy, or in the newborn infant. Let us now consider how to prevent external harmful conditions that might occur after the immediate neonatal period.

Specific infections

The outlook for children's health has been altered for the better with the availability of reliable vaccines and their use worldwide. In the United Kingdom the DHSS has produced guidelines for a programme of immunisation organised by the community health service and carried out in welfare clinics, GP surgeries and, for older children, in schools. It is important for the well-being of all children that efficient and safe immunisation procedures should be taken up by 90% of the child population and this is the aim of the World Health Organization for all European children by 1990. The current programme is shown in Table 5.3

The take-up of diphtheria, tetanus and poliomyelitis is likely to be satisfactory, particularly now that an abbreviated schedule has been introduced. Measles is less well accepted, although it is 95% effective, and pertussis is viewed with some apprehension owing to continuing controversy with regard to possible brain damage in a very small proportion of cases. Both measles and whooping cough are serious illnesses in young children, causing a significant number of permanent respiratory or neurological complications, in some cases death, and their

Table 5.3 Recommended immunisation schedules

Disease	Method of immunisation	Age at immunisation
Diphtheria Tetanus (Note 1) Pertussis	Injection	1st: 2 months 2nd: 3 months 3rd: 4 months
Poliomyelitis	Oral	As above
Measles Mumps Rubella	Injection	1–2 years
Tetanus Poliomyelitis	Injection Oral	At school entry (5 years)
BCG	Intradermal	13 years
Rubella (Note 2)	Injection	10–14 years
Tetanus Poliomyelitis	Injection Oral	On leaving school On leaving school

Note 1 Diphtheria/tetanus is given in a few cases where there are contraindications or the parents refuse the pertussis element.
Note 2 This will be discontinued when children have been previously immunised.

prevention is an important matter. There are some contraindications to giving some vaccines, clearly set out in DHSS pamphlets, but where these are not present parents should be encouraged to take up all types of immunisation that are offered. In their paper, Senturia & Peckham (1987) make the point that 'lack of clear professional directives is likely to lead to confusion on the part of parents and may be a major factor in parental non-compliance. . . [which is]. . . probably due to confusion rather than objection'. Physiotherapists are professionals who may be consulted by parents and it is important that they should have an objective understanding of the possibilities, so that when questioned they can rationally discuss the pros and cons with the mother and, wherever indicated, encourage compliance.

Accidents

Much morbidity and mortality in childhood can be eliminated by sensible accident prevention: in the home (including child-resistant drug containers and control of non-accidental injuries), at school and on the roads. This subject is covered in more detail in Chapter 13.

SUMMARY

This chapter attempts to cover, in outline only, present practices in child health; in itself it is only a summary It explains how the services for children in the community are organised for care and surveillance from conception to adult life. At the present time many changes are taking place and these will continue as long as our horizons of knowledge of disease, disability and need are extended. Physiotherapists will continue to find challenge and reward in taking part.

REFERENCES

Cameron R J (ed) 1982 Working together: Portage in the U.K. NFER/Nelson, Windsor

Curtis-Jenkins G 1977 Surveillance of preschool children in general practice. In: Drillien C M, Drummond M B (eds) Neurodevelopmental problems in early childhood. Blackwell, Oxford, p 93–109

Drillien C M 1977 Developmental assessment and developmental screening. In: Drillien C M, Drummond M B (eds) Neurodevelopmental problems in early childhood. Blackwell, Oxford, p 44–92

Drillien C M, Drummond M M (eds) 1983 Developmental screening and the child with special needs. Heinemann, London/Lippincott, Philadelphia, p 18–23

Francis-Williams J 1977 Psychological assessment. In: Drillien C M, Drummond M B (eds) Neurodevelopmental problems in early childhood. Blackwell, Oxford, p 110–125

Giles J, Nye M 1987 Amniocentesis. Update May 15: 1171–1175

Griffiths M 1985 Assessment. In: Griffiths M, Russell P (eds) Working together with handicapped children. Souvenir Press, London, p 29–37

Hall D M B (ed) 1989 Health for all children. A programme for child health surveillance. Oxford University Press, Oxford

Kingston H M 1989 ABC of clinical genetics. British Medical Journal, London

Leschot N J, Wolf H, Verjaal M et al 1987 Chorionic villi sampling: cytogenetic and clinical findings in 500 pregnancies. British Medical Journal 295: 407–410

Levitt S 1984 Child development and the therapist. In: Levitt S (ed) Paediatric development therapy. Blackwell, Oxford, p 1–12

MacFarlane J A 1980 Child health. Grant McIntyre, London

Moore J R 1973 Comprehensive assessment. In: Griffiths M I (ed) The young retarded child. Medical aspects of care. Churchill Livingstone, Edinburgh, p 29–49

Naylor E W 1985 Recent developments in neonatal screening. Seminars in Neonatology 9: 232–249

Senturia Y D, Peckham C S 1987 Preschool immunisation: the importance of achieving adequate uptake. Children and Society 3: 198–209

Sheridan M D 1973 Children's developmental progress from birth to five years. The Stycar sequences. NFER, Windsor

Tandy A, Bax M 1987 AIDS: health education in schools. The role of the community child health services. Children and Society 2: 148–156

Wood B S B 1970 A paediatric vade mecum. Lloyd Luke, London

World Health Organization 1986 The growth chart. World Health Organization, Geneva

This section covers those conditions, diseases and disabilities that form the scope of paediatric physiotherapy. Information is given on the features, causation and prognosis of the major disorders of childhood, and the principles of management are outlined. Chapter 6 covers the neonatal problems and subsequent chapters cover respiratory, cardiac, neurological, neuromuscular, sensory, orthopaedic and metabolic disorders. The various aspects of childhood trauma are described, and the subject of accidental injury and child abuse is introduced. Chapter 16, on learning and behavioural problems, completes the section.

SECTION 3
Problems and disorders in childhood

6

Neonatal problems and the neonatal unit

A. Parker

INTRODUCTION

About 10% of neonates will have problems that necessitate admission to a Neonatal Unit (NNU). Approximately 3% will require intensive care including ventilation. Reasons for admission to a NNU are:

- low birth weight
- perinatal problems
- congenital abnormalities.

Low birth weight (LBW)

About 40% of infants who are admitted to a NNU are preterm — less than 32 weeks' gestation — and weigh less than 2500 g. Some infants are born at only 23–24 weeks' gestation and may weigh as little as 450 g.

The cause of preterm birth is often unknown but there is an association with deprived socio-economic circumstances. There are more specific causes such as:

- antepartum haemorrhage
- cervical incompetence
- multiple pregnancies.

More mature infants may be of low birth weight (LBW) due to intrauterine growth retardation (IUGR). Causes of this include:

- placental dysfunction
- smoking

- intrauterine infection, e.g rubella
- chromosomal abnormality.

Perinatal problems

Perinatal problems are those that occur at or around the time of birth, e.g. birth asphyxia, meconium aspiration. Birth asphyxia accounts for about 10% of admissions to a NNU.

Congenital abnormalities

About 10% of infants admitted to NNU will have congenital abnormalities, e.g. congenital heart disease (see Chapter 7 Respiratory Conditions and Cardiothoracic Disorders), diaphragmatic hernia.

PROBLEMS AND MANAGEMENT OF LBW INFANTS

Respiratory problems

The functional and structural differences between the respiratory systems of neonates and older children or adults, which make them more susceptible to respiratory problems, are summarised below. These problems are compounded in preterm and LBW infants.

- *High larynx*, which enables the neonate to breath and swallow simultaneously up to the age of 3–4 months. This makes neonates obligate nose breathers, any nasal obstruction greatly increasing the work of breathing (Purcell 1976).
- *Lack of structural support* and the small diameter of airways mean that these can be easily blocked, leading to atelectasis.
- *Lungs are less compliant*, but the chest wall is more compliant, therefore neonates have to work harder to ventilate their lungs.
- *Less alveolar surface area* — this increases rapidly in the first year of life and continues up to about the age of 8 years.
- *Horizontally positioned ribs* and weak intercostal muscles mean that neonates are predominantly diaphragmatic breathers.

- *A reduced number of type 1 muscle fibres* in the diaphragm means that it is more liable to fatigue.
- *Irregular breathing patterns* often lead to apnoea. The more preterm the infant the more irregular the breathing pattern.
- *Increasing the rate* rather than the depth of breathing compensates for respiratory distress.
- *Infants preferentially ventilate the upper lung* when positioned in side-lying (Heaf et al 1983). Adults preferentially ventilate the *lower* lung.

The main cause of respiratory distress in the preterm infant is the respiratory distress syndrome (RDS). This is caused by lack of surfactant in the immature lung. Surfactant is the phospholipid alveolar lining that lowers surface tension and allows the lung to expand more easily. Surfactant appears in the lung at about 20 weeks' gestation, the amount present increasing slowly until the lung becomes functionally mature at about 34 weeks.

RDS presents within a few hours of birth with:

- sternal and costal recession
- grunting
- tachypnoea (respiratory rate more than 60 per minute).

Treatment

Treatment is supportive, maintaining the infant in a stable condition until the lungs are able to produce surfactant efficiently. This usually takes 36–48 hours. Treatment includes avoidance of hypoxia, which hinders surfactant production, by:

- keeping the infant warm
- minimal handling
- oxygen (O_2) therapy.

The use of artificial surfactant, instilled directly into the lungs to reduce the severity of RDS, is not yet widespread. The exact dosage, timing and type of infants it helps is still being evaluated (Morley 1991).

Less severely affected infants may only require humidified oxygen via a headbox, a clear plastic box placed over the infant's head. Humidification of the inspired gases is essential to prevent drying and thickening of secretions. Humidifiers are usually heated and can be used with or without ventilators. Water temperature should be 37°C minimum to optimise humidity and reduce bacterial growth.

Assisted ventilation. Infants with severe RDS may require intubation and ventilation. Endotracheal tubes may be nasal or oral (Fig. 6.1) and are uncuffed to reduce the risk of tracheal stenosis. This means that the tube may easily be displaced and that there is also a possibility of aspiration of milk or vomit around the tube.

Modern ventilators are able to provide all forms of assisted ventilation and may be pressure- or time-cycled. Pressure-cycled ventilators give pressure-limited ventilation, with the volume that is delivered being dependent on lung compliance and the amount of air leakage around the uncuffed endotracheal tube. Time-cycled ventilators deliver preset pressure for a selected length of time. The ventilator delivers a continuous flow of gas so that the infant is able to breathe spontaneously between ventilator breaths.

Intermittent mandatory ventilation (IMV) and continuous positive airways pressure (CPAP) are the most commonly used forms of assisted ventilation, with intermittent positive pressure ventilation (IPPV) being used only for severely affected infants. IMV is really a slow form of IPPV — the infant receives a preset number of breaths per minute at a preset pressure but is also able to breathe spontaneously between the ventilator impulses. The number of breaths per minute is gradually reduced as the infant's respiratory condition improves.

CPAP may be used to wean an infant from the ventilator or may be the first-line treatment of those infants with less severe RDS. The patient breathes spontaneously against a continuous positive pressure, which may help in keeping the airways patent. CPAP can be delivered by endotracheal tube, nasopharyngeal tube or nasal prongs. One disadvantage of the last two is gaseous abdominal distension.

Maximum pressures used in all forms of assisted ventilation (IPPV, IMV, CPAP) will depend on the size of the infant and severity of the RDS. Regular blood gas measurement ensures that the minimal amount of assisted ventilation is given to produce satisfactory blood gas levels.

Continuous oxygen monitoring may be facilitated by the use of transcutaneous oxygen monitors (TcO_2) or pulse oximeters.

TcO_2 monitors are a non-invasive way of measuring the partial pressure of arterial oxygen (PaO_2) in the arterialised capillaries through the skin. Electrodes with a heating element are placed on an area of thin skin, e.g. the abdomen, and oxygen is detected by a sensor within the electrode. The sensor is heated to 44°C so the electrode needs to be resited every 4 hours to prevent burning. A digital display shows the PaO_2.

Pulse oximeters measure the infant's arterial blood saturation. Saturation is defined as the proportion of oxyhaemoglobin in the blood. The sensor consists of two parts, which are taped on opposite aspects of the hand or foot. One part emits red light of two different wavelengths and the other part detects how much of this light has been absorbed by the tissues. The percentage difference in absorption between the two wavelengths correlates with the oxygen saturation.

Complications of assisted ventilation

Pneumothorax. This may occur spontaneously in 1% of full-term infants, but occurs mainly in LBW infants with poorly compliant lungs who require positive pressure ventilation.

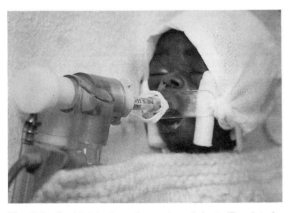

Fig. 6.1 Oral intubation of a preterm infant. (Reprinted by permission of Faber and Faber Ltd from Cash's textbook of chest, heart and vascular disorders for physiotherapists, Patricia A Downie (ed).)

A large tension pneumothorax will usually cause rapid clinical deterioration, which requires emergency drainage by chest drain. Pneumothorax has also been noted in very LBW infants with chronic lung disease following perforation of a bronchus by a suction catheter (Vaughan et al 1978).

Pulmonary interstitial emphysema (PIE). This occurs when gas leaks out of an alveolus and tracks along the bronchovascular bundle, where it is trapped, forming interstitial pockets of gas. It may be asymptomatic but in severe cases it may cause a steady deterioration of blood gases. Fast rate ventilation is used for these infants and if very severe PIE is present then needle scarification, followed by chest drain, is used.

Sub-glottic stenosis. This can occur in some infants following prolonged intubation, and leads to upper airway obstruction. Stridor is often present and severely affected infants may require tracheostomy until the airway has increased sufficiently in size to allow adequate ventilation.

Retinopathy of prematurity (ROP). This is a condition in which the delicate capillaries in the retina proliferate, leading to haemorrhage, fibrosis and scarring of the retina. In the most severe form this may result in permanent visual impairment. The cause is unknown but prolonged periods of hyperoxia (partial pressure of arterial oxygen (PaO_2) above 16 kPa) is thought to be a major predisposing factor.

The fundi of infants at risk are regularly examined and if vascular proliferation is seen then cryotherapy with liquid nitrogen is performed.

Bronchopulmonary dysplasia (BPD). This is defined as being present in infants who:

* are dependent on respiratory support at one month
* have an associated abnormal chest radiograph.

There is widespread destruction of terminal bronchioles and alveoli, which are replaced by areas of collapse, emphysema and fibrous tissue. There are many infants, however, who may be oxygen-dependent and have abnormal chest radiographs without fitting the exact definition of BPD and the term chronic lung disease of

prematurity (CLD) is now more commonly used to describe these patients. The exact cause of CLD is unknown but it is thought to be mainly due to prolonged mechanical ventilation, especially with high pressures and high inspiratory oxygen. The incidence varies between 4 and 40%, depending on gestational age, the more preterm infants being more at risk. Infants are ventilated with pressures that are kept as low as possible, while maintaining adequate gases, to try to prevent the onset of CLD.

The use of drugs such as steroids, bronchodilators and diuretics as treatment for CLD is still being evaluated.

Infants suffering from CLD may need supplementary oxygen for many months, until their lungs have had a chance to recover and grow. During this time there is an increased risk of viral chest infections and obstructive airway disease. Some infants never recover and need increasing amounts of oxygen, leading to the development of cor pulmonale and eventual death.

Temperature control

LBW infants have difficulty in maintaining their body temperature. They have a large surface area and a small body mass and easily lose heat through the skin by evaporation and radiation. They also have a smaller proportion of brown fat in comparison with full-term babies and thus they can rapidly become hypothermic. Some effects of hypothermia are acidosis, hypoglycaemia, increased oxygen (O_2) consumption and decreased surfactant production. Therefore it is *vital* to maintain body temperature.

Management

Infants should be kept in a thermoneutral environment, i.e. the temperature at which O_2 consumption is minimal in the presence of a normal body temperature. This will vary according to the patient's gestation and weight.

To maintain a thermoneutral environment infants are nursed in incubators — enclosed units of transparent material with port-holes in the sides for access — or under radiant warmers — open-topped units with radiant heating devices.

These allow free access and space for infusions and tubes but their disadvantages are convective heat loss and insensible fluid loss. Heat shields are used to reduce radiant heat loss and the ambient room temperature is kept high, at 27–28°C.

Infection

The preterm infant is particularly vulnerable to infection — the skin is very thin, easily damaged and infected, and cellular and humoral defences are impaired.

An organism that may cause only a minor problem in an adult may cause an overwhelming infection in a neonate, e.g. septicaemia and meningitis, both of which can, of course, be fatal.

Management

The most important means of preventing and reducing cross infection is by scrupulous hand-washing by all staff members and visitors. Regular use of an alcohol-based antibacterial solution, e.g. Hibisol, for the hands is also necessary.

Visitors to the unit are usually kept to a minimum, i.e. parents, grandparents and siblings, and anyone with an infectious disease, e.g. gastroenteritis, respiratory illness, boils, etc. should be excluded.

Prompt treatment of any infection in the baby with appropriate antibiotics is usual to prevent infection becoming severe and life-threatening.

Jaundice

Physiological jaundice is common in the normal, full-term infant, appearing after 2 days and usually disappearing by 7–10 days of life.

The jaundice is due to a raised blood level of unconjugated bilirubin, which gives the characteristic yellow skin colour. Unconjugated bilirubin is lipid-soluble and easily diffuses through brain cell membranes, particularly the basal ganglia. This can lead to a condition called kernicterus, which is characterised by athetoid cerebral palsy (see Chapter 8 Disorders of the Central Nervous System), deafness and mental retardation. Occasionally it may be fatal. Preterm infants are particularly prone to developing jaundice and run an increased risk of subsequent kernicterus. Jaundice can also be severe in infants with rhesus incompatibility.

Management

Daily serum bilirubin levels are measured in blood taken by heel prick from jaundiced infants. Treatment consists of phototherapy, where the infant is exposed to lightwaves of 400–500 nm, which oxidise unconjugated bilirubin into harmless derivatives. The use of eye-shields reduces the theoretical risk of eye damage.

In severe cases, exchange transfusion may be required. In this procedure blood is withdrawn from the infant in small amounts of 5 or 10 ml and replaced by donor blood until twice the infant's blood volume has been exchanged.

Periventricular haemorrhage

Periventricular haemorrhage (PVH) is a major cause of cerebral damage and death in the LBW infant. It occurs spontaneously in at least 30% of infants weighing less than 1500 g, but particularly occurs in those infants who have suffered episodes of hypoxia, hypotension and apnoea. It is most frequent and tends to be most severe in the smallest and least mature babies.

The haemorrhages arise from the fragile capillaries of the extremely vascular germinal layer in the floor of the lateral ventricles. Fluctuations of PaO_2, $PaCO_2$ and blood pressure leading to marked variations in cerebral blood flow will cause capillaries to rupture and bleeding to occur into and around the ventricles.

There are four grades of severity:

1. Bleeding into floor of the ventricle.
2. Bleeding into the ventricle — intraventricular haemorrhage (IVH).
3. IVH with dilation of the ventricle.
4. IVH and bleeding into the cerebral cortex around the ventricle causing areas of ischaemia.

Regular cerebral ultrasound scanning of infants indicates the presence of PVH and whether it is extending.

Management

Infants with Grade 1 and 2 PVH are often asymptomatic, require no treatment and have a good prognosis.

Infants who survive a Grade 3–4 haemorrhage may develop hydrocephalus and many will have some degree of neurological handicap. Patients with severe hydrocephalus will require shunt insertion and those with fits will require long-term anticonvulsant therapy.

Prevention of PVH is directed towards minimal handling of infants at risk and avoidance of hypoxic and hypotensive episodes.

Periventricular leucomalacia

Periventricular leucomalacia (PVL) may occur on its own or be associated with PVH. Ischaemia of the brain adjacent to the ventricles may produce destruction of tissue and hence cystic change. There is an association with development of cerebral diplegia.

Management

Management is directed towards prevention by minimal handling as, once PVL is present, nothing can be done. Regular monitoring is important to ensure that early intervention is given as necessary.

Feeding

All neonates lose weight in the first few days of life, especially those born preterm. Adequate calorie intake and weight gain are important to avoid hypoglycaemia, persisting jaundice and delayed recovery from RDS.

Management

Feeding should be commenced early, either orally, in those who can tolerate it, or intravenously.

Preterm infants cannot suck satisfactorily and have impaired swallowing and imperfect cough and gag reflexes, so that most will need to be fed nasogastrically until these reflexes develop. Feeding bolus feeds this way can increase respiratory distress due to:

- abdominal distension
- nasal obstruction by nasogastric tube.

Pooling of milk in the stomach can also lead to regurgitation and aspiration. Continuous infusion of milk using a syringe pump avoids some of these problems and in infants with respiratory problems, orogastric rather than nasogastric tubes may be used.

Healthy LBW infants can be put to the breast even when being fed nasogastrically. This encourages development of the sucking reflex and aids attachment between the mother and the infant.

Infants may be fed with their mother's expressed milk, although this does not contain sufficient vitamins, iron or phosphorus for preterm infants. Additives should be given or the infant should be fed on preterm formula milk preparations. Dietary phosphate deficiency can lead to 'rickets' of prematurity unless sufficient additives are given.

Necrotising enterocolitis

Necrotising enterocolitis is a serious disorder that occurs mainly in preterm infants. The cause is unknown but predisposing factors include:

- presence of umbilical arterial or venous catheter
- episodes of hypoxia and acidosis
- infection
- severe IUGR.

The infant becomes pale and unwell, with abdominal distension. X-ray shows dilated loops of bowel and, in severe cases, may show free gas in the peritoneum due to perforation of the bowel wall.

Management

Treatment is initially conservative, with gastric aspiration, intravenous nutrition and antibiotics. In some cases laparotomy may be required with resection of necrotic bowel.

Handling

Handling a sick neonate in any way will cause

their condition to deteriorate, usually by making them hypoxic.

Management

Handling should be minimal and procedures such as chest physiotherapy should only be given when necessary, and not as routine.

PERINATAL PROBLEMS AND MANAGEMENT
Birth asphyxia

This is defined as delay in establishing respiration after birth. Modern obstetric practice means that only about 10% of infants suffer from birth asphyxia but in a few this might be severe enough to require admission to a SCBU.

Asphyxia may occur due to:

* occlusion or prolapse of the umbilical cord
* uncoordinated hypertonic uterine contractions
* placental separation leading to antepartum haemorrhage
* malpresentation including breech delivery.

Asphyxia is more common in infants suffering from IUGR and in the preterm.

Apgar score

The usual way of assessing severity of asphyxia in the neonate is to use the Apgar score (Table 6.1). This grades five clinical features with scores from 0–2 at 1 minute of age. Apgar scores are repeated at 5, 10 and 15 minutes to indicate the success of the resuscitation and the degree of asphyxia. The best indicators of severity are the heart rate and the onset and type of breathing. The need for resuscitation is largely determined by these.

Severe asphyxia can lead to heart failure, CNS damage and renal failure.

The severity of CNS damage may range from cerebral oedema to subdural or subarachnoid haemorrhage. Long-term neurological sequelae are difficult to predict in the early days and even severely asphyxiated infants occasionally may make a reasonable neurological recovery.

Table 6.1 The Apgar score (Apgar 1953)

Clinical feature	Score		
	0	1	2
Heart rate	0	<100	>100
Respiration	Absent	Gasping or irregular	Regular or crying lustily
Colour of trunk	White	Blue	Pink
Muscle tone	Limp	Diminished	Normal
Response to oral suction	Nil	Grimace	Cough

Management

The infant will need careful monitoring over the first days. Careful control of fluid and electrolyte balance is necessary in these infants, particularly when renal failure is also present.

Convulsions of varying severity, which may occur in some infants, need to be treated by drugs such as phenobarbitone, diazepam or phenytoin. Long-term anticonvulsant therapy may be necessary.

Birth trauma

Birth trauma, e.g. severe bruising, fractures and nerve injuries do not usually require admission to a NNU but may be seen in an infant who also has birth asphyxia.

Brachial plexus lesions are the most common injury and can occur after difficulties with delivery of the shoulders, when the injury is likely to follow lateral traction of the neck. When the upper roots (C(4), 5, 6, (7)) are affected, the arm hangs limply by the side, internally rotated with the elbow extended and the wrist flexed (Waiter's tip position). This is known as Erb's palsy. Occasionally, in severe lesions, the diaphragm may also be affected.

Injury of the lower roots (C7, 8, T1) causes wrist drop and flaccid paralysis of the hand — Klumpke's paralysis.

Recovery usually occurs in both cases but may take months.

Management

Physiotherapy management consists of advice to

parents on dressing and handling and also making splints for wrist drop (see Chapter 19 Treatment Methods).

Meconium aspiration

This mainly occurs in full-term infants who become hypoxic due to a prolonged and difficult labour. Hypoxia causes the infant to pass meconium into the amniotic fluid and to make gasping movements, so that some of the meconium is drawn into the lungs. The irritant properties of meconium can cause a chemical pneumonitis and predispose to bacterial infection.

Management

If the mother's liquor is meconium-stained, a paediatrician should be present at the delivery to suck out the infant's airway as soon as the mouth is free to prevent further aspiration when the first breath is taken. Once delivered the infant may need to be intubated for further suction. A severely affected infant may need to be ventilated. Treatment also includes antibiotics and vigorous chest physiotherapy as soon as the infant is stable, to aid removal of any remaining meconium plugs. If physiotherapy is not commenced early enough, the lung becomes consolidated and physiotherapy is then ineffective.

CONGENITAL ABNORMALITIES AND THEIR MANAGEMENT

Only infants with severe congenital problems will need to be admitted to a NNU.

Diaphragmatic hernia

Diaphragmatic hernia is a congenital abnormality where loops of bowel herniate through the diaphragm into the thoracic cavity, most commonly on the left side. The incidence is 1 in 4000 births. The abnormality may be diagnosed antenatally by ultrasound or the infant may present with respiratory distress. A chest X-ray will show abdominal viscera in the thoracic cavity. Pulmonary hypoplasia is associated with this condition, as the abdominal viscera occupy the space normally occupied by the growing lung.

Management

Treatment involves endotracheal intubation followed by emergency surgery as soon as the infant's condition is stable. The abdominal viscera are pushed back into the abdominal cavity and the defect in the diaphragm is sutured. The infant will usually need postoperative ventilatory support because of the pulmonary hypoplasia. Mortality is about 50%.

Oesophageal atresia

In this congenital malformation the upper end of the oesophagus finishes in a blind pouch. There may also be a tracheo-oesophageal fistula (TOF) from the lower part of the oesophagus into the trachea. The incidence is 1 in 3500 births.

The infant presents shortly after birth with respiratory distress due to the inability to swallow oral secretions, which then overflow and are aspirated into the trachea. The acid stomach contents may also be regurgitated through the distal fistula into the lungs, resulting in atelectasis and pneumonia.

Management

Surgical correction is usually attempted as soon as possible. Pre-operatively the airway should be kept clear by continuous suction of the upper pouch and the infant should be nursed head up to prevent reflux of gastric contents through the TOF.

In most cases surgical treatment consists of primary anastomosis of the oesophagus with correction of the TOF. In some cases, where the gap between the ends of the oesophagus is too large, primary anastomosis is not possible, so a feeding gastrostomy is formed with anastomosis being carried out at a later date.

Postoperatively the patient may need to be ventilated for several days and is again nursed in the head up position. If chest physiotherapy is required it should be given in this position for the first few days. Care must be taken not to extend the neck as this may put additional stress on the anastomosis. In the non-intubated patient, pharyngeal suction must be used cautiously to avoid passing the catheter into the oesophagus, thus damaging the anastomosis.

At least 50% of infants with oesophageal atresia will have other congenital abnormalities.

Meconium ileus

This is a condition where thickened meconium causes blockage of the colon and ileum. The infant presents with abdominal distension, vomiting and failure to pass meconium. About 96% of patients with meconium ileus have cystic fibrosis (CF); 12% of patients with CF present this way.

Management

The obstruction can sometimes be relieved by an enema but laparotomy is often necessary, with formation of a temporary ileostomy. A sweat test will be needed to diagnose CF and chest physiotherapy should be started as soon as the diagnosis is confirmed, unless indicated earlier (see Chapter 7 Respiratory Conditions and Cardiothoracic Disorders).

GENERAL PROBLEMS OF INFANTS IN NNU

Parental–infant attachment (bonding)

It is now accepted practice in maternity units for parents of normal infants to have physical contact with their infants immediately after birth and for some hours afterwards. Unfortunately, in the case of an infant who needs to be resuscitated and transferred to the NNU, this is not usually possible (Fig. 6.2).

The effect of early separation on subsequent parent–child relationships is controversial. Many psychologists believe that parental–infant (especially maternal) contact in the first hour after birth is crucial to avoid future 'parenting disorders' but others feel that socio-economic factors are far more influential (see Chapter 23 Parents and Children).

It is generally agreed that any possible sequelae of early separation should be minimised as far as possible.

Box 6.1 Methods to minimise the effects of parent–infant separation

• Where it is known antenatally that an infant will need to be admitted to a NNU the parents should be taken to visit the unit and meet the staff. Some hospitals routinely offer all mothers a visit to the NNU as part of antenatal classes.

• Most NNU have a booklet that explains the equipment in use and introduces staff members. This should be given antenatally where appropriate, or as soon after birth as possible. A book is also available for older siblings.

• Mothers should be allowed to hold their infants before they are transferred to the NNU whenever the condition of either allows.

• When the infant is being transferred to another hospital for special care, if possible the mother should also be transferred.

• Fathers should be allowed to visit the NNU once the infant is settled and should be given a full explanation of the infant's condition.

• Polaroid photographs of the infant should be sent to the mother as soon as possible. Mothers experience a great feeling of loss when the infant is taken away after birth and photographs can help to alleviate this.

• If the mother is confined to bed on the postnatal ward the more mature, stable infant may be able to visit her there.

• Parents should be allowed unlimited access to the NNU and be actively encouraged to visit and telephone whenever they wish.

• The infant's condition and presence of electrodes, drains, tubes, etc. should be carefully explained to the mother prior to her first visit.

• Parents should be encouraged to touch their infants, no matter how ill they are, and should be allowed to cuddle them once they are well enough to be handled.

• Infants should be given their mother's expressed breast milk and be encouraged to feed from the breast when their condition allows.

• At all times unit staff should be prepared to discuss the infant's condition with parents fully and truthfully.

• As the infant improves parents should be encouraged to take part in his care but this should never be forced upon them.

• A few mothers (and fathers) will wish to stay with their babies during most of their hospitalisation but most will at least wish to do so later on. When the time comes, mothers should be allowed to room in with their infants for a few days prior to discharge.

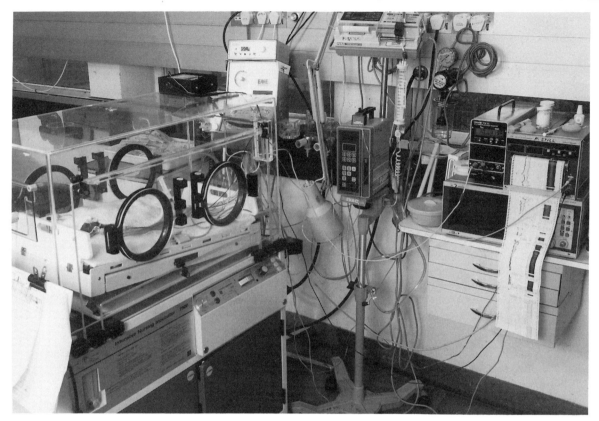

Fig. 6.2 Equipment used in a neonatal intensive care unit. (Reprinted by permission of Faber and Faber Ltd from Cash's textbook of chest, heart and vascular disorders for physiotherapists, Patricia A Downie (ed).)

If these measures are carried out then the stress and guilt that parents, especially mothers, feel when their infants are admitted to a NNU is minimised.

Unit staff should continue to support parents once the infant has been discharged, e.g. encouraging parents to visit the unit or to telephone if they are worried.

Adaptation to the extrauterine environment

Birth is a traumatic event for all infants, a change from the warm dark environment of the uterus to the bright outside world. Those infants who, in addition, require admission to a neonatal unit experience many unpleasant stimuli (Table 6.2). To minimise these stressful stimuli many neonatal units employ the following:

Table 6.2 Contrasts between the 'in utero' and 'in incubator' environments

In utero	In incubator
Balance and movement stimulation	Infant static on hard surface
Periods of activity/inactivity related to mother's routine	Haphazard handling and painful stimuli
Constant temperature	Variable temperature
Sounds — mother's voice, heartbeat, respiration, bowel sounds	Sounds — ventilator, incubator doors opening/closing
Gentle/absent light	24-hour light

• Infants are nursed on a sheepskin or bean-bag. This provides a softer surface and help to reduce moulding of the soft skull.

• Parents are encouraged to caress their infant and unpleasant stimuli such as heel pricks are kept to a minimum.

• When possible, lights are turned off or dimmed at night.

• Noise is kept to a minimum. The average ambient noise intensity in an intensive care nursery is 65 decibels (the same as in a busy street). The noise level inside an incubator is 63–64 db, banging on the top of the incubator increases this to 89 db, and closing a port-hole to 96 db. Sudden loud noises cause a drop in PaO_2, an increase in intracranial pressure and an increase in heart and respiratory rates. Staff should attempt to close port-hole doors gently and avoid placing equipment on top of the incubator.

THE ROLE OF THE PHYSIOTHERAPIST IN THE NEONATAL UNIT

There are three areas in which physiotherapy plays a role:

• respiratory care
• mobilisation and positioning
• neurodevelopmental delay.

Most NNUS do not have full-time physiotherapists, so education of nursing staff in physiotherapy techniques is a major part of the physiotherapist's role (Parker and Downs 1991). New staff to the unit should be taught individually as part of their orientation programme and there should be regular sessions for discussion and update with all nursing members.

Respiratory care

Chest physiotherapy and suction have a crucial role in the respiratory care of infants on a NNU. The main indication for chest physiotherapy (CPT) and suction is removal of secretions but hypoxia, bradycardia, arrhythmias, trauma and bronchospasm may accompany these techniques so it is essential that a thorough assessment is made prior to each treatment. There are few studies investigating the effectiveness of CPT in preterm infants, and many of these are not applicable to the very low birth weight infants nursed in neonatal units (Downs and Parker 1991).

Respiratory assessment

Respiratory assessment will follow along the lines set in Chapter 17, but some additional points to note for neonates are as follows:

• medical records
• birth history
• Apgar scores
• course of illness from birth to present time.

Verbal reports from medical and nursing staff. These should include:

• recent respiratory problems
• how the infant tolerates handling, e.g. does:
  — TcO_2 drop dramatically?
  — the infant become bradycardic or apnoeic?
  — the inspired oxygen concentration need to be increased prior to treatment?
  — the ventilation need to be increased prior to treatment?
• is the infant properly rested since the last handling episode?

Charts. These should note:

• Temperature — if less than 36.5°C then delay treatment, if possible, until the infant has warmed up.
• Trend of PO_2 from blood gases and its correlation with TcO_2.
• Oxygen saturation.
• Trend of PCO_2 — this may gradually increase if the endotracheal tube (ETT) is becoming occluded with secretions.
• Incidence of self-limiting bradycardias (SLB) — an increase in SLBs may be an indication that suction is needed.
• Incidence of apnoeic spells — an increase may mean accumulation of secretions.
• Result of last suction.

Observations. These should include:

• signs of respiratory distress
  — recession
  — nasal flaring
  — grunting
  — stridor

- skin colour
  - pale — sepsis? anaemic? respiratory distress?
  - cyanosis — unreliable sign in neonates as cyanosis only appears when the infant is very hypoxic (PaO_2 20 mmHg)
  - redness — normal colour of newborn full-term infant
- breathing pattern
  - tachypnoea — respiratory distress
  - apnoea.

Auscultation. This is very difficult to interpret in the newborn, especially in the LBW infant. The sound of water bubbling in the ventilator tubing can be referred to the chest and mimic or mask breath sounds. Referred sounds from the ventilator can also manifest themselves as strange squeaks and crackles.

When the infant is breathing spontaneously it may be difficult to hear any breath sounds, because LBW infants breathe so shallowly.

Touch. In the same way that referred sounds can be heard by the stethoscope, referred crackles can also be felt by the fingertips. If loud coarse crackles can be felt all over both lung fields, then water may need to be emptied from the ventilator tubing.

Crackles due to the presence of secretions are much easier to feel in LBW infants.

Physiotherapy management

Indications for chest physiotherapy and suction

1. Increase and/or retention of secretions due to:
   a. long-term intubation, i.e. more than 36–48 hours when mucosal irritation by the endotracheal tube causes increased secretions, which may be easily removed by suction alone
   b. meconium aspiration — for removal of remaining meconium plugs and increased secretions due to chemical irritation of mucosa
   c. postoperatively — as in older child
   d. pneumonia — chest physiotherapy is useful in the productive phase but of no benefit when the lung is consolidated (Graham & Bradley 1978)
   e. chronic lung disease — when secretions are the main problem, rather than airway collapse or wheeze.
2. Lung collapse due to mucus plugging — a common problem due to small diameter airways. The right upper lobe is particularly affected.

Contraindications to chest physiotherapy

- Severely ill unstable infant
- Pulmonary haemorrhage.

The latter may occur spontaneously or following surfactant therapy. Suction only should be given as necessary to keep the airway clear until brown, old blood-stained secretions are being aspirated when physiotherapy techniques may be used to assist clearance.

Contraindications to postural drainage

- Head down tip:
  - periventricular haemorrhage
  - recent cranial surgery, e.g. shunt insertion
  - recent tracheoesophageal fistula repair
  - abdominal distension.

The head down position causes a rise in intracranial pressure and can also increase respiratory distress, as neonates are primarily diaphragmatic breathers. Preterm infants are usually habitually nursed in the head up position to improve their PO_2 (Thoresen et al 1988).

Most infants like the prone position and tolerate it well. However, they should not be placed in the prone position when they have an umbilical arterial catheter, anterior chest drain or severe abdominal distension.

Precautions of postural drainage

- Reduced tolerance in the unwell infant
- Preferential ventilation of upper lung in side-lying, e.g. infant with non-ventilating right lung due to mucus plugging

— PO_2 in prone 56 mmHg (7.5 kPa)
— PO_2 in left side-lying 22 mmHg (3 kPa) therefore the patient is treated in prone until sufficient secretions are cleared for the infant to tolerate left side-lying.

Manual techniques

Percussion. In neonates and LBW infants percussion may be applied to in three ways:

1. Tenting — using 3–4 fingers of one hand, slightly elevating the middle finger.
2. Contact heel percussion — percussion using the thenar and hypothenar eminences.
3. Cup-shaped objects, e.g. face mask with soft plastic or foam cuff.

Percussion should be done over clothing or a towel except when using a face mask. The face mask has been shown to be a well-tolerated method of percussion (Tudehope & Bagley 1980) (Figs 6.3 and 6.4).

Shaking and vibrations. These should be carefully applied using only the fingertips. Neonates have very compliant chest walls so vibrations can be very effective at removing secretions in infants breathing at a normal rate. However, vibrations are not so useful in infants who have a very rapid respiratory rate due to the short expiratory time. Precautions in the use of percussion and vibrations include:

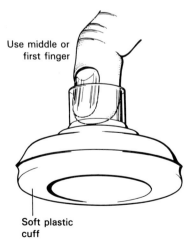

Use middle or first finger

Soft plastic cuff

Fig. 6.3 Bennett face mask for chest percussion.

• osteoporosis or rickets
• bruised damaged skin
• presence of chest drain
• thoracic incision
• bronchospasm.

Manual hyperinflation. This is not a technique usually used in the treatment of LBW infants because of the high risk of pneumothorax. It may be used cautiously in the full-term neonate in certain circumstances, e.g. postoperatively but should not be used as a physiotherapy technique when alveolar hyperinflation is a problem, e.g. after meconium aspiration.

The type of bag used in a SCBU is usually the self-inflating type, which is attached to a pressure manometer allowing the operator to be aware of the pressure he is generating.

All other precautions that apply to older children also apply to neonates.

Suction. Indications, effects and complications are the same as for the older child. Particular applications for neonates are:

• Clearance of nasal secretions is very important in neonates because they are obligate nose breathers.

• Nasopharyngeal suction can cause bradycardia and apnoea in neonates (Cordero & Hon 1971).

• Care must be taken with nasopharyngeal suction in infants with stridor as this can aggravate laryngospasm, particularly following extubation.

• Pneumothorax can occur in preterm infants with severe underlying lung disease due to perforation of segmental bronchi by suction catheters (Vaughan et al 1978). To prevent this, suction catheters should only pass 1 cm beyond the end of the endotracheal tube.

• Suction pressure should be as low as possible whilst still being effective. Suction pressures needed will depend on the size and type of catheter used.

• Size 6 and 8 FG catheters are the most useful; size 5 FG and below are often too small to remove thick secretions effectively. The diameter of ET tubes is usually too small for any catheter larger than a size 8 FG. Ideally, the suction catheter should be half the

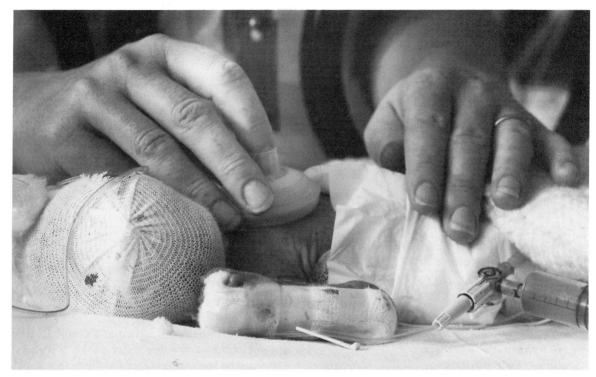

Fig. 6.4 Percussion of a preterm infant's chest with a Bennett face mask. (Reprinted by permission of Faber and Faber Ltd from Cash's textbook of chest, heart and vascular disorders for physiotherapists, Patricia A Downie (ed).)

diameter of the ETT although this may not always be possible. Size 6 FG catheters will need a higher negative suction pressure to be as effective as a size 8 FG catheter.

• A diluent such as saline is essential to loosen secretions in a LBW infant who is intubated with a size 2.0 or 2.5 ET tube. It may not be necessary when a 3.0 or 3.5 tube is used, providing humidification is adequate (Drew et al 1986). The amount of saline to be instilled prior to passing each suction catheter is dependent on the size of the infant:

— 0.45–2.5 kg   0.3–0.5 ml
— 2.50–4.5 kg   0.5–1.0 ml

• When saline is instilled into the very small bore endotracheal tubes then complete blockage of the tube may result; the infant immediately becomes apnoeic and bradycardic. The saline should be quickly removed by suction and the infant allowed to recover. This event may be avoided by instilling the saline via a suction catheter, which also ensures that

it reaches further down into the bronchi. A catheter is filled with saline from a syringe, which is left attached as the catheter is passed into the tracheal tube. The required amount of saline is then delivered and the catheter removed without applying suction. An alternative method of suctioning has been described by Downs (1989).

Procedure for chest physiotherapy

1. Prepare all equipment:
   a. suction catheters
   b. gloves
   c. saline.
2. Ensure vacuum suction is working and set at correct pressure.
3. Check monitors and note baseline values for that infant, also heart rate, respiratory rate (ventilator rate), TcO_2 (Table 6.3). It is inadvisable to begin treatment if the PaO_2 (as

Table 6.3 Baseline values for vital signs in infants

	Heart rate per minute	Respiratory rate per minute	Blood pressure mmHg
Preterm	120–140	35–45	70/40
Full-term	100–140	35–40	80/40

indicated by TcO_2) is less than 60 mmHg (8 kPa), unless the infant has chronic lung disease and is normally hypoxic. The inspired O_2 and/or ventilation can be increased until the PaO_2 reaches an acceptable level — 70–80 mmHg (9.5–10.5 kPa). Care must be taken not to allow the infant to become hyperoxic.

4. If necessary, and appropriate, the infant's position should be changed and time allowed for the PaO_2 to recover. The incubator doors should be kept closed between handling episodes to prevent the infant becoming hypothermic.

5. The appropriate amount of saline should be instilled if the infant is intubated.

6. Percussion and vibrations can be given if necessary; in some patients suction alone will effectively remove secretions.

The infant should be re-assessed after recovery and if there are still indications for physiotherapy then positioning, saline, percussion, etc., as appropriate, should be carried out until all secretions are cleared, providing the infant can tolerate this. Oral and nasal suction should then be carried out.

Once saline has been instilled the TcO_2 monitor will register the falling PaO_2. The length of the physiotherapy treatment depends on how soon this falls to an unacceptable level. Some infants deteriorate so rapidly that saline should be instilled *after* physiotherapy immediately before suction. Physiotherapy should be discontinued when the PaO_2 drops to 50–55 mmHg (6.5–7.5 kPa) and the infant should be suctioned. This will cause a further drop in PaO_2 to 40–45 mmHg (5–6 kPa) or even lower in a very unstable infant, and the infant must then be allowed to recover until the PaO_2 returns to pretreatment

levels. If the PaO_2 is slow to increase then the inspired O_2 and/or ventilation may be carefully increased.

A review of the treatment, i.e. how the infant tolerated the treatment and the amount and type of secretions, should indicate when treatment is likely to be necessary again.

Treatment should only be given when indicated, and not as routine.

Mobilisation

Unlike older children and adults, passive movements are not routinely required in the LBW infant. Preterm infants are hypotonic and over-vigorous passive handling can damage joints that are poorly protected by lax ligaments and hypotonic musculature.

LBW infants are often not paralysed and sedated for ventilation for long periods, as they are usually treated with IMV or CPAP and therefore can move and breathe actively.

Gentle passive movements may be required in full-term infants with peripheral neuropathies or birth injuries such as Erb's palsy.

Careful passive movements may be needed in infants who have had 'drip burns'. These occur when an intravenous infusion leaks into surrounding tissues, often around a joint, e.g. wrist, ankle or elbow. This causes inflammation of the tissues, resulting in ulceration, fibrosis and scarring. Particularly damaging are the preparations for intravenous nutrition, e.g. Vamin — an amino acid preparation — and Intralipid — a fat emulsion. Regular observation of infusion sites is essential as a severe burn can develop in only 15 minutes. Treatment consists of elevation of the affected limb to reduce oedema and daily dressings with a cream, such as Flamazine, to keep the burn clean and moist and to encourage healing.

During this time, regular gentle passive movements are necessary to maintain joint range and prevent contraction of healing tissues. Drip burns are extremely painful and infants may become hypoxic and bradycardic when joint movements are carried out. Severe drip burns may require skin grafting.

Positioning

A full-term infant spends the last 4–6 weeks in utero in a flexed position due to its increased size and decreased amount of liquor allowing less room for movement.

A LBW infant who has been born preterm does not experience this flexion and so exhibits an extended posture. These infants are often more stable in the prone lying position, which also accentuates extension of the hip and shoulder girdles. The LBW infant often goes on to develop retracted shoulders, externally rotated hips and everted feet.

When infants can tolerate position changes, nursing staff are encouraged to nurse them in alternate side-lying and a flexed position with shoulders forward and hands in midline. If nursed in prone a roll is placed under the hips to improve posture (Downs et al 1991). When the infant is lifted out of the incubator or cot the flexed position is maintained as much as possible. Swaddling in a small blanket or sheet is good for maintenance of the flexed posture but cannot usually be used for infants who require close monitoring. Mothers are shown how to manage infants in this way and are encouraged to continue the same techniques at home after the infant's discharge. Some units use bean bags or water beds and pillows to try to prevent postural deformity, but the use of these has not been fully evaluated (Cubby 1991).

Neurodevelopmental delay

Infants who have suffered birth asphyxia and periventricular haemorrhages may need to be seen by a neurodevelopmental physiotherapist. These infants will need individual assessments before deciding on the optimum treatment programme.

Ideally, the physiotherapist who will be treating the infant after discharge should be involved as early as possible.

In these infants, treatment in the early stages is minimal and consists of advice on handling and positioning to mother and nursing staff.

The optimum time for assessment and treatment is when the infants are awake, alert and content.

If infants are cold, tired, hungry or miserable then treatment should not be attempted (see Chapter 22 Planning for Progress).

The use of stimulation programmes in these infants is controversial. The LBW or preterm infant may already be overstimulated due to the amount of noise, light and handling it is receiving. Signs of overstimulation and stress include gaze aversion, vomiting and hiccups.

CASE STUDY

The case history below illustrates the role of physiotherapy in the treatment of an LBW infant:

Infant born at 26 weeks' gestation
Weight 800 g
Delivered by emergency caesarian section for fetal distress, mother in preterm labour
Infant immediately intubated and resuscitated at birth
Apgar score
— 2 at 1 minute
— 2 at 2 minutes
— 5 at 10 minutes
Blood gases PaO_2 40 mmHg, $PaCO_2$ 70 mmHg
Infant sedated, given IPPV
— rate 60 breaths/minute
— pressures 28/2 cm H_2O
— inspired O_2 60%

Day 1–2

Infant becomes severely hypoxic when handled or taken off the ventilator. Suction therefore carried out approximately 8-hourly to ensure patency of endotracheal tube.

Day 3

Infant's condition slightly improved. Sedation discontinued, infant weaned onto IMV 40 breaths/minute. Pressure 25/2 cm H_2O, inspired O_2 50%. Infant breathing spontaneously in between ventilator breaths. White secretions now being aspirated from endotracheal tube. Suction increased to 4–6-hourly when indicated. PaO_2 still drops when infant handled. Cerebral ultrasound scan shows Grade 2–3 PVH.

Infant tending to be nursed prone as gases are better in this position, but is occasionally turned onto side.

Day 4

Infant jaundiced — commenced phototherapy. Intravenous infusion in left hand tissues causing oedema of hand and ulcerated area over dorsal aspect left wrist. Hand elevated and burn dressed. Gentle full range wrist and finger movements commenced and given as tolerated by nurses approximately 4-hourly during the day following initial assessment by physiotherapist.

Day 5

Infant's general condition static but ETT secretions are now thick, yellow and difficult to clear with suction alone. Sputum specimen sent for culture and antibiotics commenced. Chest physiotherapy commenced.

Assessment

IMV 40 breaths/minute, inspired O_2 50%, pressure 26/2
PO_2 58 mmHg, PCO_2 55 mmHg — gases gradually deteriorating
heart rate 130, temperature 36.8°C
TcO_2 readings correlate well with blood gases.

   Attending nurse reports that the infant still becomes hypoxic with handling and requires inspired O_2 to be increased before treatment is commenced. The infant is lying in the prone position. Crackles are heard and felt bilaterally. The breath sounds equal.

Treatment

- inspired O_2 increased to 60% — minimal effect on PaO_2
- infant left in prone as does not tolerate position change
- not tipped head down due to PVH
- saline 0.5 ml instilled
- percussion with face mask over chest
- vibrations to both lungs
- PaO_2 dropped to 43 mmHg
- infant suctioned — small amount of thick yellow secretions aspirated
- PaO_2 down to 36 mmHg
- inspired O_2 increased to 75%
- PaO_2 slowly recovers back to pretreatment level.

Infant re-assessed

- more coarse crackles, especially over left side
- breath sounds equal

- treatment as before
- suctioned — small amount thick yellow secretions
- PaO_2 continued to drop dramatically
- infant develops bradycardia
- infant rapidly hand-bagged with 100% oxygen — no improvement
- poor air entry — airway blocked?
- saline 0.5 ml instilled
- infant suctioned — large, thick, yellow plug removed
- infant hand-bagged — PaO_2 rapidly recovered, heart rate returned to normal
- infant put back on ventilator
- PaO_2 up to 78 mmHg
- inspired O_2 turned down to 60%

Infant re-assessed:

- few coarse crackles heard and felt centrally
- breath sounds equal
- 0.5 ml saline instilled
- suctioned — removed loose yellow/white secretions
- PaO_2 drops to 55 mmHg but recovers quickly.

Infant re-assessed:

- no crackles heard or felt
- breath sounds equal
- inspired O_2 turned back to 50%.

Blood gases taken 20 min after treatment finished show PaO_2 68 mmHg, $PaCO_2$ 45 mmHg.

Treatment

Chest physiotherapy and suction continued as necessary over the following few days, i.e. when crackles present or gases deteriorating. Frequency of treatment varied, depending on need, from 2-hourly to 4-hourly.

Day 8

Secretions white and easy to clear with suction so chest physiotherapy discontinued. Infant now tolerating handling better so position changed more regularly from prone to alternate sides and occasionally supine.

2–5 WEEKS

Infant spent 5 weeks on ventilator. Chest physiotherapy required at times when secretions not cleared with suction alone. Wrist burn healed well with no resultant problems.

Infant moved from intensive care area to special care area still requiring 30% oxygen.

Mainly nursed in alternate side-lying with shoulder forward and hands in midline.

During his awake, alert periods, mother and nurses were encouraged to handle and talk to the infant and eye contact was encouraged. The community physiotherapist was contacted as there was concern over infant's developmental progress due to his PVH. The community physiotherapist visited the unit to assess child and to meet and develop relationship with mother. Mother was shown how to prevent infant pushing back into extension.

Infant was gradually weaned off oxygen over the next 3 weeks and oral feeding was encouraged.

14 weeks

Infant discharged home aged 14 weeks, feeding well and gaining weight.

Community physiotherapist continued to see infant after discharge.

REFERENCES

Cordero L, Hon E H 1971 Neonatal bradycardia following nasopharyngeal stimulation. Journal of Paediatrics 78: 441–447

Cubby C 1991 Cranio-facial deformity in preterm infants. Paediatric Nursing 3(2): 19–21

Downs J A 1989 Endotracheal suction: A method of tracheal washout. Physiotherapy 75(8): 454

Downs J A, Edwards A D, McCormick D C et al 1991. Effect of intervention on development of hip posture in very preterm babies. Archives of Diseases in Childhood 66(7): 797–801

Downs J, Parker A 1991 Chest physiotherapy for preterm infants. Paediatric Nursing 3(2): 14–17.

Drew J H, Padoms K, Clabburn S L 1986 Endotracheal tube management in newborn infants with hyaline membrane disease. Australian Journal of Physiotherapy 32(l): 3–5

Graham W, Bradley D 1978 Efficacy of chest physiotherapy and intermittent PPB in the resolution of pneumonia. New England Journal of Medicine 299: 624–627

Heaf D P, Helms P, Gordon I, Turner H M 1983 Postural effects on gas exchange in infants. New England Journal of Medicine 308: 1505–1508

Morley C J 1991 Surfactant treatment for premature babies — a review of clinical trials. Archives of Diseases in Childhood 66: 445–450

Parker A, Downs J 1991 Chest physiotherapy in the neonatal intensive care unit. Paediatric Nursing 3(3): 19–21

Purcell M 1976 Response in the newborn to raised upper airway resistance. Archives of Diseases in Childhood 51: 602–607

Thoresen M, Cowan F, Whitelaw A 1988 Effect of tilting on oxygenation in newborn infants. Archives of Diseases in Childhood 63: 315–317

Tudehope D I, Bagley C, 1980 Techniques of physiotherapy in intubated babies with the respiratory distress syndrome. Australian Paediatric Journal 16: 226–228

Vaughan R S, Menke J A, Giacoia M D 1978 Pneumothorax: a complication of endotracheal tube suctioning. Journal of Paediatrics 92(4): 633–634

FURTHER READING

Anthea 1986 Special care babies (a book for siblings). Octopus, London

Harvey D, Cooke R W, Levitt G A (eds) 1989 The baby under 1000 g. Wright, London

Redshaw M E, Rivers R P A, Rosenblatt D B 1985 Born too early. Oxford University Press, Oxford

Roberton N R C 1986 A manual of neonatal intensive care, 2nd edn. Edward Arnold, London

Vulliamy D G 1986 The newborn child, 6th edn. Churchill Livingstone, London

7

Respiratory conditions and cardiothoracic disorders

V. Bastow

In this chapter the respiratory conditions of childhood are discussed together with the respiratory problems associated with cardiac abnormalities.

RESPIRATORY CONDITIONS OF CHILDHOOD

Asthma

Clinical features

Asthma is characterized by spasmodic attacks of wheezing and shortness of breath. During an attack a baby may display some or all the signs of increased respiratory muscle activity — flaring nostrils, sternal paradox and rib recession — depending on the degree of airway constriction. In the older child with a severe attack the wheezing may be heard without a stethoscope and the child may appear pale and frightened and be unable to speak in sentences. However, the severity is variable and in some children wheezing may only be obvious after, say, a sudden burst of exercise or following a minor respiratory tract infection, which may precipitate a 'wheezy' cough. Parents may report that the child's sleep is disturbed by periods of nocturnal coughing. The prevalence of asthma in children has been difficult to determine because of a reluctance to label a 'wheezy' child as having asthma. However, figures of around 15–20% of children are suggested and most asthmatic children will have had at least one episode of wheeze before the age of 7 years. About 50% of children with very mild asthma appear to have 'grown out of it' by adolescence and remain free in early adult life (Phelan 1982).

Medical management

The medical management of asthma in children is similar to that employed in adults, being based on the use of steroids and bronchodilators (although the immature beta-receptors of children under 1 year may render beta-agonists not particularly effective). However, the choice of delivery method is very much dictated by the age of the patient. A nebuliser may be necessary to administer inhaled drugs to a baby or toddler, and this method is usually used in an older child during a moderate or severe attack. The spacer inhaler device (nebuhaler or volumatic), with a face mask, may be used in babies and toddlers, and without the mask in older children of between 3 and 5 years. For these children the principles of suck, breath-hold and breath out can be taught in preparation for using patient-activated inhalers such as rotahalers, diskhalers and spinhalers. These devices are accepted by most children and are easy to carry in their school bag or pocket. However, as with any patient the inhalation technique must be checked every few months and corrected if necessary.

The accurate coordination of aerosol firing and inhalation needed when using a metered dose aerosol inhaler means that it is rare for a child below 10 years to use this method accurately.

Physiotherapy management

The physiotherapist has a limited role in the management of childhood asthma. Few childhood asthmatic attacks are provoked by bacterial infections and so postural drainage is rarely indicated. The ward physiotherapist may be the person who monitors peak flows of inpatients and who teaches and checks on inhaler techniques.

Breathing exercises. Breathing exercises are of doubtful value in most children. However, the older child who appears stressed and anxious may benefit from relaxation techniques that may incorporate breathing exercises.

Exercise programmes. Exercise programmes have not been shown to have a beneficial effect on respiratory function in asthma, but there may be some psychological benefit. The parents of children with asthma often restrict the child's participation in active sports — particularly where it is exercise that provokes an attack — and this can cause the child embarrassment amongst their peers and may also have a detrimental effect upon physical fitness. By teaching inhaler usage prior to exercise and following simple rules for warm-up and wind-down periods, the child can often participate fully in the most rigorous of sports. Swimming in particular may be of benefit to

---

Box 7.1 The coffee-cup technique for drug inhalation.

The coffee-cup technique, as described by Henry et al (1983), is sometimes useful in children (Fig. 7.1). A metered dose aerosol is placed into a hole cut in the base of a polystyrene or plastic coffee cup, and the open end of the cup is placed over the child's nose and mouth in the small child, or mouth only, with gentle pinching of the nose, in the older child.

The aerosol is fired and the mist remains in the cup whilst the child breathes in and out for about 10 seconds. Further single puffs are then delivered until the prescribed quantity is delivered. This can be a useful 'emergency' technique when away from home or when not in a position to use an electric compressor and nebuliser.

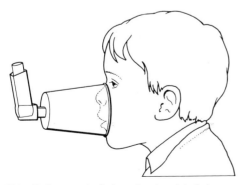

Fig. 7.1 Coffee-cup technique for drug inhalation.

asthmatic children, as it seems to produce less exercise-induced bronchospasm. Hopefully, by careful advice and training, children (and their parents) can learn to enjoy sport along with their peers.

Bronchiolitis

Bronchiolitis is the most common disease of the lower respiratory tract in infants and is caused by inflammatory obstruction of the small airways. It occurs during the first two years of life with the peak incidence at 6 months. The majority of cases occur during winter and early spring.

Clinical features

The cause is viral with respiratory syncytial virus (RSV) being implicated in more than 50% of cases, although parainfluenza virus, adenovirus and *Mycoplasma pneumoniae* have been associated with some epidemics. There is often a family history of recent minor respiratory tract illness.

The disease is characterised by marked wheeze and cough, often with sneezing and nasal discharge. The respiratory distress may be quite severe, with tachypnoea, dyspnoea, flaring of alae nasi and increased use of the accessory muscles of respiration. The child often has feeding difficulties. Bronchiolar obstruction due to oedema, mucus and cellular debris reduces airflow, particularly during expiration, leading to air trapping and hyperinflation. The smaller the child the more severe the obstruction tends to be. Approximately 30% of affected infants develop patchy consolidation on chest X-ray.

The diagnosis is made on the clinical symptoms, although this may be supported by demonstration by immunofluorescence of the RSV in a nasopharyngeal aspirate.

Medical management

Treatment of this condition is mainly symptomatic with attention to oxygenation, hydration and nutrition in the infant who is too distressed to feed adequately. Minimal handling by staff and parents is generally advised as disturbing the infant may increase the respiratory distress.

Oxygen therapy can be monitored using an oximeter and at least 85% saturation should be achieved.

Physiotherapy management

Physiotherapy has not been shown to produce any benefit in the management of these children even where there is radiological evidence of collapse/consolidation (Webb et al 1985). The physiotherapist can help by obtaining the nasopharyngeal aspirate for viral studies and may supervise the nasal suction needed to clear the often copious mucus, and hence facilitate breathing and feeding.

Bronchiectasis
Clinical features

This is a chronic disease characterised by dilatation of the bronchi, due to inflammation, progressive fibrosis and destruction of the bronchial tissue, affecting a bronchopulmonary segment, a lobe or whole lung. In children it may be congenital but is most commonly seen in patients with cystic fibrosis. It may also follow the inhalation of a foreign body, or bacterial or viral pneumonia. In a few patients it is associated with sinusitis and dextrocardia (Kartagener's syndrome) or, because of abnormal ciliary action, in the immotile cilia syndrome. It may follow measles or whooping cough that has been complicated by lobar or segmental collapse. The child with bronchiectasis may have a history of repeated chest infections with a chronic productive cough and breathlessness on exertion. Foul-smelling breath (halitosis) and finger clubbing may also be present.

The diagnosis is usually made on the clinical signs and radiological appearance, but sometimes a bronchogram may be performed to define the areas involved if surgical treatment is being considered. In children bronchography requires a general anaesthetic, unlike adults when sedation is usually adequate.

Physiotherapy management

Where there are few symptoms with minimal

secretions, regular physiotherapy treatment is not indicated unless the diagnosis of cystic fibrosis has been made. The parents should be advised to encourage exercise and be told that if the child's cough becomes worse then there may be a need to start regular postural drainage. This may also be necessary during viral illnesses such as colds, when the child may be less active and the cough more troublesome. When symptoms are troublesome and if the child is producing sputum on most days, then regular postural drainage with the active cycle of breathing techniques should be introduced and any necessary equipment, such as postural drainage wedges or tipping tables (Figs 7.2 and 7.3) supplied. Where the bronchiectatic area is localised to a specific segment or lobe, postural drainage positions specific to them should be used. With more widespread involvement generalised postural drainage may be adequate.

Medical management

Some patients with bronchiectasis show airway reversibility. The use of bronchodilator drugs prior to postural drainage may aid expectoration.

When the bronchiectatic area is confined to one segment or lobe surgical resection may be beneficial. In this case pre-operative physiotherapy may help to clear the accumulated pus and so reduce the chance of spill-over into the unaffected lung during surgery.

Cystic fibrosis

Cystic fibrosis is the most common inherited disorder affecting one in 2500 live births.

Clinical features

Cystic fibrosis is characterised by an increase in the viscosity of the mucus produced throughout the body and an excessive production of sodium chloride from the sweat glands. The pancreatic ducts become fibrosed and this impairs the secretion of pancreatic enzymes, which interferes with the digestion and absorption of fats.

The disorder may present in three ways.

1. Meconium ileus — an obstruction of the intestine in the newborn due to the presence of sticky meconium in the bowel, which may require surgery.

2. Failure to thrive — many affected babies present with inability to gain weight despite an apparently adequate food intake. This is due to the pancreatic deficiency and may be

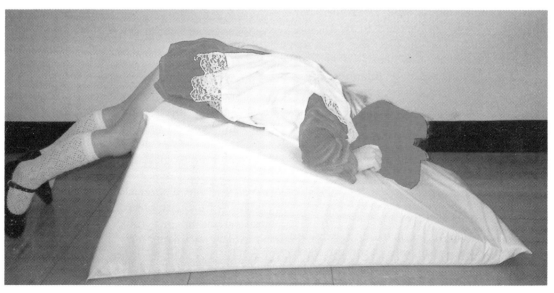

Fig. 7.2 Postural drainage: foam wedge (PVC-covered).

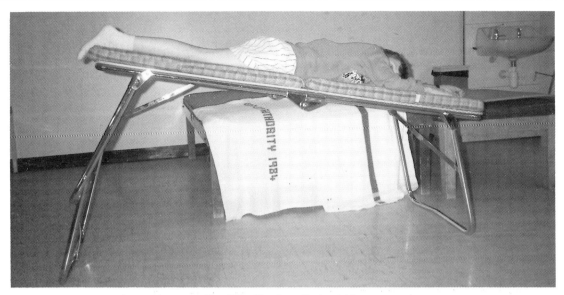

Fig. 7.3 Chesham tipping table.

associated with bulky, foul smelling greasy stools (steatorrhoea).

3. Respiratory disease — recurrent chest infections.

The diagnosis of cystic fibrosis is confirmed by a positive sweat test — sweat sodium concentration in excess of 60 mmol/litre.

Life expectancy for the child with cystic fibrosis has improved considerably: developments in pancreatic enzyme replacement therapy have improved the patient's nutritional state and antibiotic therapy has reduced the damage caused by superadded infection (particularly with *Pseudomonas*). Many patients will survive into their twenties and with the increased success of heart/lung transplant surgery, this technique may be used more often in severely affected patients. Research into the genetic abnormality responsible for the disease may lead to more effective treatment in the next decade.

Medical management

Nutritional management. The nutritional management of cystic fibrosis aims at improving the digestion and absorption of fats and fat soluble vitamins. Fat malabsorption occurs because of the reduced secretion of the appropriate digestive enzymes and treatment consists of administering the enzyme orally with each meal. Until recently the enzyme supplements available were only partially successful in increasing the absorption of dietary fat and some restriction of fat intake was necessary to avoid steatorrhoea, which hampered the provision of adequate calories. However, the newer enzymes Creon and Pancrease have resulted in a more liberal diet with less need to reduce fat content in the food. Despite this, many cystic children are underweight and of small stature for age and it appears that they need to eat 120–150% of the recommended calorie intake for their age. Salt and fat soluble vitamin supplements may be needed to compensate for the increased salt loss in sweat, and the impaired fat absorption.

Drug therapy. The two most common organisms found in the sputum of cystic fibrosis patients are *Staphylococcus aureus* and *Haemophilus influenzae*, both of which usually respond to oral antibiotic therapy. However, *Pseudomonas aeruginosa* eventually appears in the child's sputum, especially those who have suffered frequent respiratory infections, and this is almost invariably impossible to eradicate completely. Intravenous antibiotics are usually required, which necessitates a period of hospitalisation from 7 to 14 or more days. Some centres have developed a regimen of short hospital admissions and continuation of parental antibiotic therapy at home. This may not always be possible, particularly if there is concern about the efficacy of home physiotherapy treatment, although it has the advantage of the child's being able to continue schooling.

Inhaled antibiotics are increasingly being used and should be given after the chest drainage sessions. Due to the high viscosity of the antibiotics it is necessary to employ a high output compressor unit giving a flow rate of approximately 8 litres/minute (Fig. 7.4). To prevent the exhalation of antibiotics into the room atmosphere, and hence reduce the chance of antibiotic-resistant bacterial strains developing, it is desirable to use a nebuliser with a T-piece, one-way valve and exhalation pipe, which should be positioned out of the window (Fig. 7.5).

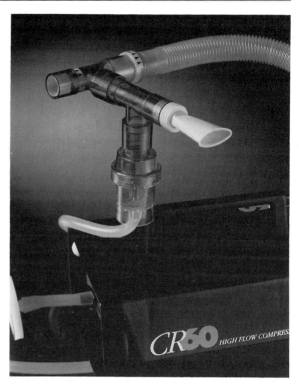

Fig. 7.5 Antibiotic 'T' system. (Reproduced by kind permission of Medic-Aid Ltd.)

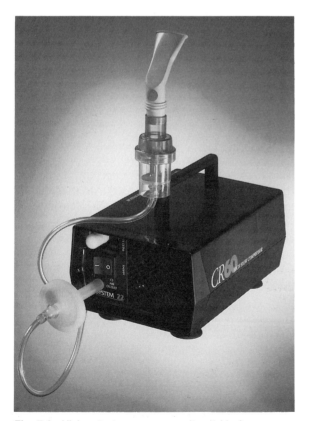

Fig. 7.4 High output compressor unit suitable for nebulising antibiotics. (Reproduced by kind permission of Medic-Aid Ltd.)

Bronchodilators (usually beta-2 agonists) are effective in approximately 40% of cystic fibrosis patients, and regular monitoring of pulmonary function and reversibility will help identify these subjects. In some patients bronchodilators may only be required during an infective exacerbation, so it is useful to perform pulmonary reversibility tests both during an exacerbation and when back to 'normal'. Nebulised bronchodilators may be of more help during an exacerbation because of the larger drug dosage administered and the additional humidifying effect of the diluent. However, when using nebulised bronchodilators the child will need to spend an extra 10–15 minutes receiving this prior to postural drainage, and this may not be acceptable when the child has to reach school on time or is wanting to play with friends. As an alternative, a rotahaler, turbohaler, diskhaler or metered-dose aerosol inhaler is quicker to use and can be carried in the pocket or satchel. It is, of course, essential to check regularly that the child is using any inhaler device correctly.

Physiotherapy management

Daily chest physiotherapy must become part of the cystic child's routine from diagnosis and this should be carried out even in the absence of respiratory symptoms.

Postural drainage. The institution of regular treatment soon after diagnosis helps to establish the postural drainage routine before the child can say 'No', and it helps the parents to focus on the chest so they notice any change early and can respond accordingly. It is important that both parents learn the physiotherapy techniques, and desirable if others involved in the child's care do too, so that the parents can have a break away from the routine.

Twice-daily treatment is sufficient for most children but those with severe chest problems may require three, four or more treatments daily. Should the child develop an upper respiratory tract infection or cold, then the frequency of treatment should be increased to try to prevent a chest infection developing.

The young baby up to about 15 months can be treated on the parent's knee, but beyond this age a small, high-density foam wedge with PVC cover is often useful and a large foam wedge is needed from about 4 years old to 8 or 9 years old (see Fig. 7.2).

After this age most children and adults appreciate the comfort of a postural drainage table, e.g. the Chesham Tipping Table (see Fig. 7.3). The more comfortable the child is during the treatment the more he is likely to cooperate and the more regularly treatment will be performed at home.

In the baby and toddler the physiotherapy is passive, relying on gravity and percussion techniques to aid drainage.

Breathing exercises. From about 3 years of age the child should be encouraged to participate in his treatment with 'tummy' (relaxed or diaphragmatic) breathing, deep breathing and coughing. Expectoration should be encouraged as early as possible to facilitate bacteriological examination of the sputum. The forced expiration technique (Pryor & Webber 1979) is best introduced around 4 or 5 years and the child encouraged to participate in the active cycle of breathing techniques with a view to achieving total independence in his early teens.

By the age of 9 or 10 years the child should be able to start taking some responsibility for his own treatment — perhaps starting with one drainage position and gradually including others as he becomes competent at independent drainage. It is usually still necessary for the parents to supervise the drainage sessions to ensure that the child does do all he should, and also to show that they are still interested in helping — even if only in a passive role. Many parents find it difficult to adopt the passive role after perhaps many years of being so actively involved, but with the encouragement and support of the physiotherapist the child and family can be helped towards sufficient independence to allow school outings, holidays and overnight stays with friends, and eventually complete independence from parental involvement.

Review of therapy. Frequent review of the chest condition is essential to ensure that the physiotherapy techniques are achieving the desired effect: the postural drainage positions may need to be changed as the disease advances. In babies treatment should include the apical segments of the upper lobes but as the child achieves a more upright position, this may not be so necessary and this drainage position may be discontinued if no clinical signs or symptoms relate to the area. The older child is susceptible to developing middle lobe or lingular lobe involvement requiring specific postural drainage, and the teenager and young adult often needs attention to anterior segments of the upper lobes and the middle and lingular lobes.

Exercise programmes. No single form of physical exercise is 'good' or 'bad' for the child with cystis fibrosis and each child should be encouraged to pursue the activity he or she enjoys the most, be it swimming, cycling, gymnastics or walking the dog! At some point in their lives the falling respiratory capacity will dictate less energetic exercise and it can be depressing for a child to fall behind friends or to be constantly put in goal to freeze in solitary confinement! It is important, therefore, to discuss sport and exercise tolerance with the school and if necessary explore other activities such as table tennis and snooker, which may be less strenuous. Swimming may be rejected during teenage years because of self-consciousness about small stature and chest deformity. Also, public swimming baths are often too cool for thin bodies and they may complain of feeling cold very soon after entering the water.

Management of childhood illnesses. Children with cystic fibrosis, like any other children, may have to undergo surgery such as appendicectomy or tonsillectomy, and in addition they are prone to the development of nasal polyps, which may occasionally require surgical removal. With planned surgery it is desirable to admit the patient a few days before surgery to enable a full respiratory assessment to be carried out and where necessary to allow a period of intensive physiotherapy.

Terminal cystic fibrosis. The child who has reached the terminal stages of cystic fibrosis may pose a dilemma for the physiotherapist. So much of the child's contact with the physiotherapist has concentrated on postural drainage and chest clearance techniques, which may no longer be deemed necessary. For the child's and the family's sake it may be important to continue seeing the child, but with less emphasis on an effective treatment and more emphasis on symptomatic and psychological support. Humidification may help the dry mouth and nose, and gentle chest drainage in the position of maximal comfort for the child may be helpful. Suction is distressing and should be avoided. Our efforts are best employed in helping the child to die with dignity and in the least distressing manner for his family.

Inhaled foreign body

Foreign bodies such as toys, beads, coins and food particles may be inhaled by children. Peanuts are the most notorious offenders and tend to lodge in the right middle lobe bronchus.

Clinical features

Any inhaled object may cause widespread inflammation, and in some patients may act like a one-way valve, allowing air to enter the segment or lobe on inspiration (as the airways widen) but obstructing the expiratory airflow when the airway narrows. This may result in obstructive emphysema developing with a hyperinflated segment or lobe.

The child may present at the hospital soon after inhaling the object, particularly if the inhalation was followed by choking and respiratory difficulty. However, some children will inhale objects unobserved and it may be many days or weeks before the problem presents, by which time a large area of the lung may be pneumonic and abscesses may have formed.

Medical management

Removal of the object at bronchoscopy under anaesthetic is urgently indicated. However, complete removal may not be possible because of the small calibre of the airways, because the object may be friable and difficult to grip, because there has been a considerable delay before diagnosis and because the object may break up and the smallest fragments may not be reached by bronchoscopy.

Physiotherapy management

Physiotherapy may help following bronchoscopic removal where there is pus, atelectasis or remaining fragments in the hope of dislodging them. It may be necessary to continue drainage and re-expansion techniques for some time and the treatment can often be continued at home after suitable instructions to the parents. In occasional cases full recovery does not occur and the child may be left with a bronchiectatic area.

Pneumonia

Clinical features

The aetiology of pneumonia in a child is similar to that of adults, with bacteria and viruses the usual causal agents and fungi and aspiration occasionally being implicated; it may follow an upper respiratory tract infection that 'goes to the chest'. Fever, shortness of breath, cough (often unproductive) and pleuritic pain together with grunting respiration may occur at the onset of the pneumonia. The diagnosis may be difficult to make in a child as he may present with symptoms that do not immediately suggest a chest problem, e.g. diarrhoea, vomiting and abdominal pain — the latter due to referred pain from the pleuritis along T6–12. Diagnosis is normally achieved following physical examination and chest X-ray, sometimes aided by sputum culture and microscopy.

Medical management

Antibiotics or antifungal therapy is instituted as soon as the diagnosis is made and, where possible, when the causative organism has been isolated, although antibiotic therapy is often instituted before sputum or blood culture results are available. Occasionally severe illness may require oxygen therapy or even assisted ventilation. Empyema is occasionally seen as a complication of pneumococcal or staphylococcal pneumonia and may require surgical drainage via thoracotomy.

Physiotherapy management

Physiotherapy may be of little benefit in lobar pneumonia except where there is previous underlying lung disease, such as cystic fibrosis, or where complications such as lung abscess or atelectasis may have developed. In the presence of underlying lung disease the length and vigour of physiotherapy treatment must take into account the illness of the child and his ability to tolerate treatment. High levels of humidification may help to liquefy and hence clear mucus. The physiotherapist's skills may be called upon to help obtain a sputum specimen helpful for the diagnosis.

Where surgical drainage of an empyema has been necessary, physiotherapy should be given as for thoracotomy procedure (see p. 112), bearing in mind how ill the child may be.

Atelectasis following empyema, pneumothorax or as a complication of pneumonia itself, requires treatment with re-expansion encouraged by inspiratory effort, incentive spirometer, 'blowing' games such as 'bubbles' and 'ping-pong' football, all of which encourage deep inspiration prior to blowing, and postural drainage to assist the removal of mucus plugging if implicated. Parental involvement is important as treatment may need to continue at home.

Whooping cough (pertussis)

This highly infectious disease may occur at any time during childhood, even in the first few weeks of life, but it is most severe in infancy.

Clinical features

The infection causes necrosis of the surface epithelium of the respiratory tract, which then becomes covered by thick mucopurulent exudate. The bronchi and bronchioles may become blocked by this exudate, which may lead to segmental or lobar atelectasis. If this persists then there is a risk of bronchiectasis occurring.

During the acute stage, the child characteristically has paroxysms of coughing in an attempt to clear the airways of the exudate. The paroxysms may last for up to 30 seconds, during which the child becomes red or even cyanosed. Eventually the child takes a deep breath in when the characteristic 'whoop' is heard. This may be followed by vomiting.

Medical and physiotherapy management

During the stage of acute paroxysms, physiotherapy is not indicated as it may induce more paroxysms by loosening the mucus and exudate in the large airways. Sometimes sedation may be prescribed, which will occasionally allow for physiotherapy techniques to be implemented without producing paroxysmal coughing. The main value of physiotherapy treatment is when segmental or lobar atelectasis is present as shown on the chest radiograph. The right middle lobe is affected most frequently. Because collapse may persist for some time, the parents may be required to perform physiotherapy at home. Techniques to encourage re-expansion of the collapsed area should be used, such as percussion, shakings and expansion exercises. It may take several months before the child has completely recovered and the parents will need support and encouragement through this long convalescent stage. Occasionally resolution is not complete and the child may develop bronchiectasis (see p. 99).

Tracheo-oesophageal fistula and oesophageal atresia

This condition affects about 1 in 3000 babies.

Clinical features

The condition is characterised by persistent frothy mucus in the pharynx, causing the baby to 'blow bubbles'. When the atresia (narrowing) is associated with a fistula, feeding the infant results in the passage of the feed directly into the lungs (Fig. 7.6C) or, if the fistula is from the distal stump of the abnormal oesophagus, gastric acid refluxes into the lungs (Fig. 7.6A). In Figure 7.6B, where there is no fistula, the fluid will overspill from the oesophagus into the trachea. The result of any of these abnormalities is the development of pneumonia. With the H-type (Fig. 7.6C), distension of the abdomen may be produced by the passage of air via the trachea and fistula into the oesophagus and stomach.

Medical management

In every case surgery is required, the anomaly corrected usually by a right thoracotomy with end-to-end anastomosis of the oesophagus and division of the fistula. Where the gap between distal and proximal stumps of the oesophagus is too great for an end-to-end anastomosis, a gastrostomy may be performed and the final anastomosis delayed, either until the oesophagus has developed sufficiently, or until a colonic transplantation can be performed at a later date. Occasionally a cervical oesophagostomy has to be performed to drain the swallowed saliva.

Physiotherapy management

These babies usually require physiotherapy. When the aspiration has produced pneumonia

A Atresia with distal fistula (70%)

Site of fistula

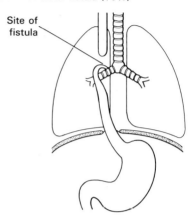

B Atresia without fistula (10%)

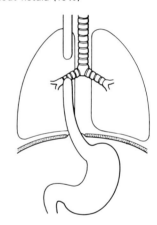

C 'H' or 'N' type (20%)

Site of fistula

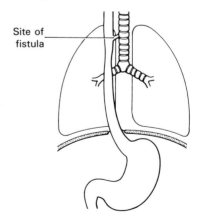

Fig. 7.6 Tracheo-oesophageal fistula and oesophageal atresia. (A) Atresia with distal fistula (70%). (B) Atresia without fistula (10%). (C) 'H' or 'N' type (20%).

(frequently with right upper lobe involvement) pre-operative treatment may be indicated. To prevent further aspiration and gastric reflux, the baby should be nursed head up, and this posture should be maintained throughout the physiotherapy treatment. Percussion, vibration and suction are the techniques generally needed, with constant monitoring of the baby's oxygen requirements.

Postoperative treatment will also be necessary, and again the head up posture may be required. The position of thoracotomy should be noted to avoid percussion or shakings directly over the wound. To avoid perforating the anastomosis with a suction catheter the level of the anastomosis should be recorded and a suitable mark at this length made on all the suction catheters. Length of insertion of the catheter via the nostril should be well within this mark, in case the catheter should enter the oesophagus by mistake.

TRACHEOSTOMY

In the last few years the introduction of plastic polymer endotracheal tubes has resulted in a reduction of the problems of tracheal irritation and stenosis associated with rubber endotracheal tubes, and so many children and adults have been able to be ventilated for much longer periods of time (in the region of 10 days to 2 weeks) without the need for an elective tracheostomy.

Elective tracheostomy

Elective tracheostomy for long-term intubation is still performed in children, particularly where there is a mechanical obstruction in the upper airway, such as congenital laryngeal web or atresia, tracheo-oesophageal anomalies and tracheal stenosis. It may also be necessary in acute epiglottitis, laryngotracheobronchitis or viral croup, where the obstruction is too advanced for naso- or orotracheal intubation. Tracheostomy is still necessary where retention or secretion is prolonged, such as may be found in the comatose patient or in neurological conditions where muscular weakness compromises respiratory function.

Types of tube

The type of tube used in children will depend on the personal preference of the surgeon. Initially a plastic tube is inserted and in the non-verbalising child may be used permanently. Silver speaking tubes have been available for a long time and have now been joined by fenestrated plastic tubes. Both of these tubes allow air to pass through the vocal cords on expiration, and hence facilitate sound production, and should be used in the child who can speak or where speech is beginning to develop. The child who has had a tracheostomy since the first year of life will almost invariably have very delayed speech and it is important that a 'speaking' tube is inserted at an early stage to encourage speech development.

Problems resulting from tracheostomy

All children with a tracheostomy need careful and regular assessment.

Tube blockage

Children with small calibre airways are at high risk of the tube blocking with sputum, and so great care must be taken to humidify the inspired gases adequately. This may be achieved in several ways, including the use of a heated water bath type of humidifier of the sort used in intensive care units for ventilatory humidification. Care must be taken to ensure that overheating of the airway does not occur and great attention must be paid to ensure sterility. The bath must be sterilised and changed regularly and sterile water or sterile normal saline must be used.

Small airway flooding

Small airway flooding is also a risk, particularly with ultrasonic humidification when smaller water droplets are produced, which penetrate further into smaller airways and may 'drown' the patient. Small condenser humidifiers are now available (Fig. 7.7). These clip on to the tube and contain a bacterial filter, which also serves

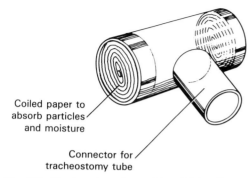

Coiled paper to absorb particles and moisture

Connector for tracheostomy tube

Fig. 7.7 Tracheostomy thermal humidifying filter.

to warm and moisten the inspired air, and so provides a more natural temperature and humidity in the trachea. However, not all children will tolerate this external attachment and will remove it as fast as it can be replaced!

Crusting

When crusting is a problem, instillation of sterile saline prior to suction is helpful and parents should be taught this technique for use at home. This method also has the advantage of facilitating catheter insertion, as the saline will act as a lubricant in the tracheostomy tube. The volume of saline instilled into the tube should be 0.20–0.5 ml and should be instilled during inspiration to ensure entry into the tube and large airway.

Suction equipment must be available and ready for immediate use as the child will frequently cough and loosen mucus as soon as the saline enters the airways. The saline should be kept at room temperature in unopened sterile vials and any saline not used should be discarded. Cool or cold saline kept in a refrigerator should not be used as it may induce bronchospasm.

During the first 72 hours post-tracheostomy a degree of bleeding must be expected and the parents and child should be reassured that this is normal. Explanation and reassurance about the procedures should also be given.

Pooling of secretions

Because of the presence of the tracheostomy tube

in the trachea the mucus-secreting cells are stimulated and produce vast quantities of mucus, which cannot be removed by the normal mechanism of the mucociliary escalator as ciliary function is inhibited by the presence of the tracheostomy tube. Consequently, these secretions tend to 'pool' in the large airways and can seriously impair air flow unless removed by suction. This over-production of mucus tends to settle down after a few days as the trachea becomes accustomed to its 'foreign invader'.

Impaired coughing

Normal coughing is impaired in these patients as they are unable to generate the large intrathoracic pressures necessary to produce a cough — normally, high intrathoracic pressures are generated against a closed glottis, which is then opened to allow an 'explosion' of air or cough.

Suction procedures

Unless the child is old enough to place a finger over the tube orifice and coordinate finger release correctly, the intrathoracic pressures will be insufficient to shear all the secretions adherent to the walls of the tube or bronchi. Because of this, regular suction of the tracheostomy tube is necessary, often in conjunction with chest drainage technique. The exact time interval between suctioning will be dictated by the rate of mucus production and will vary from child to child. The parents must be taught the suction procedure and, where indicated, physiotherapy techniques, and observed to perform them correctly on repeated occasions before discharge from hospital.

All the necessary equipment should be supplied either by the hospital or the community nursing agency and regular monitoring maintained. The child with a tracheostomy may well have feeding and swallowing difficulties because of the altered movement of the larynx during chewing and swallowing. This may result in aspiration of food around the tube and hence it is important that suction equipment is available during feeding. In the toddler, who is just starting on a mixed diet, and during the self-feeding stages, it is also advisable to ensure that the child wears a bib that will prevent food entering the tube from the mouth and chin area.

The parents should also be instructed in regular removal and thorough cleansing of the inner tube (if one is used) to prevent crusting. In most instances it is advisable for the parents to be taught to change the complete tube in case of accidental tube removal (decannulation) or tube blockage. This is normally taught by the medical or nursing staff. Routine tube changing is necessary about once a week.

RESPIRATORY PROBLEMS ASSOCIATED WITH CARDIAC ABNORMALITIES

The child with a cardiac condition will frequently present with a respiratory problem too. Generally speaking, these problems arise because of retained secretions, with or without super-imposed infection, and atelectasis. Impaired airflow caused by airway compression from engorged pulmonary vessels or increased airway fluid from pulmonary oedema are the usual causes. The main categories of conditions seen in association with these problems are:

Left to right shunts

Left to right shunts are most commonly produced by:

- atrial septal defect (ASD)
- ventricular septal defect (VSD)
- patent ductus arteriosus (PDA) (Fig. 7.8).

When the lesion is between the ventricles (VSD) or pulmonary artery and aorta (PDA) the high pressures from the left side of the heart are transmitted to the pulmonary circulation, causing vascular engorgement, which may in turn obstruct the airways. Particularly at risk are the left main bronchus, left upper lobe bronchus and right middle lobe bronchus. Until the defect has been surgically corrected there is little that can be done to lower the pulmonary vascular resistance, but continuous oxygen therapy may help by dilating the pulmonary vessels. However, the oxygen may sometimes increase pulmonary blood

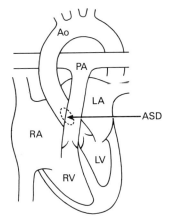

A   Atrial septal defect

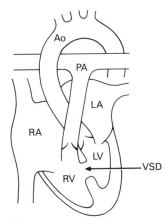

B   Ventricular septal defect

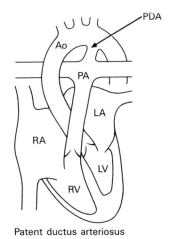

C   Patent ductus arteriosus

Fig. 7.8 Left-to-right shunts. (A) Atrial septal defect. (B) Ventricular septal defect. (C) Patent ductus arteriosus.

flow by improving cardiac contractability and so increasing the pulmonary vascular pressure. Oxygen use must, therefore, be closely monitored.

Left heart obstruction

When the left ventricular outflow is impeded, as with coarctation of the aorta or aortic stenosis (Fig. 7.9), there may be a rise in left atrial pressure if the mitral valve becomes incompetent, resulting in a rise in pulmonary venous and arterial pressure. An increase in left atrial pressure may re-open the foramen ovale between the atria, causing a left to right atrial shunt. This will

again increase the pulmonary blood flow, and yet little of the oxygenated blood will reach the systemic circulation. To increase the blood flow to the aorta, and hence systemic circulation, the infant may be treated with prostaglandins (PGE_1) to keep the ductus arteriosus open — this situation is described as being 'duct dependent'. Paradoxically, oxygen therapy may worsen the child's condition — the duct will tend to close as oxygen stimulates the sensitive cells in the duct, this being the mechanism by which the duct closes naturally during the first few hours or days of life as the infant's circulation adjusts to carrying oxygenated blood from its own pulmonary circulation. Corrective surgery will be necessary to decrease the obstruction to blood flow from the left side of the heart.

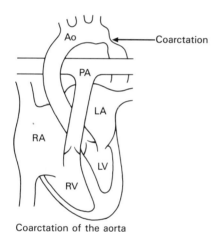

A   Coarctation of the aorta

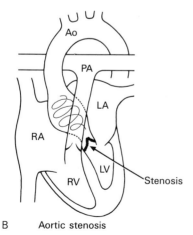

B   Aortic stenosis

Fig. 7.9 Left heart obstruction. (A) Coarctation of the aorta. (B) Aortic stenosis.

Hypoxaemic lesions

Systemic arterial oxygenation is inadequate for hypoxaemic lesions, which may be due to any of three abnormalities:

Transposition of the great vessels

The aorta arises from the right ventricle and the pulmonary artery from the left ventricle (Fig. 7.10A).

Truncus arteriosus, single ventricle or common atrium

These all result in systemic and pulmonary blood mixing within the heart (Fig. 7.10B).

Fallot's tetralogy

When there is obstruction to pulmonary blood flow and a shunt present between the right and left side of the heart proximal to the obstruction (Fig. 7.10C).

In these situations increasing the inspired oxygen levels (FiO_2) to 100% will increase the blood oxygen levels, but only by a small amount, as the pulmonary blood flow increases and worsens the intrapulmonary shunt.

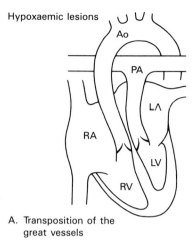

A. Transposition of the great vessels

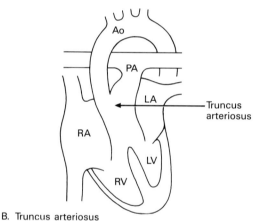

B. Truncus arteriosus

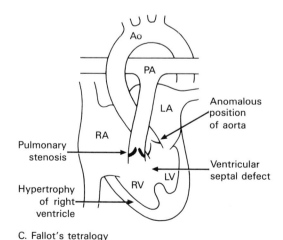

C. Fallot's tetralogy

Fig. 7.10 Hypoxaemic lesions. (A) Transposition of the great vessels. (B) Truncus arteriosus. (C) Fallot's tetralogy.

Vascular anomalies

Abnormalities of the intrathoracic blood vessels occasionally result in compression of the trachea and bronchi. This may be found with vascular rings, anomalous innominate and pulmonary arteries, pulmonary arteriovenous malformations and congenital obstruction to venous return. The symptoms may include stridor and respiratory distress, particularly when feeding, and may result in retention of airway secretions and atelectasis.

Physiotherapy treatment

The techniques employed to treat the problems of retained secretions (with or without infection) and atelectasis have been described previously (p. 108). However, in cardiac conditions the length of treatment and technique used may need to be modified. Optimal cardiac and respiratory function is frequently obtained in the 'head up' position, in which case treatments should be carried out in this position too. Discussion with nursing and medical staff on the indications and contraindications for additional oxygen therapy should take place before commencing treatment in case cyanosis is induced or worsened. The child's condition should be closely monitored throughout the treatment and afterwards for a short while to ensure that this does not worsen. Further details of assessment procedures and treatment principles are covered in Chapter 17 (Common Assessment Procedures) and Chapter 19 (Treatment Methods).

THORACIC SURGERY

Thoracic surgery in children is not uncommon and in the majority of cases is performed to correct cardiac anomalies. This may be by either a closed procedure or an open procedure requiring cardiopulmonary bypass. Thoracotomy may also be performed for lung surgery.

Closed cardiac surgery

This is performed for the following reasons:

1. To correct the constriction caused by a coarctation of the aorta using a dacron graft.

2. To ligate a persistent patent ductus arteriosus.

3. To perform pulmonary artery banding to increase the pulmonary artery pressure and so improve pulmonary blood flow as a temporary measure in ventricular septal defect until corrective surgery is carried out.

4. To improve aortic or pulmonary artery blood flow by diverting blood from the subclavian artery (the Blalock–Taussig shunt diverts blood from the left subclavian to the pulmonary artery and the Waterston shunt directs blood from the right subclavian to the ascending aorta).

The approach for closed surgery is normally via a left posterolateral incision through the fourth interspace.

Open cardiac surgery

Open cardiac surgery is necessary when a defect is present within the heart and direct vision is essential for the surgery. The heart and lungs are temporarily bypassed by a 'heart and lung machine', which oxygenates the blood and pumps it round the systemic circulation. The main indications for this type of surgery are Fallot's tetralogy, transposition of the great vessels, pulmonary atresia, pulmonary stenosis, aortic stenosis and ventricular or atrial defects. In the majority of cases the approach will be via a median sternotomy incision, although in some instances a right or left thoracotomy may be preferred.

Lung surgery

Thoracotomy for lung surgery is sometimes necessary in children. Thoracotomy may be performed for:

- lobectomy in localised bronchiectasis
- pleurectomy or pleuradesis in the child with repeated or persistent pneumothorax
- pleural decortication following empyema that has failed to resolve with more conservative management
- open lung biopsy for diagnostic purposes.

Pre-operative physiotherapy

The physiotherapist should be familiar with the surgical techniques employed by the surgeon in order to outline the procedure to the child and/or parents with an explanation of the physiotherapist's role.

A thorough assessment of the child should be made with particular attention to underlying chest or mobility problems (see Chapter 17 Common Assessment Procedures). Pre-operative chest clearance may be indicated and treatment planning should take into account any cardiac condition and be modified accordingly. In the older child a rehearsal of breathing exercises, huffing, supported coughing and arm, leg and trunk exercises is very important. Bubbles and incentive spirometry can help to ease the child's anxieties and give the parents a useful role to help them all through a difficult and worrying time. The pre-operative visits by the physiotherapist will also help establish a good relationship with the child and thereby increase cooperation in the recovery period.

Postoperative physiotherapy

In some units it is the policy to nurse children in the immediate postoperative period in the intensive therapy unit. Other units reserve this for the open-heart patients and for particularly poorly children. Wherever the child is nursed, the surgeon's preferred postoperative routine must be adhered to.

Assessment

The physiotherapy assessment should pay particular attention to the incision site, position of chest drains, blood pressure, breath sounds, chest X-ray and cardiac state. Wherever treatment is indicated, this is best timed after analgesia, unless a continuous infusion system is in use when, hopefully, pain will be at a minimum.

The infant and young child

The infant and young child often do not require any treatment: shoulder and trunk movements are often not inhibited and the main discomfort may be from the chest drains. However, should there be a problem with retained secretions positioning and suction alone (in the intubated child) will often be sufficient to clear any secretions. If this is not sufficient then gentle percussion and vibrations may be used with caution, particular care being taken to avoid the incision site. The head down position should also be avoided as this is generally contraindicated in the immediate postoperative period.

The older child

Older children may require more treatment as they will often restrict inspiration and suppress coughing for fear of experiencing pain. Much reassurance is required, and gentle persuasion to join in with the treatment. If postural drainage is indicated, modified positions will often be necessary to avoid the head down posture. Turning the child into side-lying may not always be possible, as side-lying on the thoracotomy side is frequently very painful. Adequate support of the thoracotomy or sternotomy is often not possible as the child is fearful of anyone touching the incision site. When able, the child should be encouraged to support his own wound. As in the infant, any percussion or vibratory techniques should be used with caution and modified as necessary.

Inspiratory and expiratory games

With such restriction on treatments, a lot of emphasis must be placed on inspiratory and expiratory games, such as blowing bubbles and tissues, and using the incentive spirometer or blow-bottle. Once the child is free of drips and drains and allowed to gently mobilise around the ward, rapid improvement is frequently noticed in the respiratory condition.

General exercise

Shoulder, thoracic and postural exercises are often necessary in the older child. Games may be the mainstay of treatment to encourage arm and shoulder movement, particularly post-thoracotomy. Encouragement to rest the arm on pillows in a progressively more abducted position for the shoulder may help the very reluctant child to move his arm away from his side.

Duration of hospitalisation

The duration of hospital stay will vary from child to child, depending on the surgery and speed of postoperative recovery. For the more simple procedures in the relatively well child, the stay in hospital may be as short as 4 or 5 days, with the child returning for suture removal at around the tenth day. Wherever possible, children return home as soon as deemed fit enough and with appropriate advice to parents where necessary to continue physiotherapy at home.

REFERENCES

Henry R L, Milner A D, Davies J G 1983 Simple drug delivery system for use by young asthmatics. British Medical Journal 286: 2021
Phelan P D 1982 Asthma in children. Medicine International 1(22): 999–1002
Pryor J A, Webber B A 1979 An evaluation of the forced expiration technique as an adjunct to postural drainage. Physiotherapy 65: 304
Webb M, Martin J, Cartlidge P, Ng Y, Wright N 1985 Chest physiotherapy in acute bronchiolitis. Archives of Diseases in Childhood 60: 1078–1079

FURTHER READING

Campbell T, Ferguson N, McKinley R G 1986 The use of a simple self-administered method of positive expiratory pressure in chest physiotherapy after abdominal surgery. Physiotherapy 72: 498–500
Davies H, Kitchman R, Gordon I, Helms P 1985 Regional ventilation in infancy. New England Journal of Medicine 313: 1626–1628
Gaskell D, Webber B 1987 The physical treatment of cystic fibrosis. Cystic Fibrosis Research Trust Publications, Bromley

Gregory G A (ed) 1982 Respiratory failure in the child. Management of respiratory failure of cardiac origin. Churchill Livingstone, London, ch 6

Heaf D, Helms P, Gordon I, Turner H 1983 Postural effects on gas exchange in infants. New England Journal of Medicine 308: 1505–1508

Kendall L 1987 A comparison between adult and paediatric intensive care. Physiotherapy 73: 495–499

Kipling R M, Grace A 1988 Tracheostomy. Hospital Update May: 1641–1649

Parker A 1987 Paediatric and neonatal intensive therapy. In: Cash's textbook of chest, heart and vascular disorders for physiotherapists, 4th edn. Faber & Faber, London, p 295

Young C S 1984a A review of the adverse effects of airways suction. Physiotherapy 70: 104–106

Young C S 1984b Recommended guidelines for suction. Physiotherapy 70: 106–108

Young C S 1988 Airway suctioning: a study of paediatric physiotherapy practice. Physiotherapy 74: 13–15

8

Disorders of the central nervous system

S. Bedford   I. McKinlay

INTRODUCTION

In this chapter the two major handicapping conditions of childhood are considered — cerebral palsy and spina bifida. Their causative factors, manifestations and the management and treatment approaches are described. The common factors influencing treatment in both disorders are then discussed. The chapter ends with an analysis of the nature of the associated condition of epilepsy.

CEREBRAL PALSY
S. Bedford

INTRODUCTION

Disorders of the central nervous system are the result of either abnormal development of the central nervous system or an insult to the brain or spinal cord. Cerebral palsy and spina bifida are examples that affect the sensory motor activities of the child.

The term 'cerebral palsy' covers a group of conditions in which affected children have a lack of neurological control of their movements. 'Cerebral palsy is a disorder of movement and posture due to a defect or lesion of the immature brain' (Bax 1964). An arbitrary age of onset before 3 years is usually assumed. The neurological lesion in cerebral palsy is not progressive, although variations and changes occur in the way in which the disorder manifests and develops in individual children. These changes are due to a number of factors, including maturation of the brain, body growth, muscle imbalance, and the child's movement and postural habits.

CAUSATION

In the past, single risk factors have been cited as possible causes of cerebral palsy. However it is now thought that a number of factors exist in the majority of cases.

These factors may be prenatal, perinatal or postnatal.

Prenatal factors

Familial predispositions

In a few cases there may be a direct inheritance of the condition, e.g. familial spastic diplegia and ataxic diplegia. More commonly there may be an inherited vulnerability to other risk factors (Stanley 1984).

Maternal influences

A number of diseases and disorders acquired by the mother may put the child at risk, e.g. rubella, cytomegalovirus, toxoplasmosis and toxaemia; the chronic maternal use of alcohol, or drugs may also be a factor. Complications of pregnancy may change the quantity or quality of blood supply to the developing brain, e.g. placental problems such as insufficiency, which may cause the fetus to be retarded in growth.

Cerebral malformations

These occasionally occur in the early months of gestation, when they are likely to cause extensive damage to brain function.

Prematurity

Prematurity is one of the most common risk factors, especially when associated with birth weights below 2500 g, or with babies who are small for gestational age. The latter is usually the result of intrauterine retardation of growth. The factors associated with the greatest risk of developing cerebral palsy are to be born too soon or too small (Hagberg & Hagberg 1984).

Perinatal factors

The perinatal period is described as the time between the onset of labour and the seventh day after birth.

Breech presentation

As breech presentations may have cord complications or birth trauma, and be associated with asphyxia, they must be considered as a factor.

Birth asphyxia

Asphyxia, especially when severe, has been associated with both term and preterm babies who later develop cerebral palsy.

Neonatal jaundice or kernicterus

This is not such a common factor as it used to be, as it can be more successfully prevented and treated. It is associated with choreo-athetosis.

Postnatal factors

Postnatal factors are those arising after the seventh day and up to 2–5 years of age, depending on the views of the clinician of the upper age limit for the designation of cerebral palsy. In less affluent populations, such as India, it may account for 25% of cases, but for just 6–11% in other countries. Infants, especially boys in the first year of life, are most at risk. A wide range of postnatal factors exist, accidents and infections of the central nervous system being the most common (Table 8.1).

ADDITIONAL COMPLICATIONS

Besides movement difficulties, children with cerebral palsy may have additional handicaps:

Table 8.1 Postoperative causative factors in cerebral palsy. Western Australia Study (Blair & Stanley 1982)

Factor	Percentage
Accidents Motor vehicle and other	22.5%

Infections
  Meningitis
  Encephalitis
  Influenza
  Measles
  Septicaemia
	62.9%

Cerebrovascular accidents Spontaneous or postoperative	4.5%

Anoxia
  Suffocation
  Post epileptic
  Near drowning
	7.9%

Malnutrition Aborigines	2.0%

Speech problems

Speech problems may be due to cerebral impairment, resulting, for example, in problems of verbal comprehension or expression. Or they may be due to difficulties of articulation, or lack of environmental stimulation.

Epilepsy

See p. 144

Visual problems

Squint or strabismus is fairly common in children with spasticity, while children with ataxia often show nystagmus — when the eye repeatedly moves quickly laterally, then more slowly returns to its normal central position. Some multiply handicapped children may also have lesions in their visual cortex, which cause varying degrees of perceptual blindness. Hemianopia and tunnel vision may occasionally occur.

Hearing problems

Children who have had damage in utero as a result of maternal rubella, which should now be fairly rare, often have hearing problems, such as a lack of acuity or deafness in specific frequencies.

Learning problems

Some children with cerebral palsy have generalised learning difficulties, which may vary in degree, but which are sometimes severe. Other children may have specific learning difficulties, such as perceptual problems.

Perceptual problems

Kinaesthetic memory is the ability to memorise movements using proprioceptive sense, and appears to depend on practice of movement. Children born with spasticity or athetosis have poorer kinaesthetic memory than normal children, but children with athetosis tend to have less difficulty than those with spasticity, possibly because they are able to move more, even though their movements may be involuntary.

CLASSIFICATION OF CEREBRAL PALSY

Cerebral palsy can be classified according to a combination of a number of factors:

- tonus variations
- distribution of tonus changes
- severity
- type.

Tonus variations

One of the main features in determining types of cerebral palsy is muscle or postural tone, where tone is defined as: 'the sustained contraction of living muscle subserving posture and movement' (Woods 1975). If a persistent increase in resistance to passive stretching is greater than occurs in normal muscle, then that muscle is said to be *hypertonic*. If the resistance to passive movement is lower than normal, then the muscle is *hypotonic*. If increased resistance lessens abruptly with a 'clasp knife' quality, it is termed *spasticity*. *Rigidity* or *plastic hypertonicity* is considered to be present if there is a sustained increase in resistance in all directions. This rigidity is said to be more like very severe spasticity with co-contraction than the rigidity associated with midbrain lesions, hence the term plastic hypertonicity (Bobath 1980). With *athetosis* tone may quickly change from hypotonia to normal, or even to hypertonia, giving an instability to posture, and to movements that are jerky and lack grading. The classification of dyskinesis is sometimes used to cover choreo-athetosis and dystonia. Postural tone tends to be persistently low in *ataxia*.

Hypotonia in the early months of life may eventually turn to hypertonia and spasticity as the brain matures; or to athetosis or ataxia. It may also indicate other conditions, e.g. muscular dystrophy, mental handicap or delayed development without any perceivable disorder, which may have a familial base.

One difficulty with using tone as a factor is that there is no scientific means of measurement, it is a subjective assessment (see Chapter 17 Common Assessment Procedures).

Distribution

In most cases the trunk and the neck are involved, as well as the limbs.

Hemiplegia

'Hemiplegia' is used when one side of the body is affected, including the trunk, and possibly the neck as well as limbs. The adductors of the legs are not usually particularly spastic. Generally, children with hemiplegia have spasticity, but occasionally they may have athetosis.

Diplegia

'Diplegia' is used when the legs are more affected than the arms. However, the severity of the extent to which the arms are affected may vary from mild to moderately severe. The terms tetraplegia or quadriplegia may be used by some people if the arms are more than mildly affected, and it may be necessary to establish a common understanding of terminology in any discussion. Spastic diplegia is the most common

form of diplegia, although some children have a degree of hypotonia. More rarely, ataxic diplegia occurs, when ataxia as well as spasticity is present.

Quadriplegia or tetraplegia

'Quadriplegia' and 'tetraplegia' are used when all the body is involved, and when the arms are as severely or more severely affected than the legs. 'Double Hemiplegia' is used by some clinicians, when the two sides of the body are unequally affected, with the arms as severe or worse than the legs. Other clinicians may use the term where the adductors of the legs do not show increased spasticity, as is common in ordinary hemiplegia (Woods 1975). Children with quadriplegia may show spasticity and/or athetosis.

Severity

It is possible to define severity as the person's ability or inability to perform tasks, irrespective of whether the affected parts are participating or not. In physiotherapy it is more usual to quantify severity according to how severely the affected parts are handicapped. For example, with spasticity the degree of hypertonicity that the child demonstrates may be graded as mild, moderate or severe.

Types of cerebral palsy

Young children with cerebral palsy experience varying degrees of delayed development in different parts of their body. The more affected parts will have most delay. Developmental delay can result from:

- the effect of pathology on the body, which makes movement difficult and lacking in variety
- some degree of mental handicap
- lack of opportunity and motivation to move as often as they might do.

The pathology of the various types of cerebral palsy affects each child differently, although tonic reflex activity often occurs in both spasticity and athetosis.

Spasticity

In the first 4 months of life most children who later develop spasticity have normal tone, although they may occasionally have hypotonicity. Gradually they acquire increased tone as they develop (Bobath & Bobath 1975). However, severely handicapped children with spastic quadriplegia may show hypertonicity by the age of 4 months.

Children with moderate spasticity may have difficulty moving their affected parts, other than in limited spastic patterns. Total patterns of flexion and extension may be present and the child will lack the ability to move one part of a limb, say, the foot, without moving the rest of the limb in a similar way. Their memory of movement, and hence their movement habits, tend to be limited to these abnormal movement patterns, and to abnormal compensatory patterns, unless they can learn otherwise. They lack variety in their movements.

When severe spasticity is present, agonist and antagonist groups of muscles are both severely affected, co-contraction is present and active movement may be impossible or very limited.

Athetosis

The word athetosis means 'without fixed position'. Children with athetosis have difficulty in maintaining a posture, they show involuntary movements and they have difficulty in grading movement. For example, they may move from standing to sitting very quickly, and are unable to stop at any stage of the movement. They may be unable to separate eye from head movement, and often do not look at what they are trying to reach and grasp. They may learn to use an asymmetric tonic neck reflex (ATNR) before the age of 12 months, in order to try to reach for objects. They may later use the reflex for activities such as walking. This will lead to stereotyped patterns of movement without the capacity for modification and variety. Generally their arms are more affected than their legs.

Children with athetosis may have involvement of the muscles of their face, which may make them grimace, and in infancy they often have early sucking and feeding problems. Speech problems will often be present. In infancy children with athetosis tend to be 'floppy' and have a delay in acquiring head and trunk control; the athetosis may not manifest until after they are 1 year old.

Ataxia

Ataxia is the least common of the cerebral palsies, with unsteadiness of movement, imperfect balance, walking with a wide base and, at times, intention tremor. The term truncal ataxia is sometimes used when the trunk lacks stability.

The types of cerebral palsy are summarised in Table 8.2. As well as the classic types of cerebral palsy described in Table 8.2 there have recently been a number of young children with cerebral palsy who do not fit into any category. Many of these children are premature babies of very low birth weight with less than 30 weeks' gestation. Some have mixed abnormal tone, including a dystonic element, but they are neither classically quadriplegic nor dystonic athetoids; other children have low tone proximally and high tone distally, often with dystonia on effort. In this instance dystonia refers to extreme changes in tone through a very wide range (Bryce 1990).

MANIFESTATIONS OF CEREBRAL PALSY

Cerebral palsy may manifest in a number of ways.

1. Poorly developed postural reflex mechanism, often with delay in acquiring head control, balance, righting reactions and a lack of trunk rotation.

2. Abnormal tone, postures and movements, which limit the child's ability to perform movements normally and with variety.

3. Neonatal reflexes may be retained for a prolonged period, for example, reflex standing and walking.

4. Difficulties in varying total movement patterns, and in isolating movement to individual body parts.

Table 8.2 Types of cerebral palsy

Type and Distribution	Tone	Movement
Spasticity Hemiplegia Diplegia Quadriplegia	Tone in early months, normal or low. Hypertonicity in some who are later severely affected. Older children, normal or hypertonic at rest, depending on severity. Tone increased by: quick stretching, excessive effort or anxiety, associated reactions, movement in patterns of spasticity, tonic reflex activity. Severe cases show co-contraction.	Lack of selectivity. Inability to isolate movement to one part of the body. Poor variety of movements. Movement tends to be in total patterns of flexion and extension and abnormal compensatory patterns. Some use neonatal patterns of movement, e.g. reflex walking. Poor balance reactions. In severe cases movement is nil, or limited to mid-range.
Athetosis Quadriplegia Face may be involved Hemiplegia occasionally occurs	Infants floppy with poor head and trunk control. Older children at rest, tone hypotonic or normal. Choreo-athetosis. Large involuntary movements of limbs, with low tone and instability of shoulder and hip girdles. Athetosis with tonic spasms or dystonic athetosis. Tone shows large changes from hypotonic to hypertonic. Tonic reflex activity occurs. Athetosis with spasticity. Spasticity usually in legs, with generalised athetosis. Tone and abnormal movements increased by: anticipation of movement or speech, too much effort, excessive stimulation, anxiety, insecurity of position, tonic reflex activity.	Feeding and speech problems. Difficulty maintaining a posture. Lack of co-contraction and postural stability. Involuntary movements. Unstable sitting. Movement in extremes of range. Lack of mid-range control, with inability to stop at any stage of the movement (Grading). May not look at what they are reaching to grasp. Intermittent spasms.
Ataxia Quadriplegia	Tone usually hypotonic. Ataxia may be associated with athetosis or spasticity. Truncial ataxia: term used if trunk unstable.	Unsteadiness of movement. Imperfect balance, wide walking base. May have intension tremor, dysmetria and nystagmus.

Table mainly based on information from The Bobath Centre

Abnormal postural tone

Hypertonicity occurs because there is an increased sensitivity of the muscle spindles, which respond excessively to stimulation. The extent of this over-reaction may be less obvious when the body is at rest, and the state of arousal and degree of anxiety is low as, for example, when a young child is being nursed by its mother. Experiences that heighten arousal and/or anxiety are likely to increase the strength of the spasticity, but this will vary in different children. Unexpected loud noises or excitedness, or anxiety arising from feeling and being insecure are likely to increase tone.

Anticipation of speaking, or moving, may, for children with athetosis, increase tone. Similarly, the way therapists and carers approach children, their tone of voice and their attitudes can affect the child's reaction and tone. Infants may not react favourably to loud laughter and understanding how individual children react to people is helpful during therapy.

Hypertonicity is also increased by undue effort being put into an action. Associated reactions were first described by Walshe (1923), and later by Bobath (1966) and are particularly marked in children with hemiplegia. When running, or strongly moving the sound arm, the affected arm becomes stiffer (Fig. 8.1). When children with diplegia or quadriplegia raise their heads when lying prone, their extended legs may stiffen. This is less likely to occur if their legs are previously placed in an abducted, outwardly rotated position.

Stiffness may also increase in an affected limb because that limb is being used with too much effort. However this is not covered by the definition of associated reaction.

For each child there is an optimum level of effort required to perform any movement effectively. Getting the degree of effort correct, and positioning the limbs away from spastic patterns, can help to prevent spasticity from increasing.

Basic patterns of spasticity

Although the distribution of tone is not constant, generalisations, which may be called basic patterns of spasticity, are documented.

Arms

Spasticity is usually strongest in the flexors of the arm, with retraction and depression of the shoulder girdle, adduction and inward rotation of the shoulder, flexion of the elbow, wrist and fingers, adduction of the thumb and pronation of the forearm — a total flexor pattern of the arm (Fig. 8.2). Occasionally, some children may demonstrate protraction of the shoulder girdle, marked inward rotation of the shoulders, extended elbows and pronation of the forearm.

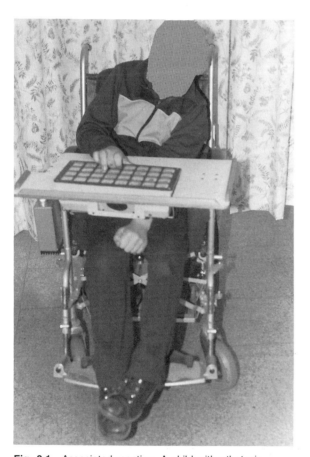

Fig. 8.1 Associated reaction. A child with athetosis using a communication board. Note the associated reaction in the left hand and leg.

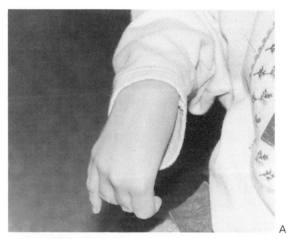
A

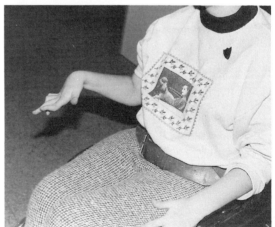
B

Fig. 8.2 Patterns of spasticity in the hand. (A) Spasticity with flexed wrist and fingers with thumb in palm. (B) Athetosis with flexed wrist and elbow during attempt to extend fingers.

Legs

The extensors of the legs are usually most affected. The hamstrings, as hip extensors, are affected, which may in turn limit knee extension. Inward rotators and adductors of the hips, knee extensors, plantor flexors of the feet and flexors of the toes are also affected — a total extensor pattern (Fig. 8.3).

The state of tone in the trunk influences tone in the extremities. For example, if the side flexors of the trunk are shortened, the arm flexors will show increased tone.

Modification of the basic patterns of spasticity

A number of factors can alter the basic patterns of spasticity:

- tonic reflex activity
- habitual postures and movements
- gravity
- the result of orthopaedic procedures.

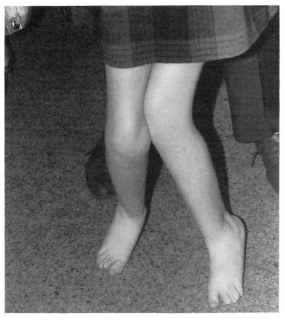

Fig. 8.3 Patterns of spasticity in the legs. Note the adducted hips with inward rotation, plantar flexed left ankle, limited knee extension and pronated feet.

Tonic reflex activity

The tonic reflexes described in the chapter on child development (see Chapter 4 The Developing Child), are often not integrated into higher activities and therefore affect the tone and posture of those children with cerebral palsy. Multiple factors affect the child simultaneously, and it may not be possible to isolate particular reflexes and determine which is responsible for a child's tonus state.

The tonic labyrinthine reflex. This reflex is stimulated by gravity acting on the position of the head, in relation to the horizontal plane. When some children with quadriplegia are lying prone, with head resting on the surface, the stimulation of the labyrinths may cause total flexion, yet the same children in supine-lying might be in total extension (Fig. 8.4).

Tonic neck reflexes. These occur in response to the position of the child's head relative to the trunk.

The asymmetrical tonic neck reflex (ATNR). This is more frequently seen on one side of the body than the other, in any one child. When the head is turned to one side, there is increased tone in the extensors of the arm to which the child looks, and an increase in the flexors of the other arm (Fig. 8.5). This may be visible, or only apparent

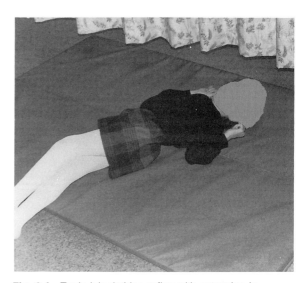

Fig. 8.4 Tonic labyrinthine reflex with extension in supine. Note retraction of shoulders.

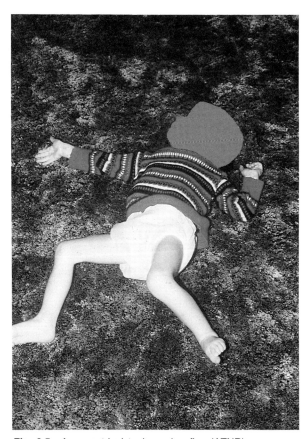

Fig. 8.5 Asymmetrical tonic neck reflex (ATNR).

by handling, when the limbs are passively flexed and extended. It is usually most easily demonstrated when the child's head and trunk are extended. Children with quadriplegia who persistently look to one side only, often accompanied with an ATNR, may develop gross asymmetry of the trunk and windswept legs. As the child looks to one side, the neck and trunk on the occiput side are usually side-flexed, which can lead to a scoliosis. The pelvis on the flexed side is often rotated forward, in both supine-lying and in sitting. The leg on that side (usually the left) inwardly rotates and adducts and, if persistently practised, may lead to a sublocation or dislocation of the hip. The other hip is usually outwardly rotated. This condition is most marked in supine-lying and it is advantageous to find alternative positions. Forward rotation of the pelvis should be corrected, and persistent one-sided head turning discouraged in all positions.

Symmetrical tonic neck reflexes. The effects of this reflex may be apparent in some children with severe quadriplegia. When placed on all fours with head extended, the arms straighten but the legs are very flexed; but with a flexed head the arms collapse. The legs are less flexed than before, but probably not extended, as they may also be under the influence of tonic labyrinthine reflexes in this position. Sitting badly towards the front of a chair with head flexed, severe cases show a flexed trunk, flexed arms with clenched hands with thumbs either inside the palms or adducted. Attempts to open the hands are likely to meet increased resistance. The legs are extended and adducted with plantar flexed feet and flexed toes.

Habitual postures and movements

If children with spasticity persistently use one position or one form of movement for a long period of time, an imbalance of tone can develop leading to deformity.

Normal infants crawl for a few seconds only, followed by possibly pulling up to standing. Children with spastic diplegia and some of the more able quadriplegics, may persistently use flexor patterns of movement such as crawling or 'bunny hopping' for long periods (Fig. 8.6); they may also sit for extended periods. This may easily result in permanently flexed legs, and the child will lack sufficient extension to stand with straight legs. Similarly, the persistent use of asymmetrical postures and movements can lead to deformity. When left to their own devices, infants with hemiplegia, usually bottom-shuffle very asymmetrically using their able side (Fig. 8.7). Crawling instead of bottom-shuffling in children with hemiplegia can lead to better use of arm and leg.

Gravity

Gravity provokes tonic labyrinthine reflexes, as explained above. It can also affect postures and the tone sustaining those postures. If weight is put on the front of a neonate's foot, the leg extends in a rigid column using the positive supporting reaction. Pressure on the pads of the

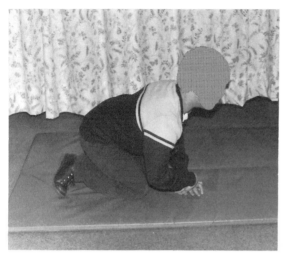

Fig. 8.6 Child with spastic quadriplegia crawling/bunny hopping.

foot created by gravity, stimulate this response. This reflex standing may not be integrated in children with cerebral palsy, and is encouraged when children are allowed to stand on plantar flexed feet, thus making the legs stiffer.

Result of orthopaedic procedures

Operations and plastering procedures can in-

fluence the distribution of tone (see Chapter 12 Orthopaedic Aspects of Childhood Disorders and Chapter 19 Treatment Methods). For example, a child with spastic diplegia may stand with plantar flexed feet. Following either tendo Achilles lengthening or plastering to correct plantar flexion, it may be found that the extensor tone has decreased, so that the child now stands and walks with bent knees (Fig. 8.8).

FACTORS INFLUENCING TREATMENT

Movement problems

A number of movement problems can be considered when planning treatment:

1. Spasticity in antagonists limits the ability of agonists to move.
2. The use of spastic patterns to move will limit the variety of movements that children can accomplish.
3. There is a tendency to move in total patterns of flexion and extension.
4. There is difficulty isolating movement to one part of the body. It may not be possible to move the eyes without moving the head,

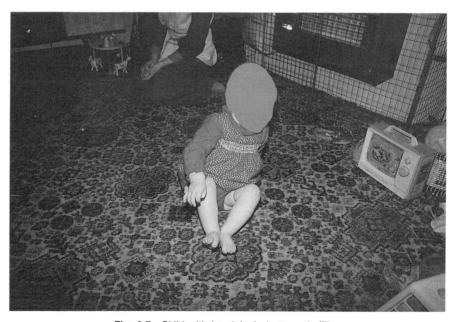

Fig. 8.7 Child with hemiplegia bottom-shuffling.

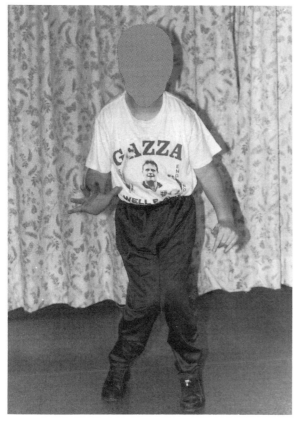

Fig. 8.8 Decreased extensor tone in standing following tendon Achilles lengthening.

the head without moving the body or the limbs without moving the body or the head.

5. Movement of one part of the body influences movement in other parts of the body.

6. Children compensate with their more able limbs, at the expense of developing their affected parts.

7. Children with athetosis can move, but their movements lack control and grading. They also lack a stable base; maintaining a posture or position is difficult. They need stability of head position, shoulder girdle, trunk and hips.

Control of jaw, lips and tongue

Feeding

Feeding and speech are closely related, as both require coordination of tongue, lips and jaw. It is therefore particularly important to establish correct early feeding. If possible, infants should be observed feeding; enquiry may not be enough, as mothers may not appreciate that anything is wrong. Young babies with cerebral palsy, and in particular athetoid babies, may have difficulty suckling. Older infants may continue to use early reflexive suckling and have difficulty taking food from a spoon or mug. They have not learned how to volitionally use their jaw, lips and tongue satisfactorily (see Chapter 20 Living Skills and the Environment). Total extensor patterns may include an open mouth; flexor patterns may include a closed mouth.

Speech problems

Articulatory difficulties can arise with children who are not using their lips, tongue and jaw correctly in a coordinated way. They may be more able to use their oral structures in some body positions rather than in others. Physiotherapists will need to work with speech therapists on this.

Drooling

Drooling is present in about 12% of children with cerebral palsy. This is a distressing condition that is not socially acceptable; the child may be persistently wet, and have unpleasantly smelling clothing. Treatment may be surgery, behaviour modification or oral motor training. Children with cerebral palsy differ from normal children in their frequency of subconscious swallowing; they may also have inefficient and uncoordinated swallowing and poor synchrony of lip closure (Harris & Purdy 1987). There is no evidence that they have an increased flow of saliva.

Feeding, speech and drooling problems all have similar basic causative factors, and may all be present in the same child.

Using the eyes

Some babies who are multiply handicapped may have damage to their visual cortex and be unable to appreciate the sensations their eyes transmit to their brains. These children have some degree of *cortical blindness*, and although they may later develop some vision, in the early days they have no eye contact with their mothers. They also lack experience in learning to recognise the subtle cues used in body language, including facial expression. Development of communication skills may also suffer if the child cannot fixate and follow objects, including the mother's face. This can occur because of poor head control, or when children have difficulty tracking with their eyes.

Many children with cerebral palsy have strabismus, or squint, which may hamper their perceptual development. Children with athetosis have difficulty in verbal communication and may use eye pointing as a means of communication. However, they often have difficulty moving their eyes separately from their heads (Fig. 8.9). These children may use ATNRs when reaching, and will therefore probably not be able to look at objects when they pick them up.

Poor head control

Poor head control may vary in degree, from not being able to hold the head in alignment with the trunk, to not being able to move it independently of the trunk. Severely handicapped children with unstable heads may stimulate a Moro reflex if their heads fall backwards.

It is difficult to seat a child with poor head control successfully, so that he can see well, and the temptation may be to tilt the seat backwards. However, in this position little that is useful can be seen and the child will not be able to visually explore his environment (Fig. 8.10). Sitting in a tilted back chair has also been shown to increase tone. Good head control is essential as a foundation for the development of most motor skills. Children with poor head control often have poor postural tone and tend not to like prone lying, yet it is in this position that the child may develop more extensor tone and stability. Prone standers can be useful in these cases.

Reduced shoulder girdle stability and arm control

Poor shoulder girdle stability and arms with insufficient tone are not able to support the body or protect it from falling. This can result from low postural tone, from a lack of co-contraction in the shoulder girdle and from inadequate arm extension, when flexor spasticity dominates. Where symmetrical tonic reflex activity influences motor behaviour, e.g. in a crawling position with head extended, the arms may be straight, but if the head is flexed the arms will bend. Generally, there is difficulty outwardly rotating, abducting and elevating arms, extending elbows and supinating forearms.

Stable shoulders and good arm function are necessary for such skills as dressing, transferring from one position to another, toileting, as well as mobility (using walking aids and wheelchairs), getting into and out of vehicles and for leisure

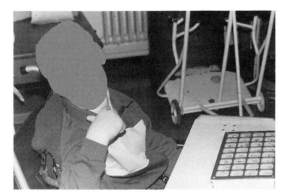

Fig. 8.9 Child with athetosis and poor speech. Note difficulty in looking towards, and reaching for communication board.

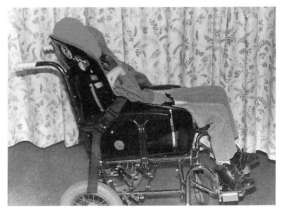

Fig. 8.10 Child with spasticity and poor head control in chair with insert to tilt backwards. Note poor field of vision which results.

activities such as swimming. Shoulder girdle stability also influences fine motor skills. This is particularly important for children with choreo-athetosis, and if their shoulder girdles are stabilised they are likely to use their hands more effectively (Shepherd 1980).

Difficulties with hand use and fine motor control

Many children with cerebral palsy have poor hand function. Their wrists tend to be flexed with ulnar deviation, fingers flexed with the thumb either adducted or inside the palm. It may only be possible to open the fingers by using a flexed wrist (Fig. 8.11). The less disabled child, with comparatively good hand use, may be clumsy with poor eye–hand coordination and perceptual problems resulting in poor manipulatory skills.

When babies with cerebral palsy are unable to use their hands, they cannot play with their own bodies — take their fingers to their mouths or put their hands together — and fail to learn about their bodies. They also lack opportunity to learn eye–hand coordination.

Children with spasticity use their hands very little, and therefore they have poor kinaesthetic memories of movement. The movements that do take place use mainly flexor patterns. As flexion is associated with pressing down on the supporting surface this is not helpful in the performance of manipulatory skills such as writing.

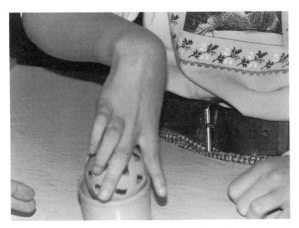

Fig. 8.11 Opening the fingers using a flexed wrist.

Athetoid children may find it difficult to bend their extended arms and to open their fingers to grip an object.

Poor trunk stability and lack of trunk rotation

Most children who have poor trunk stability also lack head control and will have the problems mentioned under that heading (see p. 126).

Balance is difficult without trunk stability. For example, unsupported sitting on the floor may require support from one or two hands for a prolonged period, thus preventing the use of the hand for manipulatory skills. This may affect choice of handedness. With poor trunk stability it is likely that the child will sit with a rounded back, and may develop a kyphosis.

Children with poor trunk control who sit asymmetrically on a chair, especially with a round back, are at risk from developing a scoliosis.

Children with spasticity commonly lack trunk rotation, leading to difficulty in rolling and in sitting up from the floor. It may also restrict balancing that utilises trunk rotation.

Stable sitting and standing

Sitting

Sitting requires the ability to keep the back extended with flexed hips. Some children find this difficult and may need practical help to keep their buttocks at the rear of the seat. In particular, children who show symmetrical tonic neck reflexes find this difficult.

Athetoid children also find sitting difficult, as they lack stability and balance in sitting and their legs may shoot out unexpectedly, hitting trays or tables. Ideally, they should learn to control these involuntary movements themselves, but sometimes fixation is given, to allow them to learn other tasks.

Children who find sitting balance difficult may need to use two different chairs until they can balance fairly automatically. One is used for learning to balance, the other provides more support and is used whilst the child is to perform other skills, such as self-feeding, writing, or even speech without having to think about balance.

Standing

To stand, a child needs adequate extensor tone to hold them up against gravity and the ability to maintain that tone with plantigrade feet. Children with diplegia and spastic quadriplegia find this difficult, and tend to use a total extensor pattern, with plantar flexed feet. Even when a good position is possible, balance has to be learned and this, except for children with hemiplegia, is difficult. Most are unable to protect themselves if they fall backwards, either with protective stepping or arm extension backwards. They also have a narrow standing base. Moderately and severely handicapped children with spastic quadriplegia are unlikely to stand without support, and may need a prone stander (Fig. 8.12), standing frame or support for their legs, such as leggings or ankle foot orthoses.

Walking and mobility skills

Even when standing and balance have been learned, in order to walk and move one leg separately from the other children must be able to:

1. transfer weight laterally when standing from one leg to the other. This requires forward rotation of the pelvis and extension of the hip and knee on the weight-bearing side;

2. flex the moving leg while keeping the supporting leg extended;

3. take the moving leg forward, without allowing the pelvis to come forward on that side, and at the same time leave the supporting leg behind.

Children with diplegia may find all these movements difficult. They may compensate for their difficulties by using their trunks, either by bending sideways to alternate sides or by bending their trunks backwards, then flexing them forwards.

When using a walking aid, the child may swing the pelvis and side forward together with the leg, which therefore crosses over in front of the supporting leg. The legs may be bent, partly because of difficulty sustaining sufficient extensor tone but also because of a fear of falling backwards.

Children with hemiplegia may not bear weight equally on both legs and they may walk with their affected leg plantar flexed at the ankle, or flex their hips and hyperextend their knees to try to get their heels down. They often walk with unequal length strides. Children with athetosis, who have sufficient stability in standing and who learn to control their own spasms and remain free from deformities may learn to walk at a much later age than is usual for children with other forms of cerebral palsy.

To walk independently for appreciable distances children with cerebral palsy need to:

- balance, and keep their weight within their supporting base
- walk without their spasticity increasing with the effort of walking
- be able to save themselves from falling with protective stepping (Wilson 1988).

Children unable to walk independently need appropriate aids. Some that are held in front of the body, e.g. walking sticks, tripods, elbow crutches and rollaters, encourage the child to use flexor patterns of the arms, body and legs, and need to be used with care (Fig. 8.13A and B). Others, which are pushed with straight arms, e.g.

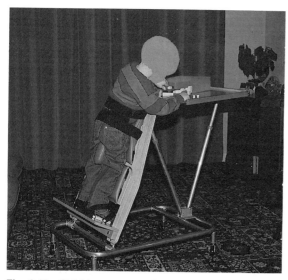

Fig. 8.12 Child in prone stander.

a ladder-back chair, are less likely to encourage the child to use a flexed posture. An alternative is the recently introduced postural control walker which, with the handgrips at the side and either two or four wheels, keeps the trunk more upright (Fig. 8.13C and D). Children need to be discouraged from walking too quickly in a bad walking pattern with an aid, as habits are difficult to change.

Movement sequences

Sequential movements require the child to remember a sequence of things in a set order,

and can cause problems for some children, especially if they have poor short-term memories or if they are unable to 'rehearse' by quickly repeating to themselves what they have to do before they forget.

Long-term treatment aims

The long-term treatment aims in cerebral palsy are to develop a variety of normal or near normal movements and simple skills appropriate to the child's stage of development, condition and potential, that will form the foundation for more difficult functional skills (Table 8.3).

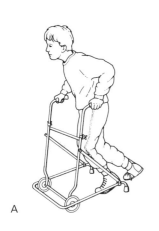
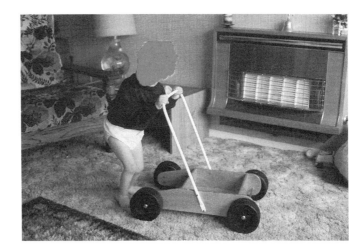
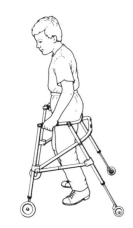
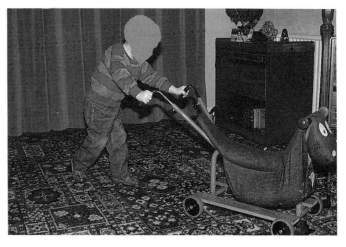

Fig. 8.13 Use of walking aids. (A) and (B) Note the flexor pattern of arms, body and legs. (C) and (D) Note the improved extension with straight arms and extended legs.

Table 8.3. Treatment aims with cerebral palsy

General aims
Prevent and treat deformities
Normalise tone
Encourage symmetry and two-handed activities
Facilitate and encourage near normal and normal movements and functional skills
Initially limit compensation by using the less affected parts
Try to improve the more affected parts

Treatment aims for children with spasticity	Treatment aims for children with athetosis
Decrease spasticity	Increase stability of head, shoulder girdle, trunk, and hips
Discourage abnormal movement and postures	
Encourage dissociation of total patterns	Encourage the holding of positions with a minimum amount of involuntary movement
Use optimal levels of effort	
Avoid positions that may stimulate tonic reflex activity, including persistent head turning to one side	Develop grading of movement
Use inhibitory techniques	

SPINA BIFIDA
S. Bedford

INTRODUCTION

The term 'spina bifida' is used for congenital malformations of the spinal vertebrae when the two halves of some spinous processes do not fuse together. In the most severe form there is involvement of the spinal cord and its coverings.

Three main types of spina bifida can be described:

• spina bifida occulta
• spina bifida cystica meningocele
• spina bifida cystica myelomeningocele.

Together with two associated congenital abnormalities of the cranium:

• cranium bifida
• anencephaly.

Spina bifida occulta

Outwardly there may be no evidence of the underlying defect except, in some instances, a hairy patch or unusual dimple or thickening on the lower back. Although there is no defect in the spinal cord, neurological signs may sometimes occur in the legs as the child grows. Radiography may detect a defect in some vertebrae.

Spina bifida cystica

There are two types of spina bifida cystica:
   Meningocele. An external cystic swelling containing cerebrospinal fluid and meninges protrudes through the malformed vertebrae. The spinal cord is intact and there is usually no sensory or motor defect. They most commonly occur in the cervical region.
   Myelomeningocele. This serious form of spina bifida cystica is unfortunately the most common. It is considered in detail on page 131.

Cranium bifida

A malformation of the occiput is present, with outward protrusion of either the meninges (meningocele) or part of the brain (encephalocele). When the protrusion is small and contains only the meninges, the prognosis is usually good, but when it is large and contains brain tissue it is less good. The child may develop spasticity and his vision and intelligence may be affected (Lorber 1968).

Anencephaly

Anencephaly is a neural tube defect associated with spina bifida in which the skull and brain are severely malformed. Babies with this defect may be stillborn or survive only for a very short time.

SPINA BIFIDA CYSTICA
Myelomeningocele

In this form of spina bifida a part of the spinal column is severely malformed and the spinal cord and nerve roots are also involved and protrude, together with the meninges, in a cystic swelling on the surface of the back (Fig. 8.14). This is

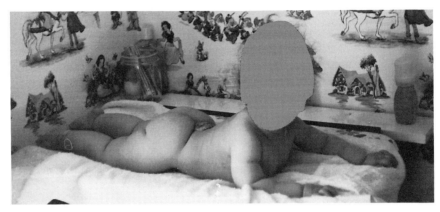

Fig. 8.14 Child with myelomeningocele

usually covered by a thin delicate membrane, or occasionally skin. Infection to the central nervous system is a serious problem, particularly if there is an open wound or when the covering membrane is very fragile. Myelomeningoceles can occur on any region of the spine, but are most common in the lumbosacral and thoracolumbar regions.

Incidence

The incidence of spina bifida cystica varies between countries, but it has been fairly common in Britain and in 1966 the incidence was about 2 to 3 per 1000 births, with regional variations. It is now probably much lower, in part because of improved antenatal screening but also as a result of improved diet or dietary supplements such as Pregnavit, which have been recommended by some authorities for women thought to be at risk and are taken before conception. Although it is thought that there has been some selection of cases for 'back repair' operations in a few hospitals since the early 1960s (Anderson & Spain 1977), since the 1970s this selection of cases has probably been more widespread. Therefore, many of the children who now survive are less handicapped than previously, although some children are still severely handicapped.

Manifestations of spina bifida

Children with a myelomeningocele are likely to experience some of the following problems,

depending on the severity of the lesion and the region of the spine affected:

- some degree of flaccid paralysis with sensory loss
- incontinence of bladder and bowel
- about 80% will also develop hydrocephalus
- learning difficulties, general and specific, which may particularly be associated with hydrocephalus
- many have a low average intelligence, clumsy hand function and visuoperceptual problems
- some have additional congenital abnormalities to their urinary, alimentary and skeletal systems, e.g. club feet, cleft palate
- children with spina bifida may also be born with deformities of the legs and feet, which may be due to muscle imbalance or be the result of intrauterine pressure on flaccid legs.

The distribution and severity of paralysis

The severity and distribution of the paralysis will depend on the spinal level of the lesion and the severity of the damage to the spinal cord.

Spinal level of lesion

Myelomeningoceles can occur at any level but

are most common in the lumbosacral region, in most cases some degree of flaccid paralysis is likely to result (Table 8.4). Occasionally, parts of the spinal cord below the lesion have some spinal reflexes intact, usually without cortical control. This results in some muscle groups being spastic, whilst others remain flaccid.

Severity of lesion

The damage caused by a myelomeningocele will be much greater than that caused by a meningocele, but even with the former lesion the damage to the cord can vary. In some instances the damage may be slight, but in severe cases the cord is completely destroyed below the level of the lesion. In other cases it may affect the two sides of the body unequally, and in extreme cases one leg may be affected and the other not.

The motor handicap and its consequences

The effect of the lesion on motor activity will not only determine the possibilities the child has for movement but will also affect circulation and the

Table 8.4 Distribution of paralysis in spina bifida

Level of lesion	Extent of paralysis or paresis
Cervical	Uncommon, usually partial. Arms and finger movements may be impaired. Sometimes spasticity in all limbs.
Thoracic and lumbar Above L4	Flaccid paralysis usually involving all leg muscles.
Lumbar Between L4 and S1	Some function in hip flexors, adductors, knee extensors. If lesion severe, paralysis of all other leg muscles, including hip extensors, knee flexors, producing a flexion deformity of the hips.
Sacral Between S1 and S3	Good function in hip flexors, adductors, knee extensors, and dorsiflexors of feet. Hip extensors, knee flexors may be weak. Plantar flexors of feet probably paralysed.
Sacral Below S3	Paralysis unlikely. Incontinence a probability.

strength of the leg bones and will determine the type of deformities that may arise through muscle imbalance.

Movement

Thoracic lesions above L3, if complete, will lead to a total paralysis of the legs and the child will also have weak trunk muscles, making independent sitting very difficult. The lower the lesion the better the trunk activity is likely to be and the less the paresis of the legs.

Circulation

Because of paucity of movement and lack of vasomotor control, circulation is very poor with blue, cold limbs and a tendency to chilblains. In extreme cases, because of the lack of awareness of the sensation of cold, frostbite may occur. Lesions such as pressure sores, ulcers and abrasions usually take a long time to heal.

Fractures

Bones of the legs are liable to fracture extremely easily, particularly following long periods of immobilisation after orthopaedic operations. The child and his carers may be completely unaware of the fracture.

Deformities

Unless there is a total flaccid paralysis or the disability is very slight, deformities all too easily occur because of muscle imbalance. With lesions between L4 and S1, hip flexion and hip adduction, together with extension of the knees, develops as a dominant position of the legs which may lead to permanent deformities. Muscle spasticity may also lead to imbalance and deformity. Deformities such as scoliosis may develop as a result of the persistent use of asymmetrical postures and positions that encourage constant shortening of some structures. Gravity also plays its part (see Chapter 12 Orthopaedic Aspects of Childhood Disorders).

Sensory effects of the handicap

The child is likely to have both a sensory and a

proprioceptive deficit in those parts of the body normally supplied by the damaged cord.

Sensations

Children will lack sensations of touch, pressure, temperature and pain, and will be unaware when they suffer trauma. They may not know to move from a hot water bottle, kettle, or radiator that is burning them, and will not feel uncomfortable from continual pressure. The latter is particularly likely to occur where bony prominences are only covered by skin, and where they take weight (Fig. 8.15). Deformed, insensitive feet need a lot of care when they take weight and great care has to be taken with new calipers, ankle foot orthoses (AFOS), boots and other appliances.

Proprioception

Children also lack proprioceptive feedback from muscles and joints in areas supplied by the damaged cord. Because of lack of tactile kinaesthetic feedback, they will rely on visual input only to develop a sense of body awareness of their affected parts.

The lack of information from the affected parts may make righting the body difficult; for example, in sitting up straight.

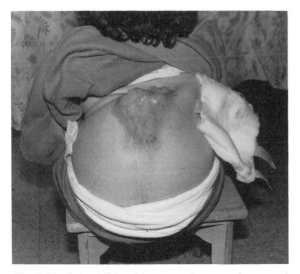

Fig. 8.15 Spina bifida — bony prominence only covered by skin. Note severe scoliosis.

Bladder and bowel control

The majority of children with a myelomeningocele have incontinence of the bladder, and often of the bowel as well. The bladder has two sources of neurological control:

1. A nerve supply from the sacral part of the spinal cord, which induces contraction of the bladder, and relaxation of the sphincter muscle.
2. Voluntary control from the brain, once a child is toilet trained.

Both sources may be affected in children with spina bifida. Children may not feel when their bladders are full, nor do they feel themselves passing urine.

Three types of incontinence have been described in children with spina bifida (Lorber 1968):

1. Overflow incontinence from a distended bladder. This is the most common problem and it has the most serious consequences.
2. A small proportion of children have an open sphincter to their bladders, and constantly dribble even when the bladder is comparatively empty.
3. A few children can automatically empty their bladders, but they have no knowledge of it occurring.

With 'overflow incontinence', the bladder fills and distends, but as there is no innervation to the bladder to cause it to contract, there is a constant slow dribble of urine as the bladder overflows. This has three serious effects for the child:

1. Infection of the bladder and possibly the kidneys; infection is more common in girls than boys.
2. Back pressure of urine from the bladder to the kidneys, which may damage the kidneys and ureters.
3. The possible social problems for child or young adult who is constantly wet with urine and wearing nappies should be considered.

Coping with incontinence

Some children who have overflow incontinence may be taught to periodically express their bladders, by pressure downwards and backwards on the lower abdomen. This may successfully keep the child dry if the time periods between expressing are accurately estimated. Ilial loop bypass operations were much used in the past, especially with girls, but are now less common. Boys may be fitted with a penile urine collector. Recently, self-catheterisation has been learned by older children and rhythmical tapping of the abdominal wall has been taught, as a means of inducing flow and emptying the bladder. These newer methods of control have led to some older children and young people needing only a small protective pad, which has improved their way of life. Cleanliness of any equipment used in the various methods is essential, and must be understood by the child.

Regular urine tests are essential, as urinary and kidney infections are responsible for a lot of serious illness in children with spina bifida.

Children are unlikely to have any voluntary control of the lower bowel, and it is therefore unlikely that they will learn normal bowel evacuation. However, some children who have been taught regular habits are able to empty their bowels at specific times of the day. Others may need to rely on suppositories, or enemas.

Incontinence is a great problem for these young people, who are often very concerned about it. It not only lowers their self-esteem, but can be a barrier to their forming social relationships.

Hydrocephalus

In hydrocephalus there is an excessive amount of cerebrospinal fluid in the ventricles of the brain and the increased pressure causes the cranium to increase in size; 75–80% of children with myelomeningocele are either born with hydrocephalus or develop it later. The severity may vary and some minimal cases may not require treatment. The head circumference of children with spina bifida is measured at birth, and daily during assessment, to see that it keeps within nor-

mal limits. Other signs of hydrocephalus are tense or bulging anterior fontanelle, separation of sutures and downturning of the eyes (Kapila 1977). To confirm a diagnosis, brain scans and procedures to measure the pressure of cerebrospinal fluid are undertaken.

Severe and prolonged pressure may cause damage to the tissue of the brain, even when treated by shunts. In many children this is associated with a degree of intellectual impairment, probably specific learning problems, and clumsy hand function. Some children may also have spasticity in muscle groups not directly affected by the spina bifida.

The Arnold–Chiari malformation. Sometimes tissue from the cerebellum descends through the foramen magnum and is damaged.

Treatment of hydrocephalus

Although some children with hydrocephalus have been treated with drugs (Lorber 1972), most are fitted with a Spitz–Holter or Pudenz shunt.

The Spitz–Holter shunt has a compressible tube that can be used as a pump, usually situated under the skin behind the right ear (Fig. 8.16). The shunt allows liquid to flow from the brain when the pressure is sufficiently high, but not in the reverse direction, thus helping to control the hydrocephalus. One catheter is in the right lateral ventricle, the other in the right atrium or peritoneal cavity.

As the child grows it is often necessary to replace the original catheter leading to the atrium with a longer one. A shunt may need immediate attention if it does not function properly or if there is sepsis. Parents are taught to watch for symptoms of raised intracranial pressure, which might arise from a faulty valve. These are, 'irritability, drowsiness, refusal of food, vomiting, squint or coma' (Kapila 1977). If the child starts to show these signs, the parents will probably have been told to contact the hospital immediately, although they may also have been shown how to test the valve. Some parents find that constantly being concerned about whether a valve is functioning or not is very stressful.

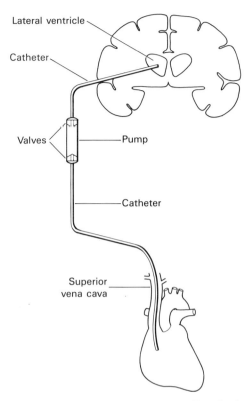

Lateral ventricle

Catheter

Valves

Pump

Catheter

Superior
vena cava

Fig. 8.16 Diagram of Spitz–Holter shunt. The distal end is shown draining into the superior vena cava; it may also be positioned to drain into the peritoneal cavity.

MANAGEMENT AND TREATMENT OF SPINA BIFIDA

The management and treatment of children with spina bifida is dictated by the needs of the child, which result from the manifestations of their disability.

The arms

Children with spina bifida need to compensate with their arms for the poor motor control of their legs and trunk. Strong arms are a great asset for daily living activities such as:

- helping young children without trunk stability to sit
- using hand-operated mobility aids, e.g. a prone trolley, wheelchair or crutches
- periodically rising from the seat of a chair, to relieve pressure on the skin

- transferring from seat to toilet, bed, or car seat
- standing up from the floor, or from a wheelchair.

Exercises to strengthen the arms are an important part of treatment and include:

- wheelbarrows, providing the legs are supported at thigh level; the less able will also need support under the abdomen or chest.
- long sitting on the floor, with hands on blocks each side of the trunk
- extending the arms to lift the seat off the floor
- press-ups with pillows under the knees and feet.

Strong arms are also useful for leisure activities such as swimming, archery and weight training, which in turn will further strengthen them.

Poor sitting balance

Many children with spina bifida have a poor sitting balance, especially those who have a severe high lesion.

Causes

A number of factors contribute to poor sitting:

1. Weak trunk muscles lack dynamic stability; they are unable to allow adjustment of posture to occur while at the same time providing stability.

2. Paralysed legs are not used as a counterbalance to movement in the upper body.

3. Lack of sensation from the lower trunk, buttocks, legs and feet means that there is no proprioceptive and tactile feedback from the base formed by the feet and buttocks. The information that normally makes us conscious or unconsciously aware of equal weight distribution on the two sides of the body, thus helping us to sit up straight, is not received.

4. A large head caused by hydrocephalus

may make head and trunk control while sitting difficult, especially in young children.

Infants and very young children with spina bifida have poor sitting balance, especially when sitting on the floor. When a child continues to need to support itself with one or both hands he may have little opportunity for learning manipulatory skills and for developing eye–hand coordination. This may possibly affect the child's choice of handedness and will also interfere with using two hands together in midline.

From an early age children with spina bifida should be encouraged to adopt positions in which they can indulge in two-handed play, e.g. prone lying over a small roll of carpet or over a wedge, or a chair with a tray and a back support so that they can reach forward.

To improve sitting balance. Head control must be improved if sitting balance is also to improve. The extensors of the back must be strengthened and balance exercises used, e.g. sitting astride the legs of the therapist, or astride a roll; sitting on a stool, low plinth or the floor. Activities that use rotation must be practised, e.g. rolling — getting from prone lying to sitting or hitching along a bench. Children and their conditions differ and activities should be selected and graded according to the needs of the individual child.

Special seats, or wheelchairs with moulded seats or inserts, which provide adequate support for the trunk, are necessary. When moulded seats are first used, pressure is placed on areas not used to stress. Regular relief from pressure is therefore necessary, and inspection of the skin is required (Settle 1987).

Trunk

Deformities

Some children may have a pronounced kyphosis at the site of the original vertebral deformity, which adds to the problems the child may have in sitting and makes fitting some orthopaedic appliances difficult. The back can easily be damaged by friction and pressure and care has to be taken to avoid bruising and lesions of the skin.

Scoliosis is common in older children and may eventually require some form of orthopaedic stabilisation (Fig. 8.17). There is a need for vigilance in the child's management to try to prevent this need from occurring. Muscle imbalance is a great problem and is most marked in those cases where the damage is very asymmetrical.

Lack of motor power

The back, especially below the lesion, will be weak and in high lesions this may make independent sitting very difficult. Head and trunk control will be late in developing, therefore arms need to be strengthened to assist with sitting and efforts must be made to improve head control.

Care must be taken to see that the child sits and stands with a good symmetrical posture, and that support is given to the back if necessary.

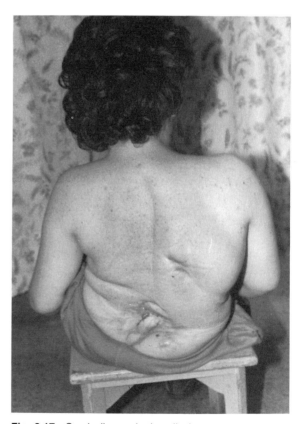

Fig. 8.17 Surgically repaired scoliosis.

Severe cases will require a seat moulded to the shape of the child's back.

Legs

Deformities

A child born with deformities of legs or feet may benefit from early passive stretching (which must be done with the orthopaedic surgeon's approval) and possibly from some form of splinting, which may help to correct the deformity (see Chapter 12 Orthopaedic Aspects of Childhood Disorders and Chapter 19 Treatment Methods). Talipes equinovarus may be treated with strapping or splinting, or with surgery, depending on the technique preferred by the orthopaedic surgeon. Great care needs to be taken of the skin when using strapping.

As the children get older, if they are to stand well it is important for them to have plantigrade feet. Where there is danger of feet being pushed into equinus, pressure from bedclothes should be avoided. Regular passive stretching is undertaken if toes are flexed or there are other possibilities of deformity occurring. Suitable footwear should be used. Some will require orthopaedic surgery.

Flexor deformities of the hips may be treated with stretching and nursing in prone over the parents' knees or on the floor in prone lying. The adductors may also require stretching.

Dislocation of the hip may be congenital or may be the result of muscle imbalance, such as that which may occur in lesions between L4 and S1, when there is unopposed flexion and adduction of the hip with a shallow acetabulum.

Children in danger of flexor deformities of the hips should avoid using long sitting for prolonged periods, for example, with a Chailey chariot — a prone scooter would be better and could be used for alternate periods with the chariot.

Older children with less severe lesions and who walk independently must also be kept under review. There is a danger that flexion deformities of the legs may develop through the effects of gravity pulling them down, especially if they put on too much weight.

Orthopaedic surgery plays a major role in correcting and preventing deformities in these children, but splints and regular stretching, correctly done, may be helpful in preventing deformities (Shepherd 1980).

Lack of motor power

A muscle assessment is important before commencing treatment. In infancy, and without a complete flaccid paralysis, movement may sometimes be promoted by stimulation of muscle groups by brushing, tickling or stroking. Where movement is present in the agonists only, care must be taken that muscle imbalance does not lead to deformity. It is important that the ability to extend the hips is preserved if the child is to be mobile on his feet. The child may need to spend periods in prone lying, or use a prone trolley, standing frame or swivel walker.

Loss of sensation

Parents need to be warned of the dangers of burns from hot kettles, radiators and baths; also the need to protect against cold, pressure and the trauma that can occur with a child dragging bare, insensitive feet or legs over a rough or hard surface. As the children get older, they must be taught to look after their own bodies; pressure sores, burns and chilblains must be guarded against. Pressure, particularly over bony prominences for long periods of time, may cause trophic ulcers. When lying in bed, the lower part of the back, and the backs of the heels are susceptible to pressure. A sheepskin, or a substitute that can be easily washed if the child is frequently wet, may be used for the back and sheepskin or foam slippers may be used for the heels. The chair seat needs to be padded with a fleecy cover, or a cover made from stretch cotton towelling, which can be regularly changed. The child should be taught to push up from the seat to relieve pressure. Standing for periods each day also relieves pressure. Appropriate support, e.g. swivel walker or standing frame may be required, but care needs to be taken that other parts of the body are not now subject to pressure from the standing frame. Standing is also helpful for urinary drainage, bowel function and to help diminish the number of spontaneous fractures (Butler et al 1982).

Special antipressure cushions such as the inflatable Roho cushion (Fig. 8.18) and cushions filled with silica gel or polystyrene 'beans' can be used when there is a special need, for example, if a pressure sore is threatening. Trainers and fleecy-lined boots are useful, but care needs to be taken when they are new. Orthoses, calipers and other orthopaedic devices must fit properly and need to be put on with care.

Sores can take a long time to heal and may mean time off school. Children must be taught to examine their own bodies daily with the help of a mirror, and be shown how to recognise the early stages of pressure sores. Carers should regularly check until the child is capable of doing this thoroughly itself. Children must also be taught how to look after their own hygiene, which is particularly important if they are incontinent, not only for health of their skins, but for social reasons. Poor hygiene can interfere with the formation of friendships.

Alternative forms of mobility

A child who cannot walk unaided, or whose walking is very limited, may require one or more aids.

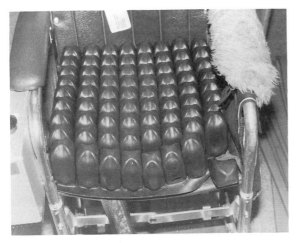

Fig. 8.18 Roho cushion.

1. A preschool child may require help to get around the house. A Chailey Chariot or Shasbah trolley, prone scooter or York Hill-type chair are useful. If they cannot stand unaided, then either gaiters, ankle or knee foot orthoses, which may be reinforced with carbon for extra strength, calipers or a swivel walker may be used, depending on the degree of handicap.

2. Parents will also need a suitable wheelchair to take the child out. If the parents do not have a car, and need to use public transport, then the chair needs to be one that the child can be lifted out of, easily folded and taken on to the transport. This is not an easy task, especially if there are young siblings as well.

3. Older children will also need a means of getting about school, and outside, independently.

Children who need total leg appliances may be fitted with a swivel walker, which allows the use of both hands. Calipers with crutches or walking sticks may also be used and, as the child gets older, Orlau hip guidance calipers or reciprocal gait orthoses can be fitted and used with elbow crutches or a walking frame. Reciprocal gait orthoses keep the legs in a good position and assist reciprocal movements of the legs (Fig. 8.19). They can remain on while sitting in a wheelchair, but have to be removed for self-catheterisation (see Chapter 21 Aids and Appliances). Protective helmets are advisable for some children when walking, as a safety measure.

As children get older, many opt for using a wheelchair, either hand or electrically operated. Because of the wide choice that is now available, expert advice should be obtained on what will be most suitable for that individual (see Chapter 21 Aids and Appliances).

Learning problems
General intelligence

Although some children with spina bifida have above average intelligence, most have learning difficulties, especially where hydrocephalus is

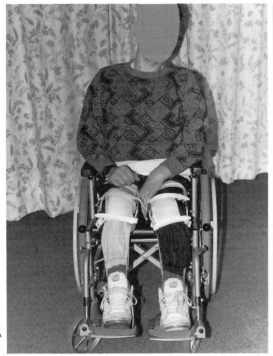 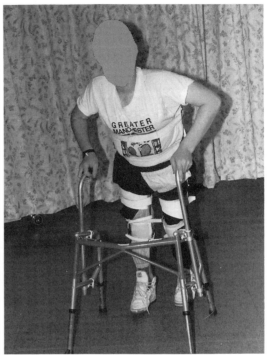

A   B

Fig. 8.19   Reciprocal gait orthosis. (A) Seated. (B) Walking.

present. In intelligence tests, verbal scores tend to be higher than performance scores.

Hearing

Hearing loss is uncommon and auditory perception or the ability to discriminate between sounds is good. However, some children seem to be hypersensitive to certain sounds, e.g. vacuum cleaners.

Use of language

Children with spina bifida often have good verbal memories and can learn the rules of grammar satisfactorily. However, it is only the more intellectually able who score well on comprehension and the appropriate use of language (Anderson & Spain 1977). Children with spina bifida have been considered to talk a great deal — using the cocktail party syndrome, or hyperverbal behaviour — often without really comprehending what they were saying; 40% of 6-year-olds with spina bifida showed this syndrome (Spain 1974).

They tended to be children with a shunt, whose intelligence was lower than average.

Visual perception

Goldberg (1968) described visual perception as: 'the ability to recognise and use visual stimuli and to interpret these stimuli by relating them to previous experience'.

Children with spina bifida have a high incidence of occular defects, in particular, squint, which may affect their perceptual abilities. Many are poor at eye–hand coordination and at differentiating figure from ground (Anderson 1975). They have also been shown to be poor at spatial performance skills and have an inability to appreciate spatial relationships. They tend to be poor at skills such as bead threading, fastening buttons, catching a ball, using scissors, number work and writing. They may also have difficulties with activities that need to be done in sequence. As well as perceptual problems, many have actual impairment of the motor control of their hands, for example, they have difficulty touching individual finger tips with the thumb of the same hand. Many are slow to develop a preference hand and more are left handed than would be expected. Children with hydrocephalus are more likely to have the above educational problems (see Chapter 16 Learning and Behavioural Problems).

Circulatory problems

Circulatory difficulties not only lead to cold limbs, with prospect of getting chilblains or frostbite, but to the skin breaking down more easily to pressure. Sores, ulcers and other skin lesions are more difficult to heal. Children may not be aware that their limbs are cold and they have to be taught how to look after their bodies, by regular daily examination, and by wearing appropriate clothing. Until children are proficient enough to do this, carers need to examine the limbs regularly. Two pairs of stockings, a thin pair underneath and a woollen pair on top, and warm shoes or boots lined with lambs wool may be needed in cold weather, together with trousers or slacks.

COMMON FACTORS INFLUENCING TREATMENT

Although the following factors influencing treatment are common to both cerebral palsy and spina bifida, individuals may not be adversely affected by all, or indeed by any of them and, when they are, the degree may vary from mild to severe.

The long-term treatment aims are to develop functional skills that will provide a degree of independence which is in keeping with the child's potential (Tables 8.5 and 8.6). For some severely handicapped older children it may only be possible to aim to maintain the functional level already attained. However, the following aspects should be included in all physiotherapy programmes:

- increased experience of movement
- prevention of deformities
- extension of the time scale for learning

Table 8.5 Treatment aims in spina bifida

Aims
Treat and prevent deformities
Strengthen arms and improve hand function
Improve head control, trunk control and balance
Encourage early standing and mobility using adequate aids
Provide guidance on management, and supervision of the provision of equipment

- encouragement of body image and perceptual abilities
- respiratory management
- promotion of stamina and endurance
- improvement in concentration and learning skills
- enhancement of decision-making and planning
- encouragement of social skills
- preparation for life.

Table 8.6 Treatment systems and methods

Condition	Treatment	Cross-reference to chapter
Cerebral palsy	Bobath approach	18
	Conductive education	18
	Hydrotherapy	19
	Vibration	19
	Serial splinting	19
	Feeding	20
	Dressing	20
	Computer technology	20
	Orthoses	21
	Seating	21
Spina bifida	The clumsy child	16
	Exercise and activity	19
	Hydrotherapy	19
	Individual learning programmes	19
	Wheelchairs	21
	Orthoses	21
	Seating	21

This table is not intended to be all-inclusive and only indicates treatment systems and methods for consideration. Bobath techniques are valuable when facilitating movement in the child with spina bifida and exercise is essential for the child with cerebral palsy. Respiratory management is an ongoing factor in therapy at all times.

Increased experience of movement

'Life is movement' (Sandow 1919). Movement is important not only for well-being but also for physical and cognitive development. Piaget (1953) stressed this when he described the sensorimotor stage of development. Any neurological condition that diminishes the possibility of movement, and hence of interaction with the physical and social environment, is likely to interfere with a child's physical, intellectual, emotional and social development. Furthermore, this need to interact with one's environment is not limited to infancy, but extends throughout life.

Many preschool handicapped children cannot get around inside the house by themselves; they get about outside even less. In a Greater London Council study on children with spina bifida, only 40% of 4-year-olds were able to walk outside sufficiently well to go to the shops (Anderson & Spain 1977). Movement experience both indoors and outdoors gives knowledge about space and about moving in space. It also provides a better bodily awareness and extends the child's experience of his environment.

When walking is not possible, or is limited, experience may be extended with tricycles, Chailey chariots, wheelchairs, and other aids to mobility.

Prevention of deformities

The causes of deformities have been previously outlined and muscle imbalance and inefficient management of children's postural positions are common to both spina bifida and cerebral palsy. The prevention of deformity is particularly important in the preschool years, but deformities may still occur or get worse throughout life, particularly during periods of rapid growth. They may get worse when the child leaves school, as frequently there is no adequate physiotherapy provision.

Prevention of deformity is central to treatment. Deformity cripples and prevents the development of movement and function, taking away the possibility for the children to develop to their full potential. Deformities make caring for the severely handicapped more difficult and as children get older, chest deformities arising from scoliosis diminish respiratory function, and other deformities such as windswept legs, may become painful. Gross deformities can also be cosmetically unsightly and a barrier to social interaction.

Consistently good management, keeping the child's weight down, together with physiotherapy techniques and the selective use of orthopaedic appliances and surgery can do much to prevent deformities. Once acquired they are difficult to treat satisfactorily.

Extension of the time scale for learning skills

Young disabled children who lack neurological control need adequate time to react to handling, e.g. when being picked up and carried they need to be given time to adjust to new positions and to learn from the experience. Research studies have shown that 50% of children with spina bifida, especially those with a shunt, were much worse in time-controlled, manipulative tests than normal children (Anderson & Spain 1977). Most children with cerebral palsy have even poorer neurological control of their hands.

Ample time has to be allowed when skills are being learned but, once learned, the prolonged time it takes to perform tasks like dressing and handwriting may be a handicap in certain situations, e.g. to cope in a mainstream school, or to obtain and keep a job. Therefore, in a 'learning situation' it can be to their advantage to practise skills against the clock, and in different contexts. They may be able to undress fairly quickly in a quiet corner of a clinic, but how do they cope in a cloakroom with noisy children around?

Encouragement of body image and perceptual abilities

Reduced body image, poor eye–hand co-ordination and perceptual difficulties are often present in children with neurological disorders. This may be largely due to lack of preschool sensorimotor experience. Infants need to:

• use their eyes fixating and following objects

- use their hands to explore their bodies
- use their hands to reach, grasp and manipulate objects.

If young children need to use their hand(s) for support while sitting on the floor or in a chair, they need positions and chairs that support them and leave both hands free to manipulate. They also need toys and suitable materials to play with (Norris undated, Riddick 1982).

Parents of handicapped children may need to be taught how to play usefully with their children and given explanations why this is important.

Older children also need opportunity and encouragement to practise arm and hand movements and skills. Catching and throwing bean bags and balls can be enjoyable and useful, even when sitting down.

Respiratory management

Respiratory problems are common, partly because the respiratory muscles may be involved but also because of the lack of taxing exercise to make them breath deeply. Absence from school may be reduced by:

- avoidance of unnecessary exposure to infection
- prevention of chest deformities
- physiotherapy chest care
- activities tailored to their ability, that encourage improved, deeper breathing (see Chapter 19 Treatment Methods).

Promotion of stamina and endurance

Many handicapped children tire easily and lack stamina and endurance, which will adversely affect their chances of succeeding in situations such as holding down a job and enjoying leisure activities.

Stamina and breathing can be improved by progressively working at:

- suitable physical education
- swimming
- energetic wheelchair activities, e.g. wheelchair dancing.
- high repetition weight training for stamina

- modified aerobic exercise groups.

The present fitness cult should offer an incentive to disabled children and adults to participate in fitness activities, if time, supervision and facilities are available (See Chapter 19 Treatment Methods).

Care needs to be taken with children who have cerebral palsy, to ensure that excessive effort does not make them stiffer and less able.

Improvement in concentration and learning skills

Children with neurological damage are often easily distracted, reacting to inessential tactile, auditory and visual stimuli, while finding it difficult to retain attention on items that are relevant, particularly if the task is demanding.

In a school situation, Anderson & Spain (1977) suggest that structured behaviour modification can be helpful. Many neurologically handicapped children answer questions impulsively. They can be taught to:

- reflect
- talk the problem over to themselves
- then give an answer.

Enhancement of decision-making and planning

Frequently these children are poor at making decisions and at planning. One possible reason for this is that adults constantly make most of the decisions for them. Young handicapped children should be encouraged to make choices; older children should make more important decisions and then plan how to carry them out.

Encouragement of social skills

A study of 119 handicapped adolescents by Anderson et al (1982) said that parents tended to describe their children as being shy and withdrawn. Few met friends outside school hours or went out in a group. Having a severe handicap or being immobile made them less likely to have friends and to mix with others. The severely handicapped children were also less likely to be given independence and responsibility by their parents. Of the children reviewed, only 21% seemed to have a satisfactory social life, while many others were unhappy about their social opportunities. Many also had psychological problems of depression, anxiety and lack of self-confidence.

It is important for these young people's happiness, that they develop social skills. They also need the mobility and opportunity to meet people.

Preparation for life

Research has highlighted some of the difficulties facing young handicapped people. Workers, such as Anderson et al, looking at large numbers, have published similar results. There is a lack of services to help the handicapped after leaving school. Once they have left the paediatric medical service, few see consultants or therapists. Many become less mobile and more deformed and have inadequate, poor-quality wheelchairs and lack adaptation of kitchens and access for wheelchairs. Some now lack the 'high tech' communication equipment they used at school.

It was felt that possibly 50% of pupils could have been more independent if they had been taught social and independence skills before leaving school. Anderson et al felt that parents could have allowed adolescents more independence and responsibility.

A small number of disabled individuals, with encouragement from others, have had the courage, motivation and audacity to break through the barriers of behavioural expectations, that society holds for them. Severely handicapped people have married, had children and become grandparents; others have skied, ventured abroad by themselves, succeeded as writers, painters and doctors, while others have had enjoyment and fulfilment from other forms of achievement. But this has not been the majority, although some have obtained a job, others lack the drive or capacity to either get to work, or to hold the job down. Others stay at home and watch television.

The treatment and management of children with neurological disorders is prolonged and needs a large team. Most parents, given knowledge and encouragement, can provide considerable help, especially in the preschool years. They in turn require support. As well as 'basic' physiotherapy and management, it is possible to help in the global development of the child, e.g. by encouraging decision-making and functional independence. This need not entail an increase of treatment time, just a little understanding of the total needs of the child and his family, and a slight adjustment in approach.

THE EPILEPSIES
I. McKinlay

INTRODUCTION

In the last 30 years nearly 100 epilepsy syndromes have been described in infancy, childhood and adolescence (O'Donohoe 1985, Roger et al 1985, Aicardi 1986, 1990). Advances have been made in investigation, treatment and management. The pathophysiology, genetics and prognosis are better understood but the disorders are still the subject of stigma not associated with some other chronic sicknesses such as diabetes, renal failure, heart disease or cystic fibrosis. Diagnosis is still difficult and errors are common.

It is not enough to offer reassurance that most children with seizures are healthy in other respects, or that many children grow out of epilepsies. Chronic disabilities affect a sufficient proportion of children with seizures to reinforce prejudices. The onset of a seizure may be alarming and unpredictable. It has been described as: 'a brief excursion through madness into death' (Taylor 1989). Even brief seizures involve a loss of voluntary control. It is not possible to judge whether a seizure will be brief until it has ceased.

Health professionals may become familiar with a wide range of seizures and feel confident about their management on professional territory, but an unexpected seizure in a close friend or relative, or when no treatment facilities are available, may be another matter. It is easy to understand why most parents think their child is dying when they witness a first seizure and recall of the episode is often vivid many years later.

TYPES OF EPILEPSY

Epilepsies are recurrent episodes of brain dysfunction with altered consciousness associated with abnormal electrical brain discharges, which may be detectable by electroencephalography (EEG).

Three-quarters of all people with epilepsies have the onset of their condition in childhood. The symptoms and signs associated with these episodes of abnormal brain discharge are called seizures, which may be generalised or partial.

Generalised epilepsies

Generalised epilepsies include absences, myoclonus, infantile spasms, tonic, clonic or akinetic seizures. By far the highest incidence is in the first two decades or in old age. EEG shows synchronous bilateral discharge or diffuse abnormalities.

1. Absence (petit mal) is a transient loss of consciousness, usually for a few seconds.
2. Myoclonus is a jerking of the muscles.
3. Infantile spasms are brief nodding attacks, with flexion of the trunk, during the first year. They are sometimes preceded by an upwards movement of the arms. Often a series of these will occur at times of reduced alertness.
4. Tonic seizures are episodes of stiffening, often with flexion of the arms and extension of the legs and trunk.
5. Clonic seizures cause rhythmical jerking of the face, trunk, arms and legs. These may be preceded by a tonic phase (tonic–clonic seizures or grand mal).
6. Akinetic seizures cause a loss of postural tone.

Partial epilepsies

Initial symptoms depend on the part of the brain affected: epigastric sensations, hallucinations, memory disorders, dreamlike states, flashing lights, tingling or twitching of parts of the body (aura). EEG shows localised brain discharge. Partial seizures may become generalised.

Benign epilepsies

A number of seizure disorders, in addition to febrile convulsions, remit spontaneously. These include (Roger et al 1985):

- benign idiopathic neonatal convulsions
- benign familial neonatal convulsions
- benign myoclonic epilepsy in infants
- benign partial epilepsies in childhood
- benign epilepsy with centrotemporal spikes
- benign epilepsy with occipital paroxysms
- benign epilepsy with affective symptoms
- benign partial epilepsy with extreme somatosensory-evoked potentials
- photosensitive epilepsy
- benign partial seizures of adolescence.

Knowledge of these disorders allows doctors to give an optimistic prognosis while children may have frequent seizures. Treatment may be effective while symptoms persist.

Malignant epilepsies

There are three 'malignant' epilepsies of childhood (Brown & Livingstone 1985):

- Ohtahara syndrome
- infantile spasms (West's syndrome)
- Lennox–Gastaut syndrome.

They are severe, largely unexplained epileptic encephalopathies, which respond poorly to treatment and are associated with lifelong mental retardation in at least 80% of affected children.

Ohtahara syndrome

Ohtahara syndrome (Clarke et al 1987) begins in the first few days after birth. There is a high mortality rate in infancy and early childhood.

Infantile spasms

The main features of West's syndrome are:

- onset around 4–6 months

- infantile spasms
- hypsarrhythmic EEG (high voltage and severely disorganised) (Fig. 8.20)
- response to steroids so far as seizures are concerned
- high risk of subsequent mental retardation
- autism
- episodes of minor status epilepticus with myoclonus and low genetic recurrence risk (1% unless the child has tuberous sclerosis and has an affected parent or sibling).

Lennox–Gastaut syndrome

Lennox–Gastaut syndrome has an onset between 2 and 6 years. Many children who have had Ohtahara syndrome or infantile spasms go on to have Lennox–Gastaut syndrome. The condition accounts for 70% of children with intractable epilepsy. Episodes of minor status epilepticus, staring, jerks and falls are characteristic. The EEG shows slow spike and wave discharge. Drugs are disappointingly ineffective and benzodiazepines given over a period of time can cause deterioration. The condition can persist into adult life without the child reaching a state of brain maturation capable of inhibiting it.

Status epilepticus

This is a continuous or serial seizure lasting more than 30 minutes without recovery of full consciousness. It requires urgent treatment and, where a seizure lasts for more than 5–10 minutes, preparation should be made to seek medical help. Seizures that last for longer than 30 minutes may cause brain damage.

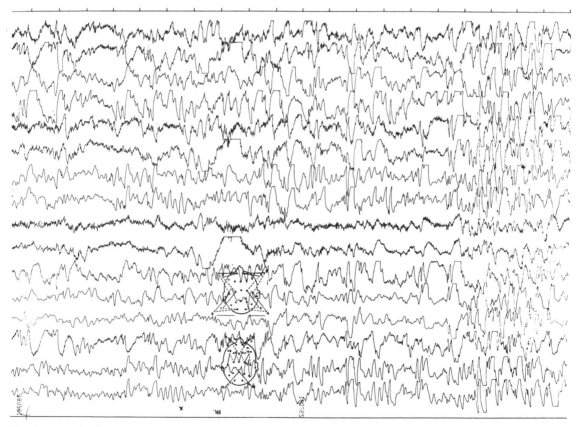

Fig. 8.20 An EEG pattern for a child showing hypsarrhythmia. Note the severely disorganised pattern and the irregular high voltage activity.

NON-EPILEPTIC SEIZURES

Seizures can be confused with a variety of other types of childhood episodes.

Differential diagnosis

- Breath-holding may result in children going blue and passing out.
- Vertigo (giddiness) may cause loss of balance, particularly in children who have had ear infections.
- Syncope (fainting), even in infants, can be caused by unpleasant or unexpected sensations, including nausea or painful bumps, and the description of precipitants and marked pallor in the attacks is very helpful.
- Night terrors, in which the child seems to wake up in an agitated state, often shaking, sweating and talking nonsense, can be alarming because the child (who is asleep, although the eyes may be wide open) will not be comforted.
- Overbreathing (hyperventilation) can cause stiffening of the limbs, especially the hands and feet.
- A low blood sugar can cause children to behave strangely. This occurs most commonly in diabetic children who have missed meals but can also affect young, thin children.
- Masturbation in infants and young children may be confused with seizures.
- Cardiac arrhythmias can cause seizures in children, though these are not common.

Simulated seizures

Older children may occasionally simulate seizures and inducing blackouts by the Valsalva manoeuvre may occur in epidemics in a school. Parents may:

- give false descriptions of seizures in their children to obtain attention for themselves
- induce seizures in children, e.g. by pinching their noses
- induce drowsy states by giving them sedatives.

About one-quarter of the children referred to specialist clinics with a provisional diagnosis of epilepsy turn out to have alternative diagnoses.

Febrile convulsions

The most common cause of convulsions in childhood is acute febrile illness, usually associated with upper respiratory tract infection. One child in 25 will have at least one of these, usually between 6 months and 3 years, with a peak in the second year. Fewer than one-fifth have their first febrile seizure after 3 years.

The earlier the first febrile convulsion, the more likely it is to be complex and the greater are the risks of recurrence, of epilepsy in later childhood and of learning difficulties in school. There is no evidence that febrile convulsions damage children's brains unless they last longer than 30 minutes; 80% of prolonged seizures are first seizures. Peak vulnerability of the left hemisphere is waning by the second year, while vulnerability of the right peaks at around 3 years. Girls pass their peak of maximum incidence at a younger age than boys. This is consistent with differences in brain maturation.

Reflex syncope is quite common in febrile illness and is not considered as a febrile convulsion. Although febrile convulsions are indistinguishable from epileptic seizures in their various focal and generalised forms, they are by convention excluded from the usual classifications of epilepsy; this is because of the trigger of fever. Most children grow out of them by school age and there is debate as to whether anti-epileptic prophylaxis (as opposed to emergency treatment) is effective (Nelson & Ellenberg 1978, Newton & McKinlay 1988, Wallace 1988, McKinlay & Newton 1989). Most experts now believe that such prophylaxis should only be used exceptionally.

Two-thirds of parents witnessing the child's first febrile seizure think the child is dying. Advice is given on management of recurrence (1 in 3 risk) and of febrile illness.

DIAGNOSIS
History

An accurate history is invaluable. Part of the

function of taking a family history is to try to understand what a diagnosis of epilepsy means to the family. It may be that a relative is believed to have been 'put away' because of epilepsy or to have 'died in a fit'. Therapists or other professional staff who witness possible seizures should note their observations and parents should be informed what to look out for.

Observation

- Circumstances, e.g. sitting in the dentist's chair, standing in a queue on a hot day, subsequent to a blood test.
- State — waking, sleeping, between the two, excited, frightened.
- Precipitants — an unexpected bump, a loud noise, going to be sick, watching television, vigorous exercise.
- Medication — insulin, antihistamines, tricyclic antidepressants, phenothiazines, isoniazid, withdrawal from barbiturates.
- Presentation — shout/choking, head turned to one side, twitching, complaint of dizziness or tingling or flashing lights, fall.
- Appearance — pale and sweaty, flushed, blue, blotchy.
- Associations — vomiting, incontinence, talking nonsense, bumping into furniture, purposeless searching, undressing, tongue thrusting, bleeding from the mouth. Pulse felt?
- Affected parts — whole body, face, limb.
- Movements — stiffening, twitching, jerking.
- Duration — can be hard to judge during the attack — seconds/minutes?
- Recovery — immediately back to normal, confused, complaining of headache, paralysed limb, unable to speak, asleep.

Examination

Physical examination

A general physical examination is made, noting in particular skin rashes on the face, trunk or limbs; poor growth — height, weight and head circumference; eye signs — malformation, retinal scars; pulse and heart sounds; enlargement of the liver/spleen could show the cause.

Neurological examination

Neurological examination is mainly to look for focal signs, especially when partial seizures are being considered or when trying to explain associated disorders, e.g. skin lesions in tuberous sclerosis. Not all focal brain pathology gives rise to focal neurological signs (e.g. temporal lobe lesions). However, if pyramidal tract signs are found in association with poor growth, e.g. asymmetry of hands or feet, it is likely that the pathology is of long standing — mild cerebral palsy rather than an evolving tumour.

Investigations

Electroencephalography (EEG)

The best known investigation for epilepsy is the EEG, which helps determine seizure type. Electrical activity from the surface of the brain is recorded and after amplification the activity is written out on paper or stored on tape.

Ambulatory recording. Miniaturisation of electronics allows a pre-amplifier to be glued to the scalp and connected to a cassette recorder worn on a belt. Brain electrical activity is recorded while the child is at home, in school or moving about (ambulatory recording). The leads can be concealed by the hair and under a jumper. The cassette has an event marker button, which can be pressed when an incident occurs. When the tape is played back in the laboratory it stops automatically at times when the event marker has been pressed.

Sleep recording. Because some seizures are state-dependent and only occur during sleep, ambulatory techniques may pick up nocturnal seizures at home. If more information is required a more detailed recording may be made in the laboratory while the child is asleep. This technique is called 'sleep recording'.

Activating techniques. Two routine activating techniques are used to provoke brain dysrhythmias:

1. A flickering light or a rapidly alternating chequer board is placed in front of the child's face. This is called photic stimulation.

2. The child is encouraged to take deep breaths for a couple of minutes as hyperventilation can provoke seizure discharge.

If it is thought that the child is having reflex syncope (after explanation to the parent) the child is induced to close the eyes and both eyeballs are pressed on firmly, using the thumbs. In susceptible individuals ocular compression will commonly reproduce the seizure. The EEG shows brief cardiac arrest followed by slowing of brainwaves.

EEG evidence is only supportive of a diagnosis. Some people with epilepsy may have a normal EEG in the laboratory (Fig. 8.21). Conversely, epilepsy-like discharges in healthy people are five times more common than in people with epilepsy.

However, if a normal record is obtained within minutes or a few hours of an episode it is unlikely that a diagnosis of a major generalised seizure would be made (Tables 8.7 and 8.8).

Computerised tomography

Computerised tomography (CT) scan, which is a specialised X-ray technique, is not a routine test for children with seizures as the results rarely influence management. However, when a surgical solution is being considered in a child with partial epilepsy and consistent focal EEG abnormality a high resolution scan may be very helpful (Fig. 8.22). CT scan is sometimes useful in genetic counselling when clinical examination gives an uncertain result.

Magnetic resonance imaging

Magnetic resonance imaging (MRI) is not widely

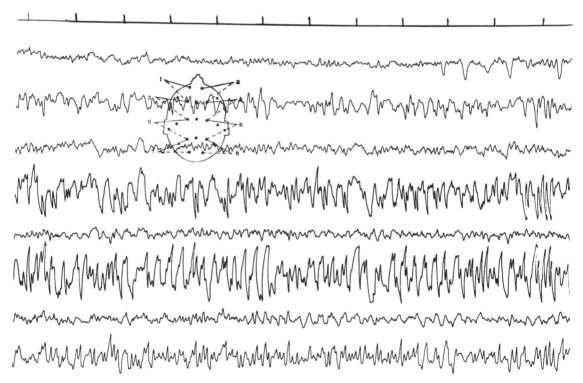

Fig. 8.21 EEG of a child with left hemiplegia and epilepsy. Note the asymmetry of the reading with right hemisphere abnormalities showing on leads 2, 4, 6 and 8. Leads 1, 3, 5 and 7 show normal readings. Although the record shows continuous abnormalities the child only had seizures every month or so.

Table 8.7 EEG findings: 130 children in Salford (1975–1989) with cerebral palsy but no history of epilepsy

Type of cerebral palsy	Normal	General dysrhythmia	Focal slow waves	Focal spikes sharp waves	Generalised 'epileptic' discharges
Hemiplegia	21	19	3	3	2
Spastic quadriparesis	19	12	1	0	3
Spastic diplegia	14	8	0	2	2
Athetosis	12	3	0	0	0
Ataxia	2	4	0	0	0

Table 8.8 EEG findings: 55 children in Salford (1975–1989) with cerebral palsy and epilepsy

Type of cerebral palsy	Normal	General dysrhythmia	Focal slow waves	Focal spikes sharp waves	Generalised 'epileptic' discharges
Hemiplegia	2	8	9	6	4
Spastic quadriplegia	3	4	3	0	0
Spastic diplegia	1	4	0	2	1
Athetosis	2	2	0	0	1
Ataxia	0	1	0	0	0

available. It is an expensive investigation but has the merits of not using X-rays and of showing little distortion as the result of bone (base of skull). It has given clear images for some patients with unusual disorders but its place in the investigation of the child with troublesome epilepsy is still the subject of research. It has not, unfortunately, increased the information available on the more intractable forms of epilepsy.

Biochemical tests

Metabolic causes of seizures include low blood glucose, low calcium, amino acid disorders and enzyme defects, including pyridoxine dependency in infancy. However, routine biochemical tests have a low yield. Some children with mental retardation due to chromosome defects have seizures. Subacute sclerosing panencephalitis, a late consequence of measles infection, can present with seizures. Affected children have high levels of measles antibody in cerebrospinal fluid and serum and show a typical EEG pattern (regular generalised high voltage, slow wave discharges).

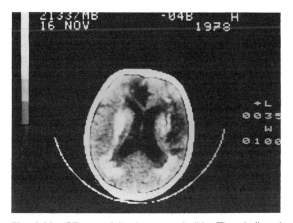

Fig. 8.22 CT scan following encephalitis. The skull and scarred (calcified) areas of brain show a white image. The enlarged ventricles and atrophic areas show a black image whilst the remaining brain gives a speckled grey image. The child had severe and frequent seizures.

TREATMENT
During an epileptic seizure

All staff treating or teaching children who may

have seizures should understand the principles of first aid. Risks of harm during seizures from sharp surfaces, fires and radiators, stairs, water, etc. should be avoided. The child should be treated calmly and quietly. If the child is unconscious the airway should be protected by placing the child in the recovery position (Fig. 8.23) until the seizure ends. During recovery the child should be reassured and kept quiet. Some children need to sleep it off or may experience a headache.

In some partial seizures the child may move about in a confused way. Occasionally the behaviour may seem aggressive but this has a 'robotic' quality and is not difficult to manage. Quiet supervision and prevention of accidents are the principles of care.

Status epilepticus

It is not necessary to seek urgent medical help unless the seizure is prolonged. Seizures which last longer than 30 minutes require urgent treatment, and if a seizure has lasted for more than 5–10 minutes preparation should be made to seek medical help. A doctor should be called to the child, or the child taken to a doctor, ensuring that the child's airway is protected en route. It is wise to alert the doctor or casualty department that the child is on the way so that treatment can be started on arrival. Diazepam solution is usually given, intravenously or rectally (a commercially available rectiol called Stesolid is available). Alternatively, paraldehyde can be given intramuscularly or phenytoin can be given intravenously.

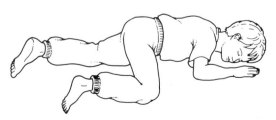

Fig. 8.23   The recovery position.

Prophylactic anti-epileptic medication

The main medical treatment for children with epilepsy is the use of anti-epileptic drugs, of which the most commonly used are carbamazepine (Tegretol) and sodium valproate (Epilim). Carbamazepine needs to be introduced gradually, as it can cause dizziness and nausea. A few children develop severe skin rashes and although desensitisation is possible the drug is usually stopped. Sodium valproate can cause indigestion and should be taken with food. Paradoxically, it is sometimes associated with excessive weight gain. Very rarely it can cause liver failure.

Phenobarbitone

Phenobarbitone is the cheapest and most widely available anti-epileptic drug worldwide, but it has a high risk of side-effects and is not a good choice for first-line treatment of children. It can cause troublesome hyperactivity and irritability.

Phenytoin (Epanutin) is an effective drug that is sometimes used in status epilepticus. It is still useful for maintenance treatment for some children. However, it is associated with a high risk of the following side effects:

- hairiness
- swelling of the gums
- loss of balance
- interaction with other drugs

Primidone (Mysoline) is a derivative of phenobarbitone and is little-used for children. Ethosuximide (Zarontin) is an effective drug for absence seizures and can also be used for unusual epilepsies, although it often causes indigestion or visual problems.

Benzodiazepine

Drugs such as nitrazepam (Mogadon), clonazepam (Rivotril) or clobazam (Frisium) may be used for children with severe seizure disorders, especially those involving myoclonus. They are sedative, however, and often cause irritability or ataxia. As with other anti-epileptic medication there is a risk of making seizures worse, for example, in the long-term treatment of Lennox–Gastaut syndrome. These drugs are presumed to suppress inhibitory mechanisms. Their use is associated with increased bronchial secretion and increased production of saliva, which can be a problem for children with cerebral palsy who have increased risk of chest infection and drooling.

Any child with epilepsy whose intellectual ability, posture or balance seems to be deteriorating, who seems to be losing weight or to be lethargic, irritable, hyperactive or depressed may be showing side-effects to anti-epileptic drugs. Occasionally, children thought to be dying may be restored by a treatment change.

New drugs

Recently two new drugs have been introduced: lamotrigine and vigabatrine. These should be used under the supervision of a paediatric neurologist in a regional centre.

Exceptional treatment

Some unusual remedies are used for children.

Hormonal treatment

Adrenocorticotrophic hormone (ACTH) can be very effective in stopping the seizures of children with infantile spasms. Although it stimulates secretion of high levels of steroids, it is associated with marked weight gain, irritability and sleeping disorders. It does not usually affect the intellectual outcome (up to 90% of affected children are mentally retarded and some become autistic).

Diet

Children with severe seizure disorders that do not respond to conventional anti-epileptic therapy may respond to a diet that is very high in fats or oil and low in carbohydrate (ketogenic diet). This needs a high level of parental commitment but can be worth it.

Pyridoxine

Another empirical strategy worth considering for children who are doing badly on conventional treatment is to use high doses of pyridoxine.

Pyridoxine (vitamin B6) may have a dramatic effect on newborn infants with an inborn error of metabolism (pyridoxine dependency). In older infants and children, transfer from a conventional anticonvulsant drug to pyridoxine may be associated with improvement in seizures. It is difficult to know whether this indicates benefit from withdrawal of the former or a positive effect of the latter, but the tactic is worth considering for children with unexplained refractory seizures.

When treatment fails it must be acknowledged. Children may be better off taking little or no medication (Taylor & McKinlay 1984).

Alternative treatment

Parents may be so desperate to rid their child of seizures that they will pursue remedies for which no scientific justification exists. Examples are changes of diet to avoid foods to which the child may be allergic, Dubard music therapy, aromatherapy, hypnosis, homeopathy, herbs and unprescribable preparations. Sometimes the child improves — possibly through relaxation or stimulation or possibly because the anticonvulsant therapy, which was making things worse, is stopped.

Behavioural treatment

It is possible for children to learn to recognise the symptoms at the start of a seizure and to use cognitive strategies or physical distractions to prevent the seizure from continuing. Examples include doing mental arithmetic, reciting poems, imagining pictures, sitting on a hand or singing. Generally these are too difficult for children under 7 years (developmentally or chronologically).

ASSOCIATED DISABILITIES

Those who advocate the case for understanding epilepsy tend to stress that people with seizures are otherwise perfectly 'normal'. If individuals do have other disabilities they are described in terms of the other disability. Charities for people with epilepsy consider that they would lose many of their supporters if they were seen to be identified closely with the needs of those people with mental retardation, autism or cerebral palsy who also have epilepsy. People with epilepsy who have been damaged by severe head injuries seem to be disowned even by the services for those with mental retardation.

Down's syndrome

Epilepsy affects 2% of children with Down's syndrome, as against 0.2% of the general child population. A study of 154 pupils with severe learning difficulties in special schools in Salford (McKinlay 1989) showed a prevalence of epilepsy of 34.4%. The rate was 26.7% for those under 10 years of age and 39.4% for those over 10 years of age. The prevalence in children with severe mental retardation in institutional care was 68.5%.

Cerebral palsy and autism

One-third of the 106 children with cerebral palsy in Salford either have or have had epilepsy (McKinlay 1989). A similar proportion of children with autism or Asperger's syndrome develop seizures. Typically, the onset or recurrence may be in adolescence.

Severe disabilities associated with seizures occur sufficiently frequently to reinforce the alarm already present in parents of newly diagnosed children.

Behaviour problems

Some parents and teachers may be anxious that normal discipline may provoke seizures, but they should be disabused of this. Children with epilepsy tend to be anxious, quiet and withdrawn rather than aggressive or prone to conduct disorders. If they behave badly there is no question of allowing epilepsy to be an excuse, provided that the psychological components of seizures are understood.

Learning difficulties

Although many children with epilepsy are of average or above average intelligence, there is a greater likelihood of them having learning difficulties, including clumsiness, than other children. There has been much discussion of the possible association of specific learning difficulties with epilepsy and no doubt this does occur (Addy 1987, McKinlay 1989).

The part played by medication has probably been exaggerated and it is likely that subclinical seizure activity is at least as important. Although some anti-epileptic therapy is sedative, effective treatment can also make a child more alert by suppression of seizure discharge.

LIVING WITH EPILEPSY

Psychological aspects of management are as important as drug treatment. Ensuring that the affected child or adolescent and the family understand epilepsy and its treatment is vital. One consequence of the onset of epilepsy in a child is that undue dependency and anxiety can dominate family relationships. Children who are bored or unhappy are likely to have more seizures than children who are occupied and encouraged. Excessive restrictions in case anything goes wrong are counterproductive (see Chapter 23 Parents and Children).

School

Maximal attendance at school and acquisition of qualifications is particularly important for children with disabilities. Making sure that school placement is appropriate and that teachers know what they can do to help repays the time taken. Restrictions on the school curriculum to avoid accidents, should be minimised. For example, a child with epilepsy is more likely to fall away from a lathe or laboratory experiment than to fall forward. A child should not normally be sent home after a seizure.

The British Epilepsy Association publishes information for teachers and runs regular training courses. An education package for teachers is available from the National Society for Epilepsy.

Sport

Children with epilepsy are more likely to drown from inability to swim than from a seizure. Cycling is a hazard for all children and allowing this in safe circumstances only is prudent. Children and adolescents who are prone to seizures but lead an active life could wear an inscribed pendant or a bracelet saying that the wearer experiences epilepsy. These are available from the Medic-Alert Foundation and the SOS Co. Ltd. Showers, rather than baths, may be best for active young people of an age when washing is unsupervised. Occasionally a bathroom/toilet door may need to be adjusted to open outwards and it should be able to be unlocked from the outside in an emergency.

Coping with prejudice

Confusion can frequently be caused by the terminology used: fits, seizures, convulsions and epilepsy may be used interchangeably. In lay terms, fits or convulsions may refer to seizures with involuntary movements, but temper tantrums may also be referred to as fits. Parents also refer to 'turns', 'do's', 'blackouts', 'wobblers', 'attacks' and other euphemisms. To avoid confusion it is essential to obtain a clear description to distinguish between seizures and other phenomena.

Children who have seizures may be called 'eppy' or 'spaz', as a reflection of prejudice about a condition affecting a small minority. The teaser is not likely to have connected the conditions of epilepsy and cerebral palsy. 'Epileptic' may be used pejoratively to describe a person rather than a seizure. For instance, play may be made of the term in the press if an individual has committed an offence, as if little else could be expected of such a person.

People who have not had seizures but who are seen as evil may be described as epileptic, and historically epilepsy was ascribed to demonic possession. Some affected women were considered to be witches and were treated with great cruelty. Taylor (1989) describes a patient who had had seizures for a number of years but who claimed triumphantly that he had been wrongly diagnosed as 'epileptic' before his brain tumour was detected.

CONCLUSIONS

Fits, faints and funny turns in childhood present common problems for health services. Their significance ranges from the trivial to the disastrous and treatment may be successful or ineffective. All cause concern for families and others involved in the care of children. The key to success is accurate diagnosis, appropriate treatment and sensitive counselling for the affected children and their families.

REFERENCES

Addy D P 1987 Cognitive function in children with epilepsy. Developmental Medicine and Child Neurology 29: 394–397

Aicardi J 1986 Epilepsy in children. Raven Press, New York

Aicardi J 1990 Epilepsy in brain-injured children. Developmental Medicine and Child Neurology 32: 191–202

Anderson E M 1975 Cognitive and motor deficits in children with spina bifida and hydrocephalus: with special reference to writing difficulties. Unpublished PhD thesis, University of London

Anderson E M, Spain B 1977. The child with spina bifida. Methuen, London

Anderson E M, Clarke D, Spain B 1982 Disability in adolescence. Methuen, London

Bax M 1964 Terminology and classification of cerebral palsy. Developmental Medicine and Child Neurology 6: 295–297

Blair E, Stanley F J 1982 An epidemiological study of cerebral palsy in Western Australia 1956–1975. Developmental Medicine and Child Neurology 24: 575–585

Bobath K 1966 The motor deficit in patients with cerebral palsy. Spastics International Medical Publications. William Heinemann Medical Books

Bobath K 1980 A neurophysiological basis for the treatment of cerebral palsy. Clinics in Developmental Medicine 75. Heinemann, London

Bobath B, Bobath K 1975 Motor development in the different types of cerebral palsy. Heinemann, London

Brown J K, Livingstone J 1985 The malignant epilepsies of childhood: West's syndrome and the Lennox–Gastaut syndrome. In: Ross E, Reynolds E (eds) Paediatric perspectives on epilepsy. John Wiley, Chichester

Bryce J 1990 The changing face of cerebral palsy. British Association of Bobath-trained Physiotherapists Newsletter 7

Butler P B, Farmer I R, Poiner I, Patrick J H 1982 Use of the Orlau swivel walker for the severely handicapped patient. Physiotherapy 68(10): 324–326

Clarke M, Gill J, Noronha M, McKinlay I 1987 Early infantile encephalopathy with suppression bursts: Ohtahara syndrome. Developmental Medicine and Child Neurology 29: 520–528

Goldberg J K 1968 Vision, perception and related facts in dyslexia. In: Keeray K A, Keeray V T (eds) Dyslexia diagnosis and treatment of reading disorders. C V Mosby, St Louis, p 90–109

Hagberg B, Hagberg G 1984 Prenatal and perinatal risk factors in a survey of 681 Swedish cases. In: Stanley F, Alberman E (eds) The epidemiology of the cerebral palsies. Clinics in Developmental Medicine 87. Blackwell Scientific Publications, London

Harris S P, Purdy A 1987 Drooling and its management in cerebral palsy. Developmental Medicine and Child Neurology 29(6)

Kapila L 1977 Primary treatment of spina bifida. Physiotherapy 63(6): 184–185

Lorber J 1968 Your child with spina bifida. Association of Spina Bifida and Hydrocephalus

Lorber J 1972 The use of isosorbide in the treatment of hydrocephalus. Developmental Medicine and Child Neurology, Supplement 27, p 87

McKinlay I A 1989 Specific learning difficulties and epilepsy. Education and Child Psychology 26: 822–827

McKinlay I A, Newton R W 1989 Intention to treat febrile convulsions with rectal diazepam, valproate or phenobarbitone. Developmental Medicine and Child Neurology 31: 617–625

Nelson K B, Ellenberg J H 1978 Prognosis in children with febrile seizures. Pediatrics 61: 720–727

Newton R W, McKinlay I A 1988 Subsequent management of children with febrile convulsions. Developmental Medicine and Child Neurology 30: 402–416

Norris (undated) Choosing toys and activities for handicapped children. Toy Libraries Association, London

O'Donohoe N V 1985 Epilepsies of childhood, 2nd edn. Butterworth, London

Piaget J 1953 The origins of intelligence in children. Routledge and Kegan Paul, London

Riddick B, 1982 Toys and play for the handicapped child. Croom Helm, London

Roger J, Dravet C, Bureau M, Dreifuss F E, Wolf P 1985 Epileptic syndromes in infancy, childhood and adolescence. John Libbey Eurotext, London

Settle C M 1987 Seating and pressure sores. Physiotherapy 73(9): 544–547

Shepherd R 1980 Physiotherapy in paediatrics, 2nd edn. Heinemann, London

Spain B 1974 Verbal and performance ability in pre-school children with spina bifida. Developmental Medicine and Child Neurology 16: 773–80

Stanley F 1984 Perinatal risk factors in the cerebral palsies. In: Stanley F, Alberman E (eds) The epidemiology of the cerebral palsies. Clinics in Developmental Medicine 87. Blackwell Scientific Publications, Oxford

Taylor D C 1989 Psychosocial components of childhood epilepsy. In: Hermann B, Seidenberg M (eds) Childhood epilepsies: neuropsychological, psychosocial and intervention aspects. John Wiley, Chichester

Taylor D C, McKinlay I A 1984 When not to treat epilepsy with drugs. Developmental Medicine and Child Neurology 26: 822–827

Wallace S J 1988 The child with febrile seizures. Wright, London

Walshe F M R 1923 On certain tonic or postural reflexes in hemiplegia with special reference to so-called associated movements. Brain 46(2)

Wilson J M 1988 Selecting and using posture walkers for children with cerebral palsy. Totline 14(2): 15–16

Woods G E 1975 The handicapped child. Assessment and management. Blackwell Scientific Publications, Oxford

FURTHER READING

Aicardi J, Chevrie J-J 1986 Children with epilepsy. In: Gordon N S, McKinlay I A (eds) Neurologically handicapped children: treatment and management. Blackwell, Oxford

Brett E 1991 Paediatric neurology, 2nd edn. Churchill Livingstone, Edinburgh

Chadwick D, Usiskin S 1987 Living with epilepsy. Macdonald Optima, London

Department of Health and Social Security 1969 People with epilepsy. HMSO, London

Department of Health and Social Security 1986 Report of the working group on services for people with epilepsy. HMSO, London

Fukuyama Y 1985 Epilepsy bibliography, 5th edn. Books and monographs (1945–1984), Kyowa Hakko Kyogyo, Tokyo (Available from the Department of Pediatrics, Tokyo Women's Medical College)

Hoare P (ed) 1988 Epilepsy and the family: a medical symposium on new approaches to family care. Sanofi UK Ltd, Manchester

Hopkins A 1985 Epilepsy: the facts, 2nd edn. Oxford University Press, Oxford

Jeavons P M, Aspinall A 1985 The epilepsy reference book. Harper and Row, London

Jeavons P M, Bower B D 1964 Infantile spasms. Clinics in Developmental Medicine 15. Heinemann, London

Kuijer A 1978 Epilepsy and exercise. Thesis: University of Amsterdam

McKinlay I A 1989 Therapy for cerebral palsy. Seminars in Orthopaedics 4: 220–228

Millichap J G 1968 Febrile convulsions. Macmillan, New York

Ounsted C, Lindsay J, Richards P 1987 Temporal lobe epilepsy: a biographical study 1948–1986. Clinics in Developmental Medicine 103. MacKeith Press/Blackwell, Oxford

Reynolds E H, Trimble M R 1981 Epilepsy and psychiatry. Churchill Livingstone, Edinburgh

Ross E, Chadwick D, Crawford R 1987 Epilepsy in young people. John Wiley, Chichester

Sander L, Thompson P 1989 Epilepsy: a practical guide to coping. The Crowood Press, Ramsay, Marlborough

Sillanpaa M 1973 Medico-social prognosis of children with epilepsy. Academic dissertation, University of Turku. Acta Paediatrica Scandinavica, Supplement 237

Sutherland J M, Eadie M J 1980 The epilepsies: modern diagnosis and treatment. Churchill Livingstone, Edinburgh

Trimble M R 1989 Chronic epilepsy: its prognosis and management. Wiley, Chichester

Trimble M R, Reynolds E H 1988 Epilepsy, behaviour and cognitive function. Wiley, Chichester

Wood C 1985 Epilepsy and mental handicap. Round Table Series 2. Royal Society of Medicine Services/Labaz Sanofi UK, London

9

Developmental delay

M. Clegg

INTRODUCTION

Many paediatric therapists will have had a child referred to them with the term 'developmental delay' written on the form as a diagnosis. This is an all-encompassing term usually used to describe a baby or young child who is slow in attaining his normal developmental milestones. A definite diagnosis such as Down's syndrome may account for this, but more often there is no apparent reason. This chapter aims to identify the more common causes of motor delay other than those caused by cerebral palsy, spina bifida and neuromuscular conditions, which are dealt with in Chapters 8 and 11. In some cases the delay may be thought initially to be caused by prematurity or failure to thrive for social reasons, but further observation and assessment may prove otherwise. Advance in such tests as brain scans, can now determine the presence of damage.

RECOGNISING DEVELOPMENTAL DELAY

Observation and accurate record keeping are essential if developmental delay is to be recognised (see Chapter 17 Common Assessment Procedures). The 'quiet' baby can often be one who is not receiving and acting on the normal cues from the environment. This in turn may lead to fewer cues and responses being given by the mother, who thinks how lucky she is to have such a quiet baby. However, this reaction may then be followed by seeds of doubt as she becomes both more aware of a lack of response and uncertain as to how to interest and play with her child.

The pattern of awareness on the part of the parent may vary. Delay in a first-born child may not be noticed because the parents do not know what to expect, whereas with a second or successive child, the parent may block the possibility of any problems from his or her mind.

It must be remembered that it is the baby or young child who controls the speed of development, which is a period of progress and achievement resulting from the constant interaction between the baby and its mother. The environment is thus initiated by the baby. From this interaction, motor development begins, together with the basic skills of communication and socialisation. If the baby does not initiate his needs correctly or in a progressive way then the process of the child's development will become stilted and slow down, and the developing responses introduced by the higher centres will be slow in developing. In Figure 9.1 a 10-month-old baby with Down's syndrome is beginning to correct his head in line with gravity, but has not yet developed a sideways parachute reaction with his arms, although he is no longer showing a startle reaction as he goes off balance.

Low muscle tone, as seen in the floppy baby, may be a reason for difficulty in performing a motor function, or indeed holding his head well enough to allow it to turn to a sound. Thus, he does not appear to respond enough to reinforce his mother's interest and she ceases to provide the stimulus. Similarly, such a baby will not begin to support himself in this upright position because the hypermobility of joints resulting from poor muscle tone produces lax ligament structures and consequently lack of stability. The baby is unable to support himself against gravity (Fig. 9.2).

Most people are aware that children develop at different rates and that comparisons can be unhelpful. For this reason it is important to remember the very wide variations of the normal. Occasionally developmental delay may prove to be a benign hypertonia, hypotonia, or delayed maturation of the central nervous system. However, persistence of the delay must cause concern and careful observation should be undertaken in an attempt to recognise whether the delay is within the boundaries of normal motor patterns or showing signs of divergence.

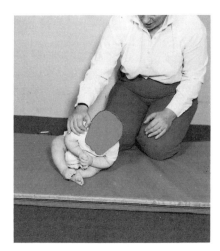

Fig. 9.1 A 10-month-old baby with Down's syndrome. Note the head is aligned with the body but there is no side-ways saving reaction (from the Department of Medical Photography, Wordsley Hospital, Dudley Health Authority).

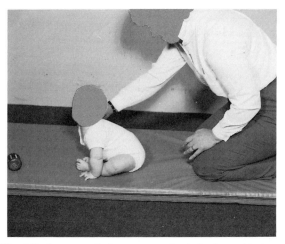

Fig. 9.2 Low muscle tone means the baby is unable to support his back and trunk in an upright position (from the Department of Medical Photography, Wordsley Hospital, Dudley Health Authority).

Divergent patterns in development or developmental delay?

The Oxford dictionary describes 'delay' as a hindrance or something being put off, and 'deviant' as a circuitous or erratic route. Both these words may describe a slowness in development, but common usage infers that with deviant or divergent development there is usually a specific cause. However, many children who are delayed may also show a deviance in the way in which they are achieving their developmental milestones.

The way in which developmental skills are achieved can be a prognostic indicator of future development progress. It can often indicate the presence of a pathological cause for this delay (Table 9.1). Divergent patterns in development usually show evidence of abnormal pathology and the retention of primitive reflexes may be related to cerebral palsy. With developmental delay primitive reflexes are not retained and, although slow, developmental patterns are along normal lines.

Divergent patterns in development

In Figure 9.3 the child is showing increased tone in the lower limbs when placed on her tummy and lifting his head with upper trunk. There is difficulty in pushing up on to extended arms. These problems are caused as a result of damage

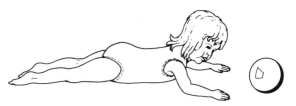

Fig. 9.3 Deviant patterns in development: increased tone in legs and an inability to push up on the arms.

to the motor cortex. Figure 9.4 shows a child learning to walk but with a pattern that deviates or diverges from normal.

Developmental delay

A delay in development may also be seen in Figure 9.5, where the child is pulled to sit but has a slight head lag. There does not seem to be any noticeable cause for this, i.e. increased extensor tone. Figure 9.6 shows the same child in prone lying. He has the ability to lift his head in midline from the floor but is not yet pushing his body up. The tone in his legs appears normal and the conclusion drawn would be that developmental patterns appear to be along normal lines but slow and delayed.

It must also be remembered that whilst many quite normal children show variation within their development they never show deviance. The most common variation may be the child who bottom-shuffles before walking, and only learns

Table 9.1 Divergent patterns of development

Arms	
Reach and grasp with	— flexed head and trunk
	— inward rotation of arms
	— pronated forearms
Inability to put hands together in supine	— shoulders retracted
	— shoulders laterally rotated
	— elbows flexed
	— arms resting or supporting surface
Legs	
No isolated ankle or knee movements	— total pattern of leg extension and/or
	— total pattern of leg flexion
Child held in standing	— inward rotation of hips
	— adduction of hips
	— extended knees
	— plantar flexed ankles
	— inversion of foot

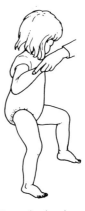

Fig. 9.4 Deviant patterns in development: high stepping gait pattern and abnormal weight distribution. The child is not preparing her balance correctly.

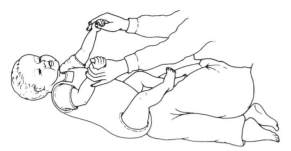

Fig. 9.5 Developmental delay: head lag when pulled to sitting, but tone in the lower limbs is normal.

to crawl when fully mobile in the upright posture (Fig. 9.7). A point to remember with bottom-shufflers is to check that they can crawl once they have learned to walk; do not assume that this will happen automatically.

MEASURING DELAY

How is delay measured? Although it is useful to use developmental charts as a check list, it is unfortunate that developmental progress is so often measured and described as a set series of actions that a child is expected to achieve and perform within a certain time span (see Chapter 4 The Developing Child and Chapter 5 Practices in Child Health).

Identifying slight delay

A sense of security must not arise because the profile from the developmental check list looks alright. This may happen for a number of reasons:

- the 'cogs' of the developmental progress have suddenly matched the chronological age

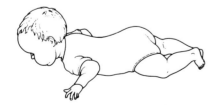

Fig. 9.6 Developmental delay: child not yet able to push up on arms and raise body. Note the normal tone shown in the legs.

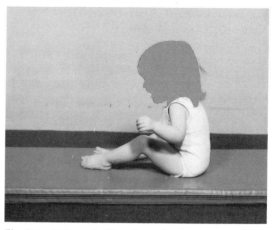

Fig. 9.7 Bottom-shuffling (from the Department of Medical Photography, Wordsley Hospital, Dudley Health Authority).

- 'cues' have been picked up
- the task is being performed abnormally.

The delay may be so close to the 'normal' that at certain times there is an overlap. During this process the next stage of development may start to emerge, since any one stage never works in isolation but always in concert with the areas before and those to come, i.e. those achieved and those ahead. If the child continues to be delayed then these overlaps will become less frequent, as the chronological age of the child grows ahead, faster than his emerging motor development.

Normal development

During the learning process, the baby repeats movement patterns over and over again, practising until he has perfected them. The first time a skill is achieved there is often a look of surprise, whereupon the baby will repeat the movement almost as if to say 'Did I really roll over?' He then tries again and may or may not achieve the same movement.

Suspected delay

A baby suspected of delay can achieve a motor movement but does not subsequently practise it, and therefore the consolidation of the developmental skill does not take place. Many weeks may pass before another attempt is made to perform the same movement.

Factors in measuring delay

When measuring for delay a number of questions should be asked. How a child performs a movement can be of more importance than whether or not he can do it (Table 9.1).

'*What*'. Observing the reason for movement can be an indicator of whether or not the movement is purposeful or aimless and whether the child is practising the movement to learn its function and then making use of the learning; or whether it is aimless and non-directed.

'*Why*'. A child may move:

- as a result of an abnormal reflex stimulation
- in response to his development progress and a normal postural reaction
- in response to some external stimulus and excitation.

A baby rolls towards a toy he wants to reach, but in just the same normal developmental period, he may sit, shake his hands, and stiffen his legs in the exciting anticipation of a chocolate button.

'*When*'. The age at which a movement begins to emerge compared to the time at which it ought to appear will be dependent upon the baby's maturity rather than his chronological age. It is important to allow for any degree of prematurity so that the outcome of any motor assessment will be accurate. Progress should be measured against the span of the child's own development and not only against that of chronological development charts.

In a normal infant no movement is done in isolation from another. Each skill overlaps with the movements that develop before and after it and demonstrate the interlacing of the maturing nervous system. The normal child is beginning to pull to standing before sitting balance is perfected; he does not 'wait' to achieve one skill before moving on to the next. A baby who will show a delay in his development can often only perform a movement in isolation from another movement. In other words, he is unable to initiate a movement in response to handling or to recognise when a movement may lead to an achievement.

COMMON CAUSES OF DELAY

Listed are some of the common causes:

1. Prematurity and hospitalisation. These may include such things as respiratory problems and anything that necessitates a prolonged stay in hospital during the early months of life.
2. Failure to thrive.
3. Specific sensory deficit.
4. Abnormal body proportions, particularly a large head, which may only be a 'familial' feature not an abnormality.
5 Down's syndrome.

Prematurity and hospitalisation

Respiratory problems can result in the necessity during the early months to keep the baby free from infections; overprotection on the part of the parents may hinder both physical and social development. Fear of the child's catching a cold can result in constant picking up and a level of attention that does not allow the baby to develop an interest in play or concentration on toys. Hyperactivity may develop later on and is often combined with hypertonia when mobility is achieved, resulting in a considerable delay in walking.

Developmental delay can also be caused by the prolonged hospital stay following a premature birth, reducing the parental bonding to the extent where the mother may also be reluctant to cuddle and handle her baby, and therefore slowing development.

Illness and surgery

Prolonged stays in hospital because of illness or the need for surgical intervention may cause a delay in motor development. The most common cause of hospital admission is probably congenital heart disease. The delay will be proportional to the severity of the lesion and the energy the child has (see Chapter 7 Respiratory Conditions and Cardiothoracic Disorders).

Congenital dislocation of the hips will also hinder motor progress because of the need to stabilise the hip joints in the correct position for a long period of time. Movement and its progress require both freedom and energy.

Therapeutic advice in handling and stimulation is helpful in all cases of this sort (see Chapter 12 Orthopaedic Aspects of Childhood Disorders).

Prematurity

Babies born prematurely are low in birth weight and, depending on the extent of prematurity, usually remain in Special Care Units until weight gain is such that they may go home. With advances in technology and medical science we are seeing more and more premature babies, some of whom have survived from as early as 24 weeks. Most of these babies do very well, and develop normally. Some, however, may sustain brain damage, some may become oxygen-dependent and some may become delayed due to an early lack of bonding with the parents or because of parental anxiety at caring for a precious and often longed-for baby (see Chapter 6 Neonatal Problems and the Neonatal Unit).

In the case of suspected brain damage a scan may be done to determine permanent lesions, the result of which will give clear indication of the level of outcome of the motor problem. The treatment and therapeutic handling will be adjusted to accommodate the problem and promote development.

Some premature babies will have difficulty with the adjustment and monitoring of blood gas levels required due to the underdeveloped lung tissue. This will require oxygen and a few babies remain oxygen-dependent for some months. This in turn will cause a failure to thrive and the baby remains hypotonic and lazy in his responses. Because these babies are nursed to a large extent on their backs, they develop a 'frog-like' posture and stiffness may occur at the hip and shoulder joints. The arm retraction and the low muscle tone also delay eye–hand coordination (Fig. 9.8). Developmental therapy and suitable positioning should be implemented.

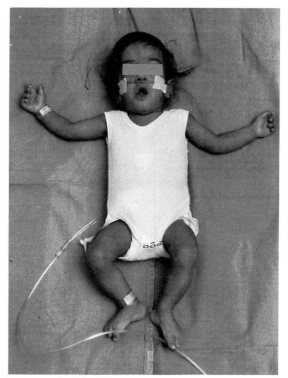

Fig. 9.8 8-month-old baby, born at 24 weeks. Note the shoulder retraction (from the Department of Medical Photography, Leicester Royal Infirmary).

Failure to thrive

Social and emotional deprivation, as well as the more straightforward poor feeding skills, may cause a delay in motor development. A mother may not know how and what to feed her baby or how to play with him. The interaction that takes place during nappy changes, bathing and feeding do not occur, because the task itself is too great (see Chapter 20 Living Skills and the Environment). The emotional stress within the family may lead to an irritable baby causing rejection on the part of the mother, and so the inevitable cycle of events leads to a motor delay. Much of this type of problem has been alleviated in recent years, as awareness has risen with the development of the primary health care teams. The 1989 Children Act (see Chapter 25 Legal Aspects in Paediatric Physiotherapy) will further raise this awareness of the child's needs for developmental progress.

Some babies and young children may show delay because of social deprivation although, if of normal intelligence, most will overcome this with entry into nursery and early educational intervention through schemes such as Portage. If such a delay continues, then other causes may be looked for.

Specific sensory defect

Development of vision and hearing are important factors when considering the level of a child's development. Vision has long been considered the most important input for normal development (Sarksen, Levitt and Kitsunger 1984). It is rarely obvious that a young baby has a sensory loss, and being unable to hear or see can severely interfere with the stimulation provided naturally by the mother and her interaction with her baby so vital for normal development (see Chapter 14 Sensory Disorders: the Deaf and Blind Child).

Hearing

Often some weeks or months may have passed before it is recognised that a child may have a visual or hearing problem. Hearing deficit may be picked up earlier than vision mainly due to the fact the some more obvious primitive reactions, e.g. the Moro reflex, can be in response to sound. Motor development can then be monitored and adequate stimulus should prevent any delay, providing that loss of hearing is the only problem.

Vision

Vision can be much more difficult to assess and the extent of the visual defect has a considerable bearing on its ease of detection.

The child's motor development may already have fallen behind due to the gradual demise of the normal activities between mother and baby. Lack of response leads to disappointment in the parent and a slowing of enthusiasm to stimulate the baby. The baby may be very quiet and unresponsive, or may be very irritable and not easy to pacify. This in turn may lead to a disturbance in the bonding process with the mother. Some

parents may respond by becoming overprotective, not allowing the baby to progress in his development for fear of self-injury. This is particularly so in the case of a blind child.

If the deficit is purely sensory, then there should be no reason why motor skills will not develop, although probably later than normal, and somewhat clumsily. However, often these deficits are combined with other problems and the resulting delay in development more complex.

Abnormal body proportions

Some families have characteristic features. One example is a child who has a large head in proportion to the rest of his body. The weight of the head can make it difficult to control until the muscles become stronger and the overall growth brings the body parts more in proportion. Lack of head control leads to a motor delay because control initiates early motor movement with the development of the normal postural reactions. Normal development may be slightly later in appearing.

Down's syndrome

The motor delay seen in Down's syndrome has attracted considerable study. The most significant feature to be seen is the marked degree of hypotonia and the very late development of normal postural tone. In most cases the tone remains low throughout life. Combined with the hypotonia is the continuance of the primitive reflexes beyond the normal time expected. These combined features cause different lengths of delay in the motor development of children with Down's syndrome, with large variations.

A study of Table 9.2 will identify the development milestones for Down's syndrome children, compared to the average norm.

Down's syndrome children can attain most of the gross motor skills of their peers but the fine movements are often very late in appearing and remain clumsy and unrefined. This clumsiness can be associated with an interaction between poor sensory feedback, lack of postural stability around joint structures and a slower intellectual

Table 9.2 Developmental milestones for children with Down's syndrome (adapted from Cunningham 1982)

	Children with Down's syndrome		'Normal' children	
	Average age (months)	Range (months)	Average age (months)	Range (months)
Gross motor activities				
Holds head steady and balanced	5	3–9	3	1–4
Rolls over	8	4–12	5	2–10
Sits without support for 1 minute or more	9	6–16	7	5–9
Pulls to stand using furniture	15	8–26	8	7–12
Walks with support	16	6–30	10	7–12
Stands alone	18	12–38	11	9–16
Walks alone	19	13–48	12	9–17
Walks up stairs with help	30	20–48	17	12–24
Walks down stairs with help	36	24–60+	17	13–24
Runs	Around 4 years			
Jumps on the spot	4–5 years			
Fine motor activities				
Follows objects with eyes, in circle	3	1.5–6	1.5	1–3
Grasps dangling ring	6	4–11	4	2–6
Passes objects from hand to hand	8	6–12	5.5	4–8
Pulls string to attain toy	11.5	7–17	7	5–10
Finds objects hidden under cloth	13	9–12	8	6–12
Puts three or more objects into cup or box	19	12–34	12	9–18
Builds a tower of two-inch cubes	20	14–32	14	10–19
Completes a simple three-shape jigsaw	33	20–48	22	16–30+
Copies a circle	48	36–60+	30	24–30
Matches shapes/colours	4–5 years			
Plays games with simple rules	4–5 years			
Personal/social/self-help activities				
Smiles when touched and talked to	2	1.5–4	1	1–2
Smiles spontaneously	3	2–6	2	1.5–5
Recognises mother/father	3.5	3–6	2	1–5
Takes solids well	8	5–18	7	4–12
Feeds self with biscuit	10	6–14	5	4–10
Plays pat-a-cake, peep-bo games	11	9–16	8	5–13
Drinks from cup	20	12–30	12	9–17
Uses spoon or fork	20	12–36	13	8–20
Undresses	38	24–60+	30	20–40
Feeds self fully	30	20–48	24	18–36
Urine control during day	36	18–50+	24	14–36
Bowel control	36	20–60+	24	16–48
Dresses self partially (not buttons/laces)	4–5 years			
Uses toilet or potty without help (often too small to get up on to a toilet, unless a special step is available)	4–5 years			

interpretation of the requirements of movement. This hypermobility of joints can be seen in Figure 9.9.

Down's syndrome is now diagnosed at birth and early therapeutic and educational intervention is desirable to encourage maximum attainment. In recent years this early intervention has been more readily available because of raised awareness and changes in social policy.

Early developmental handling of these children will increase confidence and enhance the early development of motor skills.

Mental handicap

Increasing delay in motor development is often followed by the emergence of mental handicap. A degree of hypotonia is frequently present and

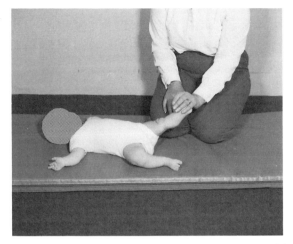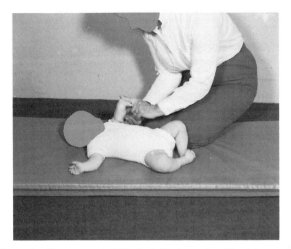

Fig. 9.9   A baby with Down's syndrome: hypermobile joints (from the Department of Medical Photography, Wordsley Hospital, Dudley Health Authority).

this, combined with the child's inherent lack of response to stimuli, can lead to a 'slow-for-milestones' baby who is sometimes also rather obese.

Careful observation on the part of the therapist may be a key factor in establishing the final diagnosis of babies who are slow to develop. The motor development will fall further and further behind as the child grows. In the author's experience it is not uncommon to find that a child who has been referred for physiotherapy and who is not walking at 15 months has a degree of mental handicap.

Providing there are no other complications, such as cerebral palsy, these children do learn to walk and achieve finer skills but, as with Down's syndrome children, are often very clumsy.

PHYSIOTHERAPY INTERVENTION

Various   therapeutic   approaches   used   in

paediatric   physiotherapy   are   discussed   in Chapters 18–22.

Developmental therapy combined with advice on management and stimulation can help provide the experiences needed for motor development. This should take place in all the environments in which the child finds himself. For this reason, a major role of the paediatric physiotherapist is to teach not only the parents, but also the other teachers and carers who have care of the child. Resources do not allow for daily input by a physiotherapist and indeed this is not desirable. The child's life should continue to be as normal as possible and his own environment should provide the input he needs. Leisure activities, such as swimming and horse-riding, can combine a therapeutic as well as social activity. This type of activity may be an introduction into taking part in normal activities for both the parents and the child.

REFERENCES

Sarksen P M, Levitt S, Kitsunger M 1984 Identification of constraints acting on motor development in young

visually disabled children and principles of remediation. Child Health Care and Development 10: 273–286

FURTHER READING

Burns R B 1986 Child development. A text for the caring professions. Croom Helm, New York

Carr J 1975 Young children with Down's syndrome. Butterworth, London

Cowie V A 1970 A study of the early development of Mongols. Pergamon, Oxford

Cunningham C C 1982 Down's syndrome. An introduction for parents. Souvenir Press, London

Drillien C M, Pickering R M, Drummond M B 1988 Predictive value of screening for different areas of development. Developmental Medicine and Child Neurology 30: 294–305

Drillien C M, Drummond M B 1977 Neurodevelopmental problems in early childhood. Assessment and management. Blackwell Scientific Publications, Oxford

Griffiths M I 1976 Development of children with Down's syndrome. Physiotherapy 62: 11–15

Illingworth R D 1983 The development of the infant and young child — normal and abnormal. Churchill Livingstone, Edinburgh

Lane D, Stratford B 1985 Current approaches to Down's syndrome. Holt, Rinehart & Winston, Eastbourne, Sussex

Sheridan M D 1973 Children's developmental progress from birth to 5 years: The Skycar Sequences. NFER Publishing Co., Windsor, Great Britain

10

Profound and multiple disability

E. Bell   J. E. Lamond

BEHAVIOUR, SELF-HELP AND REALITY
J. E. Lamond

INTRODUCTION

Profound and multiple disability is difficult to define, but the term is usually invoked to describe a child who is highly dependent, with a lack of functional skills associated with one or more physical handicaps, and an IQ of under 25 (Hogg & Sebba 1986). The majority of profoundly/multiply disabled children also have eye defects, are often epileptic and usually doubly incontinent. Most have some degree of cerebral palsy, but there are some who appear to have no physical disability, yet have profound mental impairment.

Causes

Causes of profound/multiple disability are attributed to many factors — birth injury, sex chromosome abnormality, prenatal factors, metabolic disorders, postencephalitis or meningitis, and increasingly nowadays to non-accidental injury or the results of road traffic accidents.

Presentation

The appearance of profoundly/multiply disabled people is often very deceptive, as seldom does chronological age have any bearing on physical development. What seems to be a small child may be an adolescent with adolescent feelings and moods, whilst an apparent adult retains childish habits, perhaps carrying around cuddly toys. It is an aspect of working with this group that can be both difficult and challenging.

Historical perspective

In earlier times it was usual for the profoundly disabled child to be put into one of the large institutions, to be cared for physically but forgotten by society as a whole who considered them to be an embarrassment, and it was a brave parent who insisted on keeping the child at home. Today, with more enlightened thinking and an increase in the availability of community facilities, children are no longer admitted to large institutions. Early intervention by Child Development Centres, with their core of professional staff, more back-up services for parents, increasing numbers of special schools and volunteers willing to provide parental relief, have all helped to bring about a different model of care.

Professional challenge

In no sense can the treatment of these children be described as easy, and the work to be done for the results achieved has to be viewed in terms of years, progress of any sort usually being extremely slow. In consequence, it has not been a popular field for physiotherapists to work in, although those who have done so have found the challenge rewarding. With increasing knowledge and developing technology, more interest is being aroused and there are more therapists now working with these children.

Great patience, perseverance and empathy are needed, as well as a willingness to cooperate with all other professionals working with the child. Communication between members of the professional team (teachers, nurses, doctors, social workers) and parents, if the child is living at home, is crucial to the attainment of results. In addition the emotional demands are great as instant feedback on work being done is seldom provided. Faced for the first time with a profoundly disabled child, the therapist is usually guaranteed to feel totally inadequate and then to react with 'What can I do?' What indeed?

ASSESSMENT

Assessment has to be undertaken to give a baseline from which to start planning a treatment regime. However, it must be viewed as something that is ongoing, as the initial contact with the child will usually only provide a glimpse of the real problems. Each member of the team involved in the overall care plan will make his or her own assessment and the sum of their deliberations, plus the parents' observations, will form the basis for work to be started. Continued and frequent communication and planning between all team members is important because all small changes, whether for better or worse, have to be noted and programmes adjusted accordingly.

Physical assessment

Physical assessment should cover motor and sensory disturbances, taking particular note of hand function and any gross deformities present. These deformities may manifest as:

- windswept and/or subluxated hips
- scoliosis with associated distortion of the rib cage, caused by the unequal pull of muscles
- tight flexors of shoulders, elbows, wrists and knees (Fig. 10.1).

With today's early intervention these deformities are not as common as in earlier years and may be easily recognised at an early stage. The child's nature and how he/she will react to physical handling may take months to discover.

Behavioural assessment

The children with no apparent physical abnormalities may display strange behavioural traits — hyperactivity, constant hand-flapping, self-mutilation, mouthing of fingers and hands, faeces-smearing, hair-pulling, scratching and biting being but some. Constant tearing of clothes, pulling out threads, stripping, refusal to wear footwear and overbreathing to the point of collapse are others. The causes of these are dif-

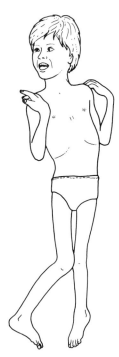

Fig. 10.1 Deformities of the profoundly disabled child.

ficult to define but may be due to anger, frustration, boredom or just attention-seeking. Again, observations from team members may provide some clue, and help from psychologists will be necessary. In all instances the approach to the children must be consistent, so that they gain some understanding of their parameters; reward and reinforcement of good behaviour is important. Continuing observation by everyone concerned plus careful record keeping will indicate improvements or otherwise.

AIMS OF THERAPY

Having made an initial assessment and tried to identify the major problems, a treatment and long-term management plan, with aims clearly stated, can be formulated. This should be realistic in the light of the degree of physical/mental impairment present. Main underlying aims are:

1. Getting to know the child as a whole — likes, dislikes, background, past history and parental attitudes are all important.

2. Establishing communication links by various means, such as eye contact, touch, voice, signing.

3. Stimulation to increase awareness of self and environment.

4. Maintenance and, if possible, improvement of any skills present, by whatever means. Particularly self-help skills.

5. Prevention of deformities using good positioning and frequent changes of position. If deformities are already present, attempt to prevent further deterioration.

6. Obtain mobility by whatever means possible.

Getting to know the child

The initial approach is very important and should be a gradual process. Sudden appearance from behind or from a blind-side can startle, whereas a frontal approach, possibly at the child's level — even if it means getting down on the floor — is more reassuring. Gaining the child's confidence is so important that it cannot be over-emphasised; at the least he is more likely to relax if he trusts the person dealing with him and, in the wider context of his treatment, is more likely to try to do what is asked of him. It can take a long time to build this type of relationship, but it is time well spent. If for some reason the therapist and child cannot relate to each other — and it does occasionally happen — some other person should take over. Parents also need to have confidence in the people caring for their child, and should feel able to discuss their problems.

All profoundly disabled people are very aware of being touched and handled but may not be able to express their feelings. Brudenell (1986) cites one boy whose pulse rate increased dramatically when picked up suddenly by someone unknown to him but, over a period of time, as the person was accepted, the pulse rate gradually dropped.

Tension can cause muscle spasm, which is painful, and stroking of the back or legs and arms can ease this, as well as building up trust of being handled. Once that trust appears to be established it is possible to move on to the next stage.

Establishing communication links

To help the child understand what is required of him, some form of communication is required, not necessarily speech. As we have already seen, touch is important, particularly to someone who is blind. For instance a tap on the cheek and lip could mean 'Open your mouth for food'; equally the child may touch someone with a hand or foot and mean 'Hello, I'm here!' (see Chapter 14 Sensory Disorders: the Deaf and Blind Child).

Eye contact

Eye contact is important because it requires a measure of concentration, if only for a few seconds, and the child learns to 'look' at a person or object within the range of his vision. Bearing in mind that vision is often defective, the range may not be great, maybe as little as 18 inches, but sometimes objects in bright luminous colours of orange or green can be seen at a greater distance. Occasionally looking at, or towards, something may be the child's only way of indicating his wishes.

Sign language

Various sign languages have been developed, but to be successful all the people the child meets should know the particular chosen language, so that he can 'talk' to them, and usually the child needs the ability to use his arms and hands with some competence.

Bliss symbolics uses a system of signs to which the child points to answer questions put to him, or to indicate what he wishes to say. If the ability to physically point is not present, a pointer fastened on a head band is sometimes used. It is rare for a child to initiate a conversation.

Voice

Voice is often the most successful means of conveying meaning, the tone used indicating command, disapproval or approbation, sympathy or joy, whilst the child can sometimes use sounds in the same manner to reciprocate. Knowledge of the child will help the interpretation of his meaning, and thus a form of communication is established over a period of time.

Whatever the communication method, it is important for everyone — parents, teachers, therapists, nurses and friends — to know how it works as it is the child's link to the world around him.

Sensory stimulation

Left to our own devices most of us tend towards doing as little as possible, and the profoundly disabled child is no exception. He needs to be stimulated to make efforts to move, learn and develop.

Vibration

A vibrator can be useful because it uses tactile stimulus to encourage movement, and this stimulus in turn can be used as a reward for effort. Vibration may be applied with a hand-held vibrator, or as a pad to sit or lie upon, the rate of the vibration determining the degree of stimulation. Some patients will make enormous efforts to touch the source; others just enjoy the feeling; a few actively dislike it. Individual methods for using vibration have been developed, for example, a specially designed slide where reward for getting up the steps was vibration at each level, and a further stimulus at the bottom of the slide! The children concerned loved it and made huge efforts to use the toy. (See Chapter 19 Treatment Methods: Vibration Therapy.)

Food and drink

Food or drink can provide stimulus. One small boy learnt to pull himself across a room for a cup of tea, when no other inducement was successful, and another girl, who was very lethargic, showed choice by physical resistance to efforts to feed her with fish.

Electronic technology

For the really immobile child, the development of electronic technology has provided some ingenious gadgets. For someone lying on the floor, an electronic beam directed across the body will be broken by any movement made. This in turn can then ring a bell or turn on a radio or tape, as reward for the effort made to move, and provides the stimulus for further effort. Brightly coloured mats with inbuilt pressure pads that play a tune or make a noise when pressed provide another incentive for movement (Fig. 10.2).

Ritual

Sometimes just the prospect of a simple ritual like being bathed or dressed causes sufficient excitement to initiate activity of some sort. Whatever is found to be successful can be explored and developed.

Environment

Research has shown that the nature of the environment has varying effects on the occupant of that environment. It is well known that warmth, soft lights and sweet music induce relaxation, but conversely loud noises, bright lights and crowds can have the opposite effect. For children with little ability to discover the outside world themselves, their environment is supremely important. Colour, textures, smells, heat, light and sound all need to be considered with a view to highlighting and enhancing awareness.

Fabrics

The fabrics that cover rolls, seats and wedges on which many children are placed is invariably

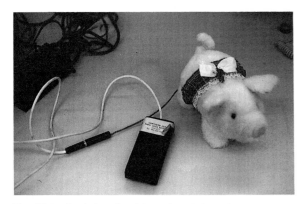

Fig. 10.2 A wedge-shaped touch switch and toy. (Reproduced by kind permission of Northern ACE.)

smooth and often brightly coloured, but towelling loose covers in different thicknesses can be used in equally bright colours and will feel warmer and are more tactile.

Toys

Brightly coloured toys are easily available and the variety is considerable, but it is well to ensure that the paint will withstand possible sucking and that the construction is strong. Soft toys are also easy to obtain, but need to be easily washable. Often home-made ones, using an assortment of fabrics, can provide variety of tactile stimulation, e.g. a doll with velvet dress, silk body, thick wool for hair, leather shoes and maybe a furry hat.

Teachers are usually expert in the making of wall collages using crinkly paper, felt, painted egg cartons, dried pulses, foil in different colours, sandpaper, and even panscrubs! Most of these materials are freely available and easily replaced if destroyed. They also provide both visual and tactile stimulation.

Mobiles can be bought or made in many colours, encompassing all sorts of subjects from animals and flowers to cars, planes or just abstract shapes. They can catch a child's attention and fascinate them, breaking up an apparently endless stretch of blank ceiling. Wind chimes hung where they catch a draught are stimulating too, because of the sound combined with movement.

Balloons are cheap, come in all colours and sizes and are easily obtainable. They can be hung from the walls or the ceiling, tied to a wheelchair or frame and the slightest touch makes them move, providing reward for effort, which is important. Some children may dislike the bang if they burst, others enjoy it.

Smell

Smell is often forgotten, but is very essential. Small animals recognise their mothers by smell, and possibly small babies also associate certain odours with Mum. Hospitals usually smell aseptic, as do dentists' rooms; homes may smell of polish or flowers, cooking or cleaning fluids, all of which have associations for a child, helping him to identify his surroundings. Many smells are pleasurable, for instance, the almost endless sorts of soap, talc or perfume, used by most people today provide a great deal of olfactory stimulation and have become part of the environment. Cooking smells can 'make our mouths water' or wrinkle our noses in dislike. Many normal children love being in the kitchen, tasting, or licking baking bowls, playing with pastry, smelling celery or spices, vinegar or cheese, warm bread or newly baked cake, bacon cooking, meat roasting, but so often disabled children are denied these simple pleasures and kept out of the kitchen. They may not be able to move, but they can watch; if they cannot see or maybe hear, they can smell and their lives are enriched as a result.

Wind is an interesting sensation. Hairdryers provide hot and cold breezes, hand-held fans give a gentle draught, electric fans provide a breeze like a hair-dryer. Wind can be seen to blow the washing on the line, or the leaves round the garden. It can be exciting even if you cannot move. One small very disabled boy taken on a speedboat trip grinned broadly when his hair blew with the speed, but cried bitterly when taken ashore.

Visual stimulation

There is much expensive and sophisticated equipment now coming on the market that provides a visual stimulation to the environment. Fibre-optic lamps with glowing, moving fronds and ever-changing colours, perspex columns filled with coloured liquid and irridescent shapes that move, oil-filled lamps containing wax that melts as the lamp gets warm and makes unending changes of shape, which are fascinating to watch. Projectors with rotating coloured discs and an oil-covered plate can make swirling coloured patterns on walls and ceilings. Rotating balls made of many small mirror facets make flickers of bright light, and all these are there to provide interest to our surroundings.

Pets

Pets are controversial in that they move, are warm, pleasant to touch and will make a noise, but they may scratch or nip, and some children are terrified of an animal when they are unable to move out of its way. Birds and fish, which are enclosed, do not pose a threat. Many homes keep caged birds and their cheerful noise and fluttering do help to focus attention, as do tanks of tropical fish. On the other hand, the experience of having more mobile pets, such as dogs or cats, can prove beneficial.

Outdoor environment

It must be remembered that the environment is not just indoors. To be outside provides a host of sensations, as already mentioned, the wind blowing washing, or trees, and grass making patterns of light and shade. Sounds of birds, insects, passing traffic of all types, maybe cows lowing or sheep bleating, all provide auditory stimulus. Fire engines, police cars and ambulances make interesting noises. A child can be taken to a zoo or a market, shops or the seaside and, whilst initially they may not appear to notice the surroundings, further visits often provoke a reaction of some kind. For an immobile child, sand is only interesting because it can be felt, poured over his fingers or toes. For the child who is able to explore it more freely it can be something that is poured or dug, or raked, or thrown and just good fun. Water is interesting for nearly everyone, whatever the disability. It allows more freedom of movement and can be invaluable as an aid to gaining confidence. Again, it is an experience that has to be introduced gradually. Inflated arm bands will help to promote a feeling of security in a swimming bath, as will polystyrene floats.

Those of us who take our environment for granted, wherever we happen to be, unconsciously assimilate the stimuli with which we are being bombarded. The profoundly disabled child, whose awareness we are seeking to increase, needs the stimulus to be greater and as varied as possible to increase the range of his experience.

Music and movement

In these days of transistors, TV, videos and tape-recorders, music is freely available, with a large choice from the jingles of advertising to the grand operas and symphony concerts. A child needs the opportunity to hear them all, and most disabled children can display their feelings in some way about what they are listening to. An unending theme of background music of any sort is seldom noticed, but music played during a quiet time, or used as an accompaniment to movement is much more noticeable, and certain sounds can be associated with certain happenings.

A wheelchair dance group for multiply disabled children, with staff pushing the chairs, can be a huge success as the movement is not only anticipated, but also the music used for each move. Many people sing to their children from infancy, which encourages the children to listen and helps the learning of tunes. Similarly, though it may take longer, the disabled child may listen and assimilate a tune, even if he cannot reproduce it. Music can be a means of communication in group work, can help to establish rhythm and is usually a source of pleasure. Rhythmical movement is easier to perform and the range usually increases with practice. Exercises to music are often easier to do, and a tune can be associated with a movement. Action songs, for the more able, are popular.

Preventing deformity

The range of equipment in use for disabled children is wide and varied, the importance of correct positioning to prevent deformity and assist movement being underlined by the number of wheelchairs, special seats and individually designed seat moulds now being marketed. What is selected is a matter of choice, but it is essential to consider:

- how a particular item will be of benefit
- is it well designed and functional?
- is it strongly constructed (profoundly disabled children can tear and damage by picking and chewing)?
- does the use justify the expense?
- can it be easily cleaned (incontinence makes this a necessity)?

Equipment for positioning

Padded rolls and wedges, side-lying boards, prone boards and moulded shapes are basic for positioning, whilst large inflatable 36″ and 44″ balls have many uses (Fig. 10.3).

Mirrors, preferably large ones, will help with the understanding of body image, provide entertainment and sometimes puzzlement — 'Is that Me?' Standing frames, both fixed and tilting, can be bought commercially or made to measure by an orthotist.

Tilting tables are extremely useful and can be used to give a different perspective by gradually tilting towards the vertical, as well as tilting downwards. Children with flexion contractures of knees and/or hips should not be raised to such an angle that they are weight-bearing, but I have found that, with the footplate removed and the angle of tilt at no more than 45°, regular use of this position for short periods does seem to reduce the severity of the contracture. For the child who can bear weight it does improve

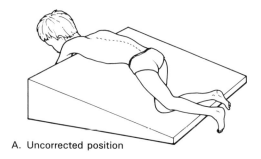

A. Uncorrected position

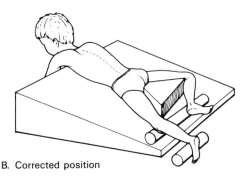

B. Corrected position

Fig. 10.3 Use of wedge with additional foam blocks to correct positioning in prone. (A) Uncorrected position. (B) Corrected position.

muscle tone and, with a table placed in front, allows hand usage. It has been noticed that some children who have had constant urinary infections improved considerably during long-term use of a tilting table, and one mother pointed out that her child had increased frequency of urine and no infection for 2 years, where previously she had never gone longer than about 6 weeks.

Equipment for movement

Large bed swings, hammocks of all descriptions, leaf-shaped swings and boat swings are freely available. They provide vestibular stimulation and relaxation. Water beds are very useful in many ways and are popular with nearly all patients, but do take up a large amount of space. Trampolines are obtainable in various shapes and sizes but should be used with some forethought — a very active child may have his energy channelled in a constructive way by the use of a trampoline, but the nervous, immobile child can be made to feel even more insecure.

In addition to the static equipment there is a huge range of specially adapted tricycles, prone trolleys, buggies, wheelchairs and push-along toys to encourage mobility. Many therapists, in conjunction with inventive parents, design one-off pieces of equipment for a particular child, or provide their own adaptation of a commercial one. For instance, a low coffee table, either square or oblong, provides a much more secure seat than a stool for a nervous child and allows the therapist room to work. If the top can be padded, so much the better.

Some centres have rooms specially constructed as totally soft play areas, with padded walls, slides, steps, hanging and vertical shapes, as well as a variety of wedges and rolls, all in very bright colours. They provide a safe play environment, but are expensive and perhaps of more benefit to the active child. Ball pools (Fig. 10.4) — padded tanks filled with bright coloured plastic balls — provide reward for movement, as they shift with each change of position, but no child should be put in a ball pool and left unattended because they may gradually sink down and disappear!

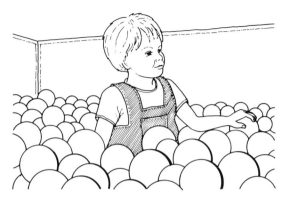

Fig. 10.4 A ball pool.

Motivation to move

The expanding field of electronics is providing much that is useful: a wide range of pressure switches can be activated by the smallest movement to control toys, lights, music, computer programmes and even wheelchairs. The possibilities are endless and proving invaluable for learning programmes. Work now being done with speech synthesisers for disabled young people is proving increasingly successful.

Most therapists also have their favourite small pocket-sized toys, used to attract a child — short lengths of chain with different sized links, a squeaky mouse, a bunch of keys, coloured ribbons or a small ball. These are useful as a talking point and help with initial contact. Teachers use many materials, paint, chalk, crayons, wooden inset puzzles of differing degrees of difficulty, musical toys, such as drums, wrist bells, maracas and rattles, stacking toys, skittles and so on, all with a view to encouraging the child's interest and will to learn and to move.

METHODS OF THERAPY

Having discussed treatment aims and the importance of rapport between therapist and child, environment and the necessity of increasing awareness, plus cooperation and communication between all staff and parents, the form of treatment or management chosen is based on the assessment and may be any of the well-known methods, i.e. Bobath or Temple Fay. More often the therapist may choose to be eclectic and use a combination of methods, most of which are discussed in other chapters (see Chapters 18 and 19 Treatment Systems and Treatment Methods). The need to set realistic targets must always be borne in mind, or the child will be discouraged from trying. It is no use to set a target of using a knife and fork if the child has no grasp and cannot hold a spoon! Holding a spoon is of little benefit with no hand to mouth movement. Whatever is done, the overall aim is to make the profoundly/multiply disabled child more aware of his surroundings, whilst being encouraged to move and explore his environment, and hopefully to gain some independence and self-help skills.

Every child needs the opportunity to achieve these aims, and workers will need continuing enthusiasm over a long period. Sometimes there is success in one area of development but not in another; often there may be setbacks through illness and very occasionally the years of work achieve little result. However, the rewards for giving the opportunity are enormous: the emergence of a personality, the achievement of each small goal, with the ensuing pleasure at the attainment of a new skill, are well worth the effort involved. Continuing research and increasing technology hold out greater hope for the profoundly disabled youngster than in any other time.

CASE STUDIES

The three case studies which follow highlight the aims of physiotherapy outlined above and describe various approaches which have been used when working with children with profound, multiple disabilities.

Objectives (see Case study 1)

Prevent self-mutilation and provide purposeful activity. Michael was provided with lightly boned arm gaiters to prevent the self-mutilation and fingering of his mouth, whilst attempts were made to distract his attention from himself. Sitting on a vibrating pad proved very popular, as did a hand-held vibrator moved over different areas of his body and, after some weeks, he would approach the therapist and drag her to

---

CASE STUDY 1

Michael, a profoundly and multiply disabled but very mobile teenager, presented with problems of:

- self-mutilation, particularly arms and face
- excessive salivation
- refusal to feed himself
- sore hands caused by constant fingering of the inside of his mouth, which had become slack and loose lipped
- not toilet-trained
- was unsociable and did not mix with others in the home where he lived.

Initial assessment showed no physical abnormalities other than an enlarged tongue and the loose-lipped mouth.

---

the vibrator. Gradually it was withdrawn as a source of distraction and used instead as a reward for purposeful and constructive movement. By this means he was induced to start throwing beanbags into buckets then retrieve them.

Encourage self-drinking and feeding. Michael was encouraged to use building blocks and simple wooden inset puzzles until gradually his manual dexterity improved, and the day came when the gaiters were removed and he was given a cup of milk to hold and attempt to drink. His first efforts were slight but over 6 months they improved considerably, particularly when it was discovered he liked cocoa.

During this time toilet training was instituted on a regular basis, success being reinforced by praise and a drink. He continued to finger his mouth if the gaiters were kept off and he had no other distractions. His drinking was continuing to improve, and he particularly enjoyed sitting with the staff when they had a drink.

To persuade him to start feeding himself proved more difficult when he refused to hold the spoon, throwing it to the floor continually. Again the vibrator was used as a reward for success, but only for a short time and under his chin. An attachment for the spoon made by the occupational therapist, kept it in his hand, and only one gaiter was removed for mealtimes. For many months he was assisted to feed himself with the spoon secured in his hand, and gradually he consented to grasp it, though still refusing to be independent. His diet was reviewed with more of his favourite food included, plus bananas, crisps, toast fingers, etc. that he could hold and eat independently. This proved more successful and he started using the spoon for feeding though, if he was stressed in any way, he reverted to food refusal.

Encourage positive activity. In the interim, various activities had been tried but Michael's concentration span was short; he was disinterested and wanted to wander away. It was then realised that he wanted to go on the large bed swing in the physiotherapy department where he was being treated. Allowed to use the swing, his pleasure was obvious and, during the time he spent on it, the mouthing stopped and the gaiters could be removed for quite long periods. Following this discovery it was decided to try a visit to the local swimming pool. At first he was very doubtful, but eventually consented to stand and splash, looking very surprised each time his hands hit the water. Further visits were made to the pool and the problem was to get him out!

Encourage contact with others. Eventually the self-mutilation had ceased, self-feeding had been instituted and a certain willingness to relate to others was becoming evident. The toilet-training was also progressing.

As he became more sociable, Michael began to point to what he wanted and his vocalisation began to have some meaning, making plain what he liked and disliked.

Outcome

After 5 years Michael was more sociable than previously, had acquired some self-help skills and was better toilet-trained than when the programme had started. The loose-lipped mouth was still something of a problem and drugs were being tried to control the excess salivation which, although improved, had not entirely ceased, causing soreness in the skin round his chin through the constant dribble. He loved being taken out in windy weather and would spin round in circles to show his pleasure.

Much of the success was due to the close co-operation of all the staff, who persevered very hard in the early days to carry out the therapist's suggestions, and were eventually rewarded by the changes that took place. The trust developed between the boy and the therapist allowed her to persuade him to undertake tasks that previously he would not attempt and, during a period when she was on holiday in the early years of treatment, he regressed, refusing to work with another person. As time went on and his confidence increased, his reliance on one person was less total, allowing for some staff changes.

It was noticed that the pleasure felt by everyone at the progress being made was reflected in the boy's attitude and general behaviour, so that he became a more acceptable member of the group in which he lived.

CASE STUDY 2

Jane, aged two, was small for her age and looked like a small baby. She was:

- blind
- microcephalic
- suffered from severe epilepsy
- was doubly incontinent
- had no self-help skills
- was bottle fed
- appeared to be very floppy with occasional twitching of her hands.

On initial assessment it was discovered that the floppy appearance was deceptive to some extent in that, when put into a prone position, she objected strongly and made attempts to move on to her side. She was also very sensitive to being handled by strangers. Her mother had never felt able to attempt anything other than bottle feeding, being frightened that the child might choke on solids. Much of the time Jane lay curled in a fetal position.

Objectives of Case Study 2

Increase tolerance to handling. It was decided to attempt to increase Jane's tolerance to handling by stroking, cuddling, talking and singing to her, followed by persuasion to active movement using her objection to being in prone as an incentive. There was also some emphasis on touching her face and mouth to prepare her for introduction to a spoon.

Eventually she accepted all of these goals, but it took nearly 3 years, as her programme was constantly interrupted by severe fits, after which she slept for long periods. She also had several urinary infections and a bout of pneumonia.

Encourage response to music. During this time it was found that Jane enjoyed music, providing it was not of the Radio 1 type, and would turn her head to follow sounds she enjoyed. Eventually it was hoped she might be able to use a pressure switch attached to her clothing to turn on a tape.

Begin spoon feeding. In the meantime the next objective was to start spoon feeding soft foods, and to try introducing finger foods like toast or sponge fingers.

Provide changes of position. We also arranged for her to have a small moulded seat insert, with harness, so that she could have another position than the variations of lying. The seat was provided but, apart from giving some support and a change of position, nothing further was achieved as Jane could not be persuaded to use her hands to actively explore toys, sand or water, and made no attempt to grasp. She tolerated some spoon feeding but made no attempt to chew in spite of repeated and prolonged efforts by the occupational therapist to teach her, but she did show preference for savoury type foods and strong dislike of fish, in whatever form, firmly shutting her mouth and turning her head away.

Outcome

The parents' marriage broke up with the strain of looking after the child, who was then taken into care. By the age of 12, repeated chest infections and minor illnesses had caused numerous setbacks for Jane and she was still extremely small for her age. In spite of continuing work to increase her awareness and instigate active movement she gradually deteriorated and finally died following a severe throat infection.

Objectives (see Case study 3)

Developing sitting balance. Initially it was decided to try putting Mary in an armchair in-

---

CASE STUDY 3

Mary had lived with elderly foster parents for all of her 11 years but, due to several moves round the country, had never had any treatment for a substantial length of time. When she first came to be assessed she screamed loudly whenever any attempt was made to touch her, at the same time hitting out in all directions and kicking her legs wildly. Her foster parents said she was:

- unable to sit and always lay on a couch at home
- spoon fed, although she spat out anything she did not like and would constantly put her fingers in the food in her mouth
- diagnosed as having a mitral valve defect in her heart, and defective vision
- mildly epileptic and doubly incontinent.

In the first instance the very caring, but exhausted, foster parents were persuaded to allow her to come into hospital for a short time, for continuous observation, when she finally calmed down. She remained in the hospital for a month, during which time her general muscle tone was noted to be good but there were signs of an incipient scoliosis, which it was felt could be left for a little while at this stage.

---

stead of leaving her lying down, but she promptly wriggled out on to the floor. She was next placed on a stool with a large bean bag behind it, in a sitting position and with the therapist firmly holding her knees down. For the first few times she threw herself backwards on to the bag but, as she was not helped up, she eventually consented to sit upright. From then on she always sat upright on a stool or straight chair, but would wriggle out of anything more comfortable.

Having made this gain she was rewarded with a chocolate button, and the therapist was rewarded by a smile for the first time!

Encourage purposeful use of grasp. The next problem was grasp. It was felt that Mary could grasp but was not willing to do so, and she also evinced a certain amount of manual dexterity in tearing her clothes and picking threads out of her jerseys. Various toys were tried and attempts to interest her in sand and water play were tried, but there was little response other than an occasional ear-splitting scream. However, arm gaiters prevented her destroying her clothes and, as she seemed to like noise, gloves that had a slot in the palm were fastened on her hands, a drumstick put in the slot and she was helped, to bang a drum. This proved a huge success. Before long the gloves were discarded and the drum would be banged loudly, with the drumsticks firmly held in her hand.

Develop self-feeding. It was time to start a feeding programme using a spoon — we already knew she had a good hand to mouth movement. The grasp of a spoon did not take long to achieve but, having done that, food was thrown far and wide and dishes pushed to the floor and broken. Discussions with the psychologist resulted in a programme of behaviour modification which, over a period of months, was reasonably effective — as long as she was being fed by the hospital or school staff. At home, in spite of much help and advice for the parents, she continued to misbehave, throwing food in all directions unless she was fed by them.

Develop standing skills. Apart from all this it was felt that she needed some work on standing and she was introduced to a tilting table, with the usual kicking and screaming, plus another development — biting. Having eventually settled down to this new experience, which gave her a different perspective, she would finger any object placed in front of her that made a noise, often discarding it on the floor, but willing to try something else. Her legs grew stronger, and the tilting table was exchanged for a made-to-measure standing frame.

Control scoliosis. By this time her scoliosis was becoming more marked and she was fitted with a Milwaukee brace which, to everyone's surprise, she accepted surprisingly well. At home she slept in a large hospital type cot and the mother reported that she was beginning to stand holding the bars whilst being dressed, so free standing holding a bar was included in her day-to-day schedule.

Outcome

Now 19 Mary can feed herself in situations away from home, no longer wears a brace and her scoliosis is controlled. She is still incontinent but is beginning to walk holding two hands. She can stand holding a bar and her behaviour has improved considerably, although she occasionally pulls viciously on any hair within reach and will bite a stranger. Work on a programme of dressing and undressing has resulted in her being able to remove her coat and hat and pull her jersey down if it is put over her head.

Her foster parents are delighted with her progress, finding that she will sit in the car without trouble, where previously she threw herself on the floor, and she is much easier to bathe because she now sits in the bath unsupported. At home, with help from the Social Services, a downstairs bathroom has been installed with a hoist to lift Mary in and out, as she is now too big for her foster parents to lift. She also sleeps downstairs.

The success of the work with Mary was largely a result of the unending perseverance of the physiotherapist, who refused to be intimidated by the noise and aggression displayed, patiently trying a large variety of ways to channel the aggression into something useful. The cooperation and support of nursing and teaching staff, plus the psychologist also played a large part. It does not appear likely that Mary will ever participate in community activities, but her behaviour is now more acceptable and she is slowly making some physical progress.

CONCLUSION

Present-day thinking, together with increased knowledge and technology, have immeasurably increased the opportunities for management and care of the profoundly/multiply handicapped, and rightly so. But the cost in terms of time, money, patience and emotional stress is high and, whilst opportunity for development has to be given, and the community at large is increasingly accepting the presence of profoundly disabled people in their midst, the very nature of the disability continues to isolate not only the child but the family. The long-term future of the people now resettled in the community is still a matter for deliberation.

POSTURE AND DEFORMITY
E. Bell

INTRODUCTION

The beginning of this chapter dealt with factors that might lead to physical deformity in children with profound and multiple disability.

This section will deal with the need to recognise the possible causes and problems resulting from incorrect positioning, and will suggest preventative action, which should become the therapeutic management for children with multiple disabilities.

THE EFFECTS OF IMMOBILITY

Everyone concerned in the daily life of a child with cerebral palsy and who may have multiple and profound handicap should be aware that the child's inability to change position will probably result in soft tissue shortening and moulding with a gradual decrease in, and ultimate loss of, range of joint movement. These can give rise to reduction or loss of function or can prevent the acquisition of function, leading to developmental delay and frustrational behaviour in the child.

Because of the nature and multiplicity of problems associated with cerebral palsy, deformities may develop as a result of the following physical factors:

- paresis
- muscle imbalance
- rigidity
- dynamic and/or congenital deformity
- spasticity
- growth
- malpositioning
- moulding and
- gravitational effects.

The child with moderate to severe cerebral palsy, who is incapable of changing position, and who displays signs of spasticity and who demonstrates unilateral head dominance may develop obliquity of the pelvis with 'windswept' hips. This may result in dislocation of the adducted, internally rotated hip and abduction and external rotation of the opposite hip. A varying and increasing degree of scoliosis may follow (see Fig. 10.1, p. 169).

Difficulties in handling may arise through time, and with growth, so that it can be almost impossible to place the child safely or comfortably in a chair (Fig. 10.5). Difficulties can also arise in feeding, dressing, changing and carrying the child, leading to anxiety before physical handling and pain, discomfort and stress during the procedure (see Chapter 17 Common Assessment Procedures).

Additional complications might be:

- pain
- loss of tissue viability
- skin lesions
- decreased respiratory incursion leading to repeated chest infections
- difficulties in feeding, swallowing and vocalisation.

Social, emotional and cognitive delays are also possible complications in the immobile child with severe physical handicap who has preserved reasoning and intellectual ability.

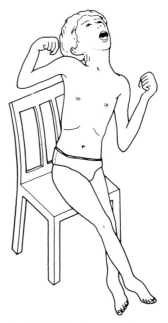

Fig. 10.5 Physical deformity preventing a child being placed safely or comfortably in sitting.

Immobility and positional deformity

There is little point in administering vigorous once-daily 'physiotherapy' sessions if the child is subsequently left in an ill-fitting chair, a sag bag or floor mat for the rest of the day (see Fig. 10.8 p. 183 — uncorrected position).

Leaving the child to assume, or, to remain in, the windswept position will have far-reaching physical effects and may compound developmental delays. It is necessary to govern position throughout the 24 hours of the day and night in the child showing signs of positional deformity and spasticity.

Children with severe disabilities resulting from cerebral palsy need to be helped both to experience and to be aware of normal movement through multiple sensory stimulation. As they develop and motor and sensory functions gradually improve, the problems of immobility are considerably reduced. Constant encouragement and support is needed so that these children gain the satisfaction of achievement and the development of skills. They learn self awareness and the world around them through exploring their own body and its relationship to their environment and its properties. Movement to music, soft play environments and use of texture described at the beginning of this chapter play a part in developing the concept of self.

When children have been provided with mobility and orthotic aids, they are encouraged to move independently and to explore, to become more alert, more physically robust and vocalisation improves. This increased motivation results in improved development, as the child is enabled to take advantage of experiential learning.

MANAGING THE MOVEMENT REGIME

The physical therapeutic regime must begin as early as 2 months old to prevent deformity and to facilitate child development. The regime should also be planned in such a way that it can be carried out continuously during a 24-hour period, 7 days a week.

It is vital that parents or carers or both receive encouragment, support and guidance to carry out the appropriate activities and positioning schedules from the earliest opportunity, before deformities and distortions arise.

Early treatment

As the deformities of the windswept position can develop within the first 10 months of life, it is advised that a regular physical management programme of the baby is established as soon as possible after birth or when a diagnosis of cerebral palsy is first suspected. The earliest possible opportunity should be taken by the physiotherapist to recognise and prevent these malpositioning windsweeping deformities.

Parental involvement

Management of the control and prevention of positional deformity should be seen in the context of the total management of a child within and by its own family.

The therapist must work towards building up a trusting and supportive but not dominant relationship with the family and should advise on management without disruption of the whole family.

Without support at home, obsessional following of the regime could cause tensions and stress, with no allowance being made for the needs of the rest of the family. Means of family support may be sought through social services, through voluntary carer groups or from the extended family.

The importance of family involvement cannot be over-emphasised because the types of deforming positions which may develop require constant attention. The way in which a child is handled and the method by which movement is facilitated can assist or greatly reduce the threat of positional deformity.

Families with experience of a 24-hour regime might help by sharing their experience with a family new to such a regime.

Parents need to be supported in their choice to follow the advised therapeutic management plan and activities. The therapist must discuss and demonstrate clearly the need for the regime described below and its role in the future welfare of the child.

THE 24-HOUR REGIME

Parents and all carers should be educated and encouraged to change the position of the child at least every 2 hours during the day and at night if possible.

A typical regime will include changes between the following positions:

- lying — including side-lying
- sitting
- standing.

The experience of movement (particularly through trunk and head rotations) is crucial to child development. Passive movements and facilitation techniques are useful in achieving this (see Chapter 18 Treatment Systems).

The child with movement difficulties needs to be placed in positions for play, feeding (Fig. 10.6), learning and communication which not only inhibit abnormal posture and deforming positions, but which encourage and enhance normal movement patterns, exploratory play and thereby promote a sense of achievement in both parents and child.

Normal gross motor developmental progression is from the establishment of eye contact, head control in midline, hand use, pulling to sit, side-lying, sitting, rolling over, prone-lying, coming up through trunk rotation into standing and walking unaided.

Frequent changes of position during the day and night not only help to prevent deformity but also mean that the child gains different sensory experiences.

Record charts

Accurate recording forms the basis of planning an effective regime of positioning to prevent and/or correct deformity.

By monitoring the range of movement a child achieves both actively and passively, a check is maintained on problems and progress. Sequential charting is used to assist detection of potentially deforming signs and situations and the development of positional deformities.

Relevant factors to record include:

- asymmetry of neck rotation (this could

A. Incorrect

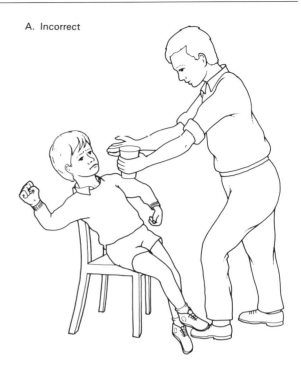

B. Correct

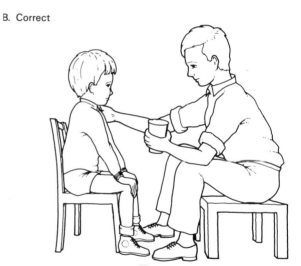

Fig. 10.6 Correct positioning for feeding. Note the level of eye contact, position of arms and feet and the placing of support of the carer's right hand. (A) Incorrect. (B) Correct.

precede a frank head preference)
- preferred head position
- presence of an asymmetrical tonic neck reflex (ATNR)
- presence and detail of scoliosis

- asymmetry of hip rotation
- windsweeping position.

Positions to encourage

The normal child moves easily and frequently from one position to another. The profoundly disabled child needs the help of parents and carers to experience these necessary changes in position.

Standing

Well-controlled standing, with the child symmetrically placed in a standing frame is an important position because full weight-bearing through the hip joints has been shown on electromyogram (EMG) to show less tonic activity than sitting or lying. Scoliosis is secondary to pelvic obliquity and hip dislocation and it is therefore most important to ensure that the pelvic and pectoral limb girdles are kept in alignment with the spine straight (Fig. 10.7). Midline symmetry, hand to mouth and hand–eye contact are to be encouraged at all times.

Positioning and movement of a child are part of the therapy programme and are enjoyably beneficial for many severely handicapped youngsters. However, care should be taken that adverse tonic activity is not precipitated, e.g. neck retraction and tonic extension of the whole arm, preventing hand to mouth, reach and grasp. Unless this abnormal posturing and the tonic neck asymmetry are inhibited through careful position-

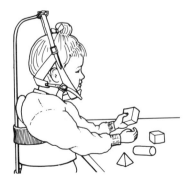

Fig. 10.7 Well-controlled standing with a symmetrical position, forearm support and head support.

ing and support, tissue shortening and uneven weight-bearing further precipitate the aquisition of positional deformities (see Chapter 18 Treatment Systems).

Sitting

Sitting is an important position because it is the one from which most children will engage in social activity and communication with others. However, even appropriate seating can present difficulties if the child stays in one position for too long and a 'sitting position' deformity may result, with flexed hips and knees.

Continuous observation is also required to ensure that the child does not slide down in the seat. The resulting shoulder retraction, neck extension, arched back and open jaw mean that all attempts by the child to reach forwards, look at a toy, or communicate purposefully will be frustrated (Fig. 10.8). Trial and error will be needed to devise the most appropriate positioning of cushions, rolls, wedges and straps to maintain a good functional position which is comfortable and acceptable to the child and which does not limit excessively already restricted movement.

Care must be taken that moulded and modular seating systems do not reinforce positional deformity and spasticity in some children (Brown & Fulford 1976) instead of being an antidote. A modular seat may be an adjunct to care and management but may not be as effective as the described positioning regime (see Chapter 21 Aids and Appliances).

Wheelchairs require individual adaptation and needs must be very carefully assessed (see Chapter 21 Aids and Appliances). As with other equipment, all straps and corrective padding must:

- maintain the desired correction
- maintain postural alignment
- maintain control of hypertonus
- ensure evenness of weight distribution.

Attention must be paid to inhibition of the stretch reflex and also to ensure that the correct proprioceptive stimulation will produce the desired motor feedback.

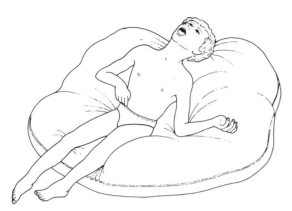

Fig. 10.8 Problems result when the child slides down in the seat. Note the position of the head, jaw and trunk and the lack of balance and saving reactions.

Table 10.1 The use of side-lying to reduce deformity

Problem	Position	Reason
Head preference to right, minimal scoliosis convex to left	Right side-lying	Discourage further head rotation scoliosis control by gravitational pull
Scoliosis convex to right	Right side-lying	Scoliosis control by foam wedge under trunk
Adductor spasticity. Legs windswept to left		Foam wedge between legs to control hip adduction and align legs with trunk

The sides of the wheelchair should be removed as much as is safe and possible to encourage self-propulsion, exploration and socialisation.

Lying

Side-lying is a particularly useful position for the correction of deformity (Fig. 10.9). Many of the effects of gravity are eliminated and it is a position in which children are able to bring their hands together, to hold a toy and make purposeful arm movements, and to establish eye–hand contact. The choice of side upon which to place the child depends on an accurate assessment and recording of the child's deformities (Table 10.1).

Foam wedges and apparatus used for positioning should be measured and recorded on the positioning chart, together with changes which are noted on regular review and reassessment.

Lying in supine should be avoided except when used to engage the child actively in activities involving arm reach and eye contact (Fig. 10.10). It can otherwise become a passive and potentially deforming position.

Positioning at night

It is accepted by many therapists that, no matter how carefully a child may be positioned and facilitated to move during the day, the positive effects of this care will be considerably reduced if the child is allowed to assume deforming postures while asleep.

Night positioning is crucial in the complete management of positional deformity and should follow these guidelines:

- obtain and maintain symmetrical alignment between shoulder and pelvic girdles
- keep head in midline with spine straight
- keep hips symmetrically abducted
- allow for some small degree of spontaneous movement within correct alignments
- ensure parents and carers are taught appropriate methods of turning the child through the night-time positions.

Individual positioning programmes should be devised for each child, with particular attention being paid to corrective positions if the child has acquired positional deformities.

Intercurrent illness

General health improves in many children who undergo this 24-hour regime, with diminution of recurrence of chest infections and the reduced need for vigorous respiratory physiotherapy and suction care.

However, when intercurrent illness, such as acute chest infections, uncontrolled epilepsy, urinary tract infection or episodes of surgery occur, it may be necessary to relax the positioning regime. This may predispose the child to the development of deformities. The attention of

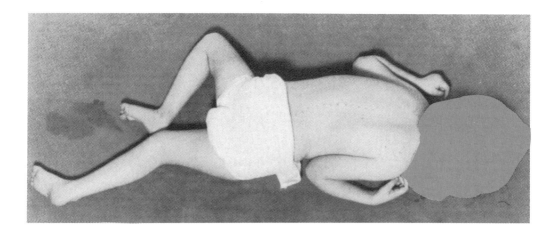

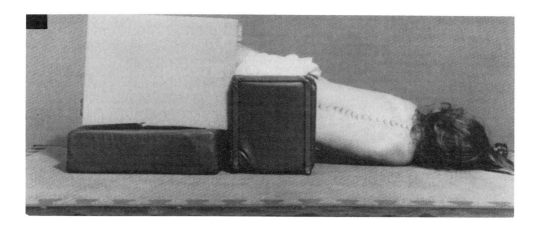

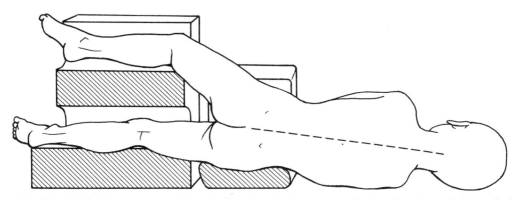

Fig. 10.9 Use of side lying to correct deformity. The U wedge is moved, effectively 'hanging-out' the scoliosis. The foot of the upper leg projects beyond the abduction block, the weight of the head thus keeping the leg in external rotation (reproduced by permission of Laurence Earlbaum Associates Ltd from Bell E, Watson A 1985 Deformity: the prevention of positional deformity in cerebral palsy. Physiotherapy Practice 1: 86–92).

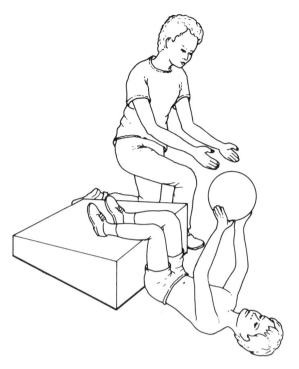

Fig. 10.10 Effective use of supine lying. Note the use of a wedge to correct pelvic alignment.

ward staff should be drawn to correct use of the child's own equipment and the choice of management methods.

Equipment

Equipment should be individually tailored to meet specific problems of each child.

The aim of lying, sitting and standing aids is to maintain a stable, well-aligned position from which a child may be encouraged to develop movement range and skills (including spontaneous postural adjustments).

Attention must be paid to the safety aspects of materials. Flame-retardant foam, fire-retardant covers which are easily washed, and non-toxic paint on wooden frames should be used.

Foam blocks are cut to shape and placed within a simple wooden three-sided box-like frame.

• For side lying — a U-shaped, angled block allowing 30 degrees of movement thereby relieving constant pressure on one point.

• Hip symmetry is maintained with a foam abduction block having channels for each leg. This allows slight knee flexion/extension and external hip rotation — the heel hanging free.

• Corrective dome-shaped pressure pads may be used to correct scoliosis. The weight and position of the topmost leg may be used for gravitational correction, whilst the spine is wedged into a corrective position with the child in side-lying.

The depth and position of the correctional wedges are determined by the degree of correction possible and the position and complexity of the scoliosis.

SUMMARY

Physiotherapists should be involved in assessment and care of children with cerebral palsy or with the suspicion of developmental abnormalities from a very early age. Therapists are responsible for helping the families to understand the problems, undertake the positioning regime and to encourage rational developmental stimulation of their own children.

The family and the care and education staff require an awareness of the importance of regular corrective positional changes, the need for facilitation of normal movement and for the encouragement of developmental skills. They need to understand the factors responsible for abnormal posture and for poor or inadequate positioning.

Cooperation of everyone concerned with the positioning and movement regime for a child should lead to minimising and helping to prevent the development of abnormal posture leading to positional deformity, thereby encouraging development and enhancing the quality of life for the child and its family.

ACKNOWLEDGEMENTS

The author (E. B.) wishes to acknowledge the advice of Alys Watson, Senior Physiotherapist, Scottish Council for Spastics, Edinburgh, in the preparation of the section on Posture and Deformity.

REFERENCES

Brown K, Fulford J 1976 Position as a cause of deformity in children with cerebral palsy. Developmental Medicine and Child Neurology 18(3)

Brudenell P 1986 The other side of profound handicap. Macmillan Education Series

FURTHER READING

Evans P, Ware J 1987 Special care provision. NFER Nelson, Windsor

Finnie N 1974 Handling the young cerebral palsied child at home, 2nd edn. William Heinemann Medical Books, London

Gordon N, McKinley I (eds) 1986 Neurologically handicapped children — treatment and management. Blackwell Scientific Publications, Oxford

Hogg J, Sebba J 1986 Profound retardation and mulitiple impairment. Croom Helm, London

Levitt S 1982 Treatment of cerebral palsy and motor delay, 2nd edn. Blackwell Scientific Publications, Oxford

McCarthy G (ed) 1984 The physically handicapped child — an interdisciplinary approach to management. Faber & Faber, London

Oswin M 1984 They keep going away. Critical study of short term residential care services for children who are mentally handicapped. Oxford University Press, Oxford

Russell O 1985 Mental handicap. Churchill Livingstone, Edinburgh

11

Neuromuscular disorders

W. J. K. Cumming

INTRODUCTION

Neuromuscular disorders in childhood are amongst the most challenging of conditions, not only from the point of view of diagnosis, but also with respect to management. Incorrect diagnosis, and/or inappropriate management may affect the subsequent course of the child's development. As many neuromuscular disorders are progressive such consequences may well prove to be irremedial and it is of great importance that the child is investigated thoroughly at the onset of the disease to ensure that the diagnosis is correctly established. Management of the child's disease is not the province of a single individual but requires a team approach where the role of the physiotherapist is often central.

THE INVESTIGATION OF A CHILD WITH A NEUROMUSCULAR DISORDER

History

A detailed history of the child's disability is the starting point of investigation. It is unusual to obtain the history in full at a single clinic visit as the parents are usually markedly anxious on first contact and may still be pondering the first few questions when subsequent questions are asked. Indeed, the relevance of some of the questions may seem obscure to them; for example, they may not understand the point of asking about delay in motor milestones when they have brought along a 9-year-old who has been suffering from the disorder for a few months only.

Ideally, therefore, the family should be interviewed again after they have had time to ponder the questions and formulate answers.

The duration of the disorder is often difficult to determine as muscle weakness may present insidiously; a child with weakness of the legs that has been apparent for a few months only, but in whom there is also a history of delayed motor milestones and poor athletic activity as compared to other normal children, will have a totally different disorder from the child who was as active as his peers until the time the parents first noticed the disability.

As many of the neuromuscular disorders are inherited, a detailed family history has to be obtained, which may include examination of relatives who, although they consider themselves to be normal, may exhibit early signs of neuromuscular disease.

Distribution of weakness

From the history, the distribution of the weakness may be classified into two broad categories:

1. Proximal — in the upper limbs, difficulties in using the arms above the head and, in the lower limbs, problems with climbing stairs, pushing up from a seat and getting out of a bath.
2. Distal — difficulties in the upper limbs with fine hand and wrist movement and, in the lower limbs, tripping or wearing out the fronts of shoes.

It will also be possible to tell whether or not the weakness is symmetrical. It is important to know if the weakness is episodic (as, for example, in periodic paralysis or myasthenia gravis), static or progressive.

Physical examination
Muscle weakness

Physical examination is undertaken to determine the pattern of muscle weakness. It appears that four patterns of weakness account for the majority of disorders irrespective of the aetiology:

1. Limb girdle (LG) (Fig. 11.1A). The majority of disorders (about 75%) exhibit an LG pattern. Weakness in LG affects the proximal upper and lower limb girdles.
2. Fascioscapulohumeral (FSH) (Fig. 11.1B). Approximately 20% of disorders have an FSH pattern. Weakness is seen in the obicularis oculi and oris and the proximal upper limb girdle. Striking weakness of serratus anterior may lead to marked scapular winging. The distal upper limb and all the leg muscles are spared.
3. Scapuloperoneal (SP) (Fig. 11.1C). This pattern affects about 4% of cases. The weakness is similar to that in the upper limbs in FSH but also involves the anterior lower leg muscles.
4. Distal (D) (Fig. 11.1D). This pattern affects about 1% of cases. The forearm, intrinsic hand muscles and anterior and posterior lower leg muscles are involved.

With disease progression the four types of presentation of muscle weakness tend to merge into a common end-stage involvement, which is at that stage indistinguishable. There is evidence from computerised tomographic (CT) scanning of muscle that the clinical subdivision into four groups is more apparent than real, as the CT scan, which reveals changes in muscle that are present prior to the development of muscle weakness, cannot distinguish between the four types of clinical presentation (Sambrook et al 1988).

Hypertrophy of muscles, commonly the gastrocnemius and soleus group, but sometimes other muscle groups, is often seen and in these cases the muscles have a firm, rubbery consistency. The degree of symmetry and selectivity of muscle involvement may help in determining the underlying disorder. Primary disorders of the muscle cell (the 'myopathic' disease) usually show symmetry without selectivity. Disorders consequent upon anterior horn cell disease (the 'neurogenic' disease) commonly show asymmetry and selectivity of involvement (Fig. 11.2).

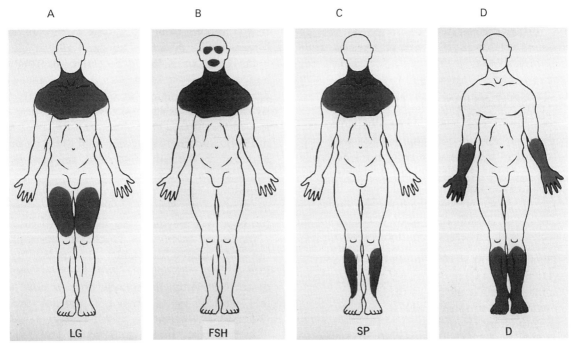

Fig. 11. 1 (A–D) Schematic representation of muscle weakness.

Other investigations

Further investigations are now required and are 'invasive'.

Blood tests

A blood sample is taken for the estimation of serum creatinine kinase (CK), which is moderately to markedly elevated in the primary myopathic disorders and mildly to moderately elevated in the neurogenic disorders. Electrophysiological investigation involves sampling several muscles with a concentric needle electrode (EMG) and the estimation of conduction velocity and terminal latency in the peripheral nerves (NCV). These techniques help to determine if the disorder lies in the anterior horn cell, the peripheral nerve or the muscle.

Imaging of muscle using CT, ultrasound or radioisotopes remains a research tool at present, but may become of considerable importance in the future, particularly in following the progression of the disease.

Muscle biopsy

All patients require a muscle biopsy to determine the pathological state of the muscle. Biopsies are commonly taken from the vastus lateralis either via a surgical incision (the 'open' technique) or via a trocar (the 'needle' technique). The preparation of muscle biopsy samples is complex and should only be undertaken in specialised neuromuscular laboratories. A detailed description of electrophysiological and muscle biopsy

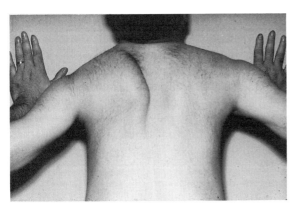

Fig. 11.2 Unilateral weakness of serratus anterior in neurogenic disease.

techniques is outside the scope of this chapter and further details will be found in the appropriate references (Barwick & Fawcett 1988, Pamphlett 1988).

CLASSIFICATION OF THE NEUROMUSCULAR DISORDERS

In the past, various eponymous titles were used for disorders that are now recognised as similar diseases. Although the increasing sophistication of investigation constantly provides new diseases, many of these are single cases or individual families. The classification below accounts for the majority of the diseases commonly seen:

- Duchenne and Becker muscular dystrophy (DMD/BMD)
- spinal muscular atrophies (SMA)
- myotonic dystrophy (MyD)
- inflammatory myopathy
  — polymyositis/dermatomyositis (PM/DM)
  — viral
  — granulomatous
  — infective
- congenital myopathy
- metabolic myopathy
  — periodic paralysis
  — glycogen disorders
  — lipid disorders
  — mitochondrial disorders
- neuromuscular junction disorders
  — myasthenia gravis (MyG)
  — congenital myasthenia
- peripheral neuropathy
  — inherited polyneuropathy.

Muscular dystrophy

Duchenne and Becker muscular dystrophy (DMD/BMD).

Aetiology

Duchenne dystrophy is the most common and most severe form of muscular dystrophy. Recent advances in the field of molecular biology have led to the identification of the gene defect in the condition (at site 21 on the short arm of the X chromosome: Xp2l) and have also identified the protein coded for by the gene — dystrophin — that is missing from the muscle membrane in all boys with the disorder (Rowland 1989).

DMD is an X-linked recessive disorder and hence the disease is expressed in the male and carried by the female who, on rare occasions, may show minor muscle weakness (manifesting carrier). It is thought that about two-thirds of cases of DMD are due to inheritance of the gene defect and that, in the remaining third, the gene defect has arisen as a new mutation.

Despite these advances in understanding of the aetiology of the disease, no 'cure' is available and the boys will inevitably die from the disease.

(Although therapy for Duchenne dystrophy is not immediately available, the possibility of introducing myoblasts, which will express dystrophin within the muscle fibre, is now possible, and is called myoblast transfer therapy (Kakulas 1990, Karpati 1990, Law et al 1988). This is a fairly major undertaking and requires immunosuppression, since it is a foreign cell. The possibility of being able to introduce dystrophin directly via gene transfer has now been shown to be feasible in the experimental animal (Lee et al 1991), though this has not yet been extended to the patients with DMD.)

Pathological features

The pathological features of DMD depend on the age of the boy at the time of biopsy. Within the first few months of life, the only abnormality in the muscle biopsy is the presence of hyaline fibres. These fibres represent damaged myofibres where, because of the presence of excess intracellular calcium (Ca^{2+}), the muscle fibre becomes irrevocably committed to cell necrosis. Initially regeneration can keep pace with necrosis, but eventually it fails, so that persisting necrosis leads to replacement of muscle fibres by connective tissue and fat. By the time the boys lose the ability to walk the muscle biopsy shows marked variation in fibre size, split fibres and replacement of fibres by fat and connective tissue. It is readily apparent that a muscle fibre that is smaller than normal, split and wrapped up in a sea of fibrous tissue, cannot exert its normal tensile strength, thus leading to muscle weakness (Fig. 11.3).

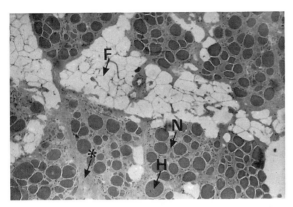

Fig. 11.3 Late stage Duchenne dystrophy (aged 9 years) showing marked variation in fibre size with the presence of necrotic (N) and hyaline (H) fibres. There is a marked excess of fibrous tissue (*) which is both endomysial and perimysial. There is replacement of muscle tissue by fat (F).

Dystrophin is one of a group of cytoskeletal proteins that stabilise the muscle membrane. The exact mechanism whereby lack of dystrophin leads to muscle fibre loss is not, as yet, understood (Barkhaus & Gilchrist 1989).

Management

Management of DMD falls into two groups:

- management of the boy with DMD
- support for the family caring for a boy with DMD.

Management of the boy with DMD. A boy with DMD will spend roughly half of his life ambulant and half in a wheelchair.

Although the disease is present from birth, as manifested by massive elevation of the CK (levels of 20–25 000, normal <120 IU/l, being common) and abnormalities in the muscle biopsy, unless there has been a previous affected boy in the family, the usual age of presentation is around 3–4 years.

The parents give a history of delay in motor milestones, with walking often delayed up to 18 months of age, and the boys rarely learn to run or hop. They exhibit the so-called Gowers' manoeuvre (Fig. 11.4A–D) when rising from the floor, where, because of weakness in the lower limb girdle, they are unable to rise normally to a standing position and 'walk-up' their legs. Examination reveals an LG pattern of weakness with characteristic calf hypertrophy.

It is at this time that the boy exhibits his best muscle strength. With advancing age, up to about 7–8 years, there is a slow progression of weakness. Contracture of the Achilles tendon develops and, unless treated by passive stretching and night-splints where indicated, the boy will 'go-off' his legs earlier than needed.

At times of growth spurts, the boy may appear to be improving his muscle strength and this, unless explained to the parents, may give them false hope. Explanations about the progressive nature of the disease must be given sensitively at this stage.

The upper limbs are involved at this stage, but to a lesser extent than the lower limbs. From the age of 7–8 years there is progressive decline in function, with the boy losing the ability to climb stairs and subsequently the ability to rise from the floor unaided. When the latter function is lost, wheelchair dependence usually occurs within 12–18 months. As the boy is losing the ability to walk it is important that mobility is encouraged and long-leg calipers are employed to maintain standing. The importance of this is that the longer the boy is kept in the upright position the more the development of scoliosis is delayed. In the majority of cases between the ages of 11–13 years the boys become wheelchair-confined. Psychologically this is often a major trauma for the family, although the boys are usually pleased at their increased mobility. As the parents have considerable contact with their physiotherapist it is usually the latter who helps the family through this time.

During the wheelchair years, particularly in the first few years, the maintenance of an upright posture by the provision of standing frames and 'clickers' is again important.

Scoliosis will develop in the majority of boys, although a few will lock in extension and thus maintain a relatively curve-free back. Although the vital capacity has started to fall before scoliosis supervenes, the rate of loss of ventilatory function increases with increasing scoliosis. For this reason orthopaedic correction of the scoliosis may be not only necessary but also desirable.

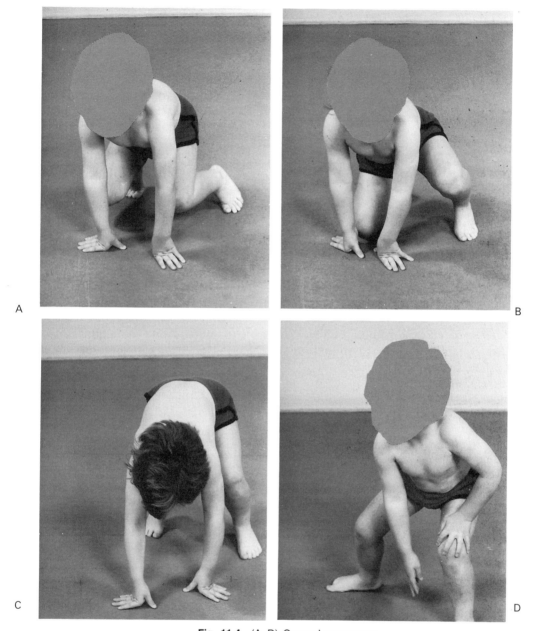

Fig. 11.4 (A–D) Gowers' manoeuvre.

During the wheelchair years upper limb function is progressively lost and increasing contractures develop at ankles, knees, hips and eventually elbows. These require constant attention. With progressive loss of lung function, scoliosis and immobility, chest infections supervene and require aggressive therapy. Breathing exercises help in this situation, as does teaching the parents postural drainage and suction techniques.

Although heart muscle is affected in DMD it is rarely a clinical problem because of the loss of mobility. However, the boy will eventually die from cardiorespiratory disease between the ages of 18 and 22. At all stages of the boy's life, therapy is directed to reducing the consequences of the disease.

Family support. The parents of a boy with DMD will require long-term help and support throughout the boy's life and often also after his death. They have to come to terms with the fact that the disease is incurable and will end in death, but that this will be many years delayed.

As the disease is carried by the female, it is vitally important that the carrier status of the mother, and also her first degree female relatives, is determined. If they are shown to carry a deletion of the gene for dystrophin at Xp2l then they require genetic counselling regarding future pregnancy. The burden of a boy with DMD in a family is great and the occurrence of a second or subsequent affected boy in the nuclear or extended family should be preventable. Easy access to a department of medical genetics, which can investigate and counsel the family, is therefore required.

Once the diagnosis of DMD has been established, the family have need of the services not only of the medical staff, but also physiotherapists, social workers, specialist and community care staff and the medical genetics department. The burden of attending several different clinics with a handicapped child, when the parents are just coming to terms with the diagnosis, can lead to resentment. Provided the mother or her first degree female relatives are not pregnant, or contemplating pregnancy in the immediate future, the involvement of other health care professionals can be delayed until the family can cope with the extra pressures.

As the boy's disability increases, the family requires advice and help in selecting appropriate aids, dealing with the local Social Services and the provision of home improvements, schooling (best undertaken in a school for the physically handicapped), holidays and the emotional demands of the boy. Only a team approach to the boy and family with DMD will help in these situations.

Becker muscular dystrophy (BMD)

This disease, which is now known to be allelic to DMD (Fischbeck 1989), may be considered as the less severe variant of DMD. The absolute level of dystrophin is reduced as compared to normal, but not absent as in DMD, and dystrophin is present in the muscle membrane although its distribution in the individual fibre is patchy (Nicholson et al 1989a, b). The disease follows the same course as in DMD, although the age of presentation is later (5–15 years) and may be delayed into adult life. The progression of the disease is much slower than for DMD with boys ambulant up to 25–45 years. Pathologically the features are similar in the two disorders but again much less severe in BMD. The same principles of management apply to BMD as to DMD.

Spinal muscular atrophies (SMA)

The SMAs constitute the second most common childhood neuromuscular disorder. The pathological features of the disease are due to anterior horn cell death, the cause of which is unknown.

Types of SMA

SMA is subdivided on the basis of age of onset:

- SMA 1 (Werdnig–Hoffmann) onset birth–12 months
- SMA 2 (Kugelberg–Welander) onset 1–4 years
- SMA 3 onset late childhood, adolescent and adult.

Excluding SMA 1, which presents as a 'floppy-infant' (Fig. 11.5), SMA 2 and 3 present as an LG, FSH or SP syndrome. As the pathological basis of the disease is in the anterior horn cell of the spinal cord, the clinical picture is that of a neurogenic disorder, i.e. exhibiting asymmetric and selective involvement of muscle. The serum CK is normal or mildly raised. EMG studies reveal signs of denervation with giant motor units.

The muscle biopsy changes in SMA depend on the age of the child and the severity of the muscle weakness.

Pathology

In the normal individual, the anterior horn cell supports the muscle fibre through its axon. The terminal portion of the axon branches and a fine

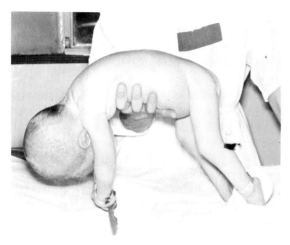

Fig. 11.5 Gross hypotonia in a child with Werdnig–Hoffmann disease aged 8 months.

twiglet of nerve attaches to the muscle at the neuromusclar junction. A single anterior horn cell supports hundreds of muscle fibres, which are distributed throughout the muscle rather than being grouped together. If an anterior horn cell dies, the muscle fibres it supports atrophy and become small, ribbon-like and atrophic. As the fibres from a single anterior horn cell are scattered in the muscle, so the atrophic fibres are also scattered. Provided the nerves close to an atrophic fibre are healthy, they can sprout and annex the atrophic fibres, which subsequently redevelop to normal size (Fig. 11.6). There are two major fibre types (Type I, Type II; slow, fast; glycolytic, oxidative) and the muscle fibre type

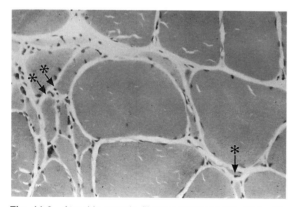

Fig. 11.6 Atrophic muscle fibres occurring both singly (*) and in groups (**).

depends on the type of the parent nerve. Normally when the nerves are scattered, the fibre types show a checkerboard pattern. As reinnervation proceeds this pattern is lost as more and more fibres of the same type occur together, showing the pattern of grouped reinnervation. When one of the nerves that, in addition to its original muscle fibre complement, has annexed large numbers of atrophic fibres, dies, then groups of atrophic fibres are seen occurring together.

This process of denervation with subsequent reinnervation of the muscle fibres forms the basis of SMA. If denervation is proceeding rapidly, with little in the way of reinnervation, then a severe form of disease results — SMA 1. The moderately severe forms seen in early childhood represent SMA 2 and the more benign forms, SMA 3, are seen in late childhood, adolescence and adult onset disease.

SMA 1 (Werdnig–Hoffmann). The child with SMA 1 is usually born floppy, with little or no muscle tone, poor feeding and often respiratory weakness. However, the disease may not present for up to 6 months, when it is recognised that the child has poor head control and is not attempting to sit unsupported. The condition is relentlessly progressive with death, from respiratory insufficiency, occurring by 2 years at the latest. No form of therapy is available.

SMA 2 (Kugelberg–Welander). This group of SMA presents a major management problem. The group is further subdivided into 2a and 2b on the basis of whether the child achieves the ability to walk. In 2a, the child shows delay in motor development and never learns to walk; in 2b there may or may not be delay in motor development but the child does walk, only to lose this ability with the passage of time.

Investigation of these children shows a mild to moderate elevation of the serum CK, giant units on EMG, and muscle biopsy evidence of denervation with incomplete reinnervation.

In SMA 2a, the child will be confined to a wheelchair at an early stage. Contracture is a major feature and requires active intervention, up to and including surgical release. Given that bone development is to some extent dependent on normal muscle pull, scoliosis is a prominent feature, with resulting respiratory difficulties. Careful attention to chest disease is therefore crucial.

Despite their severe physical abnormalities, these children have in most cases a relatively slow progression and long-term survival into adult life is common. If, however, the intercostal muscles are involved, the prognosis is poor.

SMA 3. SMA 2b and the late childhood and early adolescent forms of SMA 3 are much more benign disorders. The progression is very slow, with long periods of apparent arrest of muscle weakness. It is important, therefore, that walking ability is maintained by correction of contracture and the provision of physical aids as required. Survival to adult life is the rule, although there may be some degree of physical handicap.

The gene locus responsible for the common forms of SMA has recently been identified on the long arm of chromosome 5 (5q11.2–13.3) (Brzustowicz et al 1990, Gilliam et al 1990). However, the gene product is as yet unknown. There is a rare X-linked adult form of SMA, which is associated with gonadal abnormalities (Kennedy syndrome), in which the gene locus is on the long arm of the X chromosome.

A family history of SMA is seen in about 50% of cases. It is in this disease in particular where a careful examination of all first degree relatives is important. The manifestations of SMA 3 may be sufficiently mild that the individual considers himself to be normal. If such cases are missed, then incorrect genetic advice may be given on the basis of an isolated case when in fact the disease is inherited.

The patients with SMA 2b and 3 who, on examination, show the SP distribution of weakness have a particular risk of developing cardiac abnormalities. Cardiac conduction defects, which may require pacing, can develop at any time and a few cases develop a cardiomyopathy. The reasons for this cardiac involvement are unknown.

Myotonic dystrophy (MyD)

This disease is characterised by the presence of distal weakness and myotonia (delayed relaxation). It is predominantly a disease of adult life with the onset of myotonia in the teens and weakness in the 30s–40s. The gene defect responsible for the disease has been located to chromosome 19 (19q13.2) (Shaw et al 1989). In addition to muscle involvement, there are widespread abnormalities in other systems with the development of cataracts, frontal balding, facial weakness and wasting of the sternomastoids, cardiac involvement, poor or absent contraction of oesophagus, stomach, gall bladder (leading to gallstone formation), small and large intestine, diabetes mellitus due to end-organ unresponsiveness to insulin, and gonadal failure. The importance of recognising this disorder is that there is a congenital form of the disease, which presents at birth or early infancy. For reasons that are not understood, the congenital form of the disease is seen only in children born to mothers who have the condition. An affected mother may produce a normal child, who has not inherited the gene defect, or a child who has inherited the defect but who presents in the typical manner for the disease, but she can also produce a child who has inherited the defect which presents as a severe form of disability in infancy — congenital MyD. This sydrome is characterised by hypotonia, a curious frog-like appearance to the mouth associated with respiratory and feeding difficulty. Some infants require ventilatory support from birth. These children do not show myotonia either clinically or on EMG and confirmation of the diagnosis depends on recognising the disease in the mother. If the child survives the first few months of life, they are usually severely physically and mentally handicapped.

Inflammatory myopathy

The various types of inflammatory myopathy are as follows:

Polymyositis/dermatomyositis complex

The most common form of inflammatory myopathy seen in practice is Polymyositis/Dermatomyositis complex (PM/DM). This complex is an important group to recognise as the disorder is treatable to full recovery in most cases (Cumming 1989).

Characteristics. The disease is characterised by proximal muscle weakness, which is symmetrical and non-selective. It is often associated with muscle pain, especially with or following exercise. In DM, in addition to the muscle weakness, there is an associated rash. This is found around the eyelids, across the malar region, on the extensor surfaces of the fingers and occasionally at the elbows and the extensor surfaces of the legs. The rash is a reddish/purple discoloration and is not painful. The majority of children with PM/DM complex present with the DM variant.

History. The history is usually of a few months' duration with increasing weakness to the point of becoming bedfast in a few cases. An acute presentation is sometimes seen with the weakness developing over a few days to weeks. In these cases the muscles are usually painful to touch and are oedematous. In childhood PM/DM complex there is a much greater association with arteritis than in the adult form. The arteritis can lead to mesenteric thrombosis, lung infarcts and occasionally cerebral infarcts.

PM/DM complex may be a pure disease, but it can also be associated with autoimmune diseases (e.g. rheumatoid arthritis, systemic lupus erythematosus) or with an underlying carcinoma. These associations are rare in the childhood presentation of the disease but do sometimes occur and should therefore be recognised.

Investigation. Investigation shows moderate to marked elevation of the serum CK. The EMG studies show a mixed pattern of changes, which are suggestive but not diagnostic of the disease. Muscle biopsy is required in each case, not only to confirm the diagnosis, but also to exclude other conditions, particularly metabolic myopathies where the clinical picture may be similar.

The biopsy shows evidence of active necrosis of muscle fibres and there may be an inflammatory infiltrate around blood vessels. In addition to signs of necrosis, there is concomitant evidence of regeneration (Fig. 11.7). If the biopsy shows only the features of necrosis or regeneration then the diagnosis is unlikely to be PM/DM complex. In the more indolent forms of presentation with a history over several months, there may be evidence of fibrous invasion of the

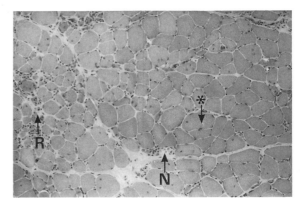

Fig. 11.7 Typical findings in childhood dermatomyositis showing areas of necrosis (N), regeneration (R) with evidence of prior necrosis and regeneration as manifested by split fibres and fibres containing internal nuclei (*).

muscle. The cause of the necrosis of fibre is probably due to an immune response with sensitised T lymphocytes destroying the muscle membrane and thus allowing ingress of excess Ca^{2+}.

Management. As soon as the diagnosis has been confirmed, which should not take more than a few days, treatment is started with corticosteroids. The dosage used is between 1.5 and 2.0 mg/kg body weight, depending on the severity of the clinical illness. The severity of the pathological process does not correlate with clinical severity. The use of immunosuppression, usually with azathioprine, is well established in treating adult disease, but its role in childhood disease is not yet established. There is evidence that the dose of steroid may be reduced more quickly in those children who are on associated immunosuppressive therapy.

These doses of steroids will frequently be associated with minor to major steroid side-effects. These have to be anticipated and treated accordingly as, if the disease is inadequately treated at the outset, there is likely to be a poor and incomplete recovery that can leave the child permanently disabled.

The best measure of recovery is sequential recording of muscle strength. Although the serum CK usually falls with recovery, in some cases it may remain elevated or even increase. If drug therapy is tailored to the CK level then excessive and unnecessarily prolonged therapy may be given with an increased risk of side-effects. If the child has gastrointestinal absorption difficulties consequent upon mesenteric arteritis, they may require nasogastric or intravenous therapy in the first instance.

On the drug schedule given above, most children show recovery to near normal muscle strength during the first 6 weeks of therapy. During this time hydrotherapy is useful. When the muscle strength is near normal, more active exercise regimes are required.

When the muscle strength is normal the dose of steroid is usually changed to an alternate day regime at the same dose level and then slowly tapered over the next 12–18 months to a holding dose of approximately 5 mg on alternate days. This dose often has to be continued for up to 3 years before the risk of recurrence of the active disease is past.

It is important to distinguish between recurrence of active disease and the development of weakness as a result of steroid therapy. In the latter, weakness is usually selective, involving psoas and quadriceps as opposed to limb girdle weakness in PM/DM complex. Repeat needle muscle biopsies are often helpful in this situation.

All patients with PM/DM complex, either during the active or recovery phase of the disease, are at risk of developing cardiac conduction defects, which therefore means regular monitoring.

Children with PM/DM complex are at greatest risk of developing calcinosis. This is commonly in the recovery phase and the calcinosis usually occurs at elbows and knees. These deposits may require surgical removal.

Prognosis. With this schedule of treatment, 85% of children will make a complete recovery and become independent, 10–12% will be left with minor disability and 2–3% with moderate disability. The disease itself is rarely fatal; when death occurs it is usually due to associated arteritic or cardiac disease.

Viral myositis

Viral myositis in children is often seen in association with influenzal infections. In this condition the child, following the viral infection, develops acute painful swelling, predominantly of the gastrocnemius and soleus groups of muscles. For reasons unknown, the disorder tends to affect children around the age of 9 years. The muscles show acute necrosis on muscle biopsy and the degree of weakness and pain is usually sufficient to render them bed-bound. Complete recovery over a period of 4–6 weeks is the rule.

Granulomatous myopathy

Granulomatous myopathy rarely presents with major muscle weakness. However, as granuloma, particularly in sarcoid, are found in muscle in 50% of cases, muscle biopsy is often used as a diagnostic procedure.

Infective myopathy

Infective myopathy is rare in developed countries, but worldwide may be the most common form of inflammatory myopathy. Localised abscesses form in the muscle; treatment is by surgical drainage and antibiotics.

Congenital myopathy

These disorders share a common clinical presentation but have varied pathological features.

The most common presentation is that of the 'floppy-infant' (see Fig. 11.5), the child who is hypotonic at birth. Some children are sufficiently severely affected to require ventilation. A less common presentation is with delay in motor milestones, where the child usually also shows slim musculature.

In the absence of a 'central' cause for the hypotonia, the majority of these children have an underlying neuromuscular disorder. Investigation with serum CK and EMG is rarely helpful, the pathological entity being established by muscle biopsy.

When SMA 1 has been excluded as the cause of the hypotonia most of the congenital myopathies are benign. Provided the children can be supported through infancy and early childhood, they usually improve to virtually normal, although they will always have slim musculature and are rarely athletic. The exception to this is Nemaline myopathy, where there is a risk of cardiac involvement, which is sometimes fatal. In the remaining disorders, if scoliosis or contracture develops, this benign prognosis is not seen.

Pathological features

The pathological features of congenital myopathy are due to arrest of normal muscle development. Normally the muscle fibre starts off as a myotube with the centre of the fibre being progressively filled with myofibres. At this stage the muscle nuclei lie centrally within the fibre. The nuclei then migrate to their normal position at the periphery of the fibre. From then differentiation into fibre types occurs, the first evidence of this being at 24–26 weeks of gestation. The fibres are initially all Type I and by birth progressive conversion of Type I to Type II occurs so that the usual ratio of 60% Type I to 40% Type II is complete by birth or soon after.

The earlier in development any delay or arrest in development of the fibre occurs, the more severe the resulting disorder. In myotubular myopathy, severe weakness is present well into adolescence but limited walking is usually possible. In centronuclear myopathy, disability is less, but is usually marked in early childhood. Both of these disorders are associated with contracture formation. There may be failure of development of one fibre type, commonly Type II (Type II fibre hypotrophy), incomplete development of a fibre type (congenital fibre type disproportion (CFTD)) or failure of the normal differentiation into fibre type proportions (Type I fibre excess). This last group is frequently associated with abnormal inclusions in the muscle fibre, e.g. Nemaline rods, central cores and other rarer disorders, e.g. fingerprint body, reducing body and curvilinear bodies. These inclusions have led to eponymous titles for the disorders, but hide the fact that they share a common aetiology.

The importance of recognising these disorders is that, although they are often disabling in infancy and childhood, they are associated with a mainly benign prognosis.

Metabolic myopathies

These disorders present as either episodic muscle weakness or a progressive myopathy of the LG type.

Periodic paralysis

In this condition there are recurrent attacks of profound muscle weakness associated with either an increase or a decrease in the serum potassium (hyperkalaemic/hypokalaemic period paralysis). Attacks of both types may start in childhood and are usually most common before the age of 30 years. In both types, there is an abrupt onset of profound limb weakness to the point where the patient is unable to move. The muscles of respiration and the cranial muscles are always spared. In the hypokalaemic type in particular, the attacks may be precipitated by a carbohydrate-rich meal, rest after exercise or by cold. In patients of South East Asian extraction, attacks of hypokalaemic periodic paralysis may be the first manifestation of thyrotoxicosis. The attacks last between 2 hours and 2 days.

Diagnosis. Confirmation of the diagnosis depends on demonstrating an elevated or lowered level of K^+ during an attack. Attacks may be provoked by either lowering or raising the serum K^+, but this should only be carried out as a planned procedure in hospital. As the disorder is usually inherited, precipitation of attacks should preferably be undertaken in adults.

Management. Treatment is either to elevate the K^+ level by potassium supplements in hypokalaemic attacks, or to lower the K^+ by diuretics in hyperkalaemic attacks.

Glycogen disorders

A detailed description of these disorders is outside the scope of this chapter and further information can be found in a recent review of the glycogen myopathies (Engel 1988). The two common disorders are:

1. Pompe's disease (infantile and childhood forms) — a progressive myopathy due to absence or depletion of acid maltase.

2. McArdle's disease — due to depletion of

myophosphorylase b, which presents as painful muscle weakness following exercise.

Mitochondrial and lipid disorders

With the advent of enzyme histochemistry, predominantly in the 1970s, there were defined a series of disorders that appeared to be characterised by excess lipid within muscle fibres. Two major types of lipid disorders seemed to occur in childhood — carnitine deficiency and carnitine palmityl transferase (CPT) deficiency. Carnitine deficiency, which presents as a progressive LG myopathy, showed massive accumulations of lipid within the muscle fibres. CPT deficiency presents with painful cramps after exercise, particularly if the child is food-deplete. The diagnosis is made by showing lipid accumulation on muscle biopsy.

It is now realised, however, that these myopathies occur as a result of primary mitochondrial dysfunction, the accumulation of lipid being secondary to the impairment of metabolism consequent upon the mitochondrial failure. This field of so-called 'mitochondrial myopathies' (Morgan-Hughes 1986) is expanding rapidly, and provides a model of collaborative research between clinicians, geneticists and basic scientists. As the field expands, so this classification will be refined with time.

Mitochondrial disorders can be subdivided into those that affect the mitochondrial respiratory chain and those that affect mitochondrial structure.

Respiratory chain disease. In respiratory chain disease there are deficiencies or absence of one of the four groups of enzymes (known as complexes I–IV) by which the mitochondrion produces energy for the cell. These disorders commonly present as rapid onset encephalopathy with marked lactic acidosis. The mitochondrial defect, which occurs in most organs, is most easily identified in muscle.

At present acute treatment is symptomatic, but the risk of further episodes of encephalopathy may be minimised by avoiding situations where the body becomes dependent on lipid metabolism for energy, e.g. prolonged fasting and particularly exercise in the fasted state.

Disorders of mitochondrial structure. The disorders of mitochondrial structure are primarily those that affect the mitochondrial genome, usually associated with a deletion of part of the genome (Harding 1991). These disorders commonly present with myopathy, although the reason for this is unknown, and there is a marked predilection for the eye muscle (Collins et al 1991). This is clinically manifest as progressive external ophthalmoplegia. Although this disorder is commonly seen in adolesence and adult life, a severe form of the disease presents in childhood. In addition to the ophthalmoplegia, there is associated retinitis pigmentosa, cardiac conduction defects and progressive cerebral and cerebellar dysfunction (Kearn–Sayers syndrome). The condition is progressive to the late teens or early twenties when death supervenes from cardio-respiratory failure.

Neuromuscular junction disorders
Myasthenia gravis (MyG)

Myasthenia gravis (MyG) is predominantly a disease of adult life but it can occur at any age. Children with MyG are in no respect different from adult patients. The disease is characterised by muscle fatigue. The eye muscles are often affected first, leading to fatiguable ptosis and diplopia. With rest the symptoms disappear and the child has to exercise the eye muscle to bring out the abnormality. The oropharyngeal muscles are affected next, leading to dysarthria and dysphagia. Limb muscles then become affected and ventilatory muscles are usually the last to be affected.

The disease arises as a result of an antibody to the acetylcholine receptor site on the post-synaptic area of the neuromuscular junction (Anti AchR-Ab). As a consequence of the antibody activity there is an increased degradation rate of the receptor.

Management. The symptoms may be improved by the administration of anticholinesterases, which prolong the action of acetylcholine at the neuromuscular junction. Plasmapheresis, which depletes the antibody load, is useful in severely ill patients and in preparation for surgery. Thymectomy is the treatment of choice and most children become asymptomatic within 6–12 months.

Congenital myasthenia gravis (C-MyG)

Congenital myasthenia gravis (C-MyG) is an extremely rare disorder that manifests in early infancy and childhood. The children often have a mild fixed weakness and develop fatiguable weakness in association with intercurrent illness. During this stage they respond to anticholinesterase drugs.

The condition is usually benign and is due to a structural abnormality of the acetylcholine receptor.

Neonatal myasthenia

This condition is seen in the newborn infants of some mothers who have MyG. Not all children are affected and there is no available means to predict if an infant will become affected.

The disease is caused by placental transfer of maternal anti AchR-Ab to the fetus. The fetus is dependent on maternal IgG, as is the infant during the first 6 weeks of life until its own IgG is fully in production. Anti AchR-Ab is an IgG type antibody and therefore, having crossed the placenta, the antibody is toxic to the fetal muscle end plates.

Mothers with MyG must be aware of the risk of producing a child with neonatal MyG. Fortunately the disease is always self-limiting within 6 weeks, although the child may be extremely 'floppy'. Treatment is with anticholinesterases.

Peripheral neuropathy

Inherited polyneuropathy

These conditions are now described under the title Hereditary Motor Sensory Neuropathy (HMSN). Although some ten disorders are recognised (Dyck 1984), only three are common: HMSN I, HMSN II and HMSN III.

HMSN I and II. Previously these have been known variously as Charcot–Marie–Tooth disease and peroneal muscular atrophy. The clinical manifestations are the same in both types, the difference lies in the underlying neuropathy. In HMSN I, NCV reveals the presence of demyelinating neuropathy this is accompanied by thickening of the peripheral nerves on clinical examination. In HMSN II the NCV reveals an axonal neuropathy.

Clinically the major abnormality is thinning and weakness of the muscles beneath the knees and the distal part of the quadriceps, giving the inverted champagne bottle appearance to the legs. There is usually an associated pes cavus foot deformity. The severity of the disorder is markedly variable.

Some patients are only aware of difficulty in obtaining footwear, whereas others have a major physical walking disability. About 10% of patients with both types also have distal weakness in the upper limbs.

Management. The disorder is only slowly progressive, if at all, but disability may be increased by inappropriate management. Contracture of the Achilles tendon is the major disability often associated with a fore foot abnormality. If the condition is not recognised surgical approaches to the foot may be undertaken with tendon transplantation to try to improve the foot deformity. However, as the muscle pull is abnormal, these procedures are of little benefit. Stretching the tendon, or even surgical slipping in selected cases, usually maintains walking ability and surgical correction of the foot deformity may be postponed until a single operative intervention can be carried out when bone growth has been completed.

In both types inheritance is autosomal dominant, and variability of expression within the family is common. For that reason the parents and siblings of an affected child require investigation.

HMSN I is associated with a gene abnormality either on chromosome 17 (17p11.2) or on chromosome 1 (1q22) (Defesche et al 1990). The gene location for HMSN II is as yet unknown.

HMSN III. HMSN III also presents in childhood. This is a severe demyelinating neuropathy that is inherited as an autosomal recessive condition. It is associated with major distal weakness in the upper and lower limbs, with hand and foot deformity. The children, if they learn to walk, are severely handicapped but have a long survival.

REFERENCES

Barkhaus P E, Gilchrist J M 1989 Duchenne muscular dystrophy manifesting carriers. Archives of Neurology 46: 673–675

Barwick D B, Fawcett P R W 1988 The clinical physiology of neuromuscular disease. In: Walton J N (ed) Disorders of voluntary muscle, 5th edn. Churchill Livingstone, Edinburgh, p 1015–1080

Brzustowicz L M, Lehner T, Castilla H et al 1990 Genetic mapping of chronic childhood-onset spinal muscular atrophy to chromosome 5q11.2–13.3. Nature 344: 540–541

Collins S, Dennett X, Byrne E, Marzuki S 1991 Chronic progressive external ophthalmoplegia in patients with large heteroplasmic mitochondrial DNA deletions: an immunocytochemical study. Acta Neuropathologica (Berlin) 82: 185–192

Cumming W J K 1989 Steroids in polymyositis. In: Capildeo R (ed) Steroids in diseases of the central nervous system. Wiley, London p 247–257

Defesche J C, Hoogendijk J E, De V M, Ongerboer de V B W, Bolhuis P A 1990 Genetic linkage of hereditary motor and sensory neuropathy type I (Charcot–Marie–Tooth disease) to markers of chromosomes 1 and 17. Neurology 40: 1450–1453

Dyck P J 1984 Inherited neuronal degeneration and atrophy affecting peripheral motor, sensory and autonomic neurones. In: Dyck P J, Thomas P K, Lambert E H, Bunge R (eds) Peripheral neuropathy, 2nd edn. W B Saunders, Philadelphia, p 1600–1641

Engel A G 1988 Metabolic and endocrine myopathies. In: Walton J N (ed) Disorders of voluntary muscle. Churchill Livingstone, Edinburgh, p 811–868

Fischbeck K H 1989 The difference between Duchenne and Becker dystrophies — editorial. Neurology 39: 584–585

Gilliam T C, Brzustowicz L M, Castilla H et al 1990 Genetic homogeneity between acute and chronic forms of spinal muscular atrophy. Nature 345: 823–825

Harding A E 1991 Neurological disease and mitochondrial genes. Tins 14: 132–138

Kakulas B A 1990 A consideration of therapeutic interventions in the light of the muscle pathology and likely pathogenesis of the Xp21.2 muscular dystrophies. In: Kakulas B A, Mastaglia F L (eds) Pathogenesis and therapy of Duchenne and Becker muscular dystrophy. Raven Press, New York p 47–58

Karpati G 1990 The principles and practice of myoblast transfer. Advances in Experimental Medicine and Biology 280: 69–74

Law P K, Goodwin T G, Wang M G 1988 Normal myoblast injections provide genetic treatment for murine dystrophy. Muscle and Nerve 11: 525–533

Lee C C, Pearlman J A, Chamberlain J S, Caskey C T 1991 Expression of recombinant dystrophin and its localization to the cell membrane. Nature 349: 334–336

Morgan-Hughes J A 1986 The mitochondrial myopathies. In: Engel A G, Banker B Q (eds) Myology. McGraw-Hill, New York, p 1709–1744

Nicholson L V B, Davison K, Falkous G et al 1989a Dystrophin in skeletal muscle. I. Western blot analysis using a monoclonal antibody. Journal of the Neurological Sciences 94: 125–136

Nicholson L V B, Davison K, Johnson M A et al 1989b Dystrophin in skeletal muscle. II. Immunoreactivity in patients with Xp21 muscular dystrophy. Journal of the Neurological Sciences 94: 137–146

Pamphlett R 1988 Muscle biopsy. In: Mastaglia F L (ed) Inflammatory diseases of muscle. Blackwell, Oxford, p 17–36

Rowland L P 1989 The transformation of clinical concepts and clinical practice by molecular genetics. In: Rowland L P, Wood D S, Schon E A, DiMauro S (eds) Molecular genetics in diseases of brain, nerve, and muscle. Oxford University Press, Oxford, p 8–23

Sambrook P, Rickards D, Cumming W J K 1988 CT muscle scanning in the evaluation of patients with spinal muscular atrophy (SMA). Neuroradiology 30: 487–496

Shaw D J, Harper P S 1989 Myotonic dystrophy: developments in molecular genetics. British Medical Bulletin 45: 439–759

12

Orthopaedic aspects of childhood disorders

J. Robb

Although this section deals with conditions occurring in childhood it is important to remember that the consequences persist into adult life and may have implications for further management. Life does not stop after epiphyseal closure.

IDIOPATHIC CLUB FOOT: CONGENITAL TALIPES EQUINOVARUS

Clinical features

The deformity comprises adduction and inversion of the forefoot and equinus, adduction and inversion of hindfoot. There is rotational deformity of the calcaneum and in severe cases subluxation of the navicular about the head of the talus. In addition, the ligaments in the posterior and medial aspects of the ankle are shortened and thickened. Apart from the obvious foot deformity there is calf muscle wasting and shortening of the foot on the affected side. It is important to exclude any other associated abnormality or congenital problem. One of the difficulties is to assess the degree of rigidity and the foot may be described as flexible or rigid (Fig. 12.1).

Incidence

The incidence in the UK is approximately 1 in 1000 live births and 2.1% for first degree relatives. There is probably a polygenetic inheritance

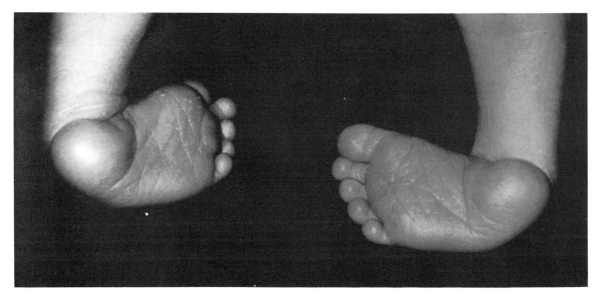

Fig. 12.1 Idiopathic club foot.

modified by environmental influences and 50% of cases are bilateral. Males are two to three times more commonly affected than females.

Cause

The cause of the condition is unknown, but two fairly recent studies on fetal embryology have provided different hypotheses.

Study 12.1   Fetal embryology and CTEV

Ippolito and Ponseti (1980) studied five fetal feet between the ages of 16 and 19 weeks and postulated a retracting fibrosis as the primary aetiological factor in club feet. Even at this early stage of fetal life extensive changes were found within the feet, in that the tarsal bones were misshapen and there was diminished size and number of fibres in the distal third of the muscles of the posterior and medial aspects of the leg and an increase in fibrous tissue in these muscles, tendon sheath and fascia.

Study 12.2

A study by Victoria-Diaz & Victoria-Diaz (1984) observed normal growth of the fetal foot. Normally at the 15 mm stage the foot lies in a straight line and at the 30 mm ($6\frac{1}{2}$–7 weeks after ovulation) stage the foot lies in equino varus and adduction. By the 50 mm stage (8–9 weeks after ovulation) there is slight equino varus and adduction. From the 15 to 30 mm stage changes are due to fibular growth and from the 30 to 50 mm stage changes are due to tibial growth and the medial foot develops during the later stages of tibial growth. The Victoria–Diazes (1984) suggested that:
• If growth is interrupted during the fibular phase a severe equinovarus foot results.
• If growth is interrupted during the tibial growth phase the result is a mild but flexible club foot.
• If growth is interrupted during the late tibial growth phase the result is a metatarsus adductus.

These two embryological studies (Studies 12.1 and 12.2) underline the extensive changes that occur in club foot at an early stage of fetal development and could also explain in part the high relapse rate after treatment.

Management

Manipulation and splintage

Most surgeons recommend gentle manipulation and splintage as initial management (see Chapter 19 Treatment Methods). This should start as soon as possible and the passive stretching and maintenance regime is best done by one person who has the necessary insight and knowledge. The organisation of such a system will vary from centre to centre but it is sometimes useful to admit the neonate to an orthopaedic ward so that the stretching regime can begin as soon as possible. Once a satisfactory position has been obtained the infant can be discharged and is then usually seen at weekly intervals for changes of splintage. The type of splintage used varies according to local preference but examples are Denis Brown splints, Jones strapping or serial plasters. The Denis Brown splint does not work as it was originally intended — as a dynamic self-manipulator — but as a static splint used to maintain correction. Strapping allows daily manipulations but plasters need to be expertly applied.

There have been few comparative studies between the various methods and probably what is most important is the consistency of technique. The sequence of correction is:

• the forefoot adduction
• the heel varus
• the equinus.

About 50% of feet will respond, indicating that the club foot is reasonably flexible. However, it is important not to produce a spurious correction by over-forceful manipulation. The foot should dorsiflex and evert beyond neutral, the heel should be in calcaneus and a rocker bottom foot, which results from dorsiflexion of the forefoot but residual equinus of the hindfoot, should be avoided.

Radiographs are helpful in assessing progress and are taken standing or by stimulated standing. Ankle equinus can be judged by the calcaneal–tibial angle and subtalar varus can be evaluated by the lateral talocalcaneal angle. Adduction at the talonavicular joint is seen by the medial displacement of the navicular. However, the navicular does not ossify before 1 year of age and so adduction can be assessed by the talar–first metatarsal angle, which should be approximately 0°.

Surgery

Operative correction is indicated once it is evident that manipulation and splintage is failing to maintain the foot. A wide variety of operations have been proposed and there is controversy as to whether surgery should be carried out at an early stage or whether it should be delayed until the foot is a larger structure.

Posteromedial release. Many surgeons now prefer to perform a one-stage posteromedial release (Cummings & Lovell 1988). The essential problem is the orientation of the talocalcaneal and talonavicular joints. The procedure consists of:

• an elongation of the tendo-Achilles
• a posterior release of the ankle and subtalar joint, including the calcaneofibular ligaments and the posterior talofibular ligament
• lengthening of the tibialis posterior tendon
• a medial release of the subtalar joint and superficial deltoid ligament
• a release of the calcaneal ligament.

In addition, extensive joint releases are necessary. The foot is usually splinted in plaster for 3 months postoperatively.

Surgery carries risks of both under-correction and over-correction, the latter resulting in a planovalgus, or stiff foot. Even after surgical correction relapses occur and it is essential to follow-up the child and most surgeons recommend some form of splintage after initial correction. A number of salvage procedures exist to deal with recurrence.

Soft tissue correction. Repeat soft tissue correction is a difficult procedure, often leading to increasing stiffness of the foot, and should be performed before bony deformity ensues. Examples of bony operations to deal with residual deformity are:

• excision of the calcaneocuboid joint
• metatarsal osteotomies
• lateral wedge tarsectomy
• triple arthrodesis.

The Ilizarov technique has also been described for correction of relapsed club foot and consists of an external distractor (Grill & Franke 1987). The aim of all these procedures is to produce a reasonably shaped foot that is plantigrade but inevitably stiff.

SCOLIOSIS

The term scoliosis indicates a curvature in the lateral plane and can be considered in the categories idiopathic, congenital or neuromuscular.

Idiopathic scoliosis

By definition, the cause of this condition is unknown. The condition consists of rotational deformity of the ribs on the convex side of the curve and there is an associated lordosis at the apex of the curve, which leads to rotational instability resulting in a scoliotic curve.

The problem is defining what constitutes the scoliosis. Most surgeons would disregard a curve of less than 5° but, generally speaking, curves above this level would be referred to a specialist. It is generally thought that there is an incidence of about 2–5 in 1000 children who have idiopathic curves greater than 20°. There is a familial pattern in idiopathic scoliosis and where there is a positive history of adolescent idiopathic scoliosis in the immediate family the probability of developing it is increased by a factor of tenfold; females are affected twice as frequently as males.

Idiopathic scoliosis is traditionally considered in three age groups:

1. Infantile, with onset between birth and 3 years of age.
2. Juvenile, which occurs after the age of 3 years but before puberty.
3. Adolescent, which occurs at puberty or shortly thereafter.

However, there is some doubt as to the existence of juvenile idiopathic scoliosis and an alternative definition of early and late onset idiopathic scoliosis has been proposed (Dickson 1985).

Infantile and juvenile idiopathic scoliosis

Incidence. The incidence of infantile idiopathic scoliosis has decreased in the UK now that more babies are sleeping prone (McMaster 1983). The condition occurs more frequently in males than in females and is usually convex to the left. The great majority of curves resolve without treatment but a smaller proportion, approximately 15–20%, may progress to severe deformity. The incidence of idiopathic juvenile scoliosis is similar to that of adolescent idiopathic scoliosis.

Management. The management of the curve is much as for adolescent curves. Extension, derotation and flexion casts have been advocated for progressing early onset curves. If spinal fusion is necessary it is best delayed for as long as possible and is inevitably a compromise between stabilisation at a relatively premature stage and foreshortening of the torso due to spinal fusion.

There has been an interest in this group of patients using surgical instrumentation without fusion to prevent the problems of foreshortening the torso but this has not proven successful.

Adolescent idiopathic scoliosis

Adolescent idiopathic scoliosis is the most common spinal deformity in children.

Diagnosis. The diagnosis is one of exclusion. Recently there has been interest in the use of school screening programmes in an attempt to identify children with curves but there is some doubt as to whether the cost involved in such screening programmes is justifiable. A large number of minor curves were discovered and the difficulty is knowing which are at increased risk of progression. There is a greater tendency to progression if the spine still has potential for growth and there is also correlation between the magnitude of the curve and the onset of the menarche (Lonstein & Carlson 1984). It used to be thought that curves did not progress after skeletal maturity but Weinstein & Ponseti (1983) have shown that curves greater than 50° at maturity are likely to progress in adulthood.

The deformity is usually detected by changes in contour of the torso. The patient is usually first aware of a prominence on the back of the rib hump and there is also asymmetry of shoulder or pelvic height. The rib deformity is due to secondary rotation of the ribs on the convex side of the curve (Fig. 12.2). Although small curves can be detected with the naked eye by trained

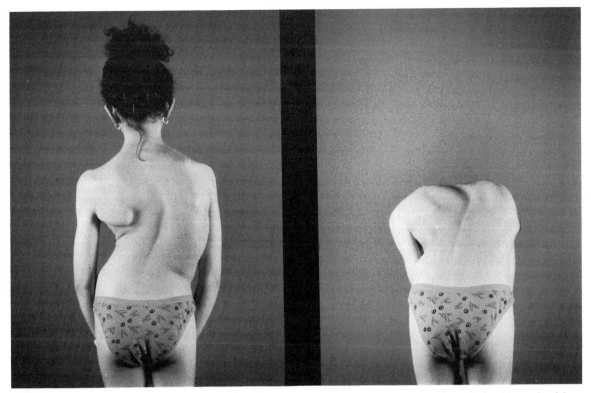

Fig. 12.2 Adolescent idiopathic scoliosis. In addition to the obvious curve, there is asymmetry of shoulder and pelvic height. The rib hump is seen better on forward bending.

observers, there has been interest recently in using other non-invasive methods of detection, such as Moire fringe photography or ISIS — integrated shape imaging system (Jefferson et al 1988). Postero–anterior X-rays of the dorsolumbar spine are required to assess the patient and a low-dose technique and screening to protect the gonads and breasts have been developed.

Management. The magnitude of the curve is traditionally measured by the Cobb angle. Those children who have curves under 20° are usually observed. There is no evidence that abdominal or back strengthening exercises have any effect on the progression of the curve.

Bracing. If the curve is greater than 20–25° and has shown signs of progression by more than 5°, bracing is traditionally used. There are a variety of braces, one of the earlier types being the Milwaukee brace, which extends from the pelvis to a ring at the base of the neck (Fig. 12.3). However, this is cosmetically unattractive and many centres now use underarm braces, the best

known of which is the Boston brace; these have also been used for thoracolumbar and lumbar curves (Fig. 12.4).

Initially it was thought that bracing would decrease spinal curvature but there is no evidence to support this. Dickson (1985) has suggested that there is no evidence that a brace alters the natural history of idiopathic scoliosis either. It is not clear how many patients comply with brace utilisation and compliance is probably poor. Other attempts at managing lesser curves have included electrical stimulation, and implanted electrodes have been used to stimulate the paraspinal muscles. There is some doubt about the efficacy of this technique in preventing spinal progression.

Surgery. Curves greater than 40° usually require surgery and the aim is to realign and stabilise the spinal deformity by insertion of metallic fixation devices and by arthrodesing the spine. The mainstay for the past 25 years has been the Harrington rod but this did not

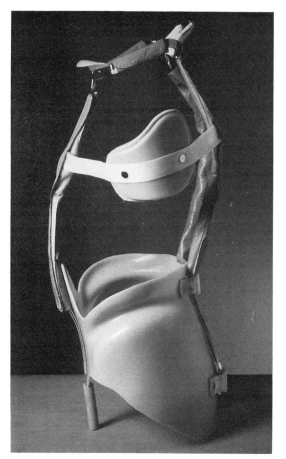

Fig. 12.3 Milwaukee brace.

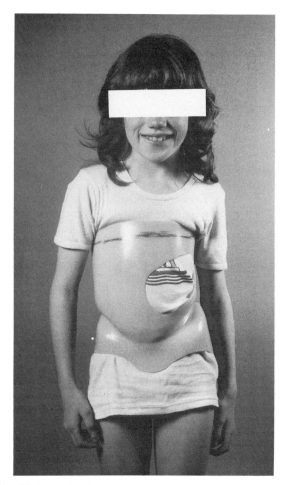

Fig. 12.4 Boston brace.

maintain correction of vertebral rotation. The lower the level of fusion for lumbar curves the higher the incidence of subsequent backache. Recent developments have been the combination of anterior and posterior surgery and newer devices for posterior fixation. For example, the Cotrel device applies transverse traction and can increase the strength of the instrumentation. The Luque system gives a very stable fixation and excellent curve correction but requires the passing of sublaminar wires, which can occasionally cause neurological injury. The rib hump, which is what the patient usually finds most unsightly, is not completely corrected by fusion, although it can be improved by rib resection (Jefferson et al 1988). Pulmonary function tests are necessary to assess the degree of pre-operative pulmonary compromise (see Chap-

ter 17 Common Assessment Procedures). A number of techniques have been used in the past in an attempt to improve the spinal deformity before surgery. These consisted of application of plaster casts and skeletal traction (halopelvic or halowheelchair).

Complications. Complications of surgery include neurological complications at the time of surgery and blood loss, and hypotensive anaesthesia is used to limit this. In the postoperative period backache can be a problem and attempts should be made to preserve the L4/5 disc space and to contour fixation rods to maintain a semblance of lumbar lordosis and to avoid a flat back. Postoperatively the spine is supported with a removable plastic jacket for 3 to 6 months, or until fusion is assured.

Congenital scoliosis

This deformity arises secondarily to malformation of the vertebral elements of the spine. It is present at birth but may not become evident until the associated truncal deformity occurs (Fig. 12.5).

Clinical features

The bony deformity can be considered as a failure of formation, e.g. a wedge hemivertebra, or a failure of segmentation, e.g. a unilateral unsegmented bar or block vertebra. A hemivertebra may be single or double. There may also be diastematomyelia — a congenital malformation consisting of a midline bony spur or fibrous septum within the neural canal. It is important to ascertain whether or not this is present as there is potential for spinal cord tethering and

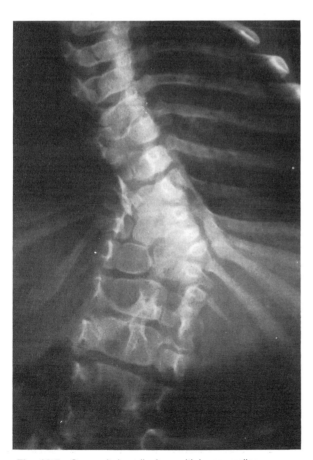

Fig. 12.5 Congenital scoliosis: multiple anomalies.

associated neurological deficit as growth continues.

Prognosis

Prognosis of congenital scoliosis depends on the type and site of the deformity (McMaster & Ohtsuka 1982). The worst prognosis is seen in the lower thoracic and thoracolumbar regions; a better prognosis is seen in the upper thoracic and the lumbar regions. From a structural standpoint, the worst prognosis is the unilateral unsegmented bar. This may be associated with rib fusion. A single hemivertebra can also cause severe deformity. Although these deformities tend to produce curves in the lateral plane it should not be forgotten that congenital kyphosis can also result from failure of formation or segmentation of vertebral bodies and can result in rapid neurological compromise.

Management

Management depends on the predicted behaviour of the deformity. Unilateral unsegmented bars and double hemivertebrae have a poor prognosis and are best treated by spinal fusion. In the young this is done on the convex side of the deformity without instrumentation; additional instrumentation is usually used in the older child. The evolution of a curve secondary to a hemivertebra is less predictable and management as for idiopathic scoliosis is justifiable.

Neuromuscular scoliosis

The following neuromuscular conditions can result in scoliosis:

- cerebral palsy
- spina bifida
- muscular disease
- Duchenne muscular dystrophy
- Friedreich's ataxia.

Curve progression is usually rapid and difficult to control by bracing, which is much more difficult in this particular group of children. The spine should not be seen in isolation and associated pelvic obliquity or contractures must also be evaluated.

Cerebral palsy

Scoliosis is common in cerebral palsy and its progression is proportional to the severity of the neurological picture (see Chapter 8 Disorders of the Central Nervous System).

Management. If the curve is progressive and threatens the child's ability to sit and other methods of containing the spine, e.g. wheelchair modifications and bracing, have failed, surgical stabilisation of the spine can be considered. Curves continue to progress even after skeletal maturity (Thomas & Simon 1988). Simple posterior arthrodesis has a higher pseudarthrosis rate than for idiopathic scoliosis and may often have to be preceded by an anterior release and posterior stabilisation with a Luque type of fixation, which has the advantage that postoperative bracing may not be required (Gersoff & Renshaw 1988). If there is fixed pelvic obliquity the fusion should be taken down to the sacrum.

Spina bifida

Several factors may contribute to the spinal deformity in spina bifida (Piggott 1980):

1. Congenital anomalies of the spine; treatment is the same as for congenital scoliosis.
2. A paralytic pattern of deformity due to muscle imbalance.
3. Cord tethering, which can contribute to the progressive scoliosis and also to a worsening neurological picture, has to be distinguished from increasing hydrocephalus.

Progressive curves in spina bifida do not respond well to bracing and usually require both anterior release and posterior surgery (McMaster 1987).

Muscular disease

There are three types of spinal muscle atrophy, which is an autosomal progressive condition with associated loss of anterior horn cells of the spinal cord. The three forms of spinal muscular atrophy are:

- type 1 — Werdnig–Hoffmann

- type 2 — chronic Werdnig–Hoffmann
- type 3 — Kugelberg–Welander.

These are very rare conditions and their descriptions are therefore not included here (further details can be found as referenced under Shapiro and Bresnan 1982a and in Chapter 11 Neuromuscular Disorders).

Surgical stabilisation of the spine is indicated with curves worse than 50° as bracing in this condition has been shown to be largely ineffective (Shapiro & Bresnan 1982a).

Duchenne muscular dystrophy

Duchenne muscle dystrophy is a sex-linked recessive disorder and children usually cease walking between the ages of 12 and 14 and then develop a collapsing type of curve (see Chapter 11 Neuromuscular Disorders) (Shapiro & Bresnan 1982c). This limits the ability to sit and also respiratory function. Braces may slow the progression but at the same time pulmonary function tests may deteriorate rapidly and may render spinal surgery impossible through pulmonary compromise even though the curve is of relatively modest proportions. In this condition the spine should be stabilised early on, either when the child ceases to walk or if the curve is greater than 25° and progressing rapidly. Fusion has to extend from thoracic vertebra two to the sacrum.

Friedreich's ataxia

Spinal deformity in Friedreich's ataxia (Shapiro & Bresnan 1982b, Labelle et al 1986) is common and parallels the severity of the ataxia. Again, bracing in this condition has been shown to be ineffective and surgery may be indicated once curves progress to beyond 50°. Pulmonary function in this condition is also compromised and has to be taken into account.

CONGENITAL DISLOCATION OF THE HIP

The term dislocation is probably better replaced by the term 'displacement' as very few infants have a dislocated hip at birth and in most with abnormal hips the hips can be subluxed or dislocated manually and in some are very unstable. These hips can be described as having a reducible dislocation or an unstable dislocatable hip.

Clinical features

In the typical displaced hip there is initial normal development of the hip joint but in an atypical dislocation there is a primary maldevelopment, which may result from a teratological dislocation or be associated with neurological disorders such as spina bifida or cerebral palsy.

In typical congenital dislocation of the hip (CDH) there is capsule laxity. The femoral head is of normal shape and the femoral neck is anteverted. Acetabular dysplasia may be primary and is thought to be an inherited defect, whereas secondary acetabular dysplasia may occur in CDH due to continuous pressure because of the abnormal relationship between the femoral head and the socket. With long-standing subluxation or dislocation secondary changes occur, and there is nearly always an angular or rotational abnormality of the acetabulum. As the femoral head displaces, the fibrocartilaginous labrum may invert and the capsule may also infold into the joint between the femoral head and acetabulum (Fig. 12.6).

Incidence

The incidence of CDH is about 1 in 1000 live births and the cause is not known, but the incidence is higher in breech delivery, in the presence of knee recurvatum, muscular torticollis and metatarsus adductus and there is a familial incidence varying between 5 and 35° (Wynne-Davies 1970).

Diagnosis

Initially it was thought that if all new-born infants were examined for CDH, early non-operative treatment might obviate the need for later surgery. However in reported series there are still cases of missed dislocation (Macnicol 1990). Ideally the evaluation of the new-born should be carried out by an experienced observer to assess hip stability.

Both the Barlow and Ortolani tests rely on capsule laxity. In the Barlow test two types of displacement occur.

1. Hips that are correctly located but can be dislocated posteriorly.
2. Dislocated hips that can be reduced into the joint.

Ultrasound (Clarke et al 1985) has become a reliable method of assessing hip stability and may reduce the subsequent need for X-ray examinations in the future. The test has the advantage that it can be carried out when the child is wearing a Pavlik harness. However, ultrasound has failed to reduce the incidence of late cases of CDH (Clarke et al 1989). A refinement of ultrasound assessment has been proposed using a stress test (Saies et al 1988).

Computerised tomography has also been used in pre-operative planning but in some centres plain radiography remains the mainstay of confirming a hip reduction.

Unfortunately, not all dislocated hips are recognised at birth and may present at a later point. Asymmetry of abduction in the infant may indicate hip displacement (Fig. 12.7). This may also become apparent when the child begins to walk and an abnormality of gait is observed, which usually consists of a unilateral limp but bilateral dislocation may not be so readily noticeable. Late untreated dislocation may unfortunately occur in children over 3 years of age.

Management

The aim of treatment is to obtain a stable and concentric reduction. Once the instability has been confirmed the infant is treated by splintage. A variety of appliances exist and it is important to avoid the extremes of any one position. Double nappies are useless. Rigid splints do not allow flexion and risk rigid abduction. Severe abduction greater than 45 to 60° risks avascular necrosis.

Pavlik harness

Pavlik harness has been advocated by many

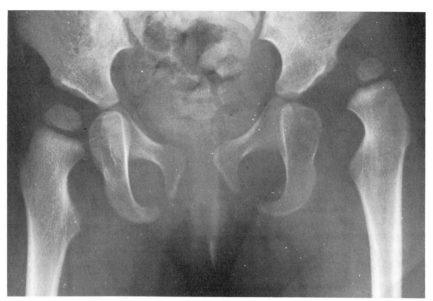

Fig. 12.6 Congenital dislocation of the hip: anteroposterior radiograph of the pelvis.

(Iwasaki 1983, Bradley, Wetherill & Benson 1987) (Fig. 12.8). This allows movement within a physiological range and avoids forced abduction but does risk medial knee instability. The position of the child within the harness is important.

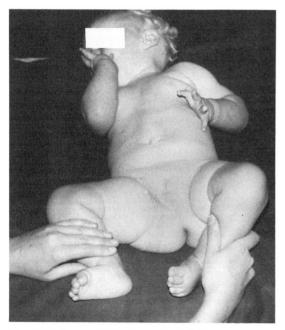

Fig. 12.7 Loss of abduction in the left hip.

The splintage is usually maintained for 3 months. The splint is then removed, the child examined and an X-ray taken or ultrasound repeated. If reduction is confirmed, the child is left free of splintage and observed until he begins to walk. If there is doubt about reduction an arthrogram should be obtained. Failure to obtain or maintain reduction is an indication for operation.

Surgery

A variety of surgical procedures has been proposed to deal with the problem according to the age of the child. Failure of initial splintage or early presentation of hip displacement can be dealt with by either closed or open reduction of the hip (Dhar et al 1990). If the hip reduces without placing the limb in an extreme position mobilisation is possible. Extreme abduction should be avoided and, if present, the soft tissue obstruction to reduction should be excised and the hip reduced by operation.

Dislocation discovered at the time of walking requires a different approach and operation is often preceded by preliminary traction to bring the femoral head down and opposite to the joint before operation. Surgery usually consists of two procedures:

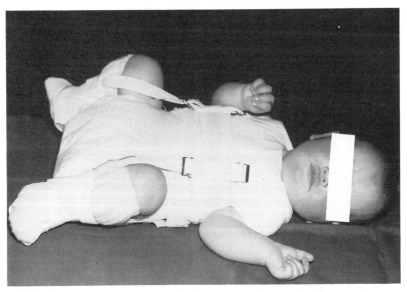

Fig. 12.8 Pavlik harness.

1. Excision of the soft tissue block to reduction, the limbus.

2. Derotation osteotomy to deal with persistent femoral anteversion.

Further development of the acetabulum is assured as it has remodelling capacity beyond 4 years, and perhaps up to 8 years, providing the femoral head is correctly located and stable. (Brougham et al 1988). Rotational osteotomy may provide such stimulus and avoid the need for pelvic osteotomy (Blockey 1984).

Should the child present at a stage where the acetabulum has not developed normally it is not always possible to provide adequate coverage of the femoral head once positioned in the socket. Pelvic osteotomy is then indicated, to provide a stable roof, which moulds over the femoral head. A Salter-type of osteotomy is most commonly used and spontaneous correction of femoral anteversion usually occurs.

The child presenting with a late untreated dislocation over the age of 3 poses a more difficult problem because more extensive surgery is required and may involve femoral shortening and then an open reduction of the hip with or without a pelvic osteotomy. Despite these procedures, late subluxation of the hip can occur and may be due to inadequate acetabular cover, to persistent femoral anteversion or to a long leg on the symptomatic side. These problems may be treated by pelvic osteotomy, repeat femoral derotation osteotomy, limb shortening or a combination of the three. Should the patient develop a subluxing hip, degenerative change may occur, even in adolescent years.

The best results of treatment for congenital dislocation of the hip are obtained by diagnosis and treatment and splintage at birth. It is still thought justifiable to reduce a unilateral dislocation, even up to age 12, but late presentation of a bilateral dislocation poses a more difficult problem. Some advocate that the situation should be accepted as it is much more difficult to obtain two symmetrical and satisfactory hips under these circumstances (Mitchell 1983).

ARTHROGRYPOSIS

Arthrogryposis multiplex congenita is a nonprogressive condition present at birth and is perhaps better termed multiple congenital contractures. It occurs in 1 in 3000 live births.

Cause

The cause is unclear as over 150 entities are

associated with multiple congenital contractures. It probably results from intra-uterine immobilisation of joints at various stages of development because of neural, myogenic or skeletal factors. Most seem to be neurogenic, e.g. due to anterior horn cell deficiency. Mechanical factors also seem to play a part as there is an association between oligohydramnios and arthrogryposis. Muscle biopsies can show abnormalities of motor endplates.

Clinical features

The condition is characterised by:

- deformed and rigid joints
- atrophy or absence of muscle groups
- diminished subcutaneous tissue
- dislocations
- intact cutaneous sensation and intelligence.

Clinically, most deformities are paralytic and there are usually associated contractures due to thickened capsule and periarticular tissues. The deformities are usually symmetrical and commonly affect all four limbs (Fig. 12.9); the trunk is often spared. The hips may be dislocated, there are contractures at the knee and talipes equinovarus. In the upper limbs there may be internal rotational deformities of the shoulder and extension contractures of the elbow. Scoliosis is common in this condition.

Management

Management of such patients includes maintenance of range of movement and preservation of joint alignment. It is helpful to record the contractures, and physiotherapy and splintage have also been claimed to give good results. Most orthopaedic surgeons find that these are transient, and that the deformity recurs.

Orthopaedic surgery has been used to restore muscle balance but recurrence is the rule due largely to inelastic soft tissues.

Tenotomies and capsulotomies followed by orthotic support to delay recurrence are usually necessary and the maximum correction that is obtained is usually that which is found at surgery. Serial casting is unhelpful.

Osteotomies do not increase joint movement but change the arc of motion to a more useful position. This is best done at maturity otherwise recurrence occurs rapidly.

As a general principle it is better to correct lower limb deformities prior to walking age but defer operations to the upper limb until the child is old enough to cooperate, usually before school entry.

In the lower limb the aims are:

- to obtain reciprocal movements at the hips
- to abolish excessive flexion contractures at the knee
- to render the foot plantigrade.

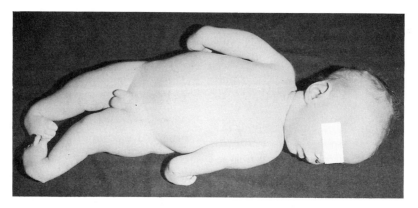

Fig. 12.9 Arthrogryposis multiplex congenita: four limb involvement.

In the severe equinovarus problem it may be necessary to perform a talectomy.

In the upper limb the aims are:

- to obtain suitable limb positioning
- to facilitate toileting and feeding (Thompson 1985).

OSTEOGENESIS IMPERFECTA

Osteogenesis imperfecta (brittle bone disease) is not common and occurs in about 1 in 20 000 live births. The cause is unknown but it is an inherited group of disorders featuring excessive bone fragility and there is evidence of a defect in collagen synthesis (Figs 12.10 and 12.11).

Clinical features

Four main types are recognised (Smith 1984):

Type 1

This accounts for 80% of cases and is an

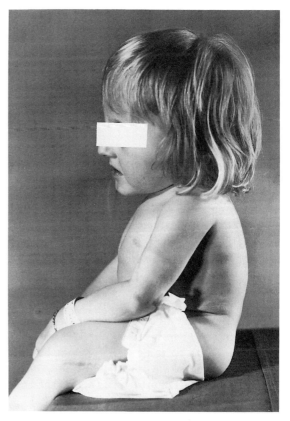

Fig. 12.11 Osteogenesis imperfecta: general appearance.

autosomal dominant disorder. The patient has blue sclerae, normal stature and deafness. There is often hypermobility of joints and dentinogenesis imperfecta.

Type 2

This is probably autosomal recessive and is a lethal form of osteogenesis imperfecta. The infant is born with multiple fractures at birth and gross limb deformities.

Type 3

This is also probably autosomal recessive but less severe than type 2. The disorder causes progressive deformation and the child may be born with fractures at birth but survives. These children often develop a kyphoscoliosis. The bones are usually very narrow but the sclerae are normal in adult life and dentinogenesis imperfecta may also

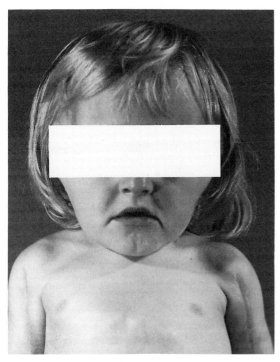

Fig. 12.10 Osteogenesis imperfecta: triangular facial appearance.

occur. These patients are often unable to walk (Shapiro 1985).

Type 4

This is autosomal dominant and rare. There is also bone fragility, short stature, normal sclerae and abnormal teeth.

Management

The cause of osteogenesis imperfecta is unknown. In mild cases fractures heal well but repeated fractures may cause deformity and necessitate intramedullary rod stabilisation of long bones, particularly in the legs (Stockley et al 1989). However, in severely affected cases walking may not be feasible and the child has to accept a wheelchair existence.

Spinal deformity occurring in osteogenesis is not really amenable to bracing as the brace itself, in a severe case, can produce rib deformity and so there may be an indication for spinal fusion in cases of progressive spinal deformity. It has been noted that if fractures occur before the child walks, 30% become wheelchair-bound.

The condition can be confused with non-accidental injury (Taitz 1987) and the recognition of a child and the parents with blue sclera or excessive joint laxity and a triangular facial appearance would confirm osteogenesis imperfecta. Radiographic evidence of wormian (multiple small bones) in the occipital region is typical of the condition.

JUVENILE CHRONIC ARTHRITIS

This is a relatively uncommon condition affecting approximately 1 in 1000 children. There has been some debate about the nomenclature and classification of the condition: in the United States it is known as juvenile rheumatoid arthritis and in Europe it is usually known as juvenile chronic arthritis. Its cause is unknown but there are a large number of non-specific immunological changes that occur in the condition.

Clinical features

Three patterns have been defined:

- systemic
- polyarticular
- pauciarticular.

These are based on the clinical manifestations seen within 3 months of the onset of the disease.

Systemic type

The systemic type accounts for approximately 20% of the children affected. The rheumatoid and antinuclear factors are usually negative and under 5 years of age boys are affected equally with girls. There is multiple joint involvement including the cervical spine. The child suffers from fever, a maculopapular rash, generalised lymphadenopathy, splenomegaly, hepatomegaly and raised white cell count.

Polyarticular arthritis

Polyarticular arthritis is defined as the involvement of five or more joints throughout the first 3 months. This pattern of involvement accounts for 50% of chronic arthritis. Females are more frequently affected than males and the condition generally occurs after the age of 4. Thirty-five per cent develop chronic joint problems and the rheumatoid and antinuclear factor can be positive in 15–20%. Hanson et al (1969) have divided this group into seronegative and IgM rheumatoid factor-positive groups, the latter usually tending to affect older children aged 9 or 10 and upwards.

Pauciarticular arthritis

Pauciarticular arthritis accounts for about 30% of cases and is defined as an arthritis of four or fewer joints in the first 3 months of presentation. This is the most common type of presentation and children tend to have chronic iridocyclitis and a positive antinuclear factor. A later onset of osteoarticular arthritis in children is likely to be associated with subsequent development of sacroileitis.

Progression of condition

The majority of children go into remission, usually after 1–2 years. Schaller (1984) has shown that

75% recover without serious permanent residual effects and Laaksonen (1966) has shown that 30% recover with complete functional capacity, 40% are left with slight residual disability and 30% are left with severe disability. The worst functional outcome is in children who have severe involvement of the hip. This is most likely in children who have the onset of the disease under the age of five and whose disease persists for more than 5 years.

Management

The mainstay of medical management is high-dose aspirin, sometimes supplemented with non-steroidal anti-inflammatory medication. Occasionally, additional treatment with gold or pencillamine is necessary if disease activity persists over a 2-year period. Frequent ophthalmic examination is necessary because of iridocyclitis. Prolonged bed-rest is undesirable although, if the child is resting during the systemic phase of the illness, care must be taken to ensure appropriate splintage and physiotherapy supervision of range of motion of joints. Prone lying is a useful technique for potential flexion contractures of the hips and knees and night splints for the wrist, knee and ankle are useful to prevent deformity. Occasionally, night skin traction can be used to maintain range of motion in the lower limbs.

Orthopaedic intervention

Orthopaedic intervention can be helpful in the overall management of these children and it is essential to view the child as a whole. Appropriate splintage for joints is helpful to prevent deformity occurring; so that, if spontaneous fusion does occur, for example, at the wrist, at least it fuses in a functional position. Synovectomy is disappointing in the long term (Jacobsen et al 1985). Tendon rupture is fortunately rare. Soft tissue surgery to abolish contractures at the hip or knee is useful to give the patient a more functional position when standing or walking and arthroplasty of the hip has been carried out with successful results in restoring lower limb function (Ansell & Swann 1983).

PERTHES' DISEASE

Perthes' disease is thought to be an osteonecrosis of the femoral head, but the cause of this is unknown (Wenger et al 1991). It has been noted that children presenting with Perthes' disease generally have short stature and one hypothesis put forward is that these children have a lack of somatomedin. Growth hormone stimulates the liver to produce this substance, which in turn stimulates DNA and RNA synthesis and collagen in cartilage. Another hypothesis is that the condition is preceded by a synovitis which causes a tamponade effect on the femoral head (excess pressure within the hip capsule), but this has not been supported experimentally.

Perthes' disease occurs four times more frequently in boys than girls and in about 10% of patients it is bilateral. The peak incidences are in boys at age 5 and in girls at age 4, and there is an incidence of 1 in 3000 live births for boys and approximately 1 in 12 000 live births for girls.

Clinical features

The child presents with a painful irritable hip and associated limp and there is usually limitation of abduction and internal rotation. It is important to differentiate this condition from multiple epiphyseal dysplasia, spondyloepiphyseal dysplasia and pseudachondroplasia, in which condition the hip is usually affected symmetrically. If both hips are involved in Perthes' disease it is usually asymmetrical and the morphology of the pelvis is normal.

Histological studies (Catterall et al 1982) have shown appearances varying from ischaemic arrest of ossification in the capital articular cartilage without infarction to multiple complete infarctions of epiphyseal bone. This confirmed the view that pathology is an osteonecrosis.

Radiographic appearance

The radiographic appearances are best seen on anteroposterior and a frog lateral view taken at 45°. There is a cycle of radiographic appearances, which have been described as stages of infarction, sclerosis and revascularisation or collapse, fragmentation and repair (Fig. 12.12). A new method of considering the three-dimensional anatomy of the proximal femur (Howell et al 1989) suggests that the femoral head and neck are in significant anteversion and true varus. Morphological changes also occur in the acetabulum (Joseph 1989) and consist of osteoporosis of the roof, irregularity of contour, premature triradiate fusion and articular cartilage hypertrophy. These changes tended to be more marked in the older child and when more than half the head was involved, and correlate with the clinical impression that the older the child at onset the worse the prognosis. Use of bone scanning is of doubtful help but the recent advent of magnetic resonance imaging has produced an interesting possibility for the assessment and classification of Perthes' disease.

Attempts have been made to classify Perthes' disease radiographically. O'Garra (1959) introduced the concept of partial and complete involvement of the head and Catterall (1971) divided these up into four groups and included 'at risk signs'. Salter and Thompson (1984) proposed a return to a simpler two-part classification based on the extent of the subchondral fracture. There is a degree of interobserver error in using the Catterall classification and many prefer to use the Salter–Thompson classification (Simmons et al 1990).

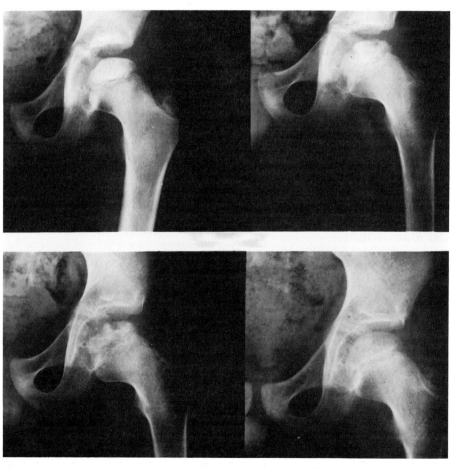

Fig. 12.12 Perthes' disease: anteroposterior radiograph of the left hip showing the sequence of changes. There has been complete resolution (bottom right).

Management

The management of Perthes' disease has to be seen in the light of the natural history of the condition (Stulberg et al 1981). The older the child at onset of disease the more likely he is to have a poor result. Many develop osteoarthrosis of the hip in later years and so very long-term follow-up is necessary to determine the outcome of various methods of management.

Most orthopaedic surgeons agree that where there is spasm and limitation of movement in the hip, rest with or without skin traction is useful and thereafter the child is either managed symptomatically or the principle of containment of the femoral head is pursued. If the femoral head can be contained within the acetabulum and moved, sphericity of the head should ensue. Groups 1 and 2 (less than half head involvement) of the Catterall classification are generally observed. The problem lies in knowing how best to manage children with group 3 or 4 (greater than half head involvement) of Catterall's classification. Management varies from observation to use of a brace, to plaster casts, to surgery to obtain containment. Patients may need to wear casts for up to a year and there is no very long-term evidence to suggest that this confers any advantage over any particular method.

Surgery

Surgery has been attempted to provide femoral head containment and there are two approaches:

1. In the USA there is a trend towards using pelvic osteotomy to obtain containment.
2. In the UK there has been a tendency to use varus derotation femoral osteotomy.

There is no very long-term information as to the efficacy of these procedures.

SURGICAL INTERVENTION IN CEREBRAL PALSY

Non-surgical aspects of cerebral palsy have been described in Chapter 8. Surgery has a part to play in cerebral palsy and can be helpful in correcting or preventing deformity, lengthening musculotendinous units and improving muscle balance across a joint, and improving walking patterns and therefore diminishing the energy cost of walking.

It is convenient to consider patients as hemiplegic, diplegic or total body involvement, although one should be aware that there are overlaps between the groups. It is also helpful to have some concept of the patient from a physiological point of view and descriptive terms such as spastic or flaccid, ataxic, athetoid or rigid are used. Knowledge of the natural history of the cerebral palsy patient is essential and it should not be forgotten that it is an incurable condition and that patterns of the cerebral palsy change with growth, adaptation of the patient to the condition and possibly after intervention. There is no good evidence that any form of splintage or physiotherapy will have a permanent beneficial effect in the long-term or prevent progression of deformity (Bleck 1990).

Assessment

The orthopaedic surgeon should be part of a team that cares for cerebral palsied children. The physiotherapist is usually the link person and is often seen as a confidant for the parents and child and an organiser of the child's various activities. It is essential to have someone who sees the child regularly so as to detect any changes in patterns of neurological impairment, as there is always a tendency for other personnel to obtain a snapshot view of the patient at infrequent examinations.

Charting range of movement

Passive range of movement and muscle charting, where possible, are very helpful in pre-operative planning and can be used to assess postoperative results. Whilst there are limitations with this approach, at least it gives a clinical record if performed by the same person and ensures that the patient is examined objectively rather than qualitatively.

Setting. Children respond and relax in familiar surroundings and a more accurate assessment of range of movement can be made if carried out by someone known to the child, usually the physiotherapist (see Chapter 22 Planning for Progress). Accurate assessment takes time and cannot be rushed, particularly when a child has a short attention span and several short examinations may be necessary. Muscle charting is difficult to perform in the presence of excess muscle tone but if the patient can cooperate broad guidelines are obtainable. It is kinder to more severely involved children and better information is obtained by examining them at their special schools or institutions in familiar surroundings rather than in an out-patient clinic.

Assessment of walking ability

Where appropriate an assessment of the child's ability to walk is essential and, if appropriate, the physiological cost index can also be measured. Although the Hoffer et al (1973) classification of walking ability was devised for spina bifida, it is also useful and simple to apply to the cerebral palsied child.

The child's walking pattern can be recorded on videotape to enable a visual assessment of patterns of gait and also to provide comparisons later. Not all centres have instrumented gait analysis. Many now feel that this is an essential part of surgical workup as neuromuscular patterns in cerebral palsy are extremely complicated to analyse and one may have a situation where two children appear to have the same walking pattern, receive the same surgery and one is worse after while the other is better (Winters et al 1987).

Instrumented gait analysis permits a better understanding of the biomechanics of gait. Two sorts of information can be obtained:

1 Kinematic, which deals with measurement of movement.

2 Kinetic, which concerns measurement of forces tending to cause lower limb movement.

An analogy is that kinematics shows what happens whereas kinetics explains what happens. In the author's practice all children who are walkers undergo instrumented gait analysis before surgery (see Chapter 17 Common Assessment Procedures). It is also essential to distinguish spasticity from fixed contracture. This is often possible without giving the child a general anaesthetic but, where there is doubt, this is an important pre-operative evaluation, as fixed deformity can be helped by surgery whereas dynamic deformity may not be and is a more difficult management problem.

Orthoses

After pre-operative assessment some patients will not require surgery but may require provision of appropriate orthoses. There is a tendency to equate the diagnosis of cerebral palsy with the provision of ankle/foot orthoses to act as a static splint (see Chapter 21 Aids and Appliances). It is better not to splint unless absolutely necessary and the decision to use splints should be taken in conjunction with an orthotist, whose skills are required to cast the child and manufacture the splint.

Ankle/foot orthoses can have profound biomechanical effects on walking and simple modifications such as altering the shank–foot angle or applying a rocker to the sole of the shoe can alter the origin of the ground reaction force and can have either a beneficial or deleterious effect on the walking pattern. Clinically, it has been widely recognised that the application of a plastic orthosis can alter gait patterns but there is an underlying biomechanical explanation for this and a greater knowledge of biomechanics and orthotic theory is to be welcomed.

Surgery

The foregoing investigations and assessments are helpful in determining what particular operation, or operations, are indicated.

Aims of management

The aim of management is to obtain the highest potential for physical and intellectual development and will vary according to the pattern of involvement. For example, a child with a mild hemiplegia may only require an elongation of the tendo-Achilles to achieve a plantigrade foot, whereas a child with total body involvement and no prospects of walking may benefit from adductor surgery to improve seating balance and perineal access for hygiene.

There has been a tendency in the past to perform one operation at a time if multiple operations are required. It is now more common to perform surgery at several levels if necessary as the above investigations can give a better evaluation of the patient. In general, in the lower extremity surgery starts at the hip and progresses distally. After surgery the child should be got up as quickly as possible using whatever aids are necessary.

Timing of surgery

In general it is better to defer surgery until the child is of a sufficient age to cooperate with any postoperative rehabilitation programme, but this is not always possible and certainly procedures to prevent hip dislocation in a child who is potentially a walker should not be deferred. Severe learning difficulties or lack of sitting balance should not be a contraindication for surgery and operations fall into two categories. Elongation of musculotendinous units or transfers can be indicated in the absence of joint deformity. In the presence of fixed joint deformity, surgery to release ligaments or perform osteotomies with or without muscle balancing procedures is indicated.

Upper limb surgery

This is not as frequently carried out as lower limb surgery and in general orthoses are poorly tolerated and usually inefficacious. Before attempting procedures in the upper limb it is essential to remember that many children have associated sensory derangement, for example deficiency in proprioception, which are permanent and will affect function irrespective of whether or not surgery has been undertaken. Surgery in the upper limb should be deferred as long as possible and procedures usually consist of positioning the arm in a more cosmetically acceptable functional position.

The shoulder. The shoulder is rarely operated on but if there is a severe internal rotation de-

formity derotation osteotomy is occasionally undertaken.

The elbow. More frequently, elbow release, consisting of bicipital and brachioradialis lengthening, is undertaken and, if there is a severe pronation deformity with associated passive supination, release of pronator teres is possible.

Wrist and finger deformities. These are the most obvious and, in a moderate deformity, musculoaponeurotic lengthening of the long flexor and tenotomies, or transfers of flexor carpi ulnaris, is possible. It is important to bear in mind that this will not necessarily improve finger function in severe deformity and if there is an unacceptable cosmetic appearance or problems with hygiene due to excessive wrist flexion, arthrodesis is possible to achieve a more cosmetically acceptable position.

'Thumb in palm' deformity. Again, this can cause problems with hygiene and operations have been designed to release the dysplastic adductor and to lengthen the flexor pollicis longus and possibly augment the abductor pollicis longus (Skoff & Woodbury 1985).

Spinal deformity

This affects patients with total body involvement more than any other group. Several types of spinal deformity occur: hyperlordosis is usually indicative of hip flexion contractures and the spine should not be seen in isolation.

Neuromuscular scoliosis occurs in over 25% of patients and can be controlled initially by the use of spinal orthoses or adjustments to seating. If the curve is progressive and threatens the child's ability to sit, surgical stabilisation can be considered and recently there has been a greater interest in performing spinal arthrodesis, even in severely handicapped children, as they will be permanently wheelchair-bound. The more severe curves require preliminary anterior release and posterior stabilisation using the Luque type of instrumentation (Gersoff & Renshaw 1988). If there is fixed pelvic obliquity the fusion should be carried out to the level of the sacrum. This is major surgery and severe retardation or handicap may present a moral quandary for the parents and surgeon.

Lower limb surgery

The majority of operations are directed towards the lower limbs. The usual hip deformities, adduction, flexion and internal rotation and their combination can cause acetabular dysplasia, hip subluxation and eventual dislocation in the more severely affected patient (Cooke et al 1989). Physiotherapy and bracing do not prevent subluxation.

Muscle releases are helpful before the onset of lateral femoral migration but, should subluxation occur, they have to be combined with a bony femoral procedure with or without pelvic osteotomy.

There is controversy as to what should be best done for those children who develop a subluxing hip and have no long-term potential for walking. The problem is twofold. In some instances there has been a fairly high rate of redislocation, even following major surgical procedures. However, although major procedures can carry the risk of redisplacement, if successful they may improve sitting balance, have a favourable effect on the spine and prevent the development of a painful dislocated hip.

Hip adduction. Excessive adduction at the hip when walking, or difficulties in perineal access, can be improved by tenotomy of adductor longus and gracilis and occasionally part of adductor brevis as well, if particularly tight. A total adductor release is contraindicated as the patient could then acquire an abduction contracture. If there is an associated hip flexion contracture, recession or tenotomy of the psoas tendon can be performed. The indication for psoas surgery varies. The patient who has hip flexion of 0° has already lost extension and has the onset of a hip flexion contracture. Because hip flexion can cause increased difficulty in walking some surgeons advocate performing psoas surgery once there has been loss of extension at the hip. Others prefer to use an upper limit of 20° fixed flexion.

Internal rotation. Excessive internal rotation of the hip can be improved by rotational osteotomy as there is no good evidence that elongation of the adductors improves internal rotation gait. The difficulty about performing derotation femoral osteotomy in the young is that the deforming forces continue to act on the immature skeleton and recurrence of the internal rotation is usually the norm. Where possible, derotation should be delayed until nearer skeletal maturity to avoid the necessity for reoperation.

Knee flexion deformity. This may be due either to spasticity of the hamstrings and relative weakness of the quadriceps or to excessive spasticity of the gastrocnemius; it is essential to determine which muscle group is causing the problem. If hamstring lengthening is being contemplated the current approach is to perform a fractional lengthening of the hamstrings. Occasionally, if the deformity is severe and cannot be corrected either by a combination of fractional lengthening and posterior capsulotomy, it is necessary to perform an extension supracondylar osteotomy to abolish the knee flexion contracture. This will not increase the range of motion at the knee but merely place the arc of motion in a more physiologically acceptable position. The knee should not be seen in isolation without carefully examining the hip and ankle.

Foot deformities. The most obvious deformity in cerebral palsy is an equinus attitude of the foot. Contracture of the triceps should be differentiated from dynamic deformity. The aim of any intervention is to produce a plantigrade foot and this may be achieved by a variety of methods to elongate the musculotendinous unit. Exercises, orthoses and serial casting do not correct equinus contracture and, if applied injudiciously, can produce a midtarsal break. The surgical pitfall is to overlengthen the triceps, thereby producing a calcaneus attitude of the foot, which is a more severe deformity than equinus. The simplest management of equinus is to provide the child with a heel raise.

Both valgus and varus foot deformities occur often in association with equinus. A reasonable indication for surgery is failure of an orthosis to maintain a proper position of the foot. Varus is the more difficult of the two to deal with but may be treated by tendon-balancing operations if the joints remain mobile, e.g. split transfers of the tibialis anterior or posterior. Fixed deformity of the heel may require treatment by a calcaneal osteotomy. Total rigidity of the foot may require triple arthrodesis (talocalcaneal, or talonavicular and calcaneocuboid joints). Hindfoot valgus responds well to a subtalar fusion and where the deformity has become rigid, triple arthrodesis again is a salvage procedure. Hallux valgus is often seen with cerebral palsy and can be treated by either metatarsal osteotomy or by fusion of the first metatarsophalangeal joint.

It is important to remember that a valgus deformity of the foot may be secondary to a valgus deformity of the knee and it is essential that the lower limb should be seen and evaluated as a whole before operating on any particular part of it (Bleck 1990).

Recovery time following even simple myotomies or tendon-lengthening procedures is lengthy and requires diligent physiotherapy support for the child. It may take many months for a child to recover from what may be a relatively minor procedure.

DUCHENNE MUSCULAR DYSTROPHY

Neurological aspects of this condition have been covered elsewhere (see p. 190) and management of this condition is palliative. However, physiotherapy plays an important role in maintaining a good range of passive movements of joints in the lower limbs and in keeping the patient as mobile as possible for as long as possible. Common deformities occurring with this condition are progressive flexion deformity at the hips, an equinovarus deformity at the feet and a collapsing type of neurological scoliosis. Surgery has a definite role to play in these deformities. Indications for spinal fusion have been covered in the section on scoliosis.

Hip flexion contracture

Once a hip flexion contracture has become significant and is contributing to difficulty in walking it is reasonable to release the hip flexor musculature. If the patient is still able to walk he should be mobilised as soon as possible, as bed-rest causes rapid deterioration in muscle strength. Hip flexor release is also useful even in the non-walking stage, as it allows the patient to sleep on his back and assist with transfers. The feet may

deform either during the walking phase or once the child becomes chairbound.

Equinovarous deformity

Equinovarus deformity can be treated by minimal surgical exposure and a tenotomy of the Achilles tendon and tibialis posterior tendons and, once again, the patient should be mobilised as soon as possible and will often require to wear an ankle/foot orthosis to control ankle position. The use of orthoses while the child is still mobile is beneficial and a thoracolumbar–sacral orthosis is often required. Once the patient becomes chairbound, underarm orthoses to control spinal curvature are ineffective.

SPINAL DYSRAPHISM

The neurological aspects of spinal dysraphism have been covered elsewhere (see p. 130) and management of the child with spina bifida involves a multidisciplinary approach (see Chapter 8 Disorders of the Central Nervous System). The UK incidence of this condition has fallen dramatically since the introduction of antenatal screening using ultrasound scans and alpha-fetoprotein determinations.

Spina bifida

Spina bifida usually involves other systemic abnormalities, particularly of the renal system. At birth it is useful to try to evaluate the neurological level and also to check on the presence of hydrocephalus and raised intracranial pressure. If the infant is likely to survive but has an open lesion (Fig. 12.13), early closure is indicated within 24 hours, and is frequently followed a few days later by the insertion of a shunt should hydrocephalus ensue. Where there is a relatively low lesion and there are particular agonist muscle groups in the lower extremities, passive stretching by physiotherapy staff to obtain a reasonable foot posture should begin at birth. Once a reasonable shape has been obtained for the foot, maintenance is often necessary using ankle/foot orthoses.

Paralytic dislocation of the hips or subluxation

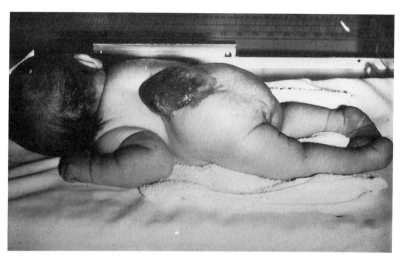

Fig. 12.13 Spina bifida: thoracolumbar lesion. Note the foot deformities.

occurs most commonly in those children who have a low lumbar lesion and is most likely to occur in a marginal walker. Hip dislocation in itself does not influence the ultimate outcome for walking and, providing reciprocal movement is possible, appropriate orthoses can be applied irrespective of whether the hip is located or dislocated. The most important factors are motivation, absence of obesity and joint contractures, and good upper limb function. A variety of surgical procedures has been advocated for neurological dislocation of the hip and depend on availability of motor units and often include adductor release and iliopsoas recession. More major procedures, such as femoral or pelvic osteotomy, may also be indicated. Surgery to relocate hips if paralysis is at L3 or above is not recommended (Drummond et al 1980).

Flexion contractures of the knee are undesirable, particularly if the child has a low lumbar lesion and is likely to walk with the aid of ankle/foot orthoses. Maintenance of motion at the knee and passive stretching of the knee are indicated but care should be taken to avoid subluxation of the knee joint during stretching in the presence of diminished or altered sensation in the joint. Where fixed flexion deformity is present surgical release of the hamstrings may be appropriate.

The foot may present in a variety of deformities due to muscle imbalance. Torsional deformities

in the lower extremities may also complicate apparent foot deformity. The aim of any treatment is to provide a plantigrade foot and the procedures undertaken will be determined by the deformity.

The indications for surgical treatment of the spine in myelomeningocele have already been covered (see p. 210).

Orthoses

Most patients who have a lower lumbar lesion and in whom there is power 5 of the quadriceps and power 4 of the medial hamstrings have the potential to walk using ankle/foot orthoses with or without an external aid. In those children with higher lesions and flail hips, early walking offers important gains over those confined to a wheelchair at an early stage, even though few continue to walk as adults (Mazur et al 1989). Patients who walked had fewer fractures and sores, were more independent and better at transferring, but early wheelchair-users were hospitalised less.

The factors affecting ambulatory status are most probably related to energy expenditure and control of obesity (Asher & Olson 1983) and a useful functional classification of walking in these patients has been provided by Hoffer et al (1973). Two orthoses have been introduced to give a reciprocal gait pattern and also to enable standing. These orthoses are: the reciprocating gait orthosis (see Chapter 21 Aids and Appliances) (Yngve et al 1984) and hip guidance orthosis (Rose et al 1983). A prerequisite before fitting such an orthosis is that there is no more than a 20° flexion contracture at the hip or the knee and the foot can be rendered in a reasonable plantigrade position. Some children may need to undergo extensive surgical operations to align the lower extremities and to abolish flexion contractures to within this range. Residual equinus or deformity in the feet can be compensated by using appropriate orthoses and, if there is a unilateral hip dislocation, limb length inequality can be compensated by an appropriate raise.

A concomitant spinal deformity can also be braced using either type of orthosis. The child needs to be assessed by an orthopaedic surgeon to determine whether or not surgery is necessary for lower limb alignment and should have power 5 latissmus dorsi bilaterally and reasonable upper limb function, cerebral function and motivation; and should not be obese. If these criteria are met orthoses may be supplied and the child then undergoes an intensive physiotherapy programme to learn how to use these orthoses. Parental support during and after training is essential for success. Long-term data on acceptability of such orthoses does not exist but preliminary experience with them suggests that they are not necessarily rejected at the time of adolescence and have the advantage of giving the individual a greater degree of autonomy.

REFERENCES

Ansell B M, Swann M 1983 The management of chronic arthritis of children. Journal of Bone and Joint Surgery 65B: 536–543

Asher M, Olson J 1983 Factors affecting the ambulatory status of patients with spina bifida cystica. Journal of Bone and Joint Surgery 65A: 350–356

Bleck E E 1990 Management of the lower extemities in children who have cerebral palsy. Journal of Bone and Joint Surgery 72A: 140–144

Blockey N J 1984 Derotation osteotomy in the management of congenital dislocation of the hip. Journal of Bone and Joint Surgery 66B: 485–490

Bradley J, Wetherill M, Benson M K D 1987 Splintage for congenital dislocation of the hip. Is it safe and reliable? Journal of Bone and Joint Surgery 69B: 257–263

Brougham D I, Broughton N S, Cole W G et al 1988 The predictability of acetabular development after closed reduction for congenital dislocation of the hip. Journal of Bone and Joint Surgery 70B: 733–736

Catterall A 1971 The natural history of Perthes' disease. Journal of Bone and Joint Surgery 53B: 37–53

Catterall A, Pringle J, Byers P D et al 1982 A review of the morphology of Perthes' disease. Journal of Bone and Joint Surgery 64B: 269–281

Clarke N M P, Harcke H T, McHugh P et al 1985 Real time ultrasound in the diagnosis of congenital dislocation and dysplasia of the hip. Journal of Bone and Joint Surgery 67B: 406–412

Clarke N M P, Clegg J, Al-Chalabi A N 1989 Ultrasound screening of hips at risk for congenital dislocation of the hip. Failure to reduce the incidence of late cases. Journal of Bone and Joint Surgery 71B: 9–12

Cooke P H, Cole W G, Carey R P L 1989 Dislocation of the hip in cerebral palsy. Natural history and predictability. Journal of Bone and Joint Surgery 71B: 441–446

Cummings R J, Lovell W W 1988 Operative treatment of congenital idiopathic club foot. Journal of Bone and Joint Surgery 70A: 1108–1112

Dhar S, Taylor J F, Jones W A et al 1990 Early open reduction for congenital dislocation of the hip. Journal of Bone and Joint Surgery 72B: 175–80

Dickson R A 1985 Conservative treatment for idiopathic scoliosis. Journal of Bone and Joint Surgery 67B: 176–181

Drummond D S, Moreau M, Cruess R L 1980 Results and complications of surgery for the paralytic hip and spine in myelomeningocele. Journal of Bone and Joint Surgery 62B: 49–53

Gersoff W K, Renshaw T S 1988 The treatment of scoliosis in cerebral palsy by posterior spinal fusion with Luque-rod segmental instrumentation. Journal of Bone and Joint Surgery 70A: 41–44

Grill F, Franke J 1987 The Ilizarov distractor for the correction of relapsed or neglected club foot. Journal of Bone and Joint Surgery 69B: 593–597

Hanson V, Drexler E, Konreich H 1969 The relationship of rheumatoid factor to age of onset in juvenile rheumatoid arthritis. Arthritis and Rheumatism 12: 82–86

Hoffer M M, Feiwell E, Perry R et al 1973 Functional ambulation in patients with myelomeningocele. Journal of Bone and Joint Surgery 55A: 137–148

Howell F R, Newman R J, Wang H L et al 1989 The three dimensional anatomy of the proximal femur in Perthes' disease. Journal of Bone and Joint Surgery 71B: 408–412

Ippolito E, Ponseti I V 1980 Congenital club foot in the human fetus. Journal of Bone and Joint Surgery 62A: 8–22

Iwasaki K 1983 Treatment of congenital dislocation of the hip by the Pavlik harness. Mechanism of reduction and usage. Journal of Bone and Joint Surgery 65A: 760–767

Jacobsen S T, Levison J E, Crawford A H 1985 Late results of synovectomy in juvenile rheumatoid arthritis. Journal of Bone and Joint Surgery 67A: 8–15

Jefferson R J, Weisz I, Turner-Smith A R et al 1988 Scoliosis surgery and its effect on back shape. Journal of Bone and Joint Surgery 70B: 261–6

Joseph B 1989 Morphological changes in the acetabulum in Perthes' disease. Journal of Bone and Joint Surgery 71B: 756–763

Laaksonen A L 1966 A prognostic study of juvenile rheumatoid arthritis. Acta Paediatrica Scandinavica 166 (Supplement): 1

Labelle H, Tohme S, Duhaime M et al 1986 Natural history of scoliosis in Friedrich's Ataxia. Journal of Bone and Joint Surgery 68A: 564–572

Lonstein J E, Carlson J M 1984 The prediction of curve progression in untreated idiopathic scoliosis during growth. Journal of Bone and Joint Surgery 66A: 1061–1071

McMaster M J 1983 Infantile idiopathic scoliosis — can it be prevented? Journal of Bone and Joint Surgery 65B: 612–617

McMaster M J 1987 Anterior and posterior instrumentation and fusion of thoraco-lumbar scoliosis due to myelomeningocele. Journal of Bone and Joint Surgery 69B: 20–25

McMaster M J, Ohtsuka K 1982 The natural history of congenital scoliosis. A study of 251 patients. Journal of Bone and Joint Surgery 64A: 1128–1147

Macnicol M F 1990 Results of a 25-year screening programme for neonatal hip instability. Journal of Bone and Joint Surgery 72B: 1057–1060

Mazur J M, Shurtleff D, Menelaus M et al 1989 Orthopaedic management of high level spina bifida. Early walking compared with early use of a wheelchair. Journal of Bone and Joint Surgery 71A: 56–61

Mitchell G P 1983 The hip: congenital dislocation. In: Harris N H (ed) Postgraduate textbook of clinical orthopaedics. Wright, Bristol, ch 4, pp 96–109

O'Garra J A 1959 The radiographic changes in Perthes' disease. Journal of Bone and Joint Surgery 41B: 465–76

Piggott H 1980 Natural history of scoliosis in myelodysplasia. Journal of Bone and Joint Surgery 62B: 54–58

Rose J K, Sankarankutty M, Stallard J 1983 A clinical review of the orthotic treatment of myelomeningocele patients. Journal of Bone and Joint Surgery 65B: 242–246

Saies A D, Foster B K, Lequesne G W 1988 The value of a new ultrasound stress test in assessment and treatment of clinically detected hip instability. Journal of Paediatric Orthopaedics 8: 436–41

Salter R B, Thompson G H 1984 Legg–Calve–Perthes' disease. The prognostic significance of the subchondral fracture and the two group classification of the femoral head involvement. Journal of Bone and Joint Surgery 66A: 479–89

Schaller J G 1984 Chronic arthritis in children. Juvenile rheumatoid arthritis. Clinical Orthopaedics 182: 79–89

Shapiro F 1985 Consequences of an osteogenesis imperfecta diagnosis for survival and ambulation. Journal of Paediatric Orthopaedics 5: 456–462

Shapiro F, Bresnan M J 1982a Orthopaedic management of childhood neuromuscular disease. Spinal muscular atrophy. Journal of Bone and Joint Surgery 64A: 785–789

Shapiro F, Bresnan M J 1982b Orthopaedic management of childhood neuromuscular disease. Peripheral neuropathies, Friedrich's ataxia, arthrogryposis multiplex congenita. Journal of Bone and Joint Surgery 64A: 949–953

Shapiro F, Bresnan M J 1982c Orthopaedic management of childhood muscular disease. Diseases of muscle. Journal of Bone and Joint Surgery 64A: 1102–1107

Simmons E D, Graham H K, Szalai J P 1990 Interobserver variability in grading Perthes' disease. Journal of Bone and Joint Surgery 72B: 202–204

Skoff H, Woodbury D F 1985 Management of the upper extremity in cerebral palsy. Journal of Bone and Joint Surgery 67A: 500 503

Smith R 1984 Osteogenesis imperfecta. British Medical Journal 289: 394–396

Stockley I, Bell M J, Sharrard W J W 1989 The role of expanding intramedullary rods in osteogenesis imperfecta. Journal of Bone and Joint Surgery 71B: 442–427

Stulberg S D, Cooperman D R, Wallenstein R 1981 The natural history of Legg–Calve–Perthes' disease. Journal of Bone and Joint Surgery 63A: 1095–1108

Taitz L S 1987 Child abuse and osteogenesis imperfecta. British Medical Journal 295: 1082–1083

Thomas K J, Simon S R 1988 Progression of scoliosis after skeletal maturity in institutionalised adults who have cerebral palsy. Journal of Bone and Joint Surgery 70A: 1290–1296

Thompson G H 1985 Arthrogryposis multiplex congenita. Clinical Orthopaedics 194: 2–3

Victoria-Diaz A, Victoria-Diaz J 1984 Pathogenesis of idiopathic club foot. Clinical Orthopaedics 185: 14–24

Weinstein S L, Ponseti I V 1983 Curve progression in idiopathic scoliosis. Journal of Bone and Joint Surgery 65A: 447–455

Wenger D R, Ward W T, Herring J A 1991 Legg–Calve–Perthes' disease. Journal of Bone and Joint Surgery 73A: 778–788

Winters T F, Gage J R, Hicks R 1987 Gait patterns in spastic hemiplegia in children and young adults. Journal of Bone and Joint Surgery 69A: 437–441

Wynne-Davies R 1970 Acetabular dysplasia and familial joint laxity. Two aetiological factors in congenital dislocation of the hip. Journal of Bone and Joint Surgery 52B: 704–716

Yngve D A, Douglas R, Roberts J M 1984 The reciprocating gait orthosis in myelomeningocele. Journal of Paediatric Orthopaedics 4: 304–10

13

Infection and trauma

P. Eckersley   M. I. Griffiths
T. Marshall

INFECTION IN BABIES AND CHILDREN
T. Marshall

INTRODUCTION

Over the past forty to fifty years there has been a dramatic reduction in infant mortality rates from 60–70 deaths per 1000 live births in the 1940s to 10–15 per 1000 in the late 1980s. Infant deaths make up 70% of the total mortality figures for childhood (0–14 years). This fall in mortality has been largely due to a reduction in mortality from infectious disease.

In the developed countries this reduction in mortality has come about through:

- Improvements in the nutrition of the population.
- Improved standards of hygiene and sanitation.
- Benefits of modern medicine including:

    — vaccination
    — improved drug treatment of infection
    — better standards of medical care.

There has also been a reduction in the virulence of some infectious organisms, e.g. the group A streptococci.

In the developed countries the common causes of infant mortality are related to preterm delivery, congenital abnormality and sudden infant death syndrome. In subsequent years accidents and malignant diseases are the most common causes of death and infection is more often a contributory cause in the already compromised child. However, in the developing countries, nutritional disorders and infection, often combined, remain the most common causes of death in childhood. A cycle of infection, often gastroenteritis leading to malnutrition, which predisposes to further infection, easily becomes established.

Despite the reduction in mortality in developed countries infection is still a major cause of childhood illness and is the most common reason for contact between a child and his general practitioner. It is important to understand that although the incidence of infectious disease has fallen in the UK there has not been the same reduction in illness due to non-contagious infection.

PREVENTION AND CONTROL OF INFECTION

Resistance to infection

The skin provides an effective outer protection against infection. Most bacteria, when placed on intact skin, are not able to cause infection. The respiratory, gastrointestinal and genitourinary systems all breach this protective outer layer and therefore have their own specialised protective mechanisms:

1. The nose acts as an efficient filter of particulate matter in the upper tract, and lower respiratory tract mucus traps particles that penetrate the first line of defence.
2. The bowel derives its protection from stomach acidity, bile, proteolytic enzymes and the established bowel bacterial flora.
3. The urinary tract derives its protection from the length of the urethra and the protective effect of regular flushing with urine.

Some bacteria and viruses have adaptations that enable them to become established despite the host's local defences. Any impairment of these natural defences will enable infection to develop. Damaged skin may become quickly infected with organisms that usually only colonise healthy skin. Bacterial respiratory tract infections are common

when mucociliary clearance is impaired, as may happen after infections that damage the ciliated epithelium, e.g. measles or whooping cough, if the cilia themselves are defective or if the mucus is excessively thick, as in cystic fibrosis. The urinary tract is more commonly infected in females, who possess a shorter urethra than males. Ascending infection will result if there is any impairment of the flushing action of urine as in urinary obstruction or vesicoureteric reflux in childhood.

Immunity

Active immunity

Active immunity may result from natural infection or from stimulation of the immune system artificially with vaccines. These vaccines may contain whole organisms, which remain live but have been made safe (attenuated), e.g. measles, mumps, rubella and BCG vaccines. Some vaccines contain killed organisms or an antigenic preparation of an organism, e.g. pertussis and cholera. Some vaccines contain detoxified toxins (toxoids), e.g. diphtheria and tetanus.

Passive immunity

Passive immunity is acquired by the fetus in the form of transplacental maternal IgG antibodies during the last trimester of pregnancy. Passive immunity may also be given in the form of an injection of antibodies, which confer temporary immunity only. Human normal immunoglobulin is used to produce protection against hepatitis A but only remains effective for 12 weeks. Human specific immunoglobulin is produced from individuals with high titres of antibodies to specific infections and may be used to provide post-exposure protection, e.g. against hepatitis B, rabies and *Varicella zoster* viruses.

Special precautions

Travellers abroad should receive the necessary immunisations and be prepared to take precautions to minimise the risk of contracting diseases endemic in the country to be visited. These include general precautions, such as drinking only bottled, boiled or purified water, peeling all fruit, washing salads in purified water and avoiding un-pasteurised milk and milk products. Swimming in lakes or slow-moving streams in Africa or Asia should be avoided because of the risk of contracting schistosomiasis. Specific precautions would include the regular use of antimalarial drugs in endemic areas and the use of insect repellents and mosquito nets.

TRANSMISSION OF INFECTION

The three main routes of transmission of infection are by inhalation, ingestion and inoculation.

Infection may be acquired either directly or indirectly in a number of different ways (Table 13.1).

SPECIAL PROBLEMS OF CHILDREN
Anatomical considerations

Respiratory infection is the most common reason for admission to hospital in infancy. Due to their small size and immaturity, infants are more liable than older and larger children to develop respiratory distress with a given respiratory infection. Consideration of the special anatomical and functional characteristics of the infant's chest and airways will help to explain this phenomenon.

Table 13.1 Transmission of infection

Method	Agent	Types
Inhalation	Droplets Particles	Whooping cough Measles Psittacosis
Contact	Fomites	Infected bedding, toys, clothes, etc
Ingestion	Contaminated food	Salmonella Hepatitis A
Insect vectors	Bites Contact	Malaria Food contamination
Inoculation	Rubbing — eyes — nose — skin	Respiratory syncytial virus Impetigo from Staphylococcus aureus Tetanus
Autoinoculation (reinfection)	Parasitic life-cycle anus/mouth transfer	Threadworms

The rib-cage of young infants is soft and compliant. During a respiratory infection, when respiratory effort is increased, infants often show dramatic sternal and costal recession during inspiration. This tendency of the chest wall to collapse inwards during inspiration reduces the effectiveness of the diaphragmatic effort. The large airways of young children are also relatively compliant and so, during forced expiration, the large airways tend to collapse and this may reduce the cross-sectional area of the airway by 50% or more.

The large airways of young children are relatively narrow compared with the total cross-sectional area of the small airways, which is relatively generous. The velocity of linear airflow in tubes is proportional to the fourth power of the radius of the tube, so it can be seen that even a small reduction in the size of a large airway of a young infant results in a disproportionately large reduction in airflow. The limitation of inspiratory and forced expiratory airflow places the young child with respiratory infection at much greater risk of exhaustion and/or respiratory failure than older children and adults.

The immune response

Young infants and children have a relatively immature and inexperienced immune system, which renders them more susceptible to infection.

In the mature individual the immune system mounts a two-pronged attack against infection. This attack consists of the humoral (antibody-related) and the cell-mediated response (dependent on neutrophils, macrophages and T lymphocytes). Transplacental transfer of IgG antibody occurs actively over the last trimester of pregnancy and gives the newborn infant a degree of protection to some of those infections to which its mother has been exposed. The infant's own IgG production increases from 3 to 6 months of postnatal life and adult levels are not reached until 6 to 8 years. The newborn infant therefore has a physiological hypogammaglobulinaemia, which persists into childhood and which is even more marked in the premature infant who may not have acquired protective levels of maternal antibody. The cell-mediated response of young infants is also immature with poor neutrophil chemotaxis and immature T lymphocyte function.

The immune system is not only immature but also inexperienced and therefore once the protection of maternally derived antibody has waned the infant will be susceptible to primary infections. It is only after an infection has been experienced that memory cells are produced and retained, within the immune system, enabling a rapid and effective response on re-exposure. Thus acquired immunity develops only gradually.

SPECIFIC TYPES OF INFECTION

Congenital infections

Congenital infections are those that are acquired by the fetus prior to birth. The result of any such infection will depend on its type and the stage of gestation. Infections at an early stage of pregnancy may result in abortion, severe malformation or disability (see Chapter 10 Profound and Multiple Disability).

Cytomegalovirus

Cytomegalovirus (CMV) is a ubiquitous virus found in blood, urine, semen, breast milk, saliva, nasal and cervical secretions. There is no known animal reservoir and infection is believed to occur by direct or indirect person to person contact.

Incidence. 40–50% of women in the UK are non-immune to CMV. 1% of seronegative mothers seroconvert during their pregnancy, indicating a primary infection, although clinically recognisable maternal infection is uncommon. 20–50% of mothers who do seroconvert will transmit the infection to their infants. Routine virology screening of infants has shown that 0.3–0.4% of infants in the UK have been infected with CMV in utero. As CMV is a virus of the herpes family it possesses the ability to lie dormant and to become reactivated. Some infants will be infected through reactivation of maternal infection rather than primary infection. These infants generally seem to be less severely affected.

Clinical presentation. The infant with the classic syndrome of severe CMV infection will be growth retarded, have evidence of myocarditis, hepatitis, pneumonitis and encephalitis and there will be haematological involvement with thrombocytopaenia and a haemolytic anaemia. The infant will therefore be jaundiced with hepatosplenomegaly. There will be a bleeding tendency and the infant will be microcephalic and suffer seizures. Only 1–2% of infants with congenital CMV infection will show this severe form of the disease. For those infants who are severely affected the long-term outlook is grim, with severe microcephaly and mental retardation, spastic tetraplegia, deafness and blindness due to chorioretinitis (and brain damage) as the likely outcome. A further 10% of infected infants may have minor or transient problems at birth. The latter group, and asymptomatic babies, are at increased risk of sensorineural deafness, learning disorders and of lower than expected IQ. It has been suggested that these more mildly affected infants may suffer progressive damage during infancy and childhood, although this is unproven and may reflect the difficulty of testing hearing and IQ accurately in the very young infant.

Congenital toxoplasmosis

Toxoplasma, a protozoal parasite, may be acquired transplacentally from mothers who have their primary infection in pregnancy. The infection may be contracted directly by ingesting poorly cooked infected meat or by indirect contact with oocysts in cat faeces or with infected soil, where the cysts may persist for several months.

Approximately 6 in 1000 women will acquire the primary infection during pregnancy, resulting in an incidence of congenital toxoplasma infection in the infants of 1–2 in every 1000 live births. Clinical infection in UK newborns is uncommon but subclinical infection more common. The clinical picture of severe illness is similar to that of the other congenital infections. Subclinical infection is associated with an increased incidence of mental retardation and visual inpairment due to chorioretinitis later in childhood. If diagnosed early, treatment with pyrimethamine and sulphadiazine may protect infants against the late effects of the disease.

Congenital rubella infection

Rubella is an acute viral infection usually of little direct consequence to the affected adult but which may cause fetal infection during a primary infection in pregnancy. Previous infection gives good protection. Rubella is frequently a subclinical infection — 26% of mothers in one study gave no history of rubella or contact with rubella during pregnancy.

Incidence. The severity of the congenital rubella syndrome increases the earlier in pregnancy the infection occurs. 90–95% of maternal rubella infection in the first 12 weeks of pregnancy results in infection of the fetus but not all infected fetuses are damaged. Infection in the first 8 weeks of pregnancy carries a 40–60% risk of fetal damage. The infant infected with CMV or rubella may continue to excrete the virus for many months after birth. Rubella virus has been isolated from cataracts excised up to 4 years of age. It is likely that the virus infection induces a defect in cell-mediated immunity, which results in continued viral excretion and for this reason these infants may remain a source of infection.

Clinical presentation. The clinical effects of the full-blown congenital rubella syndrome are similar to those described above for CMV infection. In addition rubella infection occurring early in pregnancy may cause structural abnormalities of the:

- heart — commonly persistent ductus arteriosus, ventricular septal defect, or pulmonary artery stenosis
- eyes — with cataracts and a characteristic pigmentary retinopathy
- nervous system — with deafness, microcephaly and cerebral palsy.

Prevention of congenital infections

Cytomegalovirus

An experimental live attenuated CMV vaccine has been tried on some renal transplant patients and although it does not appear to prevent CMV infection, it does appear to prevent the worst effects of CMV-related disease in these immuno-suppressed patients. New antiviral agents, active against CMV, such as Ganciclovir, have not yet been adequately assessed in the treatment of neonatal CMV infection.

Rubella

Rubella vaccine has been available in the UK for about 20 years, for most of which time the principal target was schoolgirls aged 11–13 years. One dose of rubella vaccine produces an antibody response in over 95% of individuals with little decline in antibody levels. A few recipients of the vaccine fail to produce an antibody response and some vaccinated individuals have been shown to lose their antibodies and subsequently to become infected. This loss of antibody is more likely after vaccination than after the natural infection. Women must therefore continue to be screened for rubella antibodies in every pregnancy. Susceptible women should be immunised immediately after delivery. There have been no reported cases of live attenuated rubella vaccine causing fetal infection when given shortly before conception or inadvertently during pregnancy.

Termination of pregnancy may be considered for women known to have been infected in pregnancy and thought to be at high risk of having a damaged fetus. However, a mother infected during her pregnancy will not necessarily pass on the infection to her fetus and not all infected fetuses will be damaged. Most mothers of infected infants give no history of contact with infection during pregnancy and most of those contracting such an infection will have either a subclinical or a non-specific 'flu-like' illness. Therefore, in the absence of a screening programme in pregnancy routinely testing for infections that may damage the fetus, most infections will go undiagnosed and termination of pregnancy will not be considered as an option.

Viral infections

Neonatal herpes simplex

This viral infection is usually acquired at birth. Transplacental spread, if it occurs, is uncommon.

Maternal antibodies are not protective to the baby against this infection. Active genital herpes infection at the time of delivery puts the baby at increased risk of infection, which may be as high as 50% for a mother with a primary attack and considerably lower risk — around 5% — for recurrent herpetic lesions. The majority of affected babies are born to mothers with no signs or symptoms of herpes at the time of delivery. These mothers may have asymptomatic infection or the babies may acquire their infection from medical or nursing staff or other babies. There are about 14 cases of neonatal herpes reported per annum in the UK.

Women with a history of genital herpes or in whom it develops in pregnancy should be screened weekly from 36 weeks' gestation by viral culture. Caesarian section should be performed if there is evidence of active infection at term.

Neonatal herpes may present in a localised form affecting mouth, eyes or skin, with a good prognosis. More serious infection may be localised in the CNS with meningoencephalitis, which carries a poor prognosis, or may result in widespread infection, as in the other congenital infections, with high mortality. The overall mortality is about 60%.

HIV infection in children

By the end of 1992 the WHO predicts that worldwide over one million children will be infected with HIV and over half of these will have AIDS. 80% of children will have been infected by maternofetal transmission.

Incidence. Anonymous testing of neonatal blood samples suggests the rate of HIV sero-positive mothers to be 0.02% in London, 0.2% in Massachusetts and up to 2% in some parts of New York. Vertical transmission rates, from mother to fetus, probably vary between 10 and 30%. Infected mothers in the preclinical stage appear to have a lower risk of transmitting HIV to the fetus than was suggested by early American studies, which largely concentrated on mothers with advanced disease.

Children have also been infected with HIV through the use of contaminated blood or blood products. In the UK, 20% of males with classic haemophilia are infected with HIV through the use of contaminated clotting factor concentrate. Improved screening of blood donors and treatment of blood products should reduce the risk of acquiring HIV through this route in the future.

Clinical presentation. The clinical presentation of HIV disease in children is non-specific and includes:

- failure to thrive
- recurrent chest infections
- oral candidiasis
- diarrhoea
- unexplained fever
- lymphadenopathy.

Later-stage HIV infection is a multisystem disease. Infections of the respiratory tract, gut and CNS are major hazards. HIV infection itself may cause an encephalopathy in up to 50% of children with AIDS and may affect the small bowel causing malabsorption, as well as affecting the bone marrow, heart, liver and kidneys.

Diagnosis. The diagnosis of HIV infection in young children is complicated by the persistence of maternal antibody for up to 18 months. A positive antibody test after that time implies infection. HIV may be cultured from infected leucocytes but infected children may have negative cultures. Reliable detection of HIV may be possible using molecular genetic techniques in the future.

Other laboratory tests that may help to confirm a suspected diagnosis include the development of polyclonal hypergammaglobulinaemia, reduced numbers of helper T cells and thrombocytopaenia.

Treatment. Treatment consists of vigorous supportive care. This includes aggressive treatment of infection, nutritional support with nasogastric or parenteral feeding if necessary and provision of support services. Specific treatment consists, first, of regular infusion of immunoglobulin, which reduces bacterial infections and improves weight gain, and, second, of regular use of azidothymidine (AZT) a drug that blocks viral replication but that does not eradicate the infection. The optimal dosage and timing of treatment with AZT for children has not yet been determined.

Prognosis. The European collaborative study identified a bimodal age distribution for the prognosis of HIV-infected infants. 83% of congenitally infected children showed either laboratory or clinical evidence of AIDS by 6 months of age. 26% of those infected progressed to develop clinical AIDS by 12 months and 17% died. Subsequently the disease appeared to progress more slowly. The mean incubation period for older children infected with HIV by other means is 4.7 years.

It is important to remember that one or both parents of a child with HIV are likely to be infected themselves. In addition the family may also be suffering the effects of poverty, poor housing and continued drug usage. Good community-based services are therefore of the greatest importance in supporting the child and family.

Meningitis

Bacterial meningitis remains one of the common paediatric emergencies. Meningitis is characterised by inflammation and swelling of the meninges and bacterial invasion of the cerebro-spinal fluid. Despite improvements in medical care there has been no significant reduction in the mortality over the past 20 years.

Incidence. The incidence of neonatal (first month of life) meningitis is approximately 1 per 1000 live births. The major pathogens causing meningitis in the newborn are: group B beta haemolytic *Streptoccocus* and *Escherichia coli*, with *Listeria monocytogenes* now the third most common organism in the UK. The mortality for neonatal meningitis remains high, at 20–50%, with up to 50% of the survivors showing significant handicap.

The incidence of postneonatal (1 month–1 year) meningitis is 0.65 per 1000 and between the ages of 1 and 4 years incidence is 0.16 per 1000. The incidence in the UK has increased in recent years. Children aged 4–8 weeks may be affected by organisms causing neonatal infections or by organisms common to older children.

Outside the neonatal period *Haemophilus influenzae* is the most common organism affecting children up to 5 years of age and is relatively uncommon thereafter. *Neisseria meningitidis*

(meningococcus) most commonly affects toddlers but may occur in outbreaks, affecting older children. *Streptoccocus pneumoniae* (pneumococcus) occurs throughout childhood. These organisms are commonly carried in the upper respiratory tracts of healthy, asymptomatic children and adults. It is not known why some children subsequently develop invasive disease.

Diagnosis. The diagnosis of classic meningitis, with fever, headache, vomiting, and drowsiness alternating with irritability, neck stiffness and signs of meningeal irritation, is relatively straightforward. However, in neonates and young children and in the early stages of the infection in older children, the diagnosis may be very difficult to make in the face of a number of non-specific symptoms and signs. To confirm the diagnosis a lumbar puncture is usually performed and suitable broad spectrum antibiotics started. The exact organism and antibiotic sensitivities will be confirmed after culturing of the organism for 1–2 days. Antibiotics may then be rationalised to target the specific organism.

Lumbar puncture is a potentially hazardous procedure in a child with bacterial meningitis as the majority of affected children will have a degree of cerebral oedema. The clinical signs of cerebral oedema are unreliable and so the risks of lumbar puncture must be weighed against the benefits of obtaining cerebrospinal fluid (CSF) for culture. Without lumbar puncture the organism may still be isolated as blood cultures will be positive for the causative organism in approximately 70% of cases of bacterial meningitis.

Complications. Complications of meningitis include hydrocephalus, deafness and cerebral palsy. Long-term complications are most common with pneumococcal and least common with meningococcal meningitis.

Treatment. A penicillin in combination with a third generation cephalosporin or chloramphenicol are suitable starting antibiotics. Although many antibiotics penetrate poorly into the CSF under normal circumstances most will pass freely through inflamed meninges to achieve adequate CSF levels. Chloramphenicol passes freely into the CSF at all times but is a potentially toxic antibiotic and needs to be used with caution, especially in the very young. Aminoglycosides penetrate relatively poorly into the CSF but, like penicillin, may be given directly into the CSF at lumbar puncture or by ventricular puncture if the infection does not respond to conventional antibiotic treatment.

Full supportive treatment may be required until the infection responds to treatment and will include the vigorous treatment of raised intra-cranial pressure, maintenance of an adequate blood pressure, careful observation of neurological status and early treatment of seizures.

Families and close contacts of children with meningococcal or *Haemophilus influenzae* meningitis should receive prophylactic treatment with oral antibiotics, such as rifampicin or a sulphonamide, to prevent secondary cases of the disease.

Prognosis. Nearly 10% of children with bacterial meningitis will die and permanent neurological defects or deafness may occur in up to 30% of the survivors. There is some evidence that administration of steroids may reduce the incidence of deafness following *Haemophilus influenzae* meningitis but this is not yet accepted by all authorities.

Prevention of meningitis. No vaccine is currently available for the type B meningococcus, which is responsible for around 60% of meningococcal disease in the UK. A vaccine is available for types A and C, which are more common in other countries. A vaccine to protect against invasive *Haemophilus influenzae* infection, including meningitis, appears promising in early trials and it is estimated may save up to 50 lives per year in the UK. A pneumococcal vaccine giving protection against 80–90% of the pneumococcal types causing serious infection in the UK is available. However, the vaccine has been shown to be ineffective in those children aged between 2 and 10 years who were thought to be at high risk of pneumococcal disease.

Viral meningitis

Meningitis may follow enterovirus infections such as echo, coxsackie and poliomyelitis, which occur most frequently in the summer months. Mumps and herpes simplex virus may also produce an 'aseptic' meningitis. Viral meningitis usually presents a similar, although generally milder, clinical picture to that seen in bacterial meningitis. The virus may often be isolated from throat swabs, urine, stool or CSF. Confirmation of the viral aetiology may be obtained by demonstrating a rising titre of antibody in acute and convalescent serum samples. Treatment is supportive, effective antiviral treatment with acyclovir is only available for herpes virus infections.

Respiratory infections

Acute respiratory tract infections are the most common types of infection in childhood making up 50% of all infections in children under 5 years. Children between 1 and 6 years may contract up to nine respiratory tract infections each year. The incidence of infection is increased in young children who attend child care centres or who have older siblings attending such centres (see Chapter 7 Respiratory Conditions and Cardiothoracic Disorders).

Most infections such as rhinitis, pharyngitis, otitis media and tonsillitis are limited to the upper respiratory tract. About 5% of infections affect the lower respiratory tract and are therefore potentially more serious. These include:

- laryngotracheobronchitis (croup)
- epiglottitis
- bronchitis
- bronchiolitis
- pneumonia.

Viral infections. Over 90% of respiratory infections are caused by viruses. The common viruses causing lower respiratory tract infections are: respiratory syncytial virus (RSV), parainfluenza virus 1, 2 and 3 and influenza virus A and B. Upper respiratory tract infections may be caused by all of the above viruses and also by rhinovirus, adenovirus and some enteroviruses.

Bacterial infections. *Streptococcus pneumoniae*, *Haemophilus influenzae*, *Staphylococcus aureus*, beta haemolytic streptococci and *Branhamella catarrhalis* may all be isolated from the upper respiratory tract in healthy children. As a result it may be difficult to be certain of the role played by these organisms during clinical illness.

Lower respiratory tract infections

Laryngotracheobronchitis. This infection of the larynx and lower respiratory tract is usually preceded, for 1–2 days, by an upper respiratory tract infection. Inflammatory narrowing of the glottis and subglottic region causes a hoarse voice or cry, a barking cough and limitation of airflow. Usually the respiratory difficulty is most marked when the child is upset. Signs of stridor and sternal or costal recession may largely resolve when the child is allowed to settle.

Treatment. Those children with mild to moderate respiratory difficulty are likely to settle without specific treatment within 12–48 h. For those more severely affected children oxygen may be required. Humidification of inspired air is traditional, of uproven benefit and must not interfere with careful observation of the child's clinical state. Nebulised adrenaline may produce temporary improvement in airflow by reducing mucosal oedema. Endotracheal intubation may be required for a small percentage of children (1–2%) who show signs of increasingly severe airway obstruction or who become exhausted.

Epiglottitis. Epiglottitis is an infection caused by type B *Haemophilus influenzae*, which causes acute swelling of the epiglottis and supraglottic tissues. Affected children have a short history of a sore throat, often for only a few hours, with difficulty in swallowing and increasing difficulty in breathing. On examination they are quiet, appear toxic and unwell, may be drooling saliva and usually have a low-pitched stridor, often with an expiratory component.

Treatment. These children are at high risk of acute airway obstruction and should be provided with a safe airway, preferably by endotracheal intubation by a skilled anaesthetist, as soon as possible. Prior to intubation nothing should be done which might upset the child as this may precipitate a respiratory arrest. Treatment after intubation consists of high dose intravenous antibiotics and supportive care, *Haemophilus influenzae* can often be grown from blood cultures. Extubation can usually take place within 24–48 hours.

Bronchitis. Whooping cough, caused by *Bordetella pertussis* is an important cause of bronchitis in infants and young children. The disease is highly infectious and spread by droplet infection. The infection in bronchitis is confined to the conducting airways without parenchymal lung infection. The early catarrhal stage of pertussis is followed by damage to the epithelial lining of the lower respiratory tree and the formation of thick mucoid secretions and epithelial debris. Prolonged bouts of coughing may occur and classically these may be followed by vomiting and an inspiratory whoop. Paroxysms of coughing may be triggered by eating or excitement and are common at night. The paroxysmal cough may persist for several months and may reappear during subsequent respiratory infections. Young infants with whooping cough often do not present the classic clinical picture and may not whoop, thus making accurate diagnosis difficult. Infants under the age of 3 months may become apnoeic after coughing bouts and are particularly at risk as they may not be adequately protected by immunisation. Long-term respiratory problems, such as recurrent cough and wheeze and abnormal respiratory function tests have been shown to occur with increased frequency after pertussis infection, though bronchiectasis is now an uncommon complication of this disease.

Treatment. Once the coughing phase of the illness has started treatment does not affect the course of the disease. Treatment with erythromycin is usual to reduce infectivity and may halt progression of the disease if treatment is started during the early coryzal phase.

Prevention. A full course of pertussis vaccination protects over 80% of recipients. Before large-scale introduction of pertussis vaccine over 100 000 cases were notified annually in England and Wales. In 1973, when vaccine acceptance was over 80% annual notifications fell to 2400. By 1975 vaccine acceptance had fallen to around 30% after adverse publicity concerning the efficacy and safety of the vaccine. Major epidemics followed in 1977/79 and 1981/83 with over 100 000 cases notified (in England and Wales). In 1988 vaccine acceptance had risen again to 73% and only 5000 cases were notified.

Bronchiolitis. This is the most common lower respiratory tract infection in infancy. The infection involves mainly the smaller bronchi and bronchioles. 1–2% of infants with bronchiolitis will require admission to hospital. Bronchiolitis epidemics occur in the winter months and commonly follow spells of cold weather. The respiratory syncytial virus (RSV) is the usual cause but other respiratory viruses may produce a similar clinical picture. Typically the infants most severely affected are between 1 and 6 months old. The illness starts with a runny nose and cough. The cough becomes increasingly troublesome and may be associated with wheezing and vomiting. The infant becomes progressively more breathless and has increasing difficulty feeding. On examination the infant's chest is hyperinflated and there is costal and subcostal recession. On auscultation of the chest inspiratory crackles and expiratory wheezes are heard.

Treatment. Treatment is supportive. Oxygen is supplied to maintain normal oxygen saturation. Feeds may be given by nasogastric tube or fluids by intravenous infusion. Handling should be kept to a minimum. Physiotherapy does *not* speed the resolution of the illness. 1–2% of affected children may need ventilator support for respiratory failure. Very young infants may require ventilation for recurrent apnoea.

A new antiviral drug, ribavirin, may be useful for those most severely affected infants and those infants with pre-existing cardiac or chronic respiratory conditions.

Pneumonia. Pneumonia may be defined as acute inflammatory consolidation of the alveoli or infiltration of the interstitial tissue of the lung with inflammatory cells, or both. Pneumonia may be caused by any of the viruses and bacteria mentioned above.

Clinical presentation. The child with pneumonia is usually lethargic, pyrexial and tachypnoeic. Chest examination may be unhelpful, may reveal localised inspiratory crackles or may reveal the classic signs of dull percussion note and bronchial breathing, particularly in the older child. Chest X-ray will show consolidation of the affected segment or lobe.

Chlamydia trachomatis is usually acquired at delivery as a result of undiagnosed maternal infection and may present with gradual onset of respiratory symptoms at 1–2 months of age.

Mycoplasma pneumoniae is a common cause of pneumonia in children aged 5–15 years. A flu-like illness commonly precedes the respiratory illness, which consists of a dry paroxysmal cough. Some children are more severely affected, with signs and symptoms suggestive of pneumonia. The physical signs are commonly unimpressive apart from some inspiratory crackles heard on auscultation. The chest X-ray may be more impressive, with patchy shadowing particularly affecting the lower lobes and small pleural effusions may be present.

Treatment. After the diagnosis of pneumonia has been made samples of blood, sputum, and nasopharyngeal secretions should be obtained for culture and antibiotics started. Pneumonia in young infants and children should be treated with broad spectrum antibiotics until culture results are available. Classic lobar pneumonia in the older child may be treated with penicillin alone. If a positive viral culture is obtained the diagnosis is likely to be one of viral pneumonia, even if bacteria are isolated from sputum or swabs.

Early assessment of the extent and severity of the illness is important and supportive treatment with oxygen and intravenous fluids should be given if required. Erythromycin is the antibiotic of choice for *Chlamydia trachomatis* and *Mycoplasma pneumoniae.*

Complications. Complications of pneumonias include: pleural effusion, empyema, pneumothorax and lung abscess. Pleural effusions and empyemas should be aspirated or drained with an intercostal tube if neccessary. Lung abscess may complicate staphylococcal or Gram-negative pneumonias (*E. coli* and *Pseudomonas, Klebsiella* and *Proteus* species). The possibility of an inhaled foreign body or congenital lung abnormality should be borne in mind with any pneumonia or lung abscess that does not respond promptly to treatment.

Tuberculosis. Tuberculosis (TB) is caused by infection with *Mycobacterium tuberculosis*, which may infect any part of the body. 90% of new cases involve the respiratory system. The infection is commonly spread by droplet aerosol. Transmission by this means is especially likely when the index case is sputum smear-positive for the bacillus.

The notification rates for tuberculosis in children have fallen steadily to 10 per 100 000 in 1988. The decline of TB in childhood is explained by a decline in the incidence of adult TB, the efficacy of BCG immunisation and earlier diagnosis due to contact tracing. BCG immunisation at 13 years has been standard practice in the UK for almost the past 40 years and gives 75% protection 10 years after vaccination.

Treatment. The drug treatment for proven or strongly suspected tuberculous infection currently recommended for children consists of a cocktail of rifampicin and isoniazid for 9 months with either ethambutol or pyrazinamide given in addition for the first 2 months.

Urinary tract infection

Urinary tract infection is usually caused by ascending infection with bacteria of bowel origin particularly *Escherichia coli* or enterococci. If there is impaired urinary drainage unusual organisms may sometimes be cultured from the urine. Urinary tract infection is more common in boys in the newborn period but thereafter girls predominate. 40–45% of children investigated in detail after a proven urinary tract infection will be shown to have some urinary tract abnormality. The most common abnormality found is vesicoureteric reflux, i.e. the tendency for urine to pass from the bladder back up the ureter during micturition. Reflux of infected urine to the kidneys carries the risk of pyelonephritis and later renal scarring. Current evidence suggests that it is the urine infections occurring in early infancy and childhood that are most liable to produce renal damage. Therefore all children should be referred for investigation after their first proven infection and there should be prompt treatment of symptomatic infections after samples of urine have been obtained for culture.

Treatment. There is currently considerable debate about the long-term management of those children who are at risk of recurrent urine infections. A variety of options is available, including prompt treatment of infections, long-term prophylactic antibiotics and a variety of anti-reflux surgical procedures. Enthusiasm for surgery needs to be tempered by the knowledge that vesicoureteric reflux tends to resolve spontaneously in the majority between 5 and 10 years of age and that the long-term outlook for renal function has not been shown to be improved by any surgical anti-reflux procedure.

Gastroenteritis

Rotavirus is the most common cause of gastroenteritis in children in the UK. This virus, which particularly affects infants under 2 years of age is prevalent during the winter months. Frequently symptoms of an upper respiratory tract precede the development of watery diarrhoea and vomiting. Vomiting usually lasts 1 to 3 days and the diarrhoea for up to 5 days. A variety of other viruses may produce a similar clinical picture and may be diagnosed by electron microscopy of the stools.

Bacterial causes of gastroenteritis such as *E. coli* and *Shigella*, *Campylobacter* and *Salmonella* species may produce clinical illness in children and adults. The illness may be quite severe, with prostration and offensive, bloody stools.

Treatment. Treatment of mild to moderate gastroenteritis is supportive with adequate fluid replacement, in the form of glucose and electrolyte mixture, the most important factor. The child should be admitted to hospital if fluid replacement is refused, if repeated vomiting continues, if profuse diarrhoea continues or if the child becomes dehydrated. Intravenous fluids may be needed for those children most severely affected. Measurement of the plasma sodium is important as those children who have developed hypernatraemic dehydration (plasma sodium > 150 mmol/litre) will need to be rehydrated more slowly, to avoid development of cerebral oedema. Since the introduction of modified cows' milk formula milk, hypernatraemic dehydration has become relatively uncommon, but may still occur if infants are fed over-concentrated milk. Hypernatraemia is associated with a significant risk of subsequent neurological handicap.

Some bacterial causes of gastroenteritis may be treated with antibiotics, e.g. *Campylobacter* with erythromycin, but the majority of cases of gastroenteritis require no specific drug treatment.

Prevention. The incidence of gastroenteritis in young children can be reduced by promoting continuation of breast feeding. Provision of a safe water supply is of vital importance. Careful attention to hygiene when handling and preparing food is also important.

Viral hepatitis

This term encompasses not only the acute hepatitis caused by the hepatitis A and B viruses but also the other forms of hepatitis caused by the delta agent, non-A non-B hepatitis and the hepatitis associated with other generalised virus infections, such as cytomegalovirus, rubella, EB (infectious mononucleosus) virus, herpes virus and coxsackie B virus. Some of these infections, particularly hepatitis B, delta and non-A non-B viruses, may cause a chronic hepatitis with progressive liver damage ultimately leading to cirrhosis or development of liver cancer.

Hepatitis A virus

Hepatitis A is highly contagious and spread via the faeco-oral route, usually by ingestion of contaminated food or water. The incubation period ranges from 2 to 6 weeks from exposure to the virus to the onset of symptoms, although many cases are asymptomatic or present with only mild flu-like symptoms without jaundice. Physical examination reveals an enlarged and tender liver and blood tests will be abnormal with marked elevation of liver enzymes. Confirmation of the diagnosis is usually obtained by demonstrating the presence of hepatitis A antibody in the serum. Mortality is low and chronic liver disease is not a feature of hepatitis A infection.

Treatment. There is no specific treatment during the acute stage of the disease. Preventive treatment with immunoglobulin containing high titres of antibody (human normal immunoglobulin) may be given by intramuscular injection to close contacts to control infection or to travellers going to a high risk area. The resulting passive immunity provides 85–90% protection.

Hepatitis B virus

There are 150–200 million people worldwide who are chronically infected with the hepatitis B virus. The major sources of infection are therefore either people with acute hepatitis B infection or healthy carriers of the virus. The virus is transmitted by the exchange of blood or any other bodily secretion and the incubation period ranges from 2 to 6 months. Infection may be asymptomatic or may produce symptoms similar to hepatitis A infection. Acute hepatic failure may occur in 1–2% of cases of viral hepatitis and is thought to be more common in cases of non-A non-B hepatitis. The hepatitis B virus is not itself damaging to liver cells and produces hepatitis by exciting an immune response that is responsible for the liver inflammation in the host. The reason why some people become carriers, some develop hepatitis and subsequently clear the virus, some develop hepatitis and fail to clear the virus and some develop a chronic hepatitis with increased risk of hepatocellular carcinoma is unclear.

The diagnosis of hepatitis B is confirmed by demonstrating the presence, in the serum, of antigens associated with the hepatitis B virus. A number of different antigens relating to the hepatitis B virus have been demonstrated. The common antigens in clinical use include the surface antigen (HBsAg), viral core-related antigen (HBcAg) and the 'e' antigen (HBeAg), the presence of which is related to infectivity. Persistence of these antigens is associated with the chronic carrier state with or without chronic hepatitis. Those patients mounting an effective response to the virus produce antibodies to the viral antigens which are then cleared from the serum.

Prevention. Hepatitis B may be prevented, after exposure, by intramuscular administration of specific hepatitis B immunoglobulin and is combined with vaccination. This procedure should be routine for infants born to hepatitis B-positive mothers. Without immunoglobulin and vaccination these infants have a 80–90% chance of developing the chronic carrier state if infected. Groups at high risk of contracting hepatitis B should be immunised. The vaccine is about 90% effective.

THERMAL INJURIES
P. Eckersley

Accidents are the cause of one-sixth of hospital admissions for children over the age of 1 year, and accidents in the home account for a quarter of deaths (Meadow & Smithells 1986). Of these accidents thermal injuries are of major importance and fall into two categories:

- Scalds
  — caused by hot fluids
  — result in blistering and peeling with loss of epidermis
- Burns
  — caused by direct contact with very hot objects
  — result in full thickness skin loss.

HOSPITALISATION

Thermal injuries frequently require hospital admission, especially in the case of very young children where skin loss may occur at lower temperatures. The most immediate treatment required is for shock and loss of body fluid. Intravenous fluid therapy is necessary where more than 10% of the body surface is involved. Skin loss of over 50% is invariably fatal.

The management of thermal injuries during the period of hospitalisation involves:

- correction of fluid loss
- prevention of infection
- relief of pain
- skin grafting for burns with full thickness skin loss (Meadow & Smithells 1986).

AFTERCARE

Children, who may be extensively scarred as a result of a burn or a scald injury, require a complete programme of care, for a lengthy period of time after their injuries. The care needed not only involves the physical and emotional support of the child, but also encompasses the immediate family, who often experience adjustment problems (Forshaw 1987). In this section aftercare is described in terms of:

- physical aftercare
- psychological problems.

Physical aftercare

The correct treatment of burns and scalds is aimed at:

- the reduction of scarring
- preventing disability
- reducing the need for further surgery
- producing a better cosmetic result (Mason & Forshaw, undated).

Skin condition

It is important to promote the suppleness of skin and prevent dryness. A washing and massage programme should be carried out three times daily using pure baby soap and water, followed by lanolin cream. This programme not only maintains the condition of the skin but also breaks down the collagen fibres in scar tissue responsible for puckering and skin distortion.

Skin breakdown. Scar tissue may break down more easily than normal skin and may require dressing in hospital. Care should be taken to avoid friction, knocks and sunshine on the affected area.

Pressure garments

Pressure garments are made-to-measure garments of a strong, flesh-coloured, lycra material, which produces a firm even pressure over every part of the affected area (Forshaw 1987). This pressure can prevent or reduce raised, hard areas of hypertrophic scarring.

As hypertrophic scarring may be seen as soon as 3 to 4 weeks after thermal injury, it is essential to introduce the pressure garment as soon as the skin has healed. The garment is worn for $23\frac{1}{2}$ hours each day and for up to 18 months or 2 years. It is only removed for bathing and for periods of lubrication and massage. In some circumstances additional pressure over scar tissue is necessary and to achieve this a layer of sponge is inserted under the pressure garment.

Splintage

Splints may be necessary when skin loss occurs over joints such as wrists, fingers, elbows and knees. As skin heals the scars may shrink and if corrective splints are not used, joint deformity and restricted movement may result.

Exercise and activity

Exercise is important to maintain joint and muscle function and can begin as soon as healing has occurred. Swimming can be encouraged but skin care and replacement of pressure garments must be carried out assiduously.

Psychological problems

Stress will be a major psychological problem for a child with a thermal injury and in some instances it is wise to seek professional assistance (Mason & Forshaw, undated). Guidance and counselling are necessary both to prepare children and families for discharge from hospital and to support them through the long period of treatment ahead. Psychological problems may be experienced by both children and parents.

Problems for children

Young children and adolescents will experience many difficulties from both the immediate and long-term consequences of burns. All will need positive, firm and empathetic responses from the burns aftercare team. Difficulties may include:

1. Coming to terms with a long period of wearing uncomfortable and ugly pressure garments.
2. Nightmares and fears as accidents are remembered and relived. Some children may begin to bed-wet.
3. Discomfort from dry, sensitive skin.
4. Coping with teasing, hurtful comments and the reactions of family, friends and strangers.
5. Coping with periods of hospitalisation.

All of these factors will have a considerable impact on the self-image and self-respect of the child. But most significant will be the way in which the child can be supported through, and learn to cope with a changed body image and appearance. This will involve both coming to terms with the way they look, and also with the way their skin feels.

Professional help may be needed with severe thermal injuries to enable the child to respond to the comments and questions of others, and to adjust to and understand their own injuries.

Problems for parents

The strongest reaction of many parents is one of a feeling of guilt that they were unable to prevent the injury to their child. Indeed parents are constantly reminded of the accident by their child's scarring and the nature of the aftercare treatment (Mason & Forshaw, undated).

Parents will need support to:

1. Overcome any feelings of guilt and not to blame themselves or each other.
2. Overcome feelings of shame or even revulsion.
3. Continue a lengthy and time-consuming after-care programme.
4. Support their own child.
5. Prevent overprotection or spoiling.
6. Regain confidence in themselves.
7. Overcome fears of non-acceptance and blame.

Childhood experiences

It is vital for the thermally injured child, as for any child, to experience play, companionship and exploration. It may be necessary to support a return to the community and to the school setting and both nursing and therapy staff have an important informational and advisory role in preparing for this return.

PREVENTION OF THERMAL INJURIES

There are many sources of readily available materials on preventing thermal injuries and protecting children from injury. Guidelines on prevention include:

1. Limiting the upper temperature of domestic hot water.
2. Ensuring clothing and furniture are made from flame-retarding materials.
3. Fixing fire screens, smoke detectors and pan guards.
4. Keeping hot drinks and cooking utensils out of children's reach.
5. Testing bath water before bathing children.
6. Talking to children about the dangers of fireworks, barbecues, chemical sets, etc.
7. Ensuring electric cables, pan handles, etc. are out of children's reach.

ACCIDENTS AND CHILD ABUSE
M. I. Griffiths

ACCIDENTS

Accidents are the most common cause of death in children aged 1–15 years (Table 13.2) and, for this reason alone, pose a challenge to parents, professionals and the public. In addition there is considerable morbidity amongst survivors of accidents. In particular, neurological conditions following head injury need skilled physiotherapy during the acute phase and the long-term (sometimes life-long) follow-up (Table 13.3).

This proneness to accidents is a natural attribute of children. They are energetic and adventurous and their knowledge of the relationship between cause and effect only comes with maturity. Adults who are responsible for them need to take sensible precautions to avoid unnecessary risks and need to teach children how to observe reasonable safety rules.

Most accidents are precipitated by factors in both the victim and the environment and although chance occurrences do occur the accidents would frequently have been prevented had appropriate precautions been taken (Jackson 1977).

The types of accident that occur during childhood are related chiefly to the child's age and the dangers of the environment at the time (Table 13.4). For instance, Jackson (1977) found that accidents in the home caused 41% of all the accidental deaths in the age group 0–4 years but only 7.9% and 8.7% in the age groups 5–9 years and 10–14 years, respectively. In contrast, road accidents to pedestrians represented 15% of accidental deaths in the 0–4 years age group, 50% in the 5–9-year-olds and 31% in the 10–14-year-olds. These differences are clearly related to a combination of freedom of activity and increased experience in children at the various ages, and degree of exposure to dangers in the environment. These figures take no account of fatal accidents to children who are passengers in cars: research has clearly shown that adequate restraint systems effectively protect both adults and

Table 13.2 Child mortality from accidents (from Griffiths and Wilson 1980)

Author	Leck 1975		Jackson 1977	Leck 1975		Jackson 1977
Country	England/Wales	Scotland	England/Wales	England/Wales	Scotland	England/Wales
Date	1969	1968–70	1973	1969	1968–70	1973
Age group	1–11 months	1–11 months	0–11 months	1–15 years	1–15 years	1–15 years
All deaths	7.73 per 1000 live births	9.3 per 1000 live births		0.459 per 1000 live births	0.54 per 1000 live births	
All deaths from poisoning and violence	0.72 per 1000 live births	1.5 per 1000 live births		0.153 per 1000 live births	0.21 per 1000 live births	
Ratio accidental/total deaths	1/10.7	1/6.2	1/34	1/3	1/2.6	1/3.8

Reprinted by kind permission of BIMH Publications, Stourport House, Stourport Rd, Kidderminster, Worcestershire DY11 7QG.

Table 13.3 Results of head injury (from Griffiths and Wilson 1980)

Date	Authors	Place	Number of cases	Age (years)	Type of injury	Mortality percentage	Neurological sequelae in survivors	
							Number	per cent
1967	London	Birmingham UK	120	0–15	Mainly road traffic accidents	20	25	20
1974	Jamison and Kaye	Newcastle UK	857	0–15	All except non-accidental injury	14		13
1975	Healey	USA	80	0–1	Subdural haematoma	11	22	27.5
					All	Survivors only	Significant depression of IQ	
1977	Klonoff et al	Vancouver Canada	75 39	0–9 9–15			19 8	25 20
1978	Cooper	Newcastle UK	136	Not known	Non-accidental injury	10.3	18/60	30

Reproduced by kind permission of BIMH Publications, Stourport House, Stourport Rd, Kidderminster, Worcestershire, DY11 7QG.

children. Attributes of childhood do not increase their vulnerability provided that the adults accompanying them make use of suitable car restraints.

Fortunately, only a small proportion of accidents outlined in Table 13.4 prove fatal, but all involve the child and family in traumatic emotional experiences of variable severity and sometimes in prolonged periods of treatment, which may involve separation or long journeys to hospital.

Table 13.4 Types of accidents (from Griffths and Wilson 1980)

Injury	Place	Vector	Age group (years)	'True' accident	Non-accidental injury
Head injury	Home	Falls	Usually 0–4	Common	Occasional
		Shaking (or throwing)	0–4	Rare	Frequent
		Implement used	0–4	Occasional	Occassional
	Outside	Falls	Usually 5+	Common	
		Road traffic accident:			
		car	Any age	Common	
		pedestrian	2+	Common	Not applicable
		cyclist	Usually 5+	Common	
Poisoning	Home	Domestic cleaning agents	Usually 0–4	Common	Rare
		Drugs:			
		aspirin		+	
		hypnotics			
		sedatives	0–4	Common	Occasional
		tranquillisers			
		others			
		Lead	0–4	Rare	Unlikely
Burns and scalds	Home	Fires			
		Kettles and pans	Usually 0–4	Usual	Occasional
Drowning	Home	Ornamental pools			
	Outside	Swimming pools	0–16	Usual	Occasional
		Rivers and canals			

Reprinted by kind permission of BIMH Publications, Stourport House, Stourport Road, Kidderminster, Worcestershire, DY11 7QG.

First year of life

During the first year of life comparative helplessness and lack of mobility rule out the activity and curiosity that lead older children into danger, but at the same time demand adequate standards of supervision from the carer. Falls, choking, suffocation and even drowning in the bath may occur if the child is left unattended, and at the crawling/climbing stage constant vigilance is necessary.

Sudden Infant Death Syndrome

Although not truly accidental, the Sudden Infant Death Syndrome (often referred to as cot death), has much the same stressful impact on the family as an accidental death, with the added anxiety of the lack of knowledge of a definite cause. It is the major mode of death in infants aged 1 week to 2 years (De'Ath 1990). It occurs suddenly in an infant who may have shown no signs of illness; the infant is usually found dead at home in the cot or pram. So far, no one cause has been found and extensive research is continuing to identify possible precipitating factors, to identify potential victims and to find the means to prevent a fatal outcome.

1–4 years of age

From 1 to 4 years of age the child is becoming more active, full of curiosity and heedless of danger. Most accidents happen in the home and usually involve the child's active participation. Adults must be constantly on guard against falls causing fractures, burns and scalds from children snatching unsuitable objects, poisoning, electrocution, and suffocation from plastic bags (Whittington 1977). Such accidents may be minor, major or fatal and some may have permanent consequences.

5–10 years of age

With admission to school at the age of 5 years, more opportunities for accidents are presented but at this age dangers can be explained to children and they can begin to learn to avoid unnecessary risks.

Playgrounds and play equipment need to be designed with safety in mind, and soft landings provided beneath climbing frames, slides and swings. Lessons can reinforce home training on behaviour in traffic and young cyclists can receive special instructions from the police.

10–15 years of age

From 10 to 15 years increasing freedom and leisure activities expose children to greater hazards. To some extent increasing maturity and knowledge of danger helps to balance the likelihood of accidents with the care that is taken.

Children need to be encouraged to take part in adventure holidays of all kinds, although in some of the more advanced skills training 'it is hard to exclude all element of hazard' (Hogan, 1977). However, if the course is well designed, the instructor adequately trained, and the children taught how to regulate behaviour to reduce the risk, any adverse outcomes can usually be avoided.

CHILD ABUSE

Child abuse occurs when adults who are in charge of children inflict injuries which are physical, emotional or sexual.

Physiotherapists have a dual role in this field: not only as the skilled professional who may be called upon to treat the effects of abuse but also as trained observers who may notice signs that it may be taking place and who may be able to take action to prevent permanent damage occurring.

20 times as many children in whom abuse is suspected are now notified to departments of social services or child health than was the case 10 years ago (Meadow 1989). Of these, proved cases are four or five times as common. It is not clear whether this means that there is a true increase or whether it is increased awareness: whichever is the case there is clearly a grave medical and social problem.

Physical abuse

Physical abuse (non-accidental injury) was first highlighted for professionals in the USA by

Kempe and his colleagues in 1962 and has also made headlines in this country. The tragic deaths that were highlighted represent the tip of the iceberg. It is estimated that at least 1 child per 1000 under the age of 4 years is seriously injured, and many others less severely. Injuries are inflicted by parents, siblings or other carers. The injuries are usually typical of the trauma inflicted, and are unlike the effects produced by genuine accidents.

Bruises may show the definite impression of hands or finger-tips or they may be linear, caused by beating with stick or strap. Burns may show the outline of a hot-plate or a cigarette. Single fractures may be of no significance but skeletal X-ray often reveals multiple fractures in various stages of healing. Retinal haemorrhages are diagnostic of severe shaking, and are often associated with skull fractures and possibly brain injury (Hobbs 1989).

Injuries may result in death, or in permanent neurological impairment; even in trivial injuries the psychological and emotional effect is likely to be long-lasting. It is known that many 'battered children' become 'battering parents'.

To some extent families who are at risk of causing non-accidental injuries can be identified before this has happened. The function of child protection registers is to alert health and social services of this possibility in some families. Social factors and health conditions may be precipitating causes and some can be identified in pregnancy and the immediate neonatal period. Hall (1989) comments that professional guidance, practical help, a supportive network of families and friends, helping parents in child care and development may serve to reduce the incidence of child abuse. Physiotherapists who are responsible for physical management should also direct their efforts to convince the children of their personal worth and of the security that can be offered by caring adults.

Emotional abuse and neglect

Emotional abuse and neglect may arise from lack of care for physical needs, failure to offer love and nurture based on ignorance or indifference, or sometimes overt hostility and rejection (Skuse

1989). The results may be growth failure in both weight and height, or impaired mental and emotional development. In older children severe behaviour problems may arise. Such children would not be likely to be referred to physiotherapy but it is wise for therapists to be aware that children presenting with behavioural problems or impaired growth may be subject to types of abuse.

Sexual abuse

Sexual abuse has been known to the police, paediatricians and social workers for many years but the impact of the size of the problem revealed by the Cleveland affair has raised public conscience in a highly sensitive area (Doyle 1987; Riches 1988). It has been estimated that possibly 1 child in 10 experiences some form of sexual abuse. The majority of cases occur within a family, the victim is normally a girl, and the perpetrator usually male and well-known to the child. The fatal or bizarre incidences that now make newspaper headlines are more sensational but much less common. Child sexual abuse is therefore a hidden and very secret happening, and rarely gives rise to physical signs capable of 'proof' (Bamford & Roberts 1989) (in contradistinction to physical abuse, when the typical physical signs may persist for days, weeks or, in the case of fractures, a life-time). Reliance has to be placed on the child's own story, and as it is likely to be strongly denied by adults involved, the tendency often is to disbelieve the child. Doyle (1987) however states that: 'Extensive experience now suggests that it is rare for children to make up stories of incidents of sexual abuse', and the story is often reinforced by disturbed behaviour patterns, which are often non-specific but which occasionally reveal premature sexuality or precocious sexual knowledge.

People working with children in any capacity need to be alert to these indicators and to listen and give time to the children. Doyle's (1987) paper and Riches (1988) offer extensive coverage of all aspects of child sexual abuse. Care for these children should not be seen as punishing a proven offender, but should be directed to support for the whole family. This involves not just one professional or a single interview but an ongoing, well-planned programme for each individual family, based on the type of team support envisaged in the DHSS document *Working Together* (1988).

The care and protection of abused children and children at risk is a shared responsibility. The complexities of care indicate the urgent necessity for close co-operation between agencies. Some of the pointers that might lead nurses, physiotherapists teachers, social workers or members of the general public to suspect child sexual abuse are summarised in Table 13.5. In all instances local child protection procedures should be available, understood and followed.

One further reason for physiotherapists to have some knowledge of child abuse is that it may be suffered by some of their patients. Some of the most vulnerable children are those who are most severely handicapped mentally or physically. Recent reports from America and research amongst some British paediatricans (Hobbs & Wynn 1990) have revealed abuse by staff in some residential units for handicapped children. Many of these children are unable to communicate and so symptoms of fear or withdrawal are not easy to differentiate. Close co-operation with a paediatrician who is experienced in the field is essential in such circumstances.

Table 13.5 Recognition of child abuse

Type of abuse	Signs
Deliberate injury	Multiple bruising other than on shins Bilateral black eyes Fingertip bruising on front and back of chest — indicating shaking Finger marks or hand weals on body Bite marks Cigarette burns Burns in the shape of an object, e.g. iron Scalds inconsistent with an accident Fractures
Emotional abuse	Failure to thrive Frozen awareness Self-mutilation Withdrawn behaviour Aggression Attention-seeking behaviour Unexplained under-achievement
Sexual abuse	Sudden onset wetting or soiling Explicit sexual knowledge Promiscuous affection-seeking behaviour Appetite disorders Persistent abdominal pain and headaches Fingertip bruising on knees and inner thighs Recurrent urinary tract infections Vaginal discharge

From *Child Protection Procedures*. City of Manchester Child Protection Committee (1991).

ACKNOWLEDGEMENT

The author (P.E.) wishes to acknowledge the assistance of Sister Anna Forshaw, After Care Burns Unit Sister, in the preparation of the section on thermal injuries.

REFERENCES

Bamford F, Roberts R 1989 Sexual abuse I and II. In: Meadow R (ed) ABC of child abuse. British Medical Journal, 29–36

DHSS 1988 Working together. A guide to arrangements for interagency co-operation for the protection of children from abuse. HMSO, London

De'Ath E 1990 Sudden infant death syndrome. Highlight No 94, National Children's Bureau, London

Doyle C 1987 Sexual abuse: giving help to the children. Children and Society 1: 210–233

Forshaw A 1987 The aftercare of the thermally injured child in a clinic setting. Booth Hall Children's Hospital, Manchester

Griffiths M, Wilson D (1980) Accidents as a cause of mental handicap. In: Griffiths M (ed) Prevention of mental handicap. British Institute of Mental Handicap, Kidderminster

Hall D M B 1989 Health for all children. A programme of child health surveillance. Oxford University Press, Oxford

Hobbs C J 1989 Fractures: head injuries: burns and scalds. In: Meadow R (ed) ABC of child abuse. British Medical Journal, London, pp 8–18

Hobbs C J, Wynne J M 1990 Handicapped children: vulnerability to child abuse. (Paper read at BPA conference 1990)

Hogan J M 1977 The need for adventure versus safety. In: Jackson R H (ed) Children, the environment and accidents. Pitman Medical, Tunbridge, Kent, pp 113–120

Jackson R H 1977 Setting the scene. In: Jackson R H (ed) Children, the environment and accidents. Pitman Medical, Tunbridge, Kent, pp 1–19

Mason S, Forshaw A (undated) Burns after care: a booklet for parents. Booth Hall Children's Hospital/Pan Medical, Manchester

Meadow R 1989 Epidemiology. In: Meadow R (ed) ABC

of child abuse. British Medical Journal, London, pp 1–4

Meadow S R, Smithells R W 1986 Lecture notes on paediatrics. Blackwell Scientific, Oxford

NSPCC 1989 Protecting children: A guide for teachers on child abuse. NSPCC, London.

Riches P 1988 Editorial. Children and society 2: 195–197 and 198 ff

Skuse D H 1989 Emotional abuse and neglect. In: Meadow R (ed) ABC of child abuse. British Medical Journal, London, pp 23–28

Whittington C 1977 Accidents in the home. In: Jackson R H (ed) Children, the environment and accidents. Pitman Medical, Tunbridge, Kent, pp 66–75

FURTHER READING

Arneil G C 1985 Urinary tract infection in children. British Medical Journal 290: 1925–1926

Balistreri W F 1988 Viral Hepatitis. Paediatric Clinics of North America 35: 637–669

Best J M, Banatvala J E 1990 Congenital virus infections. British Medical Journal 300: 1151–1152

Cooper C E 1978 Medical aspects of child abuse. In: Smith S M (ed) The maltreatment of children. MTP Press, Lancaster, England, pp 9–68.

Ellis M E et al 1984 Contemporary gastroenteritis of infancy: clinical features and prehospital management. British Medical Journal 288: 521–523

Gandy G, Rennie J 1990 Antibiotic treatment of suspected neonatal meningitis. Archives of Disease in Childhood 65: 1–2

Geddes A M, Lane P J L 1988 Immunisation. Medicine International 51: 2082–2089

Gibb D M 1991 HIV infection in children. Hospital Update 17: 267–281

Healey J 1975 Infantile subdural haematomas. Pediatric Clinics of North America 22: 433–442

HMSO 1990 Immunisation against Infectious Disease. HMSO, London

Jamison D L 1974 Accidental head injury in childhood. Archives of Disease in Childhood 49: 376–381

Kempe R S, Kempe C H 1978 Child abuse. Fontana/Open books, London.

Klonoff H, Low M D, Clark C 1977 Head injuries in children: prospective five year follow up. Journal of Neurology, Neurosurgery and Psychiatry 40: 1211–1219.

Leck I 1975 Paediatric aspects of epidemiology: frequency of in early life. In: Davis J A, Dobbing J (eds) Scientific

foundations of paediatrics. Heinemann, London, pp 705–757

Levin M, Heyderman R S 1991 Bacterial meningitis. Recent advances in Paediatrics 9: 1–19

London P S 1967 Some observations on the course of events after severe injury of the head. Annals of the Royal College of Surgeons of England 41: 460–479

Markovitch H 1986 Recognising whooping cough. British Medical Journal 292: 360–361

Mok J 1991 HIV infection in children. British Medical Journal 302: 921–922

Phelan P D, Landau L I, Olinsky A In Respiratory Illness in Children. Blackwell Scientific Publications, Oxford

Rudd P T 1991 Childhood immunisation in the new decade. British Medical Journal 302: 481–482

Silverman M 1988 Childhood tuberculosis in Britain. British Medical Journal 297: 1147–1148

Various authors 1981. Perinatal Infections in Clinics in Perinatology

Wharton B A et al 1988 Dietary management of gastroenteritis in Britain. British Medical Journal 296: 450–452

White R H R 1987 Management of urinary tract infection. Archives of Diseases in Childhood 62: 421–427

White R H R, O'Donnell B 1990 Management of urinary tract infection and vesicoureteric reflux in children. British Medical Journal 300: 1391–1394

Williams W O 1985 Respiratory sequelae of whooping cough. British Medical Journal 290: 1937–1940

Zuckerman A J April 1988 Hepatitis B. Hospital Update 1389–1900

14

Sensory disorders: the deaf and blind child

P. Freeman

INTRODUCTION

When a child has both an auditory and a visual impairment, and these are present from birth, a special programme of care and training is necessary to encourage and guide his development. If this programme is to be successful there must be a partnership with his parents, who will be carrying it out, and the various workers from statutory and voluntary agencies who will give them guidance. The physiotherapist will play an important role as a member of the team by developing and guiding motor and tactile skills to compensate for the loss of vision and hearing. Planning for an agreed approach and for continuity of handling is essential and must take account of the family as a whole. To understand the needs of the deaf/blind child we must first appreciate the fact that he cannot be treated as a deaf child or as a blind child; his dual disability is a unique condition and it affects every area of his development.

NORMAL DEVELOPMENT: THE ROLE OF VISION AND HEARING

By looking at the role vision and hearing play in normal development, the effect of the resultant restrictions placed on the ability to gather information, and on active and cognitive development in deaf/blind children can be assessed (Table 14.1).

Table 14.1 Sequence of eye contact and auditory discrimination

Sequence	Eye contact	Auditory discrimination
Young baby		Localises source of sound
	Stares at hands Follows object 180° side to side Fascinated by — light — movement — bright colour	Turns head to source of sound Interested in voice
	Associates touch and vision Uses vision to explore	Sensitive to — intonation — music
		Listens attentively
	Watches moving object	Reaches towards sound
	Form constancy develops	
		Joins in nursery rhymes
	Uses vision for part/whole relationships	
Older child		Acts out stories

Vision

All babies must acquire certain visual skills before their vision is fully developed (Fig. 14.1). First they must learn to look, then to use both eyes together, to focus, so they can see things at different distances, to look quickly from one thing to another and to scan a wide field to seek out what they want to see (see Chapter 4 The Developing Child). If the baby has some partial vision these skills will have to be deliberately taught. Deaf/blind children will need to be shown how to seek for what is relevant to their experiences. Sighted children learn to discriminate objects easily because they are usually within a framework that can be seen in detail, and which therefore becomes known to them. Objects are permanently there for them to see, and they come to expect them to be there. The deaf/blind child must explore the parts in order to create the whole. He must handle objects and travel between, around and with them so that he acquires mental images. These images are a prerequisite for the development of language.

Vision plays an important part in the following early learning skills.

Object permanence

This refers to the ability to know that things exist whether they are present and visible or not (Fig. 14.2). When a ball rolls out of sight the baby sees his mother retrieve and return it. This encourages a feeling of security and of knowing that things exist permanently, although the child may be separate from them. However, when a deaf/blind child throws away a toy, as far as he is concerned it has gone for ever. It is necessary to help him search for it and find it, and to make him aware that it is the same toy he threw away, and not another. Learning to search is an essential ingredient in the incentive to become mobile and explore. Without a grasp of object permanence a child does not develop good memory skills.

Cause and effect

It is by 'seeing' that a child realises that his hands can be used to get things, to do things, to manipulate tools and so achieve what he desires. It is when he 'sees' the relationship between the piece of string and the toy, that he will understand its role in getting the toy to move along. The deaf/blind child lacks these experiences, which provide the knowledge of cause and effect. Being aware of the results of his actions is as necessary as doing the activity itself. Without this awareness he will lack the interest that is the foundation for creating a sense of independence.

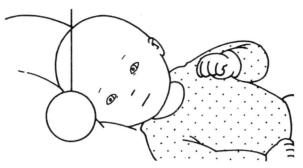

Fig. 14.1 Gassier: 'He can follow a large object through 90°'. (Reproduced by permission of Churchill Livingstone from Gassier J 1984 A guide to psycho-motor development of the child.)

Sorting

By manipulating various toys and objects and seeing their differences, similarities and functions, a child is able to sort them into categories and label them. The deaf/blind child will tend to use objects for self-stimulation if he is not shown their proper use and encouraged to classify them.

Imitation

Children acquire many of the early learning skills from seeing what others do, and in this way imitation is a great motivator. When the deaf/blind child's jaws are ready to chew, he does not have a model of the necessary actions for eating and may be frightened of textures or foods which he

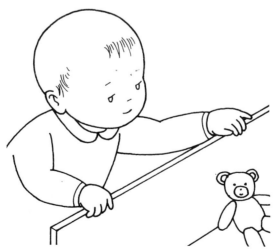

Fig. 14.2 Gassier: 'He looks for an object which is out of sight'. (Reproduced by permission of Churchill Livingstone from Gassier J 1984 A guide to the psycho-motor development of the child.)

cannot see being enjoyed by others. He may reject all but soft foods. He cannot see how others walk, so he may walk on his toes and with a downward posture of his head. The natural gestures which are part of our language (such as waving the hand for 'goodbye') are not seen by him, so communication at its most simple level is denied to him. He is unable to observe how people behave so he has no natural models for role playing, which is so important to the process of growing up.

Spatial relationships

When vision is integrated with kinaesthetic information (awareness of the movements we have made, are making and plan to make) it provides us with the ability to understand spatial relationships. By seeing, feeling and moving an object the child becomes able to recognise it from whatever angle it is seen. When the child sees objects in his path he learns to evade them automatically; he can see himself in relation to things around him and estimate whether it is necessary to move himself or to move things in varying circumstances.

Integration of all these kinaesthetic and sensory skills is critical to helping the child with a visual impairment learn how to solve problems.

Normal vision allows a child to see not only things that are part of himself and are outside him, but also things at a distance. An aeroplane in the sky has no smell and may have no sound; it can only be seen.

Hearing

Hearing plays an equally important role in enabling the child to develop various skills, especially with regard to communication and the acquisition of the spoken word (see Chapter 4 The Developing Child).

Preverbal stage

Children communicate from the time they are born, by eye contact, by crying, laughing and gesturing. They are encouraged to do this by the way others respond to them and this preverbal stage is an essential preliminary to the development of all methods of communication.

Listening

A child hears, but, during this early stage, learns to listen — to listen to sounds in general and then to discriminate between the series of complex sounds which make up the words we use. He has to learn to associate these with the objects to which they refer, remember and gradually classify them into groups (or concepts) by which they can be more easily recalled.

He also has to listen to his own sounds, so that he can approximate them to the words he hears. He is encouraged to refine these by hearing the correct word sounds which his mother and other carers give him over and over again. At the same time he gradually receives expanding sentence patterns, from which he learns how to phrase grammatically what he wants to say and how to respond to what others say to him. This too is vital. It is from the growth of and the use of language that it becomes internalised as a vehicle for thought and comprehension.

When a child hears a noise he wants to know what has made it, and this curiosity encourages him to look for it and to move to find it. Both visual and motor skills are practised. Certain sounds become warnings of danger, some, such as music, a source of pleasure, and from the human voice itself comes an awareness of emotional states such as affection, anger and discipline.

Integration of vision and hearing

Integration of the information a child receives from seeing and hearing provides a valuable cross-reference for concept and intellectual development, i.e. a sound can conjure up a visual image of its maker and vice versa.

Because of what he sees and hears, a baby's first uncoordinated movements soon become controlled, i.e. he lifts his arms towards his mother when she comes to pick him up and says to him 'Up now'. Toys and other objects he sees and hears stimulate him to roll, crawl, sit up and to walk to reach and explore them. He needs these experiences to promote the growth of physical readiness for those activities that are themselves necessary for daily living and independence. Seeing the sheer joy of a child jumping just for the sake of jumping encourages another to copy him. The deaf/blind child has little to encourage him to learn to move or to use the ability to move. It is safer for him to stay lying on his back.

PROBLEMS RESULTING FROM LOSS OF VISION AND HEARING

The deaf/blind baby needs help to fill in these important gaps in his development and intensive programmes need to be planned to help him to make use of any residual vision and/or hearing over a considerable period of time. Any information he gets without, or even with, structured activity is likely to be distorted or incomplete. It may not be enough to give him a constant picture of the world he lives in or the people around him. He will have difficulty in understanding what is around him, what is going on around him or that he is part of what is happening and has a part to play in it. He cannot be told why some kinds of behaviour are acceptable and some are not, and so it is no wonder that his actions are sometimes bizarre and difficult for us to understand.

The world of the deaf/blind child is likely to remain that of his own body. As nothing exists outside himself, there is no reason for him to explore or to communicate. People and the environment have no meaning for the child, except as they appeal to his body and fit into his pleasure world. He will lack distinction between himself and other things and will not be motivated to make relationships. He lacks the security that results from knowing how to anticipate what comes next, i.e. day follows night. There is a danger that he will become totally self-centred and resent all attempts to draw him out.

Residual vision and hearing

The presence of residual vision or hearing can be an asset, but may also be the converse. The desire to see is so strongly inborn that the need to use even a small light response can lead a child to obsessive behaviour, such as handwaving, to obtain it and to ignore every other source of stimulation. If a child has residual vision it is necessary to observe which position objects can best be seen in, whether there is a colour awareness or preference, and the strength of ambient light needed. At all times advantage should be taken of opportunities to encourage the child to look and to listen. Deaf/blind children do not often learn to speak, but they do sometimes learn to recognise and understand some spoken words (although still needing to express themselves in signs). Speech also provides other clues to communication, such as vibration, face and throat movements, puffs of air, all of which can be useful if we draw the child's attention to them.

Compensating for the losses

This picture is a very sad one. It cannot be changed by just teaching deaf/blind children to explore, to move without sight and to communicate with signs. It is necessary to recognise in detail and compensate for those areas of deprivation that occur in the early months and years of learning. Unless a firm foundation of basic information and skills is built, a child will have great difficulty in learning to learn on his own. A programme must be planned which meets each child's individual needs and those of his family. It must be begun as soon as possible. This programme has to provide information in a way that is meaningful to the child and the skills have to be broken down into steps small enough for him to achieve successfully.

ABILITIES OF THE DEAF/BLIND CHILD

The programme must progress at the pace set by the child and it must use to the full the assets he does possess.

Communication

All children have an innate ability to communicate from birth. If the deaf/blind baby fails to advance in this skill it is probably because we have failed to respond to him at the appropriate time. For too long deaf/blind children have been described as non-communicating and the fact that they communicate initially by body movements, crying and facial expression, like all babies, has frequently been ignored. When adults respond to them by meeting their needs it is necessary to let them know that it is their actions which have prompted this. It is not enough just to respond to the deaf/blind child, he must know what that response is. Later on, as he gets older, he needs to know that when others initiate a conversation he is expected to (and shown how to) make a response.

Gross and fine motor skills

Unless there is any medical reason why not, the deaf/blind baby has the same capacity to develop gross and fine motor skills as any other child. However, since he does not possess the same incentives to move and explore, he will need help and more time to achieve the milestones and exploratory skills necessary for the acquisition and use of information. It will take time and support for him to overcome his fears and to learn to move about freely and with confidence.

Tactile skills

The deaf/blind child has two hands which, through those who handle him will act as his eyes and ears. He has a body through which he can receive many clues, i.e. about people, how they feel about him (a loving hug), how they are feeling (if they are tense). Through vibration he will learn about things such as approaching footsteps, musical rhythms, differences in voice tones and spoken words, and the identity of objects, i.e. the radio, washing-machine or vacuum cleaner. As a result of having parts of his body moved and learning to imitate these in context he will develop the first simple acts of communication. An awareness of the meaning of tactile impressions on his hands and the development of fine hand and finger patterns with which to respond, will lead to the ability to sign and finger spell, a method of communication which can be as efficient as the spoken word, given time and experience.

TECHNIQUES FOR INTERVENTION
Hands-on techniques

These techniques are a means of conveying information through hand and body contact in a way that is meaningful to the child. Carers who work with the child are called 'interveners', as their task is to come between the child and the environment in order for him to learn about it.

Whilst it is not difficult to appreciate that when the intervener's hands are guiding those of the child they are communicating with him, it is not always understood that the child, through his hands, can be communicating in return. This occurs long before the acquisition of signs and finger spelling. It is important that the intervener should recognise any movements the child's hands make, however slight, that indicate that he is anticipating the next step in the activity and telling us he is ready to try to do it himself — if this is missed he may not try again and may therefore lose interest. The child's anticipatory behaviour is also a guide to the pace at which he can advance, and if this is not respected, or if pressure is given, he will become disheartened.

Each movement of the deaf/blind child will tell carers something about him. Everyone who works with the child should be trained to observe and interpret these movements and to let him know that his message has been received, otherwise he is unlikely to become a communicating person. Each gesture or action may have various meanings. A push is not necessarily an aggressive action, he might be saying 'Let me finish what I am doing' or 'I'd like to be left alone just now' or just 'I don't want to do it'. If it is not appropriate to meet his wishes, then carers must find some way of telling him why he must do what is wanted, and offer him an incentive to do it.

When interveners provide information and instruction 'hands-on', it is necessary to remember that what is being passed on is relative to the intervener's experience, which may be visual rather than tactile, and that which is a salient feature visually may not be so tactually. It helps if interveners have experience of recognising things by touch alone, recognising people without seeing them and being aware of things happening without depending on being able to see and hear. To just 'touch' a thing tells us little about it. It is through touching and moving that learning takes place (Table 14.2). It is through the intervener's hands that the child must be shown how to manipulate things, to learn what they are for and, with practice and the intervener's awareness of when to let go, to learn how to use them himself.

Use of daily routines

A baby who is able to see and hear first begins to notice things during those daily routines necessary to his well-being. It is because these happen regularly and frequently that a baby begins to pick out certain clues, links these to what is happening and then learns to anticipate them, so that the day begins to have a structure and he can start to build up a constant picture of his environment. It is necessary to provide this information in the same situations to the deaf/blind child. To the normal child slight variations do not matter, but for the deaf/blind child it is necessary to keep strictly to the routine and to the procedures within the routine activity until he has fully recognised and understood it. Variations, when they are introduced, must be linked with the old clues and must build on previous learning so that his knowledge is extended both in breadth and in complexity.

Back chaining

The deaf/blind child depends mainly on tactile and kinaesthetic experiences for recognition, memory and recall. This means learning will take place more slowly. All skills can be broken down

Table 14.2 Learning through touching and moving

Concept	Direction of movement
Shape	Over and round
Texture	Across
Weight Density Height	Up and down
Length	Along
Exploration	Around

into small stages and it is usually the final stage which is most easily remembered and learned (see Chapter 22 Planning for Progress). It is also the stage that completes the task. For this reason the final stage is often taught first through a method known as 'back chaining', so that excessive demands are not put on the child. Learning to self-feed can be given as an example. The act of filling a spoon with food, putting this into the mouth and withdrawing it empty can be broken down into a sequence of movements. The last movement of withdrawing the spoon will be the first to be learned and remembered. The help given to the child at this stage should be gradually lessened. When he can do this on his own, help is reduced at each previous stage in turn, until he has achieved the whole sequence and can feed himself (Table 14.3). As each successful stage is acquired the child must be made aware of his success, either by the carer showing pleasure or by making him aware of the difference his actions have made, i.e. the empty dish. This means that the child must have been able to feel the full dish before he began to eat!

PLANNING A PROGRAMME

Identification of developmental skills

Having identified the areas of special need, together with aspects of care and activity that are basic to its success, the individual programme itself can be planned. The main aim must be to

Table 14.3 Back chaining for feeding

Stages	Stages of skill teaching — reversed order
Stage 1	Removing spoon from mouth
Stage 2	Closing lips and removing food from spoon
Stage 3	Putting spoon in mouth
Stage 4	Raising spoon to mouth
Stage 5	Loading spoon
Stage 6	Putting spoon in bowl
Stage 7	Holding and stabilising the bowl
Stage 8	Lifting the spoon
Stage 9	Grasping the spoon handle
Stage 10	Finding the spoon

help the deaf/blind child progress through the same stages as would the unimpaired child during the first 3–4 years of life. Age comparisons are inappropriate as the deaf/blind baby cannot be expected to acquire this developmental base at the same rate as the normal child. Like many other children he may miss out some stages and may advance more quickly in some areas than others. Unless each stage is built upon the previous one, as far as possible, a good foundation will not be laid.

The programme which is set up should relate to stages of development with no reference to the age at which these should be achieved.

Starting the programme

A programme will be begun either within a few weeks of birth or when difficulties are first discovered. Whenever this happens parents will need time to come to terms with having a deaf/blind child, and should be actively involved in planning and carrying out the programme (see Chapter 23 Parents and Children). Appropriate and sensitively given information and advice will enable them to achieve a positive attitude towards the child and his future. It will also help them understand the implications of the double handicap and how to make up for this by using other learning channels. All the activities shared with the child must be pleasurable both to him and to the intervener. Whilst interveners must be aware of the underlying reason for what they do, the child must enjoy doing it, doing it with someone else and finding it rewarding in his own way.

Establishing a relationship

A good relationship with the child is basic to the success of any programme and this assumes that some form of communication occurs. Before communication can occur a baby has to know he is a person by recognising another person as separate from himself. Initially this is generally the mother, because from birth she is the person seen and heard most frequently. The deaf/blind baby's experiences are similar but he will come to recognise his mother by the way she holds him, the way she handles him during the daily

routines, by something she wears or the scent she uses, how she cuddles him, her voice vibrations as she holds him close to her. These kinds of clues will provide him with information about others who handle him. His attention can also be drawn to those things which make each person different from all other people, i.e. whether the hair is long or short, thick or thin, curly or straight, or any of the other features which give a unique identity. A deaf/blind child must feel able to trust and want to please a person before he can learn from the things they do together and it is important to reach this stage before starting a specific programme.

Once the deaf/blind child shows recognition of his mother by her handling, she can give him a more tangible clue by wearing, for instance, a brooch, which he is encouraged to touch each time she picks him up. This personal symbol is a technique which can be used by other members of the family as they begin to be involved, e.g. dad's moustache or an older sister's plaits. As the circle of people coming into contact with him widens, it will help him to identify them if they use a special way of greeting him, or wear a distinguishing symbol.

Overcoming frustration

As the child's self-awareness and awareness of his ability to influence others increases, frustration creeps in, mainly because communication lags behind awareness. It will be difficult to reason with him when he cannot have or do something he wants. It is better to keep the relationship happy at this stage by seeing that such a situation does not arise or by providing a distraction before a crisis point is reached. However, later on when he begins to act on his own but may still not have the means of self-expression, frustration can no longer be dealt with in this way. Guidelines and limits must be given and firmly adhered to. Agreed consistent responses from all who have contact with him are essential if he is to learn to control his behaviour and reconcile his desires with the demands of others. Being calm, firm and patient and having a loving 'making up' period after a battle all help to keep the relationship on firm ground. Frustration often leads to aggressive behaviour which, if it gets him what he wants, will continue. If we punish him he will at least have got our attention. The real answer lies in the development of communication.

Six-stage approach

Freeman (1985) has identified six stages which can be used to achieve mobility and fine motor coordination, and which provide a natural division for a programme. The six stages can be applied to the development of skills in:

- movement
- purposeful play
- communication
- visual training
- auditory training.

These are described in the rest of this chapter. It should be emphasised that the stages are quite arbitrary and not suitable, therefore, for assessment progress. Accordingly, they must always be adapted to meet the individual needs of the child and his family circumstances. They are, however, a starting point from which to devise additional activities which will reinforce the skills being taught and increase the child's opportunities to practise and consolidate what he has learned (Table 14.4).

Movement

Stage one. Awareness of movement

A baby's first awareness of movement is of being moved in space, having parts of his body moved and feeling movements on his body. These sensations help him to learn about what is happening. By touching his body in certain ways we can let him know when he is to be picked up or put down, go into his bath, have his nappy changed and so on. From these 'signals' he learns to anticipate what is going to happen to him and to recognise the activity that follows. We can begin to move his arms and hands in the shape of the first early signs. By caressing and massaging him when he is undressed, and his hands at *all* times, we can encourage body awareness. By

always holding him a special way for each routine he can be prepared for an activity and, by changing the hold, alerted to its conclusion.

Stage two. Motivation to move

Once the deaf/blind baby begins to learn to control his own movements interveners begin, and continue, to work with him on a brightly coloured, well-textured rug, which he will come to recognise as the signal or cue for such activities. To encourage head turning and head control, a puff of air can be blown on to his cheek on the side we wish him to turn to. This can be continued until he learns to initiate the movement himself. He can be shown how to roll by manipulation, encouraging him to complete the last bit by himself and back chaining until he can achieve the complete roll unaided. Arm movements can be stimulated when the child is lying on his back by placing a small object on his chest, such as a nice-smelling herb-bag or a vibrating toy. He can be shown how to bring both hands to the midline and touch it. He will need to be shown how to grasp and explore objects by holding them against his hand, helping him to hold them and bring them up to his face. When he is undressed stroke, pat and tickle him, rub his body with different textured things (tissue, cotton wool, etc.) and things with different consistencies, such as shaving cream or oil, for body awareness.

Stage three. Balance and exploration

It is important to do things *with* the child rather than *to* him so that he can begin to realise he can initiate and guide the activity. He must now be shown how to roll from tummy to back and how to get from lying to sitting up by manipulating those parts of his body used to achieve these skills; and he must be praised for every little effort he makes.

Sitting balance. Progress should be made towards independent sitting. The child needs to experience a variety of sitting positions, on your lap, propped up in his pram or sitting between your legs with his back to you as you sit on the floor. This is also a good 'hands-on' position when teaching such skills as dressing and

Table 14.4   The six-stage approach

Movement
      Awareness of movement
          Motivation to move
             Balance and exploration
                Initiating movement
                    Sitting to standing
                        Walking alone

Purposeful play
      Preparation
          Games involving movement
             Sitting and exploring play
                Hiding and finding games
                    Consolidation
                      Skilful games

Communication
      Signals
              Signs
                    Finger spelling

Visual training
      Visual attention
          Focus and fixation
          Tracking
              Visual coordination
                  Visual memory

Auditory training
      LISTENING
          Auditory attention
             Everyday sounds
                Vibrations
                    Distinguishing sounds
                      Complex sounds

      VOCALISING

Stage 1   Stage 6

undressing, operating toys, etc. To encourage finger awareness his palms should be held upwards and each of his fingers and thumb on each hand touched in turn whilst accompanying rhymes are sung. His hands should be guided over and round things that are round, i.e. balls of various sizes and textures, and his attention drawn to the round objects that are part of his daily life (plates, bowls, wheels of toys). Rings or bracelets can be placed on his arm and he should be shown how to remove them. It is important to show him how to transfer toys from one hand to the other and to hold two objects, one in each hand. By continuing to place small objects on his body, and by extending this to different parts, and to underneath, him he can be encouraged to find and remove them.

Environment. Now is the time to begin giving him some clues to his immediate environment and what goes on in specific rooms and areas. Parents can be advised to let him feel the pillow on his own bed, and to take him to theirs. Where he has learned a personal symbol for his parents, these could be placed on each pillow for him to feel. A strong pleasant smell could be used, which he can always experience when he goes into the kitchen. It is important to let him smell foods as meals are prepared (and taste them when possible), to feel the bubbles in the washing-up bowl and to play with safe kitchen equipment, such as wooden spoons. The bathroom or toilet should be used for potty training so that he comes to associate this room with going to the toilet and will, at a later stage, know where to go when he recognises the need for himself. He should be encouraged to help to open doors when moving from room to room and when he is carried up and down stairs the movements should be emphasised.

Stage four. Initiating independent movement

Once the deaf/blind child is sitting well he would often be content to remain in this position, but if this is allowed his world would be no more than that spanned by the forward reach of his arms. He needs to be shown how to use his body to move around by manipulating his limbs until, with regular practice, he develops the physical readiness to do it by himself. No-one moves without a reason to do so, therefore until the child has the skill and need, or curiosity motivates him, we must see that his efforts are rewarded with, for example, his favourite toy, game or food. He will need to be shown how to creep (crawl on his tummy along the floor) before learning to support himself on outstretched arms and to move his arms and legs independently. Two people may need to work with him on crawling (cross lateral), one to manipulate his legs, the other his arms.

Whenever possible the intervener should join in all activities with the deaf/blind child; crawl with him, over and beside him, roll with him, sit with him rocking sideways and encourage him to reach forwards and sideways for balance. In this way he gains information from the adult's body as to how to move his own. As an introduction to standing, he should stand facing the intervener with support and his arms gently moved up and down, showing him how to bend his knees when his hands are down. Once he begins to crawl by himself his attention should be drawn to clues which identify different parts of his home, for instance, the lino in the kitchen, different carpet textures, paving stones and grass outside. By letting him become more involved in helping in

simple ways his experiences in different parts of the house can be extended. His awareness of the outside world can also be extended by giving him toys such as a plastic windmill which he can feel going round when it is windy. Deliberately puff up slopes and run down them when he is carried and make sure people he meets give him the 'Hallo' sign. As his crawling improves, provide some obstacles for him to go over, round, through, and set up a small sequence of these for him to follow.

Stage five. Sitting to standing

This is perhaps the most difficult stage, for now he must learn how to get from sitting to standing. This needs to be broken down into a sequence of actions which build up to the skill slowly, guiding his limbs and shift of weight with him near to a chair on which there is a reward placed which he achieves once he is standing. It is important that he is shown how to reverse the sequence in order to sit down again.

When he can stand supported comfortably, with his back to you, have him stand with his feet on yours whilst you walk, rocking a little from side to side so that he begins to understand the need to change weight from foot to foot. This method can also be used to show him how to cruise round a low table by moving sideways. Walking skills can be developed further if he walks between two people who are holding his hands, by letting him push round a weighted trolley and by showing him how to use the furniture to get around and explore. The child should be encouraged to move about the house so that he begins to make a mental map of his home.

Take him walking outdoors with him holding on to you (or his pushchair). His attention should be drawn to fences, low walls and gates, curbs, autumn leaves on the path, and puddles after rain. It will be necessary to intervene directly to make him aware of the environment.

Stage six. Walking alone

The deaf/blind child will learn to walk by himself, but he will not necessarily be motivated to take advantage of the ability. Therefore, initially there must be some tangible reason for him to walk — if he walks to the toy cupboard, he must be given a toy, if to the kitchen a biscuit, so that ultimately he learns that when he wants a toy, he has to go to the toy cupboard or when he is hungry, the kitchen is where the food is kept. He first needs to get used to walking with only one hand held lightly and if he tends to swing forward or backwards to begin with a little support should be given to the shoulder of the hand not being held. Kneel behind him holding him at the hips and show him how to shift his weight from side to side and forward and backwards, so that he is taking steps in all directions.

He can now be encouraged to take his first few steps alone between two people and when he can take several steps between them successfully, he can be shown how to turn round and walk back to the other person so that he learns about balance when turning. A short 'motor' course can be organised in the garden, which will be fun and also enable him to practise all the different skills he has been acquiring.

Purposeful play

Play is a young child's best opportunity for learning and much of it is spontaneous. However, the deaf/blind child will have to be taught how to play, otherwise he may tend to resort to self-stimulation for his amusement. Play has to be initiated with him, taking advantage of the opportunities it offers to use and practise the skills he needs, for new learning, and for visual and auditory stimulation where this is appropriate.

Stage one. Preparation

In the early days, simple activities provide a preliminary to play and these should be carried out regularly for short periods, e.g. nursing the baby with his head against the carer's chest whilst talking or singing to him, rocking him.

Stage two. Games involving movement

As he gets older and more aware he needs to experience all kinds of movement through the intervener. Parents can be shown how to romp, jump, hop and dance with him in their arms. How to jog him up and down, rock in a chair with him. These activities should be stopped every now and then to see if by some movement of his body, the child indicates to you he wants to continue the game — this is a good situation for him to start communicating. When he is on your lap, with his back to you and with your hands on his, play simple nursery rhymes with actions. Games which work up to a climax should be played so that he can learn to anticipate ('round and round the garden' is a good example). Do these the same way, several times a day, so that he comes to recognise them and learns to remember the sequence of movement (which is basic to signing and finger spelling).

Stage three. Sitting and exploring play

As well as the activities discussed under Stage three of Movement, he should now be able to sit by himself in a small chair and begin to have things to explore on his own. These can be presented on a small tray. Choose objects that are bright, have good shape, different textures and some that make noises. Having different covers for the tray, e.g. vinyl for meals, black to show up toys, might also provide clues to help him recognise and anticipate the activity. Make his play rug more interesting by sewing on such things as plastic rings, large buttons, or pieces of fur, for him to discover with his feet and hands.

Stage four. Hiding and finding games

He should now be ready to play games that will help him become aware of object permanence — hiding and finding things. He should have toys that 'do' things that he can be shown how to operate himself, such as a wind-up merry-go-round, an electric toothbrush with different tops. Let him have small groups of things that have something in common to play with, perhaps all one colour, sets of things connected with a daily routine (cup/spoon/dish, sponge/hairbrush/ toothbrush) and observe whether he knows what they are for.

Stage five. Consolidation

The child will now want to spend more time moving around and toys should be put around the room for him to find. Some deaf/blind children may become hyperactive once they can move about by themselves and so it is important to watch out for boredom and to change the activity. They need to have periods each day when they sit quietly and share an activity to lessen the possibility of this occurring. Construction toys may only be enjoyed briefly as they do not have the same appeal for the deaf/blind child as to the sighted child and so it may be helpful to join a toy library to increase the variety available. Homemade things are often better, particularly if related to everyday skills, for example, a board with three or four different pockets, each with a different type of opening (zip, popper, button) into which you can put different things for him to find each day. To aid fine motor control provide opportunities for him to poke, roll, tear, push, squeeze, pat, bang, swipe, rub, punch and to pick up items of various sizes right down to the very small.

Stage six. Skilful games

Once the child is walking there are many more activities to fill his days, but opportunities must be made every day for him to sit and play by himself or one-to-one, as well as outdoors. A tricycle should be within his capability.

Sorting activities develop practical skills, as do containers with pop-on or screw tops, which he can learn to take off and put back on. Containers can be filled with items such as pasta, and he can be given things to unwrap or wrap. It is important that the child should enjoy the activities he takes part in by himself, or with the intervener. If, as well as deriving enjoyment, he is learning and practising new skills, then the aim of establishing purposeful play has been achieved.

Communication

Communication is a two-way process. Gesture and body language give important visual clues, and vocal expression important auditory clues, so that the receiver and sender of any communication can understand each other. The deaf/blind baby will need considerable help to understand what is being communicated to him, and how his attempts at communication are being received. The various signals and signs which can be used with deaf/blind children are essential to this process. Signals are those clues which we give the child to alert him to what is happening. Signs are those actions commonly used for communicating when speech is not possible and some are an extension of signals. Tapping the child's leg to let him know we want to put on his sock is a signal. Touching the baby's lips before feeding is also a signal, but this action is also used as the sign for food. Both must relate to something happening directly to the child or that he can experience by touch. He will need to have 'felt' and been shown how to make the sign himself many times before he can be expected to use it. The choice of signals and signs that are first used depends on the home environment and on observations of the child's reactions to familiar situations. Freeman (1985) gave the following suggestions for an appropriate progression:

Stage one

Signals.

- mother's and father's personal symbols, e.g. a brooch and a tie
- tap arm before picking up
- hands under child briefly before laying him down
- dabble hands in water before bathing
- touch face with towel before lifting from bath
- use cot only at night time, pram during day
- touch hips in downward direction for nappy change.

Signs. 'me' . . . child's hand touched to adult's chest 'you' . . . child's hand touched to own chest (these substitute for names at this stage).

Stage two

Signals.

- symbols for other family members, e.g. toy car for brother, toy spectacles for uncle
- pat on the head = 'good boy'
- special rug to play on.

Signs. A mother does not talk to her normal baby in single words and so they should not be used with the deaf/blind baby. Simple sentences should be used, with emphasis on the important word. By taking the baby's hand (fist probably) the following simple sentences can be signed, always saying the words at the same time.

> *Mealtimes.* 'Are you hungry?' Touch his hand to his chest (= you) then rub it in a circular movement on his tummy (= hungry).
> 'Here is your food/drink.' Touch his hand to his bottle so he knows it is there, then touch it to his chest (= your) and then to his mouth (= eat/drink).
> *Bedtime.* 'Time for you to sleep.' Touch his hand to his chest (= you) and then to the side of his head (= sleep) the side on which you are going to lay him.
> *Bath time.* 'It's bath time.' Touch his hand to his chest (= you) then rub it gently down his chest from his neck several times (= washing).

Stage Three

Signals.

- symbols or special greeting signs from people outside the family
- chair with tray for play on his own
- sits on lap for nursery rhyme play
- sits between legs on floor for instruction.

> **Signs.**
> *'No.'* (Needs to learn the meaning of this early). With the palm facing outward, move the baby's hand sharply in front of his face (Fig. 14.3)
> *'Drink.'* (Now separate from food). 'You (want) drink?' Baby's hand, shaped as if holding a cup, moving upwards to touch thumb to corner of his mouth (Fig. 14.4).
> *'Play.'* 'You (and) me play.' For play make circular movements inwards/outwards with palms of baby's hands upwards, several times (Fig. 14.5).
> *'Hallo.'* General greeting. Using one hand palm outward, make an inward/outward semicircle at shoulder height.

Stage four

The child is now ready to be shown that the movements we have been making with his hands to indicate something can also be used by him for the same purpose, i.e. asking for something he needs or to do an activity he enjoys. Also it

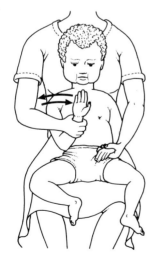

Fig. 14.3 Sign: No.

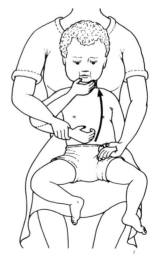

Fig. 14.4 Sign: Drink.

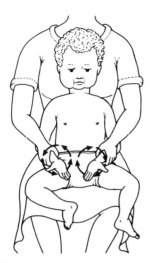

Fig. 14.5 Sign: Play.

is time for him to learn that you cannot always respond at once and that the activity cannot be continued for ever.

Signals. Many signals will occur naturally in the course of the daily routines. The child may design some of his own, i.e. running his hand up towards his neck to indicate the zip of his coat because he wants to go out. Accept these and use them, but gradually pair them with the accepted sign so that eventually this is the one the child learns to use.

Signs.
Please. Meaning 'May I have?' (later — 'Thank you'). Clasp baby's hands together, fingers over the side of each hand.

Go walking. Making a walking movement with your index and second finger down the child's wrist and on to the palm.

Going out in the car. Take the child's hands and turn an imaginary steering wheel.

Wait. The same sign as for 'Please' but now put the clasped hands down on to the child's lap with a little push, saying firmly 'Wait'.

Finished. ('No more' or 'All gone'). Hold the child's hand in the form of a fist and tap it sharply on the palm of the other.

Stage five

Finger spelling. Now is the time for begin-

ning very simple finger spelling as a means of using relationship names. Whenever he touches your special signal (brooch, tiepin or whatever) finger spell 'Mum' or 'Dad' as appropriate. Then, taking his hand, show him how to finger spell the word on to your hand so that he can advance to 'Mum play (with) me' and thereby take his first step towards symbolism.

Signs. New signs to introduce might be:
Sit down. Hands slightly over each other, palms down, press down a couple of times. Initially do this when the child is close enough to have his hands touch the thing he is to sit on.

Stand up. Palms of the adult's hands underneath the child's hands which are then moved in an upward direction (Fig. 14.6).

Want. Child's hand, palm upwards, is moved forward from the chest.

Do. Similar to the sign for 'Finished', except that the lower hand is closed as well as the upper.

Give. The 'Want' sign in reverse.

Spoon. A scooping movement upwards towards the face with one hand — this movement starting from the cupped palm of the other hand.

Biscuit. Child taps his elbow.

You can now make longer sentences such as:
Child: 'I want (a) biscuit (to) eat.'
Mother: 'Mummy give you (a) biscuit.'

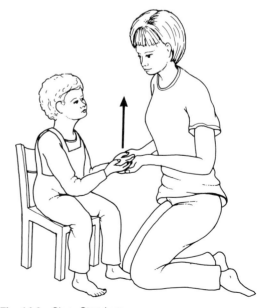

Fig. 14.6 Sign: Stand up.

It is not enough to teach the deaf/blind child to make signs, he must know what they refer to and that they are useful to him because when he makes them he gets a response. Create situations where he has a need to sign. Make sure that all who come into contact with him know the signs he responds to and use them with him.

Stage six

This is a gradual expansion of the use of signs related to the daily experiences of the child. Finger-spelt names of people can be associated with their special symbols, link words such as 'more, in, on, up, down', action words such as 'jump, run, swim', as appropriate to the child's needs can be introduced slowly. Illustrations of these can be found in the Maketon vocabulary of signs, which is related to the progressive development of signing.

Visual training

Even the smallest degree of sight can be valuable if we can teach the deaf/blind child to use it. Vision develops by being used, so it is up to us to provide visual stimulation. How much, what and where he sees has to be carefully observed first and then we have to use this information as a basis of training.

Stage one. Visual attention

To begin with, encourage the child to look at your face by wearing something bright and shiny, e.g. a disco headband, silver foil round the rims of glasses or use bright lipstick.

Stage two. Focus and fixation

Gradually start to prop the child up, with head support if necessary, so that he begins to learn about the world from the upright position (and to help counteract a preference to remain prone). Draw his attention to his hands and to yours by putting brightly coloured or reflective stickers on the tips of his fingers. Put a shiny mobile where you know he can see it (light it up with a lamp if necessary) and move him around so that he is not watching it from the same place. Shine a torch on a wall in a dark room to encourage him to fixate on it — the first of the visual skills he must learn.

Stage three. Tracking

We must provide stimulation that invites the child to follow (track) bright objects or a light source to one side and to the other side, both upwards and downwards. Use a torch beam on the wall, light up one area and when the child has noticed it, turn the torch off and move the beam to a different place. This will help him to learn to move from one fixation to another. A line of shiny or reflective objects can be placed in a line each a little further away from the child; as the torch beam is shone on each in turn the child learns to focus on objects at varying distances.

Stage four. Ocular coordination

Ocular coordination must now be encouraged by inviting the child to reach for toys to the right and to the left of him with the parallel hand, and then with both hands, so that he must look from one side to the other, crossing the midline. The distance between toys should be quite small at first. Encourage him to reach out for an object that is big enough for him to need to use both hands, e.g. a big ball, or a balloon. Blow soap bubbles and see if he can follow them and reach out and pop them.

Stages one to four are sufficient to enable the child to acquire the necessary skills to make the best use of his residual vision. They must be taught systematically and practised regularly.

Stages five and six. Visual memory

As the child progresses through these stages through other activities, it is important to make use of increasing opportunities to encourage him to 'look' at things that become available to him as he grows in awareness and mobility. If he can learn to 'see' and to retain visual images, he will use his sight, for it is the most efficient way of gathering information.

Auditory training: listening

Before an awareness of sounds is developed, let alone the ability to identify and reproduce them, it is essential to learn to listen. Vision and hearing stimulate the listening faculty, but if the sounds the deaf/blind child hears are distorted by impairment and do not stimulate his interest, he will ignore them and will not learn to listen. If he does not listen he will not be able to associate sounds with their source, he will not know that the sounds made by people are words and he will not know that he can make sounds like them and that these have meaning. It is essential that auditory training includes the encouragement both to listen and to make sounds, hoping that ultimately the two will come together so that the child is able to imitate the sounds he hears and learn to speak.

Stage one. Auditory attention

There must be something to listen to — so talk to the baby close to his ear and put plenty of emotional tone in your voice. Observe whether there is any change in his behaviour when there are any loud sounds, or perhaps if it is a woman's voice or that of a man, or music if the radio is put near to him.

Stage two. Everyday sounds

When you feel sure he is listening, observe at what distance he hears, whether he consistently shows awareness of sounds such as doors banging, the telephone bell ringing, or only high sounds or low sounds. If we can identify the sounds that interest him, a starting point will have been established. As he begins to recognise some of the routine situations, use specific phrases with emphasis on the key words, i.e. when you lay him down say '*Down* you go', when you pick him up '*Up* you come' and so on. Make sure the sounds he hears are happy and pleasant.

If he wears a hearing aid, remember it only amplifies sound, it does not make him listen. Sounds have to have meaning and be interesting if he is to remember and recognise them. It is we who have to stimulate that interest and create situations which give sounds meaning for him. Before you speak to him, get his attention by touching him on the shoulder, encouraging him to look at you and by saying 'Listen'.

Stage three. Vibrations

When the child shows that he is beginning to notice sounds let him feel the vibrations, e.g. the radio, and let him learn how to turn it on and off. When you are working with him and encouraging him to listen to specific sounds, always let him hear the sound, then no sound for a few seconds so that he has time to change from listening *to* to listening *for*. The more contrast there is between the sounds you offer, the more likely he is to notice them.

Stage four. Distinguishing sounds

Encourage him to try to locate sounds and see if he can learn to identify from, say, two noise-makers, which of the two he has heard. Show him how to take turns at using sound-makers, such as a bell, by giving one of the bells to him. He then has to be taught to listen to yours so that he knows when it is his turn to ring his own.

By this time you should know if he is beginning to recognise any of the words in the phrases you regularly use and responding to them. Even if he does, it is important to continue to sign as well as speak because he will need signs to respond to until he has speech, and this may take a lot longer to develop.

Stages five and six. Complex sounds

We need to provide and draw the child's attention to ever more specific sounds. Individual high/low, short/long, loud/soft sounds should be used, together with short sequences of these, to develop his ability to discriminate the very complex series of sounds contained in speech. We must take advantage of every opportunity to encourage him during these later stages offered by his increased activity to listen to a greater variety of sounds and to discover what makes them.

Auditory training: vocalising

To begin with the deaf/blind baby will make all the usual baby sounds. To encourage him in making and developing these sounds, copy them close to his ear. If he shows he is hearing you, encourage him to copy you and then move on to taking turns.

If he achieves this, progress to changing the pitch, and then try two sounds together, one high, one low, gradually making the difference less obvious. As each type of vocalisation is learned, encourage him to copy sounds and to take turns making them. Notice any new sounds he makes and copy these yourself. These are all links in the chain that has to be worked through slowly if he is to have the ability to use speech.

As the child becomes more skilled at controlling his sounds and approximating them to yours, continue to play the game of turn-taking, for this is the basis of communicating. Introduce some blended sounds for him to copy, like 'ba-ba-ba', 'ma-ma-ma'. Put his hands on your face to let him feel how you move your lips and face muscles to make the sounds, stressing the changes needed to make, say, 'ee-ee-ee' into 'ah-ah-ah'. As he becomes more adept at copying the sounds you make, you can bring in words that can begin to have meaning, i.e. 'Mum', 'Dad', because you can link them up with the symbols or signs he already knows. The process will take a long time and for this reason it is better to begin with the tactile method of communication as soon as possible. Waiting may perhaps mean that the child never develops a means of communication at all.

CONCLUSION

The deaf/blind child will not learn without help, but the task becomes easier once communication is established. We must recognise that the child is communicating all the time by the way he is behaving and we must become skilled in interpreting and responding to him. He, in turn, must be made to understand that our responses are directly related to his actions, i.e. that when he cries because he is hungry he is given food because he has cried, not because we happen to know it is the right time for his meal. Once he realises that by communicating he cannot only influence our behaviour but also act for himself, it is vital that we provide opportunities for him to choose how to act, i.e. to take a biscuit *or* a cake. It is all too easy to choose for the deaf/blind child, but if we do, we deny him the first essential step towards independence — which is surely our long term aim. And whilst we must be aware of the need for specific help in certain areas, we must not forget that it is the integration of sensory information, together with the ability to communicate and be mobile, that enables the deaf/blind child to use his independence.

REFERENCES

Freeman P 1985 The deaf/blind baby. Heinemann, London

FURTHER READING

Freeman P 1975 Understanding the deaf/blind child. Heinemann, London
McInnes J M, Treffrey J A 1982 Deaf/blind infants and children. University of Toronto Press, Toronto
Montagu A 1987 Touching, 2nd edn. Harper and Row, London

Royal National Institute for the Blind 1978 Guidelines for teachers and parents of visually handicapped children with additional handicaps. Royal National Institute for the Blind, London

15

Inborn errors of metabolism

J. E. Wraith

INTRODUCTION

At the turn of the century Sir Archibald Garrod introduced the concept of inborn errors of metabolism, whereby a number of different metabolic disorders with well-defined clinical, pathological and biochemical findings could be attributed to the inheritance of abnormal genes. The failure of a gene to produce normal amounts of functional enzyme can result in many different effects on an enzymatically controlled biochemical pathway, as illustrated in Fig. 15.1. An understanding of this concept is central to the appreciation of the effects of inborn errors of metabolism.

Biochemical pathways

The normal functioning of an individual is

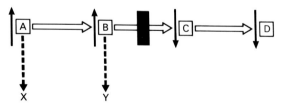

Fig. 15.1 The consequences of a metabolic block in a biochemical pathway. A metabolic block between the compounds B and C in the biochemical pathway leads to: (i) an increase in compounds A and B; (ii) a decrease in compounds C and D; (iii) the production of 'new' metabolic pathways, leading to new compounds X and Y. All of these may have an adverse effect on the individual.

dependent upon the integrity of many biochemical pathways within the cells of different organs. It is clear that there are many different possible clinical symptoms and signs that can result from a metabolic block, depending on which part of the cell or organ of the body is primarily affected. In some conditions the defect is generalised and affects all cells of the body, but in others the enzyme deficiency is limited to a particular organ, e.g. muscle in muscle glycogen storage disease (type V, McArdle's disease) (see Table 15.2, p. 273).

Although each individual type of inborn error is rare, they collectively provide many significant problems in paediatric practice. Many of the conditions require specialised laboratory investigations for diagnosis and follow-up as well as the involvement of many other disciplines to ensure the best outcomes. For this reason it is felt that referral to a regional centre specialising in the management of such children is in the best interests of patient and family.

CLASSIFICATION

A classification of some of the major types of metabolic disorder, with examples, is given in Table 15.1.

As a general rule, most of the disorders are inherited as autosomal recessives, although there are a number of important exceptions:

- mucopolysaccharidosis type II (Hunter's syndrome)
- Lesch–Nyhan syndrome
- ornithine carbamyl transferase deficiency
- Fabry's disease.

Prenatal diagnosis by either amniocentesis or chorion villus biopsy is available for most disorders. Amniocentesis involves removing a small volume of amniotic fluid at 15–16 weeks' gestation. The fluid contains skin cells from the developing infant and these can be grown in the laboratory and the relevant enzyme test performed upon them.

Amniocentesis is a safe test; the risk of miscarriage is much less than 1 in 100. The disadvantage is the relatively late stage in pregnancy it is performed, so that if a termination of pregnancy is requested due to an abnormal result,

Table 15.1 A simplified classification of some metabolic disorders

Disorders of protein metabolism
  Phenylketonuria
  Homocystinuria
  Maple syrup urine disease
  Organic acid disorders
  Urea cycle defects

Disorders of carbohydrate metabolism
  Galactosaemia
  Fructosaemia
  Glycogen storage disease

Disorders of lipid metabolism
  Familial hypercholesterolaemia
  Abetalipoproteinaemia

Disorders of trace metal metabolism
  Wilson's disease
  Menkes disease

Disorders of purine metabolism
  Lesch–Nyhan syndrome

Lysosomal storage disease
  Glycogen, e.g. glycogen storage disease type II (Pompe's disease)
  Cysteine, e.g. cystinosis
  Glycosaminoglycans, e.g. mucopolysaccharidoses
  Glycolipids, e.g. Niemann–Pick disease, Gaucher's disease, Fabry's disease
  Ganglioside, e.g. Gm1 gangliosidosis, Tay–Sachs' disease
  Sulphatide, e.g. metachromatic leucodystrophy

it has to be performed by inducing an early labour at 18–20 weeks. For this reason, chorion villus biopsy is preferred by many patients. In this test a small piece of the placenta is removed, either vaginally via the cervix or transabdominally. This test can be performed much earlier, at 8–10 weeks, and at this stage the pregnancy is usually 'private' and termination can be performed by suction curettage. The disadvantage is the higher risk of miscarriage, between 2–3 in 100 in most units.

PRESENTATION

In broad terms an inborn error of metabolism comes to notice in one of three ways:

Mass screening of the newborn population

The frequency of phenylketonuria (PKU) (see p. 269) (1 in 10 000 in the UK) and the gratifying response to a low phenylalanine diet started early in the new-born period has led to the introduction of a mass screening programme in most developed countries, which is aimed at the early detection of PKU. Depending on the type of method used for screening, a number of other conditions may be detected along with PKU. In one health region a capillary sample of blood is collected by the visiting nurse after the tenth day of life. In the laboratory the amino acids in the blood are separated by chromatography and stained by a special chemical called ninhydrin. An increase in a particular amino acid is seen as a 'dense' spot. Infants shown to have an increase in an amino acid have the test repeated and, if the abnormality is confirmed, they are seen at the unit so that venous blood can be collected for a quantitative estimation of the particular amino acid.

Some countries advocate screening for many different disorders, but it has always been necessary to justify screening programmes on economic grounds in the UK. Hypothyroidism is the only other condition that has achieved universal acceptance within the UK screening programmes. At the same time as the PKU test is performed, a sample of blood is collected on a filter paper. In the laboratory the level of thyroid stimulating hormone (TSH) in the blood sample is determined. An elevated value is found in children with hypothyroidism due to the common congenital forms of thyroid deficiency. Positive tests are followed up in a similar way to that described for PKU.

Other disorders are either too rare or the results of treatment not good enough to justify mass screening.

An acute, severe illness in the new-born period

A number of disorders, e.g. maple syrup urine disease, organic acid disorders and urea cycle defects (see p. 271), can present with a catastrophic illness in early life, leading rapidly to death or severe mental retardation in survivors if not detected and treated. The symptoms and signs are very non-specific and mimic a number of more common neonatal disorders, such as infection or asphyxia. The clue to diagnosis is a high index of suspicion on the part of the neonatal team and a willingness to investigate urgently any sick neonate for possible metabolic disease.

A subacute presentation

Those conditions that are associated with an abnormal storage of various compounds often present outside the new-born period. In lysosomal storage disease the storage occurs within a subcellular organelle, the lysosome, and these patients often present with enlargement of the liver and spleen, joint stiffness, bony deformity and neurological degeneration if the brain and nervous system are involved. In glycogen storage disease (see Table 15.2, p. 273), with the exception of type II — Pompe's disease — the glycogen is found free in the cytoplasm of the cells and is not limited to a particular organelle. However, certain organs may be predominantly affected, e.g. liver in types I, III, VI and IX and muscle in types V and VII.

It would not be possible to present all the individual inborn errors of metabolism within one chapter. The disorders chosen to be considered in more detail are the most common, or illustrate important principles in the diagnosis or management of metabolic disease. Individuals wishing to study specific conditions not discussed in the text should obtain adequate information from the reference works listed at the end of the chapter.

PHENYLKETONURIA

The most common amino acid disorder in Caucasians is classic phenylketonuria (PKU) (Fig. 15.2). This disorder is due to a deficiency of the enzyme phenylalanine hydroxylase and, as mentioned earlier, is the prototype metabolic disorder for mass screening. Plasma phenylalanine levels are consistently greater than 1200 µmol/l (normal 60–90 µmol/l) and plasma tyrosine tends to be low.

Clinical features

When untreated, the disorder leads to severe mental handicap, with an IQ score of less than

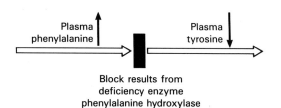

Fig. 15.2 Phenylketonuria: diagram of metabolic block.

50 in most patients. In addition, hair and eye pigmentation is unusually pale and the skin is prone to eczema.

The cause of the brain damage in PKU is not known with certainty, but the metabolic defect appears to interfere with the normal production of myelin, as well as some of the neurotransmitters.

Complications

A complication of PKU occurs in adult phenyl-ketonuric women. High levels of phenylalanine damage the developing fetus, leading to a number of congenital abnormalities, including congenital heart disease, microcephaly and mental retardation. To avoid this it is vital that PKU women return to a strict low phenylalanine diet from before conception and maintain levels of plasma phenylalanine below 400 µmol/l throughout the pregnancy.

Variants

In addition to classic PKU, there are a number of variants. These are due to deficiencies of essential cofactors necessary for the normal action of phenylalanine hydroxylase. The deficiency of these pterin cofactors is again inherited as an auto-somal recessive trait. These disorders have been labelled 'malignant' PKU as mental deterioration is not prevented by a low phenylalanine diet alone. Neurotransmitter production is critically affected in such patients and supplementation is necessary to prevent progressive neurodegeneration.

Dietary management

The dietary treatment involves the use of a phenylalanine-free protein supplement, produced either as a casein hydrolysate or an amino acid mixture, to provide the bulk of the child's protein intake. As phenylalanine is an essential amino acid, a steady intake from the diet is necessary to provide the small amount required for normal growth and development. A measured amount of phenylalanine from natural food is therefore an essential part of the diet. In addition, adequate energy from carbohydrate and fat must be provided, as well as minerals and vitamins. The artificial nature of the diet and the taste of the phenylalanine-free protein supplement are not attractive to the normal palate. Compliance with the diet is assessed at clinic visits by the dietitian and confirmed by frequent measurement of plasma phenylalanine levels.

HOMOCYSTINURIA

The biochemical defect in homocystinuria results in a failure to metabolise the amino acid methionine to cystine, due to a deficiency of the enzyme cystathionine synthase. There is a build-up of methionine and homocystine in the blood of affected patients, as well as a deficiency of cystine (Fig. 15.3).

Clinical features

Homocysteine is believed to cause the damage in homocystinuric patients; it is known to interfere with cross-linkage in both collagen and elastic fibres, impairing their natural strength. The clinical features are similar to Marfan's syndrome, with the addition that the brain is involved, leading to mental retardation and seizures in many patients if left untreated. Affected individuals are tall, with arachnodactyly; dislocation of the eye lens occurs and patients are prone to osteoporosis, leading to kypho-scoliosis. Premature arteriovenous thrombosis, leading to coronary artery disease or pulmonary embolism, is the main cause of death in un-treated patients.

These complications can be avoided with early diagnosis and treatment.

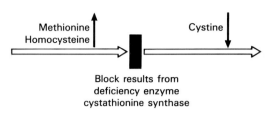

Fig. 15.3 Homocystinuria: diagram of metabolic block.

Variants

The incidence of the disorder is approximately 1 in 90 000 (Unpublished observations. Manchester, UK) and two types of patients have been described. In one group the patients improve considerably if given large doses of the vitamin pyridoxine (vitamin B6), an essential cofactor for cystathionine synthase, and these patients, termed pyridoxine-responsive, do not require any dietary treatment. Other patients are unresponsive to pyridoxine and have to be treated with a low methionine diet.

Dietary management

The principle of the low methionine diet is essentially the same as that for phenylketonuria. A small amount of methionine is essential for normal growth, the aim of treatment being to remove homocysteine from the plasma and restore cystine levels to normal. Even if the diagnosis is established after the onset of complications, there is evidence to suggest that dietary treatment at a late stage will prevent further ocular deterioration.

In all cases the diet must be strictly adhered to for life.

ORGANIC ACID DISORDERS

Organic acids are low molecular weight, water soluble, carboxylic acid metabolites of amino acids, carbohydrates or fats. A defect in the metabolic pathways involved in their catabolism leads to an accumulation in body tissues and fluids, especially urine, of these acidic compounds. Examples of this group of disorders includes methylmalonic, propionic and isovaleric acidaemias.

Clinical features

The clinical presentation of such disorders can be very variable. In the neonatal period the infant may present with apnoea and progressive neurological deterioration, leading to coma and often death. Biochemical investigation will usually show a marked metabolic acidosis, often associated with ketonuria. Infants who survive this acute neonatal presentation may present later with a similar episode of acidosis association with a minor illness, or with unexplained mental retardation or failure to thrive.

Dietary management

Some conditions respond to large doses of vitamins, but for the majority a low protein diet, together with calorie supplementation from carbohydrates, offers the only approach to therapy. Rather like very unstable diabetics, the patients require many admissions to hospital with exacerbations of ketosis and acidosis. The ultimate prognosis must be guarded.

UREA CYCLE DEFECTS

In humans the urea cycle is the main pathway of excretion of the waste nitrogen that is a product of protein metabolism. If a defect occurs within this cycle an accumulation of ammonia occurs which is highly toxic to the brain and nervous system.

Clinical features

As with organic acid defects, the clinical presentation can be very variable, but would usually include hypotonia, vomiting, seizures, coma and ultimately death. In mildly affected patients, clouding of consciousness and ataxia is common. One of the disorders of this group, ornithine carbamoyl transferase deficiency (OCT), is inherited as an X-linked disorder and the typical history obtained is of many male infants within the family dying within the first week of life. It is important to remember that some female carriers of this condition can be mildly affected and prone to attacks of hyperammonaemia if they consume a protein load.

Dietary management

An approach to treatment is to restrict protein intake to the amount necessary for growth alone. In an emergency, sodium benzoate can be administered to lower ammonia levels by converting them to the harmless compound hippuric acid, which can then be safely excreted in the urine. Despite treatment, the prognosis is poor for severely affected patients and many die, or survive with marked mental retardation.

GALACTOSAEMIA

Classic galactosaemia is due to a deficiency of the enzyme galactose-1-phosphate uridyl transferase. Affected individuals are unable to metabolise galactose, obtained from dairy products, to glucose. Galactose-1-phosphate accumulates within the cells and is extremely toxic.

Clinical features

The affected neonate becomes severely ill in the newborn period soon after the onset of milk feeds. A combination of jaundice, vomiting, lethargy, oedema and ascites occurs, and hepatomegaly and cataracts may be found on examination. The infant is prone to septicaemic illness and, if the diagnosis is not established, death from hepatic failure in the early weeks of life is common. If the infant survives the severe neonatal illness untreated, mental development is considerably affected.

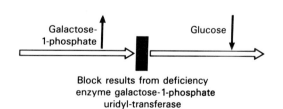

Block results from deficiency enzyme galactose-1-phosphate uridyl-transferase

Fig. 15.4 Galactosaemia: diagram of metabolic block.

Dietary management

Treatment is to remove all galactose from the diet. In older children it should be remembered that lactose is often used as in inert filling in many drugs and proprietary medicines. Despite early treatment, the ultimate results in terms of intellectual function are disappointing and many patients have IQ scores of 60–80. In addition, female patients develop hypergonadotrophic hypogonadism due to fibrous transformation within the ovaries.

Complications

Galactokinase deficiency galactosaemia rarely presents in childhood. Most affected individuals present to ophthalmic surgeons in adult life with cataracts. All patients with presenile cataracts should be investigated to exclude disorders of galactose metabolism.

A very rare type of galactosaemia due to a deficiency of the epimerase enzyme presents in an identical way to classic galactosaemia.

Again, life-long therapy is necessary for all the types of galactosaemia if complications are to be avoided.

GLYCOGEN STORAGE DISEASE

In glycogen storage disease (GSD) (Table 15.2) the inherited enzyme deficiencies lead to a disruption in the fine control of both glycogen synthesis and metabolism. It is most convenient to consider this group of diseases on the basis of which major organ is most affected by the abnormal storage of glycogen.

Liver. Types I, III, VI and IX

Children in whom the glycogen is stored mainly in the liver present with liver enlargement and fasting hypoglycaemia. Type I (von Gierke's disease) is the most severe and type IX is a mild, often asymptomatic disorder. Types III and VI are of intermediate severity. Although other metabolic problems can result from the defect in glycogen breakdown, e.g. hyperlipidaemia and lactic acidosis, it is the hypoglycaemia which is the danger to life for the severely affected

Table 15.2   The glycogen storage diseases

Type	Eponym	Enzyme deficiency	Major organ	Clinical
Ia	Von Gierke's	Glucose-6-phosphatase	Liver	Severe hypoglycaemia
Ib		Glucose-6-phosphatase-translocase	Liver	Hepatomegaly as Ia
II	Pompe's	Acid-α glucosidase	All	Lysosomal storage of glycogen cardiac failure
III	Cori's	Amylo-1-6-glucosidase (Debrancher enzyme)	Liver (muscle)	I but milder
IV	Andersen's	Amylo-1,4–1,6 transglucosidase	Liver	Cirrhosis fatal
V	McArdle's	Muscle phosphorylase	Muscle	Muscle cramps and fatigue
VI	—	Liver phosphorylase	Liver	As I but mild
VII	—	Phosphofructokinase	Muscle	As V
VIII	—	Not defined	Brain	Neurodegeneration
IXa		Liver phosphorylase kinase	Liver	As I but very mild recessive
IXb		Liver phosphorylase kinase	Liver	As I but very mild recessive

patient. Hypoglycaemic convulsions can lead to cerebral damage if the cause is not recognised and treated.

Clues to the diagnosis can be obtained by observing the response of the affected child to oral glucose or to an intramuscular injection of glucagon. The final diagnosis, however, rests on specific enzyme assay.

By providing a constant supply of glucose over a 24-hour period, either by frequent drinks or continuous nasogastric infusion of a high carbohydrate-containing solution, a considerable improvement in both clinical features and biochemical findings results. There is a tendency for the disorders to improve spontaneously during adolescence, but a number of affected adults with GSD I will still be at risk from serious complications of the disease, such as gout and hepatic adenomata.

Muscle. Types V and VII

Patients with muscle GSD have a disorder limited to skeletal muscle. Diagnosis is most often made in adult life, although many patients have a long history extending back into childhood of 'cramps' and muscle weakness on exertion. Myoglobinuria and muscle necrosis after exercise occurs in 50% of patients at some time during life.

Diagnosis is suggested by the characteristic muscle histology and established by enzyme assay on the muscle biopsy specimen. A number of patients have reported improvement in exercise tolerance when treated with a high protein diet.

Generalised Type II (Pompe's disease)

This type of GSD differs from the other members of the group as the glycogen is stored within lysosomes, due to a deficiency of a specific lysosomal hydrolase, acid glucosidase.

Affected infants present with hypotonia, hepatomegaly (liver enlargement) and progressive cardiac failure. No biochemical abnormalities such as hypoglycaemia are found on routine testing. The disorder is untreatable and usually fatal before the age of 2 years. At post-mortem there is massive infiltration with glycogen throughout the body.

WILSON'S DISEASE

Wilson's disease is an example of an inborn error of trace metal metabolism. Affected individuals develop copper toxicity due to an excessive accumulation of the metal within the body. The basic defect, which is inherited as an autosomal recessive, is not clearly defined. Affected patients are unable to excrete copper into the biliary tree and in addition have very low levels of the copper-related protein caeruloplasmin. Plasma-free copper and urinary copper levels are high in most patients.

Clinical features

The copper accumulation damages many organs, but has its most profound effects on the liver and brain. The clinical presentation may be very variable, but a combination of cirrhosis and neurological degeneration, e.g. falling school performance, ataxia, dysarthria, athetosis and spasticity, should immediately lead to copper studies. In some patients the liver disease may be fulminant, with hepatic necrosis and liver failure occurring rapidly, and in others a haemolytic crisis may be the first manifestation of the disease.

The diagnostic clinical sign, the Kayser-Fleischer ring, is a brown–green discoloration of the iris due to a deposition of copper in Descemet's membrane and is present in all patients with neurological involvement, but may be absent in those patients with predominantly liver disease.

Management

Treatment is life-long and involves trying to increase the excretion of copper from the body. D-penicillamine has been used for many years as a copper chelator, but side-effects such as skin rashes, blood abnormalities and impairment of renal function occur in 30% of patients and may be severe. Other possible treatments include other chelators as well as oral zinc.

MUCOPOLYSACCHARIDOSES

The mucopolysaccharidoses (MPS) (Table 15.3) provide a good example of the range of clinical problems that can result from a deficiency of lysosomal enzymes. In this heterogeneous group of disorders there is accumulation of mucopolysaccharide or glycosaminoglycan (GAGs) within the cell, interfering with normal cellular function. In addition, excessive excretion of partially degraded GAGs can be detected in the urine of affected patients.

Table 15.3 The mucopolysaccharidoses

Name	Eponym	Enzyme deficiency	Accumulated GAG		Comment
IH	Hurler	α-L-iduronidase	DS	HS	Severe phenotype
IS	Scheie	α-L-iduronidase	DS	HS	Previously type V
II	Hunter	Iduronate sulphate sulphatase	DS	HS	Clear cornea X-linked
III	Sanfilippo				
	A	Heparan N-sulphamidase	HS		Dementia
	B	α-D-N-acetyl-glucosaminidase	HS		May be very mild
	C	α-glucosamine-N-acetyltransferase	HS		
	D	α-N-acetyl-glucosamine-6-sulphate sulphatase	HS		
	Types A, B, C and D cannot be distinguished clinically				
IV	Morquio				
	A	N-acetyl galactosamine-6-sulphate sulphatase	KS		Normal intelligence
	B	β-galactosidase	KS		
VI	Maroteaux–Lamy	N-acetylgalactosamine 4-sulphate sulphatase	DS		Normal intelligence
VII	Sly	β-glucuronidase	DS	HS	
VIII		N-acetylglucosamine-6-sulphatase	KS	HS	Features of IV but also mental retardation

GAG, glucosaminoglycans; DS, dermatan sulphate; HS, heparan sulphate; KS, keratan sulphate.

Clinical features

As GAGs are the major component of the ground substance of connective tissue, a wide range of clinical effects can result from the different enzyme deficiencies.

All affected children are normal at birth and usually come to medical attention in one of three ways:

An unusual appearance MPS types I, II and VII

The full spectrum of the disorder is seen in MPS I (Hurler's syndrome). Affected children are short with a lumbar kyphosis, there is corneal clouding, severe joint stiffness, hepato-splenomegaly and cardiac murmurs. A persistent rhinorrhoea is one of the less attractive features of the disease. Umbilical and inguinal herniae are common and often recur after surgical repair. Most children die before the age of 10 years from a combination of cardiac and neurological deterioration. MPS II (Hunter's syndrome) shares many of these features with two important exceptions: inheritance is X-linked and corneal clouding is not a feature.

Dementia and behavioural disturbance MPS Type III

Dysmorphic features are not prominent in MPS III and, as a result, diagnosis is often considerably delayed. The clinical picture is one of severe behaviour problems, with a progressive dementia. Intense hyperactivity is common, but with age the child slows down and progressively loses skills, before dying in a vegetative state in the late teens.

There is no clinical difference between the four biochemical subtypes of MPS III.

Severe bone dysplasia MPS Types IV and VI

The majority of patients with this type of MPS disorder do not develop mental deterioration. A severe, progressive bone dysplasia dominates the clinical picture. Extraskeletal manifestations such as corneal clouding, deafness and cardiac lesions may also develop. Growth is severely restricted and patients are at particular risk from sudden atlanto-axial subluxation due to odontoid hypoplasia. Most patients survive into their thirties or forties if cervical myelopathy is avoided or treated by cervical fusion.

In all the MPS disorders, the diagnosis is suggested by the pattern of urinary GAG excretion and confirmed by specific enzyme assay on white blood cells. Prenatal diagnosis is also available for all of these conditions.

Management

Treatment by enzyme replacement using a bone marrow transplant from a compatible, unaffected donor has become increasingly popular. There is some evidence to suggest that there is a critical age before which transplant has to be performed if the neurodegenerative complications of the disorders are to be prevented. Transplant after the onset of neurological deterioration may improve the extraneurological manifestations of the disorder, but is unlikely to lead to an improvement in IQ score. This approach is also applicable in other neurometabolic disorders.

TAY–SACHS' DISEASE

Tay–Sachs' disease is a lysosomal storage disease due to a deficiency of the enzyme B-hexosaminidase. As a result of the metabolic block there is an accumulation within the cells of the nervous system of GM2 ganglioside, an essential cerebral sphingolipid. The condition occurs with an exceedingly high frequency in the Ashkenazi Jewish population, the carrier frequency in this group being 1 in 30, some 10% of the normal population. Many Jewish communities have established carrier screening programmes aimed at detecting couples who may be at risk of producing an affected child.

Clinical features

Clinically affected infants are hypotonic and have an exaggerated startle response to sound. Developmental delay becomes increasingly obvious and progressive mental deterioration from the end of the first year of life results in a state of decerebrate rigidity, and finally death at the age of 2–3 years. On examination of the fundus, the characteristic 'cherry-red spot', due to macular degeneration, may be seen. Unlike MPS disorders, there is no enlargement of the liver and spleen.

Management

Unfortunately for infants affected with Tay–Sachs' disease, there is no effective treatment. Medical efforts must be aimed at helping the family cope with the stresses involved in dealing with a child who has a progressive neurodegenerative disease.

FURTHER READING

Burman D, Holton J B, Pennock, C A (eds) 1980 Inherited disorders of carbohydrate metabolism. MTP Press, Lancaster
Holton J B (ed) 1987 The inherited metabolic diseases. Churchill Livingstone, Edinburgh
Scriver C R, Beandet A L, Sly W S, Valie D (eds) 1989 The metabolic basis of inherited disease, 6th edn. McGraw-Hill, New York
Watts R W E, Gibbs D A 1986 Lysosomal storage diseases: biochemical and clinical aspects. Taylor and Francis, London

16

Learning and behavioural problems

P. Eckersley   S. Steel

INTRODUCTION

As the child develops he gradually achieves increasing control over his environment. Each new situation he encounters will demand responses which are new, or which build on previous responses and which will require choices to be made. There is inevitably a range of fears and worries found in all children, particularly in response to strange or stressful situations (Burns 1986). Behavioural problems may result where the child is not able to make effective choices and does not interpret the environment in an appropriate way. These behaviours will not only affect his access to learning, but will have considerable implications for the physiotherapist when working on movement skills.

In this chapter the behavioural problems of hyperactivity, autism and challenging behaviours will be outlined. Educational delay and the problems of the clumsy child will also be discussed. The frustration of the child who is having difficulties with learning and with motor and perceptual tasks may well result in compensatory behaviour problems.

BEHAVIOURAL BARRIERS TO LEARNING
S. Steel

HYPERACTIVITY

What is hyperactivity?

There is a consensus of opinion amongst researchers that it is extremely difficult to diagnose hyperactivity. This is partly due to the fact that there are so many individual differences between children who may be hyperactive and they are likely to display only some of the behaviours classified under the umbrella of hyperactivity. In general, however, hyperactivity can be divided into three areas:

1. General over-activity or restlessness, where the child cannot sit still for a moment and may run about without purpose.
2. Problems in maintaining attention to a task or activity because the child lacks concentration and is easily distracted.
3. Impulsive behaviour, when the child may interrupt other children's activities or be unable to wait his turn.

That is not to say that many other children do not display these kinds of behaviour, but the significant feature of a child who is hyperactive is that the behaviour is aimless, excessive or persistent. Again, this description causes problems with diagnosis, for how persistent or excessive must a behaviour be before it is considered abnormal? Also, the tolerance levels of different adults is bound to affect their perceptions of what is hyperactive behaviour. Finally, it is important to note, as Barkley & Ullman (1975) indicated, that children who are hyperactive are not more bodily active than non-hyperactive children; the significant feature is their difficulty in controlling this activity.

Why are children hyperactive?

A large number and variety of causes have been put forward to suggest why some children are hyperactive. A major theory is that the child has suffered brain damage of some kind, though Prior & Griffin (1985) suggest that there is inadequate evidence to support this. More recently, it has been suggested that these children may be allergic to certain foods and food additives and that their behaviour is a reaction to ingestion of these substances. Prior & Griffin (1985) argued that there is little scientific evidence to support this claim, but it does appear that allergies may account for the behaviour of a small number of very young hyperactive children. It could also be argued that the current Western world pre-occupation with health and diet has enhanced the theory that diet influences behaviour. Some studies have shown increased activity in children suffering from lead poisoning, i.e. lead intake from substances containing lead in the environment. However, the extent of this research is limited. Therefore, the answer to the question 'Why are children hyperactive?' must be that no-one really knows.

The most logical current conclusion is that hyperactivity arises from a number of different factors: biological, environmental and social. A child in an optimum environment may not develop problems, whereas a vulnerable child in a deprived and/or chaotic environment may be at far greater risk.

What are the educational implications?

Many children who are hyperactive under-achieve in their learning. This is not surprising if they are unable to focus their attention on the task or activity they have been set. From a very early stage they will not benefit from play experiences if they do not stay at an activity long enough to explore its possibilities. A room set out with a multitude of activities can worsen the child's behaviour because he cannot cope with the number of options available and consequently may run around the room without purpose.

Hyperactive children can have emotional problems. They frequently display swings in mood and this, coupled with a predilection to disrupt activities, can lead to poor levels of acceptance by peers and consequently a lack of friends, even at nursery age.

Various strategies can, however, be used to

improve the child's hyperactive behaviour and learning, and these are discussed in the next section.

Strategies for dealing with hyperactive children

Medication

In the past children considered hyperactive have been diagnosed and treated within a medical model. The most likely treatment has therefore been the use of drugs, such as amphetamines, to control hyperactivity.

Diet

As mentioned previously, some attention has been focused on a change of diet as a treatment method, although there is little evidence to support this. This method prohibits any food which contains artificial flavourings and colourings. Prior & Griffin (1985) argued that a change in diet would lead to a strong expectation of a change in the child's behaviour by the family, and the child could respond accordingly. Similarly, if the diet broke down the expectation would be that the behaviour would deteriorate, and again the child could live up to this expectation.

Play activity

The use of play activity has been shown to be an effective treatment method for children who are hyperactive (Chazan et al 1983). This approach means that staff do not simply suggest an activity to the child but actively take part. During a short play session the child has the exclusive attention of an adult who praises every sign of co-operation and attention, however fleeting. Initially, a very, short period of concentration is demanded of the child. Over a period of weeks the demands are gradually increased. All distractions in the room should be reduced, with a limited choice of activity starting with one toy or activity with big results, for example, a jack-in-the-box. Gradually, the choice of activities can be increased with the understanding by the child that the activity or toy chosen must be adhered to.

Behaviour modification

This strategy for dealing with hyperactive children is based on the belief that all behaviour is learned and thus can be changed. The key to this approach is initial observation of the child, assessment and analysis of the hyperactive behaviour, the setting of a target behaviour, intervention, monitoring and recording of the behaviour and finally a re-assessment and change of intervention if necessary. Once the unacceptable hyperactive behaviours have been assessed, they can be listed in order of priority and one selected to work on. For example, it may be decided that the child will sit in his seat and complete a simple activity for 30 seconds as he is currently running aimlessly around the classroom. This child would be made to sit in a firm but gentle way with minimal attention and, on completion of the task, he would be rewarded with lots of praise and attention and allowed to run about. Gradually, the number of activities and amount of time of sitting can be increased. The behaviour is monitored and recorded and consequently an objective statement of any change in behaviour can be made. Behaviour modification must be humanely and thoughtfully used, and although many of the procedures are common sense they need to be applied in a systematic, structured and consistent way.

The advantage of both the play and behavioural approaches is that they are concerned with changing and learning new behaviours, as opposed to the medical approach of diagnosing and treating the condition.

AUTISM

What is autism?

Autism is derived from the Greek work 'autos', meaning self, and implies self-centred thinking. The term is also applied to a group of children who show extreme withdrawal, have an almost total unwillingness to communicate, and exhibit strange mannerisms before the age of 2.5 years. These children are referred to as autistic. A wide range of behaviour is often labelled as autistic but can broadly be divided into three main features (Kanner 1944):

1. A failure to develop social relationships, with strong aversive reactions to close contact with adults. As babies, these children may fail to smile socially or play social games and avoid eye contact.

2. Language impairment, usually resulting in a complete lack of speech. When speech does develop it tends to be stereotyped and full of echoed phrases.

3. Ritualistic and stereotypic behaviour such as hand flapping or obsessional attachment to an object, and insistence on a fixed routine with resistance to any change in that routine. Some perceptual experiences are ignored, for example, sights and sounds and even heat and pain, whereas others seem to become hypnotic, such as music and regular beats.

Why are children autistic?

Many views as to the cause of autism have been suggested, and some are mentioned here, but there does not appear to be any general consensus. It would seem likely that the most appropriate view is an interactional one.

It has been suggested that cold, detached and obsessional parents can lead to autism in the child, but this is not confirmed by research (Rutter 1975). Many children have suffered severe parental deprivation and have not become autistic, and if a child is diagnosed autistic, parents are only studied afterwards. They are already suffering the stresses of having a child with a handicap and the supposed differences in parents of autistic children may well be the effect of the autism as opposed to the cause.

Evidence to support brain damage as a cause of autism is not convincing, but one of the more recent theories, reported by Child (1973), is that autism is caused by a disability in interpreting sensory experiences, particularly seeing and hearing. Symbol interpretation is particularly difficult and because autistic children lack the ability to symbolise they have great difficulty in acquiring language.

What are the educational implications?

Autistic children have severe language deficits. Approximately 50% never develop intelligible speech and the other 50% have severe difficulties. Reversal of personal pronouns, for example, 'you' instead of 'I', repetitive speech and muddled word order are all extremely common. Speech is often not used to communicate but merely as a response to a stimulus. Educational achievement is often low because of these severe language difficulties, but some children do have islands of skills, for example, in music or mathematics, and some have phenomenal memories.

The Disabled Persons Act 1970 required local education authorities to provide for the education of autistic children in maintained or assisted schools as far as was practically possible. Although this provision included special schools, it was clearly intended that provision should be made in ordinary schools. However, research into understanding the complex educational needs of autistic children is still at an early stage and, because autism is a disorder in which the fundamental disabilities are in the development of language and personal relationships, there is no consensus amongst researchers as to how important it is for these children to be educated separately. Nevertheless, they have established the importance of appropriate teaching methods and the necessity for ancillary staff to provide support for teachers dealing with autistic children (Department of Education and Science 1978).

Teaching children with autism is a highly specialised field. Currently the number of specialised schools or units is fairly limited, and some of the best schools in the country are run by voluntary bodies. Public awareness of autism is due largely to the efforts of these voluntary organisations, who continue to attempt to secure a better public understanding of these children with such complex difficulties.

Strategies for dealing with autistic children

There are two main schools of thought as to the most appropriate form of treatment model for autistic children; the psychodynamic model and the behavioural model.

The psychodynamic model

The psychodynamic model focuses on factors within the child, such as neurological damage, self-image and body image, and the need for security. It seeks to effect change in behaviour by dealing directly with these factors, rather than targeting the specific behavioural problems themselves. This model is non-directive and developmental change is sought through experiential learning and play. Establishing good personal and social relationships within an unstructured environment is seen as the catalyst for change. However, a recent study of an autistic child under this treatment model (Randall & Gibb 1987) indicated that this approach can lead to inappropriate management. The child's tantrums were responded to by giving immediate and pleasant adult contact in an attempt to improve social relationships with adults, and eventually the parents concerned asked for the child to be moved to a different kind of regime.

The behavioural model

This model advocates a structured and problem-centred approach to the management of autistic children. It requires consistent management between home and school so a 24 h management regime can be set up. This approach focuses on observable behaviour, which can be identified and prioritised, and change effected by the setting of target objectives. Each objective then has a teaching programme to be used both at home and at school.

CASE STUDY

Research by Randall & Gibb (1987) used this behavioural approach with a 3-year-old child who presented with autistic behaviour. A teaching programme was set up to deal with her obsessional behaviour, which appeared to be stimulated by any toy with a circular motion. These toys were removed and her obsessional attachment to any other object was dealt with by removing that object. This would result in a tantrum. Management of these tantrums involved totally ignoring her up to the point where she engaged in physical contact with the managing adult. This adult would then remove her from the room and leave her alone until she was quiet. Both home and school followed the same procedure and the frequency and duration of the tantrums was recorded. Results indicated a significant decrease in the problem behaviours and an increase in her spoken language. Additional benefits were a continuity of management between home and school and generalising of learnt behaviour and the development of strategies for the parents to learn to manage their daughter's autism as opposed to curing it.

CHALLENGING BEHAVIOURS
What are challenging behaviours?

Challenging behaviours are difficult to define although they can be arbitrarily divided into three categories.

Self-injurious behaviour

This is often stereotyped and habitual. It can include such actions as head-banging, skin-scratching, eye-gouging and biting.

Nuisance behaviours

The child may indulge in prolonged screaming, temper tantrums, stripping or running away.

Aggression towards others

Aggressive behaviour will include kicking, biting, pulling, pushing and scratching.

Why do children present challenging behaviours?

There appear to be two main theories as to the cause of challenging behaviours:

1. That the behaviour is essentially organic in origin.
2. That it is a form of learnt behaviour under

the control of environmental or social stimuli.

Organic theorists offer in support of their argument the occurrence of challenging behaviours in children with Lesch–Nyhan syndrome and De Lange syndrome. Lesch–Nyhan syndrome is a genetic disorder and invariably children who have this engage in self-injurious behaviour at some time in their lives. Children with De Lange syndrome display both aggressive and self-injurious behaviour. Recent studies have suggested that endorphins, possibly play a role in challenging behaviours. These are opiates which occur naturally within the body and have sleep-inducing properties. Cataldo & Harris (1982) indicated that self-injurious behaviour may produce chronic raised endorphins, which contribute to the continuation of the behaviour because of reduced awareness of pain. As endorphins have addictive properties, children could self-administer them by engaging in self-injurious behaviour, which could then become habitual.

The most influential theories about challenging behaviours are those that view them as learnt behaviours. The evidence in favour of this view is overwhelming. One of the first demonstrations of the control exercised by the social environment was by Lovaas & Simmons (1969). They showed that when challenging behaviour was displayed by three children with stereotyped habitual behaviour and followed by comfort, both physical and verbal, the behaviour increased. When the behaviour was ignored it eventually disappeared. Lovaas & Simmons (1969) drew the conclusion that for these children the challenging behaviour had been reinforced by adult attention.

One of the difficulties in deciding on causes of challenging behaviours is that in any one child several factors may be involved in the origin and maintenance of the problem behaviour. For example, the behaviour could originate as an accidental occurrence and then be maintained by adult attention. Other factors, such as endorphins, could also contribute to its maintenance. The idea of a single cause of challenging behaviours is now outdated.

What are the educational implications?

Enormous energy and commitment is needed from staff to manage children who display these most distressing of behaviour problems. If the child is difficult at school, more often than not he is difficult at home as well and consequently many of these children are in residential placements. The current trend towards policies for the integration of all children with special needs into mainstream schools is causing great concern about this group of children amongst professionals. The implications of such a policy might be the creation of special units attached to mainstream schools, with children integrated in some way, and care in the community. It has been suggested that these children are the result of a failure on the part of various services because they have been badly managed in school or hostel settings, and that if the services could rise to the 'challenge' the child's problems could be dramatically reduced.

Strategies for dealing with challenging behaviours

There appear to be three main strategies for the management of challenging behaviours:

- protective devices
- medication
- behavioural treatments.

Currently, the use of protective devices is being more carefully examined, the use of medication increasingly questioned and behavioural methods have begun to investigate the function of the behaviour and to link this to programme design, rather than simply applying a set of standard procedures.

Protective devices

Faced with a child displaying challenging behaviour, most people are likely to consider the use of protective devices first, particularly if the behaviour is increasing. Often this is a necessary first step in management as the child might cause severe and permanent damage to himself or to others. Devices may be simple so that hand movements are restricted, or more sophisticated, such as arm splints or helmets. How protective devices are used has a strong influence on changes in levels of challenging behaviour. If the restraint becomes reinforcing then the behaviour may worsen, if it is aversive it may be effective in reducing the behaviour. Murphy (1985) suggested that protective devices should be viewed as an interim measure to be combined with other forms of treatment.

Medication

Despite widespread use of drugs to control challenging behaviours, particularly self-injurious ones, the benefits appear to be limited. A recent project in America, reported by Murphy (1985), demonstrated that it was possible to withdraw drugs completely from 75% of self-injurers over a 3 year period. Of these, 80% showed improvements or no change in behaviour, while the remainder were treatable by behavioural methods.

Behavioural treatments

Behavioural treatments are based on the belief that as all behaviour is learnt, it is also possible to unlearn inappropriate behaviour. In order for behavioural treatments to work it is important to first analyse the function of the challenging behaviour by systematically observing the child. Does the behaviour increase when the child is in the company of others, rather than alone, and when the behaviour is attended to? Does it occur primarily when demands are made? Does it occur when no activities are available and the environment is bare? Answers to these questions can help determine the motivation of the challenging behaviour. By looking at what happened before (antecedent) the behaviour occurred and what happened afterwards (consequence), it is then possible to devise a programme based on modifying the antecedent or the consequence. This is a particularly useful form of treatment as the emphasis is on practice rather than theory, and the programme can then be implemented by all professionals working with the child.

Intervention programmes

Once the function of the challenging behaviour has been identified, various behavioural strategies can be used when devising the intervention programme. Two approaches are considered here:

Positive reinforcement

The use of positive reinforcement is based on the assumption that the consequence of the challenging behaviour, although reinforcing, particularly if it is stereotyped or habit behaviour, is less reinforcing than some alternative stimulus available in the environment. For example, the function of the challenging behaviour in the child who rocks and chews his hand may be self-stimulatory, and it may have been established that vibration was a positively reinforcing sensory alternative. In this case the child could be provided with a toy that vibrated in an attempt to decrease the problem behaviours. However, it has been shown that using such techniques does not result in the problem behaviour disappearing permanently, and it is important that the appropriate environmental conditions are maintained.

Overcorrection

Overcorrection is a procedure which prevents the child physically from engaging in the challenging behaviour, particularly if it is aggressive, whilst at the same time encouraging more acceptable forms of behaviour through the use of graduated guidance. For example, a child might be hitting himself or others, so the arms will be restrained and then put to some positive purpose, such as playing with a toy that can be knocked or hit. However, the use of graduated guidance may require considerable force on the part of the adult in order to ensure that the child cooperates in functional movement. Overcorrection is considered ethically more acceptable than physical punishment and is believed to be more effective. The use of punishment techniques is now seen as a last resort by those dealing with children displaying unacceptable behaviour. Nevertheless, it is essential that the schedule should be clearly defined and applied consistently so that it is not used in a vindicative or arbitrary fashion. It is also important to point out that any overcorrection technique should be coupled with strong rewards for appropriate behaviour.

EDUCATIONAL DELAY

What is educational delay?

The labelling and categorisation of children was officially dropped after the implementation of the 1981 Education Act in April 1983, and all children with any kind of difficulty have since been considered to have special needs (see Chapter 25 Legal Aspects in Paediatric Physiotherapy). The debate over this continues. Ideologically it is preferable not to have sublabels for all children are different and do not necessarily fit into a discrete category. Naming a difficulty can set into motion a vast set of generalisations, biases, misconceptions and expectations that are unrelated to a child's individuality. On the other hand, saying a child has special needs does not necessarily tell you anything about that child and causes difficulties with communication between professionals when every child is simply known as a child with special needs.

However, certain categories of handicap have been retained to serve as descriptors for children's difficulties. The term 'educational delay' is used as a descriptor for children who are experiencing learning difficulties of one kind or another. Currently, professionals tend to think in terms of a range of learning difficulties from mild to moderate to severe.

Why are children delayed educationally?

Children with mild learning difficulties tend to be those children in mainstream schools who have difficulty mastering complex ideas and need clear and precise explanations and guidance. Often their lack of progress can also be affected by minor physical or sensory difficulties.

Children with moderate learning difficulties are by far the largest group of children with special needs. Although a large proportion of these chil-

dren are in mainstream schools, they also form the largest group of children in special schools. The majority of children with moderate learning difficulties come from impoverished or adverse social or educational backgrounds. This social disadvantage is often characterised by language deprivation, low parental aspirations, low parental achievement and a lack of stimulation at home. Medical factors can also be involved, such as physical or sensory disabilities, specific learning difficulties or a limited general ability in the child.

Children with severe learning difficulties are commonly referred to as mentally handicapped and there is invariably some overt evidence of abnormal brain functioning in these children. This may be due to:

1. Genetic abnormalities, for example, children with chromosomal anomalies such as Down's syndrome.
2. An adverse prenatal environment, such as rhesus incompatibility or physical damage to the fetus as a result of a fall or blow.
3. Problems during birth or adverse postnatal conditions, including meningitis.
4. Accidental brain damage, for example, in a road accident.
5. Non-accidental brain damage to battered babies.

Currently there are several factors which should contribute to a decline in the number of children educationally delayed. These include:

- improved medical care of diseases such as meningitis
- increased public awareness of harmful pre-, peri- and postnatal factors, for example, smoking, drinking and taking drugs during pregnancy
- improved nutrition of pregnant women and children
- better screening techniques
- better genetic counselling services.

What are the educational implications?

Children who are delayed educationally need to have special educational provision made for them. With the current trend towards integration it becomes more and more likely that different forms of provision will, and should, be made available to them in mainstream schools. The Warnock Report (1978), which inquired into the education of children with special needs, suggested that schools would need to make available three different types of special educational provision and that any one child might need more than one of these forms of provision. Namely:

1. A special means of access to the curriculum, which for children who are educationally delayed is likely to mean specialist teaching techniques.
2. The provision of a special or modified curriculum to help them to overcome their learning difficulties.
3. An environment in which particular attention has been paid to the social structure and emotional climate in which education takes place, which might necessitate small teaching groups or a small school.

Strategies to overcome educational delay

Professionals who work with children who are educationally delayed have a natural desire to know why a particular child is having learning difficulties. Speculation may include such things as the difficult birth, the struggle by a mother to raise the child on her own and the possibility of some brain damage. Although these factors should be taken into consideration, current trends suggest that there is a need to look at the whole child in social context. The search for a cause inevitably includes speculation about factors outside the professional's control. Ainscow & Tweddle (1979) argued that this suggests an implicit assumption that a knowledge of the cause will lead to a direct understanding of what to do about it, an approach which resembles the medical model of diagnosis and prescription. Factors such as brain damage or a deprived background will have a direct effect on a child's educational achievement, but intervention needs to focus on the teaching methods and classroom

organisation which are within the professional's control.

Curriculum-based assessment

One such approach to effectively help children who are educationally delayed starts with a curriculum-based assessment. This focuses on the child's performance in any area of the curriculum and failure to make progress is not ascribed to the child. If the child is not learning, he has not been taught the easier skills he should have mastered before moving on to the particular task he is having difficulty with. The child is assessed by a multiprofessional team so that a profile of exactly what he can and cannot do can be drawn up and strengths and weaknesses identified, and then an appropriate individual educational programme can be devised. The Warnock Report (1978) suggested a continuous cycle in which the processes of assessment and intervention are inextricably interwined (Fig. 16.1).

Individual learning programmes

The child's individual educational programme will thus specify a series of realistic short-term objectives and each teaching session is monitored and recorded so that progress can be measured objectively.

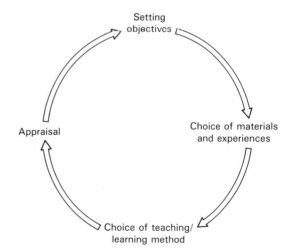

Fig. 16.1 Continuous cycle of assessment and intervention.

This approach to learning can be used with any child who is educationally delayed, whether his problems are mild, moderate or severe. The more difficulties a child has, the more detail will be required in his learning programme. Any objective set can be broken down into a number of smaller steps to make learning simpler, and obviously the extent to which the objective is broken down will depend on the extent of the learning difficulty. For example, a task such as hand washing may need to be split into a 20-step plan for a child with severe learning difficulties.

Individual learning programmes are discussed in greater detail in Chapter 19 Treatment Methods.

Experiential learning

Emphasis in the past few years has shifted away from a belief that children who are educationally delayed only learn on an individual basis. These children, particularly those with severe learning difficulties, are now being given the opportunity for experiential learning when they can bring their interests and experiences to a group or class situation and generalise specific skills they have already learnt. For example, a group of children with severe learning difficulties joining with a group of mainstream children for a physical education lesson can use the opportunity to generalise the self-help skills they have mastered. They can practise skills in dressing and undressing and washing, amongst other things.

This kind of teaching is the most difficult because it requires a high level of skill on the part of the teacher to select content which is appropriate for each child and the group as a whole, and then to involve all children equally. Nevertheless, working in a group or class allows the child to learn other things apart from the declared focus of the session, such as taking turns and how to attend.

Recent innovations in teaching children who are educationlly delayed have placed emphasis on the balance of the day between individual and other kinds of learning. They have made professionals look at the kind of programme they offer children and how effective they are as teachers in helping children to learn.

THE CLUMSY CHILD
P. Eckersley

The expression 'the clumsy child' instantly conveys a picture of a child who knocks things over, cannot catch a ball, walks into or trips over anything and everything, lets everything slip through his hands, forgets where he is meant to be or be doing, presents untidy and inaccurate work in school and is always the last to be chosen when classes are divided for team games. This is the child who frequently tries to mask his problems by becoming the classroom clown, by adopting a 'devil-may-care' leadership role or by opting out completely.

Within this picture it is important to understand that the child's problems are of an organic nature. They do not result from laziness, from lack of motivation or even from a lack of understanding of what is required. The 'clumsy' child is all too often fully aware of what he would hope to do but is aware from the start that all efforts will go awry or come to naught.

An understanding of the difficulties the child experiences from his own perspective, and in many cases an acceptance of those difficulties which do not lie in essential subjects and activities, is as important as efforts to remediate the problems.

Clumsy children show difficulties in motor co-ordination out of proportion to their general abilities (Gordon & McKinlay 1980). These difficulties frequently coexist with perceptual problems and, for a number of children, with some degree of learning difficulty.

GENERAL ASSESSMENT

A general assessment of children who experience perceptual–motor problems may reveal difficulties in a number of areas. It is necessary to identify in addition those specific problems which can be targeted for remediation.

Motor

Gross motor. Difficulties in hopping, jumping, riding a bicycle.

Fine motor. Problems with threading beads, holding a pencil, doing up buttons.

Manipulating objects. Using a knife and fork, hitting a tennis ball with a racquet, opening a door.

Balance and coordination. Standing on one leg, clapping rhythmically, moving in time to music.

Selective movement. Moving a part in isolation from the whole.

Imagination. Use of force, space and flow in movement.

Fitness. Endurance, strength and general health.

Perception

Auditory perception. Recognition of different sounds in both the environment and in language.

Visual perception. Recognition of shape and form, differentiation of foreground and background.

Sensory perception. Recognition of shape and texture by touch.

Kinaesthetic awareness. Understanding of the body's position in space and the relative position of body parts.

Spatial awareness. Understanding of the spatial relationships between objects.

Perceptual constancy. Understanding the constant shape of an object whatever the angle it is viewed from.

Learning

Sequencing. Sequencing the events which happen through the day or of a list of instructions or information.

Memory. Information remembered in context and usable from one situation to the next.

Concentration. Keeping to task, distractability.

Expressive language. Finding the correct words to describe a situation or event.

Planning. Knowing what to do next, understanding when and how, self-organisation, time-keeping.

THERAPY: A PROGRAMME OF ASSESSMENT AND INTERVENTION

The description of the therapy programme of assessment and intervention which follows is based on a six-point plan used by the author in clinical practice. Assessment and intervention are not described as separate processes, rather as interrelated elements which jointly underpin any therapy session. It is to be expected that on occasions during assessment a particular activity will prove extremely difficult, frustrating and, at times, upsetting for a child. This should be acknowledged and, bearing in mind that there is no advantage to be gained from 'practising it again', it can be helpful, and reassuring, to allow a child to exercise choice as to whether or not to work on a particular skill. Time spent discussing ways of circumventing or occasionally ignoring some difficulties can make a positive contribution to a child's self esteem and confidence. It can also form a basis for discussions with parents

The immediate aim of physical treatment is to give the child experiences which will, through sensations and movements, themselves improve motor response and skill, enhancing perceptions and thereby learning (Grimley 1980). The six elements described below are:

- understanding what is required
- an appropriate start
- an adequate performance
- memory understanding and repetition
- imagination and expression
- readiness.

Understanding what is required

Why am I here?

Children with perceptual–motor problems are usually referred for physiotherapy activities at an age when it is possible to discuss their difficulties, and their strengths, with them. Given time, and with a building of confidence, they are well able to give a picture of their own priorities for problem-solving. Remediation requires both practice on their part and cooperation. A notebook or diary for the child to keep may be helpful to record and reinforce progress. Parents and class teachers can also contribute to the overall picture, but any situation where the child is required to sit and listen to a catalogue of disasters must be avoided.

Am I ready?

If activities are to be done sitting at a table no equipment may be required but, if the session is to include gross motor activity then PE clothing or bare feet and shorts may be required. The child could be asked if he thinks any particular equipment is needed, or if any change of clothing would be appropriate. An interesting discussion may well result.

Spoken request

The child should be able to follow spoken instructions. These can range from a simple 'Put your arms up above your head' to 'Put the red brick on top of the green' to a complex 'Collect four red and two green bean bags from the cupboard on your left and go and lie on your back on the blue mat.' Each child will have a level at which the number of separate elements in an instruction make it incomprehensible. It is important to work up to, but not beyond, this level.

Visual request

This can be given in three ways:

Copy a person. The child is asked to copy body positions in a similar way to 'Simon says'. A progression in difficulty can be used for example:

- one plane patterns — both arms to the side
- two plane patterns — both arms in front
- asymmetrical patterns — one arm out, one leg bent (Fig. 16.2)
- repetition of patterns — as above, but with eyes closed (this requires the use both of memory and kinaesthetic sense).

When observing the child copying body move-

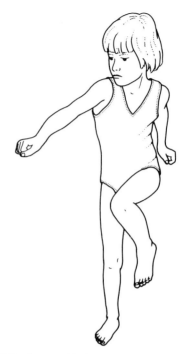

Fig. 16.2 Asymmetrical movement pattern in standing.

ments it is necessary to check whether he can move a part of the body without looking at it; some children can only put an arm out to the side if they turn their heads to that side and watch their hands. Where an asymmetrical posture has been requested the child may only be able to adopt that position by moving one arm or leg at a time. Many dyspraxic children rely on their vision to provide information that their proprioceptive knowledge cannot give (Burr 1984).

Copy a diagram or model. The child may be asked to copy a particular arrangement of bricks, a peg board pattern or the correct arrangement of knives and forks. The same hierarchy of difficulty should be followed, symmetrical patterns being easier than asymmetrical. Many children have difficulty with right/left and up/down orientation. Diagonals can be particularly problematic (Fig. 16.3).

Read instructions. It can be a progression in a treatment programme for a child to work independently through activities from a written, rather than a spoken, programme.

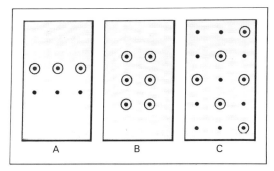

Fig. 16.3 A progression of simple to complex peg board patterns. (A) Simple, to (B) and (C) more complex.

Language used

Many of the words which are used to describe movement and pattern are difficult for the 'clumsy' child to understand. Care must be taken when analysing the extent to which a child has fully developed the concepts of:

- shape — round, square
- position — on top, at the side of
- direction — left, right, through, over
- Space — wide, narrow, tall, small
- quality — gently, slowly, smoothly.

Overload

It is essential to work in ways which consolidate skills, and introduce new ones by building progressively and gradually on existing ones. A child who can remember four components of an instruction may forget them all if given five. Being able to adopt an asymmetrical arm pattern by copying may be impossible with eyes closed.

An appropriate start

Occupying space

In order to start any activity there is an optimal place in space to occupy. The 'clumsy' child who is asked to lie on his back on the mat may lie with one half of his body on the mat and the other half on the floor. A child who has been asked to do wide and narrow jumps may stand so near a wall or furniture that the action is impossible. The same problems may be observed with drawing and writing when a child starts to draw a picture or to write a sentence either near to the right hand side of the page or at the bottom corner. The written work then 'falls off the page'.

Placing of equipment

When using equipment it is important that the relative distance between the child and the equipment to be used is appropriate for the task. Some children sit with their chairs a considerable distance from the table, with the trunk almost horizontal; others curl over their work. Activities such as pouring and building can be impossible if containers or bricks are too near or too distant. The clumsy child finds it very difficult to assess the appropriate starting distance or to understand why things have gone wrong. Discussion, reinforcement and guided analysis through trial and error should all be incorporated into the therapy programme.

Appropriate position to start in

Static or dynamic balance. Clumsy children exhibit two different types of difficulty. Some try to solve their balance problems by maintaining a stiff, rigid posture so that they can resist all forces which may disrupt that balance. Others 'give in' to any external forces and are either constantly on the move or cannot adopt and hold any static posture. A child who maintains static balance finds all running, jumping, throwing activities very difficult. The child who maintains dynamic balance finds standing on one leg or adopting a crawl position very difficult.

Movements which require a combination of the two types of position are particularly problematic. Writing requires a static shoulder girdle and a dynamic wrist and fingers. Kicking a football requires static balance in one leg and dynamic balance in the other (Fig. 16.4). It is important to build a progression of activity into the therapy programme, working on the type of balance the child finds easiest and progressing to more complex activity in positions of safety, i.e. supine lying and sitting.

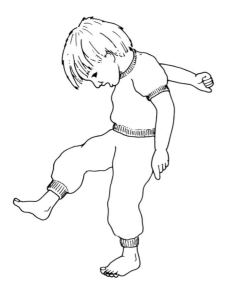

Fig. 16.4 Kicking a football: note the stable position of the left leg and the dynamic movement of the right.

Symmetry and asymmetry. When lying in preparation to perform a 'sit-up' the posture is symmetrical in a position where little balance is required. When preparing an overarm throw a complex asymmetrical posture in arms and legs is necessary with trunk and neck rotation and shifted balance. The symmetrical posture in lying can be readily understood as the easier to adopt. Similarly, high kneeling is less complex than half kneeling, wide leg standing than stride walking, and carrying a tray with a mug on it than carrying the mug in one hand.

Adequate performance

'Adequate' is an important concept. During therapy sessions the child who is clumsy is being asked to practise activities he finds difficult and perhaps frustrating. This frustration also occurs during many everyday activities, both at home and at school. In identifying the important aspects for a therapy programme, the objective should be an adequate, not a perfect, performance. If one is going to correct, it is best to correct only one fault at a time (Grimley 1980). The various elements of performance described below can be used both for assessment and for programme planning.

Coordination and balance

Direction and localisation. Problems can range from the child who has difficulties threading a bead, or posting a shape, to the child who always misjudges the space and the distance between himself and other objects or between the objects themselves. Practice in sorting shapes by feel can be helpful and should incorporate changes in size as well as shape. Sensory activities using texture can improve that body awareness which is a necessary basis for all movement. Obstacle courses can not only be fun but can also reinforce concepts such as up and down, under and over, round and through. Many school games require children to stand in lines or in circles to throw or pass things to each other. The clumsy child needs practice and discussion to work out when he is in line (Fig. 16.5) and how to position himself in a circle. Standing in line with legs wide to roll a football through to the person at the back who then runs to the front and starts again can pose many difficulties of direction and localisation. There may also be problems when remembering the sequence of the instructions.

Skills in sensory kinaesthetic localisation underpin many activities. Various assessments can be used to discover whether the child knows which part of his arm or hand has been touched when his eyes are closed, whether he can recognise a shape drawn on the palm of the hand or whether he can describe the position the arm or leg has been placed in. An awareness of unseen sensations and movements is a useful skill to develop.

Rhythm and timing. The clumsy child may not be able to clap in time to a rhythm or to move at an appropriate speed for the music he hears. When asked to repeat a movement, such as jumping, a number of times, he may become increasingly disorganised. The rhythm and flow of movement required for writing may present difficulties. It may be impossible for the child to synchronise the closing of the hands together with the arrival of a ball in order to catch it.

Flexibility and stability. Most activities require a combination of flexibility and stability between body parts. A stable shoulder girdle with

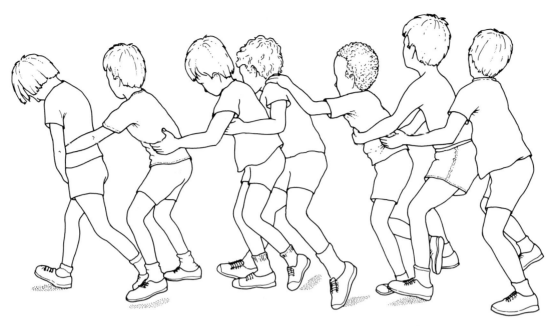

Fig. 16.5 A group of children find many ways to form a line.

flexible moving fingers is needed for writing. A door handle is grasped firmly but the wrist and elbow are flexible when a door is opened. Walking along an upturned bench requires good central stability, together with flexible arms and feet, in order to maintain balance. As movements become more complex, particularly in creative activities, practical tasks and in sport, these dynamics of changing body posture become increasingly important.

A smooth stop. The clumsy child needs an opportunity to practise the change from movement to stillness. Playing statues and games to music can be incorporated into therapy sessions, as can relaxation itself. The way in which a child stops moving naturally should be assessed during a range of activities:

1. Can he only stop running by falling down?
2. If asked to make windmills with the arms, does he stop by 'winding down'?
3. Is the child able to keep within the shape when colouring?
4. When opening and closing both hands to make a fist, can he stop one only in isolation?

A smooth stop is also needed to change the direction of movement:

- gross motor — run forwards, stop, run backwards
- fine motor — dot-to-dot patterns on paper.

The way in which an activity is finished and completed is as important as the way in which it begins.

Auditory and visual skills

Although only some clumsy children may have speech and language difficulties, auditory and visual skills should be assessed for all children referred for therapy. Games and activities for auditory and visual perception and for auditory and visual memory can add variety to the motor programme and provide an opportunity for interspersing more restful and active periods within the programme. Sound lotto, tapes of everyday sounds and clapping patterns can be used to develop auditory skills. Visual discrimination games can be found in many puzzle books and coloured bricks can be used to devise visual memory games.

Use of equipment

The child who has developed balance and co-ordination in movement will need to develop these skills so that equipment and objects can be manipulated. He can be helped to acquire a range of skills:

- fastening buttons and tying laces
- building and construction toys and games
- throwing, catching and kicking
- using scissors, knives and forks, unwrapping sweets
- tracing, drawing and painting
- carrying, pouring, sewing.

If children cannot perform these activities they will be unable to participate in age-related physical games. Those skills which confer peer group status are missing and, once again, self-confidence and esteem remain low (Russell 1988).

Memory and understanding

Movement activities are not isolated events. Most activities are built on those simple activities which form the foundation of complex ones. In order for any activity to be understood, generalised, adapted and remembered it must become part of the schema of the child.

A clumsy child may experience difficulties in a number of ways.

Repetition

Many clumsy children are unable to respond to the request 'Do it again'. This can occur with an activity they have only just completed or with a task which they did yesterday or last week. Motor memory is inadequate. It can, however, be developed by asking the child to repeat simple activities he does well and enjoys and has only just completed and then gradually progressing to the more complex and distant in time.

Description

Other children may be able to repeat a movement or point in a particular direction without being able to use description. They might say 'I did this' rather than 'I kicked the ball', or 'He went there' rather than 'He went into the kitchen'. Descriptive language may also be required when the child is asked to set out a sequence of events or to draw a picture of a place he knows well. The child who, for example, is well able to dress himself may describe pictures of the activity out of sequence. He may also be unable to draw a diagram of his own bedroom or to say whether a window is in front, behind or at the side of him when sitting in bed. However, he may be able to 'Pretend to walk over to the window' and describe the direction correctly. It is important to use descriptive language in a simple way during therapy sessions and to use description as 'topics' which underpin a therapy programme.

Failures and disasters

These will always occur. It is how the child responds to them which is important. The clumsy child, no less than anyone else, needs to know that adequate is not the same as perfect, and that everyone has difficulty with something. Some activities which are a problem can be explained and discussed. Joint plans can be agreed to achieve improvement and a contract established for activities or skills which will be practised at home. Other activities are less important either for school work or for the child personally. In this situation a joint understanding should be reached where a choice is made to accept and, therefore, ignore a particular difficulty. Sometimes, by saying 'Let's just forget about catching a ball', a considerable amount of pressure can lifted and the child remains motivated to work on another skill or activity. Choice and meaningful participation in decision-making processes are both vital for the clumsy child, as they are for all children (see Chapter 22 Planning for Progress).

Imagination and expression

Once a movement or a sequence of movements is remembered, understood and can be repeated, it becomes possible to adapt and select activities in the light of changing circumstances and situations. Success in these areas can lead naturally into an exploration of imagination and expression which, in turn, gives a quality and sense of performance to movement.

Movement in space

It is only necessary to observe a group of children in a playground for a short time to realise how large a part imagination plays in games. Children often challenge each other to more and more imaginative movements. 'I can hop' is followed by 'I can hop *and* clap' and by 'I can hop *and* clap *and* go round in a circle'. Imagination should not be defined in adult terms. 'Failures' and 'silly' actions can and do occur, but only at the end of a long sequence of experiments, and usually as a joke or to the amusement of all the children concerned. For the clumsy child, the choice of one imaginative movement may well be impossible and resorting to being a clown may seem the safest and easiest way to face the world on equal terms. It may be helpful to talk about choice and experiment in movement and to find ways of describing the actions the child is doing.

Changing the expression

Changing the expression in movement may be equally difficult. The clumsy child may not be able to select changes in expression between fast/slow, low/high, small/big or heavy/light movements (Fig. 16.6). The use of music or percussion instruments may help some children but embarrass others — they should be used with care. Other children may find it helpful to pretend to be animals or machines.

Readiness

As children grow older they gradually show qualitative and quantitative changes in motor behaviour and they steadily acquire a broad repertoire of motor skills (Laszlo & Bairstow 1985). For most children the time comes when they can perform many movements and activities automatically. The child playing football can anticipate an opponent's move, he does not have to think solely in terms of keeping his balance when

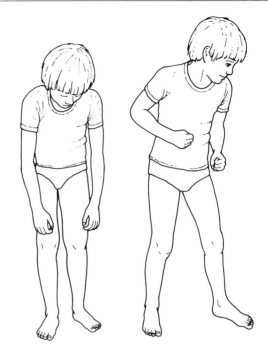

Fig. 16.6 Contrasting expression in position: a light relaxed position and a strong position with tension.

kicking a ball; during essay writing most children can concentrate on the content, it is no longer necessary to concentrate on the physical act of writing; most children can carry a cup of tea or coffee and talk to a friend at the same time. These tasks may be impossible for a clumsy child, a preoccupation with balance, holding the pen and carrying the cup are essential to avoid disaster. The clumsy child can rarely do two things at once.

A lack of confidence, lack of practice or well developed avoidance strategies may all compound the difficulties experienced by the clumsy child. Basic movement skills are never consolidated and developed. Therapy sessions should therefore incorporate:

• activities for strength, endurance and fitness
• opportunities to investigate, height, depth and enclosed spaces
• cooperative games with two or three people
• situations where decision-making skills can be used
• opportunities to enjoy movement.

CONCLUSION

'Play is necessary for motor development as well as essential to the weaving of the psychosocial milieu that is so important in developing positive self-concept and emotional stability' (Arnheim & Sinclair 1975).

It cannot be over-emphasised that the majority of clumsy children are well aware of their problems and in many instances have devised their own strategies to compensate. The therapy programme for individual skills and activities should be based throughout on the concept of an adequate performance, the child's own priorities and discussions with parents. Therapy sessions frequently develop a pattern of their own which combines an opportunity to let off steam, a contract to work on problematic areas, and an agreement to enjoy some activities which are less than perfect. The clumsy child needs to be motivated to practise those activities which he finds difficult. A supportive atmosphere, sense of humour, an ethos of partnership and a willingness to respond flexibly are essential for physiotherapists to achieve success in this field.

REFERENCES

Ainscow M, Tweddle D A 1979 Preventing classroom failure — an objectives approach. John Wiley, Chichester

Arnheim D D, Sinclair W A 1975 The clumsy child. C V Mosby, St Louis

Barkley R A, Ullman D G 1975 A comparison of objective measures of activity and distractability in hyperactive and nonhyperactive children. Journal of Abnormal Child Psychology 3: 231

Burns R B 1986 Child development: a test for the caring professions. Croom Helm, Kent

Burr L A 1984 In: Levitt S (ed) Paediatric developmental therapy. Blackwell Scientific, Oxford

Cataldo M F, Harris J 1982 Biological basis for self-injury. Analysis and Intervention in Developmental Disabilities 2: 21

Chazan M, Laing A F, Jones J, Harper G L, Bolton J 1983 Helping young children with behaviour difficulties. Croom Helm, Kent

Child D 1973 Psychology and the teacher. Holt, Rinehart and Winston, London

Department of Education and Science 1978 Special educational needs (Warnock Report). Her Majesty's Stationery Office, London

Gordon N, McKinlay I 1980 The clumsy child. Churchill Livingstone, Edinburgh

Grimley A 1980 In: Gordon N, McKinlay I (eds) The clumsy child. Churchill Livingstone, Edinburgh

Kanner L 1944 Early infantile autism. Journal of Paediatrics 25: 211

Laszlo J I, Bairstow P J 1985 Perceptual motor behaviour. Holt Psychology, Eastbourne

Lovaas O, Simmons J 1969 Manipulation of self-destruction in three retarded children. Journal of Applied Behaviour Analysis 2: 143

Murphy G 1985 Self-injurious behaviour in the mentally handicapped: an update. Association for Child Psychology and Psychiatry: Newsletter 7(2): 2

Prior M, Griffin M 1985 Hyperactivity: diagnosis and management. Heinemann Medical, London

Randall P E, Gibb C 1987 Structured management and autism. British Journal of Special Education 14(2): 68

Russell J P, 1988 Graded activities for children with motor difficulties. Cambridge University Press

Rutter M 1975 Helping troubled children. Penguin, Middlesex

This section covers the physiotherapy process from initial assessment, through intervention, to monitoring and planning for future progress. It provides an introduction to the systems and methods of physiotherapy available to the paediatric clinician. A broad range of treatment approaches, physical activities and philosophies of management are described. These can be applied to the principles of management introduced in Section 3. This section provides a basis on which to assess, make choices, plan, monitor and record an appropriate treatment regime.

SECTION 4
Physiotherapy in practice

17

Common assessment procedures

V. Bastow   M. Clegg   M. Jones L. King

INTRODUCTION

Assessment is an ongoing process which takes place throughout the period of physiotherapy intervention and forms an essential part of the planning process described in Chapter 22. Appropriate and effective intervention which is based on accurate, appropriate and effective assessment is necessary in order to:

- establish parameters for initial intervention
- agree priorities for future therapy
- monitor changes and progress
- evaluate outcomes.

In this chapter, four assessment modalities are described, which span and have implications for the range of childhood disorders encountered by the paediatric physiotherapist:

- development
- tone
- gait
- respiratory function.

DEVELOPMENTAL ASSESSMENT
M. Clegg

INTRODUCTION

The developmental assessment of a child supplies us with a considerable amount of basic information about that child. It identifies deviations from the normal developmental progress and should therefore be carried out at the earliest appropriate time, to enable early intervention. A formal developmental assessment may well follow on from the screening procedures discussed in Chapter 5 (Practices in Child Health).

PURPOSE OF DEVELOPMENTAL ASSESSMENT

This type of assessment may be used in a number of ways:

- to monitor progress as an ongoing diagnostic tool
- as a basis for planning physiotherapy intervention
- for use in explaining the child's needs to parents
- as an epidemiological record for research.

A sound assessment is an essential baseline for determining priorities when making treatment plans and considering the future management needs of the child.

True and accurate assessment of a child's developmental level is dependent upon a sound knowledge of normal development, (see Chapter 4 The Developing Child). During this assessment we observe, compare and monitor a child against a body of knowledge which is considered to be the 'norm'. If our knowledge of the 'norm' is sparse, then we are at a disadvantage. If it is extensive, we can recognise quickly anything which should give cause for concern.

Timescale

The ranges of normal development are wide, sometimes making it necessary to observe a child over a period of time, and in different environments, before drawing any conclusions. The need to do this may depend upon the reason for the assessment and is sometimes referred to as an 'ongoing' assessment.

Neurological assessment

Developmental assessment has been described as

a systematised form of observation which allows some explanation to be made of the extent of activities of the brain (Drillien and Drummond 1977).

A neurological examination of the new-born infant will normally be carried out after birth and paediatric physiotherapists should make themselves aware of what it involves, since outcomes of this screening can predetermine the future needs of a child (Table 17.1).

This early developmental testing tells us if there is normal neurological development. It may also be carried out in order to assess the maturity of the premature baby.

Assessment batteries

The most common method for developmental testing is to have a check list of the activities of a normal child spanning certain age ranges, and to check the milestones reached by the child being assessed against this (Table 17.2) (see also Chapter 6 Neonatal Problems and the Neonatal Unit).

When looking at the disorders of posture and movement in cerebral palsy, the level of ability may be seen to be dependent on the positions of lying, sitting and standing. Observational assessment should be made of the child's ability to use and adapt his posture and movement towards the next developmental stage, e.g. to adopt a lying or sitting position (Hare 1984).

Table 17.1 Examination of the newborn infant

Factors in Developmental and Neurological Assessment	
Movements	Quantity and symmetry Posture and tone
Reflexes	Moro and grasp Knee jerks and ankle clonus
Head	Measurement of circumference Palpation — anterior fontanelle — cranial sutures Examination of eyes Observation of face
Sounds	Observation of cry Cardiorespiratory function
Hips	Examination
Maturity	Assessment of level

Table 17.2 Checklist of developmental progress in sitting

Age	Activity	Achieved (√)
6 months	Sits on chair propped	√
	Sits on floor long sitting, abducted legs, supported	√
	Assists pulled to sitting	√
	Protective extension of arms forward	
8 months	Sits erect, unsteady, on floor	
	Protective extension of arms sideways	
	Rocks, equilibrium reactions begin	
10–12 months	Sits alone indefinitely	
	Goes from sitting to prone	
	Sits and pivots	
	Good equilibrium reactions	
18 months	Seats self in small chair	
	Climbs adult chair	

More specific information must include:

- gross motor skills
- fine motor skills
- range of joint movement
- muscle tone
- strength and weakness
- voluntary and involuntary movement
- coordination of movement.

Although efforts are being made to produce a standardised recording of central motor deficit with associated sensory and intellectual deficit, at the time of writing there is no one format for testing the motor skills. Some professionals may use the Sheridan Stycar Test Battery, which includes testing for vision and hearing. In common with most developmental assessment batteries, this includes assessment of:

- gross motor function
- fine motor function
- hearing and vision
- communication
- social skills
- play
- cognitive development.

If assessing for learning disorders and sensory integration, ideas for check lists of ability can be drawn from a wide range of available material. It is suggested that this type of assessment should follow on from basic central motor evaluation at school entry (Grimley & McKinlay 1977) (Table 17.3).

Children's needs

As the child grows motor development becomes more obvious, and we begin to look at what a child can and cannot do. Due regard must be taken of the parents' comments and the stimulation level of the everyday environment should be noted. The bonding and attitude of the parent can affect the developing child. To achieve the best potential for development a child needs a warm, happy, loving and secure environment. His psychological needs are as important as regular food, rest, warm clothes and sunlight. Any neglect of these needs could lead to a delay at some point of his development.

PHYSIOTHERAPY ASSESSMENT: ADDITIONAL CONSIDERATIONS

Environment

The environment in which assessments are done can affect the performance level the child achieves. The surroundings should be familiar and comfortable, giving continuity to what has gone before and thus reinforcing the child's security in the situation. This also leads to less distraction. Observation of the child's behaviour, responses and ability in a secure environment is of paramount importance. It is not always essential to obtain the hospital notes before obtaining this information. It can be useful, and sometimes

Table 17.3 Basic central motor evaluation: parameters of assessment

Parameter	Method
Balance and coordination	Heel–toe walk Walking on tiptoe
Eye–hand coordination	Standing on one leg Building tower Threading
Manual dexterity	Screwing and unscrewing Winding bobbin Simultaneous placing

Based on Grimley and McKinlay 1977

more objective, to observe and record, without the preconceptions which result from any prior knowledge.

Background information

Background knowledge must include:

- name
- age
- sex
- date of birth
- date of expected birth
- address and ethnic group
- number in family and whether natural, adopted or fostered.

Wider issues should include a brief family history and past medical history.

Working with parents

Information should be obtained in discussion with parents. During these discussions the physiotherapist should ascertain:

- how much information parents have been given about their child's condition
- how much they understand
- whether they are accepting
- how they are coping
- whether the extended family is supportive.

It will take time, sensitivity and a supportive atmosphere to discuss these issues with parents.

Professional issues

All of these issues will form core information on whether the present stage of development is within the boundary of normal child development. In order to gather this information considerable personal and professional skills are required. These skills will include listening, communicating, observing, patience, tact, making parents and child feel at ease and filtering the information being communicated. Specialist knowledge must be applied appropriately and with insight.

INTERDISCIPLINARY ASSESSMENT

In order to assess the parameters of human development described above it is necessary to adopt a holistic approach, which draws on the many professional skills of the interdisciplinary team (see Chapter 24 Team Workers). This type of in-depth assessment is done in order to plan for future needs. It may be done in parallel with an educational assessment, and therefore becomes part of the statementing process of the 1981 Education Act (see Chapter 25 Legal Aspects in Paediatric Physiotherapy). It may also take place when the child is quite young (12–18 months) as part of the action of a District Handicap Team in order to assess the necessary intervention with a preschool child and his family (see Chapter 24 Team Workers).

The paediatrician will require the help of the team to determine those deviations and deficits which may or may not be apparent at the earlier consultations.

The core format of the team may vary from district to district and extra professionals may be co-opted for specific purposes (Table 17.4).

ASSESSMENT OF MUSCLE TONE
L. King

INTRODUCTION

This section deals with the ways in which tone can be used as a factor in the assessment of handicapped, injured and sick children. Two interesting problems arise: defining terms and the difficulty of standardisation of testing due to the

Table 17.4 A typical assessment team

The core assessment team	Co-opted members
Clinical psychologist	Audiologist
Health visitor	Audiometrician
Nursery nurse	Cardiologist
Paediatrician	Child psychiatrist
Paediatric occupational therapist	Ophthalmologist
Paediatric physiotherapist	Orthoptist
Social worker	Orthopaedic surgeon
Speech therapist	Portage teacher
	Teacher of the blind
	Teacher of the deaf
AND THE PARENTS	

wide variability of muscle tone. It is hoped that the section will encourage the reader to delve deeper into this fascinating area. The Further Reading list refers to recent papers and texts of interest on these topics.

Assessment

The assessment of muscle tone is best achieved clinically at present by observation, handling and palpation. As physiological and biochemical measurement advances are made, an increased use of technology may become available (De Souza and Musa 1987) but are not, as yet, clinically appropriate.

Attitude

Evaluation becomes easier as the therapist gains experience and skill. If the therapist is anxious, the performance and the accuracy of assessment is reduced, partly because of omissions and partly because of tense handling and palpation. A relaxed therapist creates a positive environment in which patients/clients can perform optimally and also assists accuracy from a clinical viewpoint.

TERMINOLOGY

It is important to clarify a number of terms as there is often energetic discussion upon the definitions of those terms used in the field of muscle tone.

Tonus

The term 'tone' or 'tonus' as applied to skeletal muscle has acquired a specific meaning, being the 'steady reflex contraction of the muscles concerned in maintaining the posture characteristic of a given animal species' (Best & Taylor 1973). Tone has its basis in the stretch reflexes and, in the upright human being, mainly in the anti-gravity muscles (extensors). Lance (1980) has defined spasticity in strictly physiological terms as 'a motor disorder characterised by a velocity-dependent increase in tone stretch reflexes ("muscle tone") with exaggerated tendon jerks,

resulting from hyperexcitability of the stretch reflex, as one component of the upper motor neuron syndrome'. However, as Young & Delwaide (1981) point out, Lance's definition refers to the minimum positive symptom in people with spasticity and does not include other components of the upper motor neuron syndrome which are often troubling to patients, e.g. positive symptoms such as weakness and loss of dexterity. Terminology is generally used in the following way:

Hypertonicity

'Hypertonicity' is tone increased above normal levels which interferes with the accurate co-ordination of motor patterns.

Hypotonicity

'Hypotonicity' is lower than normal tone and interferes with the accurate coordination of movement.

Fluctuating tone

'Fluctuating tone' changes from hypertonus to hypotonus to normal, in any combination and sequence (such as athetosis and ballismus).

Associated movements and reactions
Associated movements

'Associated movements' are normal, involuntary responses usually occurring in situations of undue effort (for example, grimacing when lifting a heavy weight). They can be seen in young children and adults when new and difficult tasks are learned (Bobath 1983).

Associated reactions

'Associated reactions' are involuntary, unwanted, abnormal responses which interfere with normal movement, for example, a child with hemiplegia and hypertonicity may, when attempting to stand or walk, produce persistent total flexor jerks of one arm which grossly interfere with the normal pattern of movement, and with automatic balance reactions (Fig. 17.1).

Classification

Clasp knife — increased tonus

The muscle response to passive movements will be an initial resistance followed by relaxation, which allows the movement to be completed.

Lead pipe

Constant resistance to passive movement is maintained throughout the whole range. (The author has not seen this in children.)

Cog wheel

Similar to 'clasp knife' except that, after an initial resistance and release, resistance re-occurs and subsequently disappears in phases so that the muscle is extended in a series of jerks.

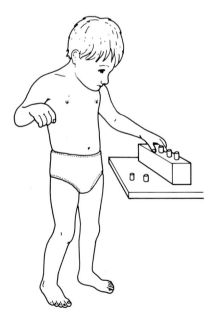

Fig. 17.1 Associated reaction in right arm of child with right-sided hemiplegia. Note flexion of the right arm and wrist and retraction of the right shoulder and hip as the child uses the left hand.

Dystonia

The dystonic child frequently shows a mixed pattern of athetosis and hypertonicity. In certain positions, such as supine lying and standing, a rigid extensor pattern occurs, with increasing extension of head and neck, shoulder retraction and strong hip adduction. At times the child appears to be locked into this position. Once the extensor component has been 'destroyed' in one body segment, e.g. flexion of the neck, the child will become 'floppy'. These extremes of tonus are characteristic.

Phenomena such as spasticity need to be identified and differentiated from other conditions such as fibrosis, ankylosis, 'cramp' secondary to muscle injury, etc.

CLINICAL EXAMINATION

This section covers examination procedure but *it is most unlikely that the therapist will gain all the information needed to record the current tonal qualities and to plan a scheme of treatment at the initial visit.* Rather, the whole picture will be collected a little at a time from a number of sessions. It should also be remembered that the picture can change from moment to moment or month to month, and it is important that the physiotherapist is ready to recognise alterations and record them as they happen. Children, therapists and relatives need to become accustomed to one another and the children need time to adjust to the unfamiliar demands placed upon them. For example, it is not necessary to take a baby from its parents' arms and unclothe it straight away at the initial visit (even though the therapist must eventually examine the baby unclothed). It may cause undue stress to the parent and baby and, as a result, the therapist may miss or misinterpret important information.

Initial observation

An example of a possible initial assessment for tone might be as follows:

Position

Extremes of muscle tonicity are fairly readily observable. Observe the position which the child habitually adopts. Often the child is carried into the room in a parent's arms. Note whether or not the child needs head support and, if so, whether he is looking around and moving his head, or whether it remains in one position (e.g. side-flexion). Observe whether the child is able to lift his head and hold it up for a reasonable length of time or whether the head immediately wobbles.

Spinal posture

Look at the neck/trunk/spinal postures. Is the neck and back rounded and unchanging or is extension available to facilitate head lift? (Fig. 17.2).

Movement

Does the child move his arms and hands symmetrically or asymmetrically? Are the movements purposeful and accurate? Does he move his legs in the same way?

Automatic balance reactions

Has he automatic balance reactions? If he is sitting on a parent's knee, watch how closely he is

held and then gently encourage the parent to reduce support and see what happens.

Child's interaction

While introducing yourself, explaining and extracting information, observe the child and his or her reactions with his parents and brother or sister. Particularly look for automatic balance and saving reactions in the child and protective actions from his relatives.

This initial observation will already have provided you with a lot of information but it will not be conclusive until you have handled the child.

Summary: Initial observation.

In summary, then, observe:
- head control
- posture
- patterns of movement
- balance reactions (gait, if appropriate)
- reluctance to move
- early fatigue
- ease with which the child changes position
- accuracy, purpose and quality of movement
- asymmetry
- associated reactions
- undue effort
- discomfort
- motivation to move
- facial expressions
- reactions and handling by parents/carers.

Ensuring that the environment is warm, light and well-ventilated and preferably with minimally distracting immediate surroundings, the child can then be appropriately unclothed. At the initial session, it is preferable for the therapist to sit back and observe whilst a parent undresses the child. Look for ease of movement, unwanted movements, primitive reflex response, etc. It is helpful for the therapist to take over at some point so that she can also feel what is happening.

Palpation and handling

Palpation

Position. The starting position used for palpation will depend upon the level at which the child is already functioning and the cooperation

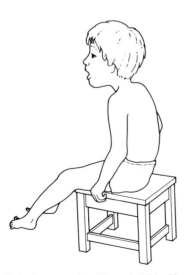

Fig. 17.2 Spinal posture in sitting of child with spastic diplegia. Note the rounded back and protracted chin, also adducted legs and reduced hip flexion.

of the child, although one can palpate in all conditions, even if the child is running around! If a
child is manifesting minimal difficulty in sitting,
it is helpful to palpate in standing; conversely, if
there are real difficulties in sitting, it may be helpful to examine them in lying. What we are
achieving here, of course, is either reducing or
increasing the base of support and centre of
gravity to alter antigravity mechanisms and thus
to test the tonal response of muscles to these
changes. It is helpful to palpate both from a static
and a dynamic position, especially if there is
minimal evidence of tonal alterations when the
child is stationary.

Selectivity. In palpation, it is important never
to test an isolated muscle or group. Always observe and palpate the whole body, checking the
agonists, antagonists and synergists in a pattern
of movement, and its effects on other parts of
the body.

Relaxed passive movements. Although extremes of muscle tonicity, whether hypo- or
hypertonus are fairly readily observable, for the
detection of smaller alterations of muscle tone,
we need to palpate and to perform relaxed
passive movements to determine changes.

It may also be necessary to perform manoeuvres to produce rapid stretch to the suspected
muscle groups. The therapist can then interpret
any resistance offered to the movement, indicating increased tone, or any excess of movement,
possibly indicating reduced tone. Remember
when performing these manoeuvres to observe
the whole body in order to detect associated
responses elsewhere.

Palpation. In palpation, feel the muscle bulk
on both sides, looking for asymmetry:

1. Does it feel flabby, soft, non-resilient and
atrophied? (atonic)
2. Does it feel soft and wasted, yet resilient?
(hypotonic)
3. Does it feel tight, tense, excessively firm,
solid, unyielding especially if put slightly on
stretch (Atkinson 1986)? This indicates
hypertonicity and in this condition the tendon
will be felt and readily observed standing out
from the underlying structures like a tight
cord.

Handling

When palpating, be aware that careless handling
may stimulate an abnormal response which is not
part of the true picture of the child and can mis-
lead the therapist. It may also cause loss of
confidence, distress or discomfort to the child.
The handling should be firm, as hesitant and
timid handling can also cause distress and discomfort. With the highly sensitive child, a 'tickle'
may have a disturbing effect and, whilst causing
amusement, will disrupt the examination.
Children with hypersensitivity may find activities
such as sand and water play and playing with
fluffy toys acutely distressing.

Reflex testing

Reflex testing is a fairly common method of assessing muscle tone and the state of neurological
pathways.

Superficial reflexes

The superficial reflexes may be tested by stimulating the skin and looking for muscle contraction
in the area, e.g. the Galant response (Fig. 17.3).
If no response occurs, the indication is that there
is either an interruption of the lower reflex pathway or a state of central shock has occurred due
to the motoneuron pools not being receptive to
stimulus. The response may be exaggerated if
spasticity is present and delayed and/or sluggish
if there is hypotonia.

Tendon reflexes

Tendon reflexes can be tested by tapping the
muscle tendon which causes a sudden stretch in
the muscle fibres. (This does not actually stretch
the tendon but creates a 'kink' in the tendon and
the resultant vibratory effect produces a stretch
in muscle fibres.)

The normal response is that the muscle fibres
contract together giving a jerk of tone in the
muscle, the most commonly known of these
being the 'knee jerk' created by striking the patel-
lar tendon.

No response indicates either sensory disruption

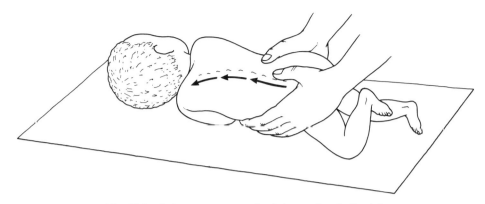

Fig. 17.3 Galant response — trunk incurvation to the left.

or an interruption of the motor pathway between the spinal cord and the muscle, indicating a flaccid muscle paralysis or a state of shock in the central nervous system (due to brain or spinal cord injury) which is often temporary.

An exaggerated response indicates hypertonicity. A pendular, oscillating response, in which the limb swings backwards and forwards several times before settling down, indicates hypotonicity.

By the time a child reaches the therapist, he has often undergone physical examination a number of times, so there is little point in tendon tapping when the child obviously has spasticity from other evidence, such as an obvious primitive reflex pattern. There are two main reasons for this. First, if we create further mass synergies (total patterns of movement) in a child who is already habitually influenced by primitive reflex activity, e.g. asymmetrical tonic neck reflex (ATNR), we are creating further feelings of stiffness, discomfort and cramp. Second, as our assessment and treatment run side by side, creating more tension in already hypertonic muscle groups, we then have to work at inhibiting what we have created before we can proceed. In hypotonia, or in milder forms of spasticity, however, tendon tapping can be valuable.

Relaxed passive movements

Points to look for:

1. Is there resistance to the movement?

2. Can the full length of soft tissue structures be obtained relatively easily?

3. Is there a lack of resistance to movement and is it easy to hyperextend joints at the end of ranges?

The relaxed passive movements should, of course, be performed both slowly and quickly to detect any difference in the response of muscles to 'slow' or 'quick' stretch. If muscles are found to be flaccid, allowing movement to occur without opposition and even permitting an excessive range of movement to occur, and the limb feels heavy due to lack of support from normal muscle action, the muscles under scrutiny may be either hypotonic or atonic. To differentiate between the two, apply quick passive movements to the joints controlled by the muscle groups. The hypotonic muscles may initiate a sluggish stretch response which is not evident in atonic muscles.

Hypertonic muscles show excessive opposition to stretch. If they are indicating spasticity, they may produce the 'claspknife' phenomenon and will oppose movements away from the primitive reflex patterns. An indication of rigidity will be stiff movements and possibly evidence of the cogwheel phenomenon.

Trunk assessment

It is surprising how few assessments of tone actually include the trunk. Since proximal tone and control usually influence distal states and, in a child, development occurs from proximal to distal, it is essential to check the trunk. A thorough assessment of the trunk should give a much clearer picture of areas in which problems lie.

Side-lying

Side-lying is useful to check elongation from the pelvis to the shoulder girdle. Is there resistance or not?

Once elongation is achieved, try:

1. Fixing the pelvis and rotating the shoulder girdle.
2. Fixing the shoulder girdle and rotating the pelvis.
3. Rotating the shoulder girdle and the pelvis in opposite directions.

This will give an impression of the proximal tone basing your evidence on the initial observation (see p. 302).

Scapular area

The mobility available in the scapular region can also be felt in a supported side-lying position, either with the child lying across the therapist's or parent's lap or, if the child is larger, on the bed, mat or plinth. Take care that the head is in a mid-position (on a pillow) and not side-flexed and that the upper leg is appropriately supported. Grasp the scapula and gently check whether or not it moves readily around the chest wall. This should be ascertained before any attempt is made to perform passive movements of the upper limbs into elevation because, if the scapula is 'fixed' by hypertonicity, the only way to achieve elevation would be by forcing protraction, with obvious consequences. It is better to mobilise the scapula and, having achieved protraction, to proceed into elevation.

Tone in the trunk can also be observed in both more static and more dynamic postures and patterns (Fig. 17.4).

Deformity and contracture

Abnormal joint positions may be produced by skeletal changes. However, abnormal joint postures may also occur with:

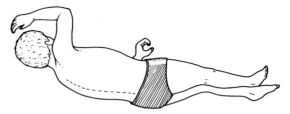

Fig. 17.4 Child with spastic diplegia — lack of rotation when rolling. Note legs, trunk and head moving in one segment, adducted legs and shoulder retraction.

- increased muscle tone
- imbalance of muscle tone.

The palpation and handling techniques already outlined are helpful in determining the causes of deformity and contracture.

Muscle wasting

This may be localised or widespread and may arise due to, for example, disuse atrophy, flaccid paralysis or long-standing spasticity.

Joint instability

This may be due to abnormal muscle pull or imbalance, low tone or congenital malformation.

It is useful to test both 'static' and 'dynamic' stability. For example, look for a hyperextended knee in standing, weight transfer and walking. With the elbow, check not just the functional activities, e.g. feeding, but also the use of the elbow in 'propping' in, for example, supported side-sitting.

Pain and discomfort

This may be due to tonal changes but may be caused by many other problems. To detect discomfort in a child who cannot speak, a useful guide is to watch for creases at the corner of the eyes. It is important to remember to indicate to the child that you have recognised his discomfort. Even the most profoundly disabled children are helped to gain confidence through the calm voice of the therapist and a reassuring, gentle and soothing touch or hug.

Discomfort or fear may be created by spasticity, when a child may complain of aching cramp, by sudden tonal fluctuations, or when he is handled too quickly without having any time to adjust. Hypotonus may also lead to discomfort, particularly where there is instability, subluxation or even dislocation at a joint. All signs of discomfort *must* be recognised, recorded and reported and it is most important to avoid creating the same discomfort again.

Crying

When children are distressed for any reason they appear to be hypertonic. In assessing muscle tone it is important that the child is as relaxed and content as possible, so the therapist should not be in too much of a hurry. Be prepared to gain a little information at a time, build relationships gradually with the child and his relatives and create a pleasant, warm environment in which to work. Try to learn as much as you can through play and activities and, when handling and palpating the child, do not try to achieve everything all at once. Children can feel very insecure if too much happens to them too quickly and they have little or no control of the situation. This may also be stressful to relatives and their anxiety can be passed on to the child.

Crying can also be a useful means of communication!

Development

Developmental delay

Children who demonstrate developmental delay *may* lead the therapist to consider the possibility of tonal change. A child with alteration of tone may demonstrate delayed automatic responses, spontaneous balance responses or even absent responses. Balance should be checked in lying and other positions, possibly using an inverted wedge or a balance board if necessary to test trunk responses.

Quality of movement

The quality of movement should also be noted. Look for:

- rhythm and speed of movement

- accuracy
- undue effort
- a reluctance to move
- signs of early fatigue
- involuntary, unwanted movements that interfere with the general quality and accuracy.

It is important to check gross motor and fine motor skills during play activities and those activities of daily living that may require more concentration and effort. Assess whether the child uses mass movement patterns or mixed patterns, as in the case of more mature coordination, but do not expect this in the new-born.

Position of head and neck

This can affect tone due to the influence of reflex mechanisms such as the ATNR or symmetrical tonic neck reflex (STNR) (see Chapter 8 Disorders of the Central Nervous System). It is usual to check from a midline position, although it may be useful to alter the head and neck position to see if alterations in tone occur beyond normal.

Speech patterns

A speech therapist should be consulted in connection with the three dimensions of speech, breathing patterns and feeding. All will have implications in the assessment of tonal alterations.

ASSESSMENT AND TREATMENT

It is important that every time the child is observed or handled an evaluation and record of his performance takes place. It is also useful to give some useful practical help and advice from the first time you meet the child and his family so that something constructive is suggested from the outset.

Check what handling or other 'treatment' influences the tone, e.g. the effect of reflex inhibiting patterns (RIPs), compression and correct weight-bearing alignment, activities in water and so on, and record the results carefully, as these will have a bearing on the future management of the child (see Chapters 18 and 19 Treatment Systems and Treatment Methods).

Timing

If possible, try to plan the assessment at a time which is suitable for the child and his family, but not just before a meal is due and not immediately after, when they tend to be drowsy. Relatives and nursing colleagues appreciate efforts to fit into their routine as much as possible.

RECENT ADVANCES

A number of different approaches to measuring and assessing spasticity are available, some using electrophysiological or biomechanical techniques, which require sophisticated and expensive apparatus, and others that look at the effect of spasticity on voluntary movement without the technology.

DeSouza and Musa (1987) discuss the different approaches to the measurement and assessment of spasticity and conclude that, at present, although the electrophysiological and biomechanical techniques are useful in the laboratory when measurements of specific physiological phenomena associated with spasticity are needed, or in attempting to determine the effect of physiotherapy, they do not, as yet, have a place in the clinical field, where a quantitative measure of the practical effects of spasticity (e.g. Oswestry Scale, Motor Club assessment) remains the priority.

ASSESSMENT OF GAIT
M. Jones

INTRODUCTION

Gait can be defined as the: 'manner of walking, bearing or carriage as one walks' (*Concise Oxford Dictionary*). Walking is the progress which is made by advancing each foot alternately, never having both off the ground at once.

Gait

The process is more precisely described by Inman et al (1981) as locomotion in which:

- the erect moving body is supported by first one leg, then the other

- the cyclic alternations of the support functions of each leg
- the existence of a transfer period when both feet are on the ground.

Rhythmical alternating movements occur in the extremities and the trunk and result in a forward movement of the centre of gravity.

An individual's gait can be regarded as unique within a specified range and is influenced by the forces of gravity acting on the variety of shapes and forms which make up the human body. It can be modified by conscious control, e.g. copying another's gait, or as a result of outside intervention. Unconscious control often reflects mood changes such as happiness or sadness. Each characteristic gait has a natural rhythm which makes optimal use of body energy.

COMPONENTS OF GAIT ASSESSMENT

In order to assess gait it is necessary to consider:

- posture in standing
- interaction of forces in walking
- basic needs for normal gait
- changes during growth and development
- essential skills for normal gait
- the gait cycle.

Posture in standing

In an easy standing position the line of gravity falls from the vertex, through the centre of gravity (approximately S2 level), through the hip, in front of the knee, in front of the ankle and within the base (Fig. 17.5). The forces exerted on the body in this position are:

- an extension force at the knee
- a dorsiflexion force at the ankle.

The posture of a child learning to stand is lordotic with a consequent alteration in the position of the line of gravity.

Interaction of forces in walking

During walking there exists a complex interaction between the forces of gravity, ground-reaction, inertia and muscle power.

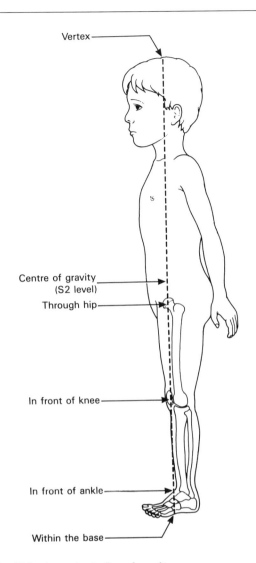

Vertex

Centre of gravity
(S2 level)

Through hip

In front of knee

In front of ankle

Within the base

Fig. 17.5 Approximate line of gravity.

Gravity

This is a constant force acting at the centre of mass of the child's body. The forces which cause rotation of the body (moment of force) will depend on the location of the centre of mass of any individual child.

Ground reaction

These are forces developed in response to the contact between the ground and the child's foot. Each step exerts a force on the ground, and a reactive force is developed in response to this.

This equal and opposite force is called the ground reacting force which supports the body movement.

The resultant effects produced by this force depend upon:

• Point of contact — the heel or the ball of the foot.
• The magnitude of the forces — the weight of the child and the changing forces of slow walking, running and jumping.
• Their line and direction — forwards, sideways and backwards.

Inertia

This is a force which resists or tends to resist any change in the state of rest or motion of the body.

The inter-relationship of these factors is of considerable importance in the accurate observation, identification and assessment of gait abnormalities, and in the prescription of orthoses which modify gait (see Chapter 21 Aids and Appliances). It is also essential that the paediatric physiotherapist has a thorough knowledge and understanding of normal child development. These skills can then be directed towards recognising variances from the norm and identifying and interpreting the abnormalities superimposed upon the normal pattern.

Basic needs for normal gait

Those factors to be considered should include both physical and psychological aspects of child development.

Motivation

Unless a child is motivated to move and explore his immediate environment he will not develop an ability to walk.

Cognitive awareness

In association with the need to move, there must be the minimal level of cognitive ability to enable the child either to work out how to move safely by imitating observed movement, or to assimilate successfully and practise trained movement.

Physical ability

In the normal child, development will be appropriate to his age and his experiences from his environment. As the skeletal structure develops so a toddler's gait will gradually alter from an initial wide-based, flat-footed, stiff-legged pattern to an adult gait at approximately 7 to 9 years. This development is related to an accommodation to changes in bodily proportions and the increasing sophistication of the neurological system.

Changes during growth and development

Body proportions

Essential energy levels and muscle power will increase as the child grows and physiological development keeps pace with skeletal development (Fig. 17.6).

Sensation for movement

The child will become increasingly skilled at using sensory information from his eyes, inner ear, joints, skin and muscle in order to progress from crawling to standing and walking (Fig. 17.7). Balance and coordination skills will concurrently develop as body image, spatial awareness and sensation reflect normal neurological maturation.

Normal gait needs:

- an intact nervous system
- efficient levers to transmit motion into action
- a desire to move and an awareness of the quality of the desired movement
- energy to fulfil the aim.

Essential skills for normal gait

The following essential features of normal gait can be related to the child's age and developmental level:

- Rise to standing — depending upon the age of the child, he will achieve this by a variety of methods including 'pull to standing', 'via half-kneeling', or 'from sitting to standing'.
- Maintain standing — this indicates control of balance and a normal response to forces of gravity.

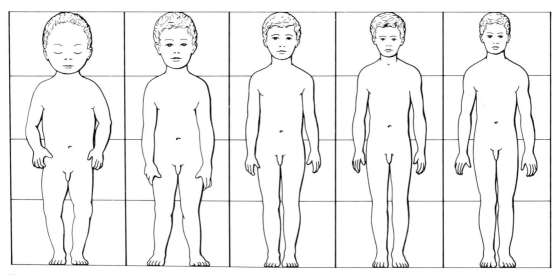

Fig. 17.6 Changes in body proportions during growth (after Sharrard 1979 by permission of Blackwell Scientific Publications Ltd).

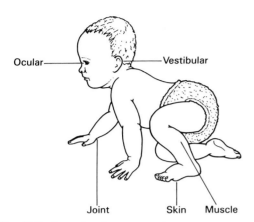

Fig. 17.7   Sensation for movement.

• Transfer weight — the child can overcome the forces of inertia in order to alternate weight-bearing between right and left side and initiate forward movement.
• Controlled movement in the desired direction — walk forward/backwards/sideways.
• Vary the speed/direction of walking as required.
• Demonstrate the ability to sustain walking — needs both stamina and repetition of gait cycle.
• Cope with obstacles, uneven surfaces and inclines.
• Climb/descend stairs — in the appropriate manner in relation to age.
• Turn around — by stepping or pivoting.

• Stop — controlled stop at will.
• Lower to resting position.

The gait cycle

Figure 17.8 provides a graphic representation of one complete gait cycle/stride. Conventionally, the cycle starts and finishes at right heel strike.

The cycle can be broken down into the two distinct phases of 'stance phase' (Fig. 17.9) and 'swing phase' (Fig. 17.10). These phases follow each other alternately when considering the leg individually, i.e. the right leg stance phase is followed by the right leg swing phase. The swing phase of the left leg takes place at the same time as the stance phase of the right.

Stance phase

There are five elements within the stance phase, or weight bearing phase:

• right heel strike
• right foot flat
• right midstance
• right heel off
• right toe off.

Swing phase

There are three elements within the swing phase, or movement phase:

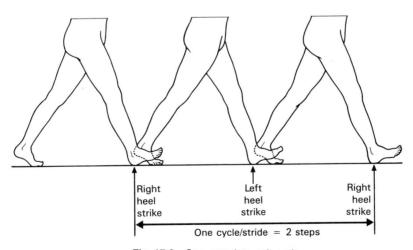

Right heel strike   Left heel strike   Right heel strike

One cycle/stride = 2 steps

Fig. 17.8   One complete gait cycle.

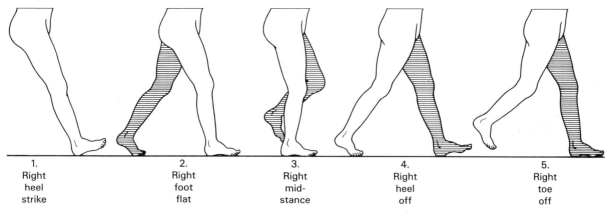

1.	2.	3.	4.	5.
Right heel strike	Right foot flat	Right mid-stance	Right heel off	Right toe off

Fig. 17.9 Stance phase.

- acceleration
- mid swing
- deceleration.

The centre of gravity of the body is displaced in two directions during movement; vertically, the highest point being at mid-stance and the lowest when both feet are on the ground, and laterally as the weight is transferred from one leg to the other.

ASSESSMENT OF GAIT

The gait of the child can only be assessed through observation over a period of time, together with a thorough physical examination and observation from all angles. In this process of assessment the child's age, developmental level and stamina must also be considered.

Preparation of the child

Ideally, the child should not be made aware of the processes of assessment. Although he will need to be suitably undressed, so that the observer can note all the relevant factors during the gait cycle, sensitivity will be needed in achieving the removal of socks and vests. The physiotherapist must be prepared for a long period of observation and assessment.

The child may be able to cooperate but unwilling to do so, or may be willing but unable to cooperate. Skill is needed in differentiating between these two situations. It could well be that the only time the child assumes his normal gait pattern is on the way out of the treatment room!

Physical examination

Prior to an observation of the child walking, it is

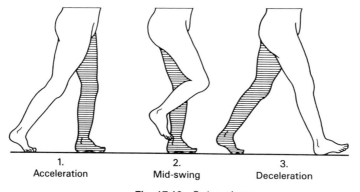

1.	2.	3.
Acceleration	Mid-swing	Deceleration

Fig. 17.10 Swing phase.

essential to carry out a thorough physical examination to assess the physical, physiological and psychological factors previously discussed. Important features will be:

- abnormal reflexes
- range of movement
- muscle power
- sensation
- fixed or dynamic deformities.

Electrogoniometers are used to provide a quantitative measure of the dynamic range of joint movement and could be useful in measuring an unused part of the range or for comparative purposes before and after surgical procedures involving joints or tendons. However, because of their bulk, they are not ideal for use with children and there is some risk of their presence resulting in inhibition of the normal gait pattern with very young children. King & Staheli (1984) advocated that when examining torsional problems of tibia and femur, attention should be paid to the angle of the feet in relation to the knees. This can be measured either by observation or by footprinting, and the evidence compared to the normal range of 0–20°, taking any secondary deformity arising from imbalanced muscle action into account.

If the initial physical examination has revealed respiratory problems or heart disease, then there may well be associated postural problems or difficulties associated with a lack of energy. Children with pathological gait have an added physiological cost (Butler et al 1984). The physical examination should therefore be extended to include:

- the distance the child can walk
- any pain or discomfort which is experienced
- callous formation
- inspection of wear on footwear.

Stage of development

It is essential that the physiotherapist assesses gait in relation to the child's age and stage of development. At birth most normal infants have increased femoral anteversion, ranging from 10–60°. During growth this decreases to the normal adult value of 15–20° (King & Staheli 1984). During the second year of life 'bow-leg' is common, as is the change to a 'knock-knee' appearance in the third year.

In a growing child with any form of muscle dysfunction, there may be periods during which bone growth outpaces soft tissue development. This can lead to a deterioration in gait which may become permanent unless treated conservatively, as described in Chapter 19 Treatment Methods (Serial Splinting) or by surgical intervention (see Chapter 12 Orthopaedic Aspects of Childhood Disorders).

Observation

Various teaching centres have their own methods of carrying out observation and assessment. At the University of New York, for example, students are taught to observe gait and label limps according to their appearance. Some suggested classifications are:

- hip-hitching;
- internal/external hip rotation;
- circumduction;
- excessive medial/lateral foot contact;
- hyperextension of the knee.

This allows for a number of observations to be grouped together for an individual child who will compensate for his disability in his own unique way.

Video recording

Video recording of play and of directed activities is useful both in subsequent analysis of abnormalities and as a record of progress for treatment evaluation. This latter function is also of value as support and encouragement for parents where progress appears to be slow. Some gait laboratories have computer-linked recording which interprets the forces resulting from ground reaction, measured when the child walks over a force plate.

Walking in isolation

It is important to remember during assessment that walking is not an activity any child carries out in isolation. He will walk whilst pushing a toy, whilst carrying a book, when holding his mother's hand and when talking to friends. Any assessment must incorporate an observation of the effect on gait of performing other tasks at the same time.

Walking outside the physiotherapy department, school or child's home will also require additional skills. Balance skills will need to be assessed, for example, when the child walks up a slope, over rough ground, or stands on an escalator.

Dynamic walking

Each child's individual style of walking has already been discussed (see p. 313). Walking is a dynamic process which incorporates coordinated movement of the whole body. Additional factors to observe are:

- rotation and side flexion of the trunk
- posture of shoulders and head
- arm swing
- ability to turn the head and observe the world
- ability to change the speed of walking, both to and from running.

Provision of aids

Where a child uses aids or appliances to walk (see p. 401), gait should be assessed with and without the aid, where appropriate. Consideration should be given to the need for the provision of aids in any form. A walking stick, rollator or splints will have a consequential effect on the gait pattern and energy expenditure.

It should also be noted that the use of such aids can in some circumstances constitute a significant psychological barrier to the child or the child's family. This may be especially evident when parents first realise that their child may never be able to walk without external assistance. This problem can arise as a result of even a well-thought-out treatment programme where parents are consulted throughout, and the physiotherapist should be aware of this and the need in these cases for family counselling.

ROLE OF THE PHYSIOTHERAPIST

An early and precise identification of gait dif-

ficulties, translated into a treatment plan, may give a growing child a better chance of overcoming or minimising the disability. This process will be aided by the development of a close professional relationship between the physiotherapist, the child and the child's parents. The parents should, where possible, take an active role in the continuous therapy programme which takes place in the treatment centre, the home and, where appropriate, the school. The maintenance of comprehensive and accurate records is essential to provide a basis of comparison and evaluation so that changes in gait patterns are identified, and treatment methods evaluated accordingly.

ASSESSMENT OF RESPIRATORY FUNCTION
V. Bastow

INTRODUCTION

The diagnosis that a child presents with can give only a general idea of the nature of the respiratory problems. For example, a diagnosis of cystic fibrosis indicates that a child has an inherited disorder which involves the respiratory and gastro-intestinal tract, each to a greater or lesser degree. In some instances, e.g. muscular dystrophy and Down's syndrome, the referral diagnosis may not suggest a respiratory problem at all but the assessing physiotherapist must be aware that the neuromuscular or cardiac problems frequently predispose the child to respiratory complications. The physiotherapist will need to assess the degree of respiratory involvement, the problems pertinent to treatment at that time and the factors that need to be considered in planning the long-term management of that patient. From this assessment a problem list can be drawn up and a treatment plan devised.

CONSIDERATIONS WHEN ASSESSING CHILDREN
Information from children

The most obvious difficulty encountered when assessing infants and children is their limited ability to give an account of their condition. The information given by the parents may also be unreliable, as they may be unaware of normality, particularly if this is their first child. Statements such as 'He doesn't cough much' must be viewed with an open mind if the family has a history of chest problems and they all cough! It may require skilled questioning to elicit relevant histories from some families.

Presentation

Young children may not complain of symptoms that would worry an older person. Pain may be ignored or normal movements and activities modified to prevent aggravating the symptoms.

The tendency to be very ill one day and almost back to normal the next is often encountered with young children.

Child development

The rapid growth and development which occurs during infancy requires consideration when assessing a child: a respiratory rate of 60 would be considered normal in a neonate and grossly abnormal in an 18-month-old (Table 17.5).

These factors must all be borne in mind when assessing the child.

STAGES OF ASSESSMENT

Assessment is carried out in a number of stages but not necessarily in this order:

- history
- general assessment
- respiratory muscle activity
- cough and sputum

- pain
- social factors, e.g. smoking
- respiratory function tests
- exercise tolerance
- auscultation
- chest X-ray.

History

A history may be obtained from one or more sources: the medical notes, the general practitioner, the health visitor, the parents or chief carers and the ward staff. The aim is to establish:

- the nature of the problem
- its duration
- whether anyone else in the family has a similar problem
- whether anything makes the problem worse or better
- whether treatment or advice has been sought from a physiotherapist before.

Note must also be made of any past medical history, including common childhood illnesses, such as measles and whooping cough, as these may have an effect on later respiratory problems. The answers to these questions should indicate the severity of the present condition and help to set the scene for the problem list and treatment plan.

The child of school age should be asked about his school:

- does he enjoy school?
- any special school friends?
- name of teacher?

Where a condition is liable to intrude into school life (e.g. the use of inhalers or limitation

Table 17.5 Normal pulse, respiration and blood pressure in children

Age	Resting pulse rate/min	Resting respiratory rate/min	Blood pressure (mmHg)
1st week	120 ± 20	$30 - 60$	80/50
2nd–8th week	110 ± 20	40 ± 10	90/55
3–12 months	110 ± 20	30 ± 10	100/60
1–6 years	90 ± 15	24 ± 5	110/65
7–12 years	80 ± 10	20 ± 5	120/70

of exercise tolerance), then discussion with teachers may help maximise the child's integration and enjoyment.

General assessment

A number of different factors must be considered:

- general appearance
- temperature
- feeding pattern
- colour
- clubbing
- posture, shape and expansion of chest
- observation and palpation of the chest wall.

General appearance

Does the child look ill? What is his colour and posture and are there signs of respiratory distress? Note should also be made of the child's size.

Temperature

In babies this may be taken rectally. The normal rectal temperature is 37.5°C, which is 0.5°C higher than an oral temperature and 1°C higher than that measured in the axilla.

Feeding pattern

Information should be available from nurses and/or parents. As infants are compulsory nose breathers they may present with an altered feeding pattern when suffering from a cold or upper respiratory tract infection, when mucus blocks the nasal passages and they are forced to breathe through their mouths.

Coughing in an older child may produce vomiting and so these children may stop eating to avoid the distress of vomiting. It may also be very difficult for an acutely breathless child to drink and the resulting under-hydration may contribute to the dry mouth and thickened secretions seen in some patients.

Colour

Observation must be made for pallor and cyanosis with constant reassessment during the

treatment of an acutely ill child, bearing in mind that skin pigmentation varies considerably between individuals.

Cyanosis is the bluish discoloration usually present when the oxygen saturation of the blood is less than 85% (normal range, 95–98%). Peripheral cyanosis is limited to the extremities, where the nail beds of the hands and feet appear bluish. Central cyanosis also involves the mucous membranes of the mouth and lips. Coughing bouts may produce cyanosis due to sudden oxygen desaturation.

Clubbing

Finger and toe clubbing may develop in early childhood where cyanotic heart disease or suppurative lung disease such as bronchiectasis, cystic fibrosis or empyema are present.

On examination there will be an increase in the longitudinal curvature of the nail and nail bed, with loss of angle at the nail and nail bed junction and a spongy sensation where pressure is applied over the nail bed (Fig. 17.11).

There may also be widening of the distal phalanx, thus making the finger resemble a club or drumstick. The reason for this alteration in finger shape is still unknown but it may partially

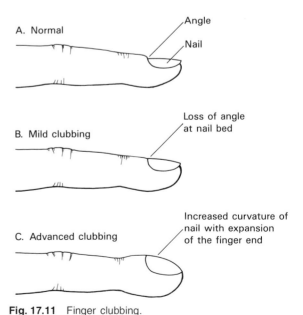

Fig. 17.11 Finger clubbing.

regress if the underlying cause is treated, e.g. surgical resection of a bronchiectatic lobe.

Posture, shape and expansion of chest

The size, shape and symmetry of the chest should be noted.

The child with a chronic chest disease may develop sternal prominence or bowing, caused by air trapping, resulting from airway obstruction. When such obstruction develops in early years it is more likely to result in an alteration of thoracic shape than in older children, due to the pliability of the ribs.

Airway obstruction in infancy may also result in permanent deformity of the lower rib cage. Vigorous inspiratory effort by the diaphragm may produce a permanent oblique depression known as Harrison's sulcus (Fig. 17.12). This is caused by the diaphragm pulling in the lower ribs along the line of muscle attachment.

Note should be made of any previous operation scar and its history obtained.

Observation and palpation of chest wall

Careful observation and palpation of the chest

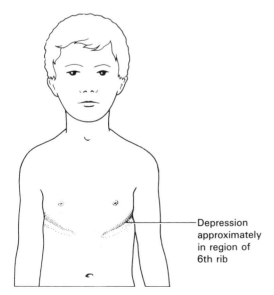

Fig. 17.12 Harrison's sulcus.

Depression approximately in region of 6th rib

wall during both quiet breathing and maximal deep breaths should reveal any asymmetry which may suggest an underlying pathology such as pneumothorax or collapse/consolidation of a lobe. Measurement with a tape measure will show total thoracic excursion but will not highlight any difference between the lungs. Tape measure recordings are difficult to reproduce accurately, either by the same person on repeated measurements or between different individuals. However, it can be a useful measurement if trying to maintain or improve thoracic mobility, as the visual feedback may encourage the child to co-operate with treatment. If measurements are to be made on a child it is probably sufficient to use only one or two sites.

Respiratory muscle activity

Airflow rate

Some of the principles governing airflow must be considered when examining the child with respiratory problems. Airflow rate is proportional to the fourth power of the radius (r^4) of the tube through which it flows (Poiseuille's law) and so, assuming a constant pressure gradient, a halving of the radius of the airways will result in a 16-fold decrease in airflow. This is particularly significant in infants, due to the small anatomical size of their normal airways.

Costal margin paradox

In the infant the ribs are virtually horizontal and there is little room for an increase in chest diameter. An increase in lung capacity can only be achieved by the diaphragm. However, the diaphragm itself is mechanically disadvantaged as its bony anchors, the ribs, are cartilaginous and pliable and the muscle lacks the curvature seen in the adult. As a consequence, contraction of the diaphragm produces an inward collapse of the lower ribs, thus decreasing the intrathoracic diameter. This is referred to as costal margin paradox, or rib recession which, if occurring over a prolonged period, may cause the permanent deformity of Harrison's sulcus.

Nostril flaring

Flaring of alae nasi (nostrils) occurs in respiratory distress in order to reduce the resistance to nasal airflow by increasing the size of the nasal apertures.

Sternal paradox

The sternum moving inwards during inspiration (sternal paradox) may also occur because the sternum is soft and flexible, allowing this movement during periods of respiratory distress.

Intercostal recession

The sucking in of the intercostal muscles during inspiration — intercostal recession — is another sign of respiratory distress.

Grunting. During normal tidal breathing in infancy the child maintains a positive end expiratory pressure (PEEP) by contracting its diaphragm and narrowing its glottis during the last stage of expiration. This ensures that the airways are kept open and so maintains the functional residual capacity and stops the alveoli collapsing. During respiratory distress these actions may be exaggerated and the child may be heard to grunt as the glottis closes and the diaphragm contracts.

Cough and sputum

A moist, productive cough may be associated with swallowing of any mucus produced; the parents or nurse may report the presence of this mucus in any vomit.

Expectoration

A child as young as 3 years of age may be able to expectorate, particularly if he has a chronically productive cough and has been taught to cough when required by parents or older siblings. However, it can be very difficult to teach expectoration to an acutely ill child with no previous cough. Vomit is sometimes the only way of assessing the colour of sputum without obtaining an aspirated sample.

Colour of secretion

The colour of expectorated secretions may sometimes give an indication of the underlying problem.

Yellow discoloration suggests the presence of bacteria, but this may be misleading as, in asthma, clumps of eosinophils can produce a yellow colour.

Green secretions suggest stagnation of infected secretions, a sign commonly seen in bronchiectasis, where secretions collect in the damaged airways. This green discoloration is thought to be caused by the release of the enzyme verdoperoxidase from disintegrating eosinophils or neutrophils. Green sputum is more frequently reported in the morning because the sputum has stagnated overnight in the airways. During the day, the colour often lightens towards yellow. Blood streaking or frank blood may also be observed and should be recorded.

Paroxysms of coughing

Several coughs occurring in rapid succession without adequate time for inspiration in between coughs, i.e. paroxysms, should be noted. Often the child becomes red in the face, or even cyanotic. A paroxysm will frequently be followed by vomiting. A child with whooping cough may be heard to inspire with the characteristic 'whoop' at the end of the paroxysm of coughing.

Pain

Pain is often difficult to assess in children. They find it hard to describe and a young child may refer to a tummy ache as a 'headache in my tummy.' Observation of the child, however, may suggest the site of his pain.

The child with pleural pain may grunt as he stops inspiration just at the point at which it becomes painful. Following thoracic surgery, the young baby may move around remarkably well with little sign of pain on breathing or arm movements. However, the older child of 3 or 4 years may display great fear and be very reluctant to move unless adequate analgesia and reassurance are given.

Social factors

Various social factors have been implicated in the aetiology of respiratory problems in the child. Recurrent respiratory tract infections and chronic cough are more prevalent in social classes IV and V. Air pollution has also been identified as a significant contributory factor in lower respiratory tract illnesses in these social classes. Overcrowding has been associated with an increase in chest illnesses, especially if a family member suffers from chronic bronchitis.

From studies in the 1970s (Milner & Martin 1985) there also appears to be a significant increase in respiratory symptoms amongst children of families with members who are heavy smokers (passive smoking). It must also be remembered that children in their early teens may be admitted to paediatric wards and they may already be frequent smokers.

Questioning of the family about their social circumstances must be handled tactfully and without prejudice.

Respiratory function testing

Peak Expiratory Flow Rate (PEFR)

This test can be used in children as young as 2, although the readings may not be reliable until the age of 5. When a child is being seen regularly it is useful to introduce him to the meter at a young age, and so familiarise him with the technique and equipment.

Low reading meters are available, registering 20–200 litre/min with a small mouthpiece.

It is usual to take three readings and record the best. As with adults, the patient with very labile airways may become progressively more wheezy as the readings are taken and the forced expiratory manoeuvres induce airway narrowing, in which case it may be judicious to take one or two only.

Vitalography

This measures the forced expiratory volume in 1 second (FEV_1) and the forced vital capacity (FVC). These measurements may be helpful when monitoring a progressive lung disorder such as cystic fibrosis or when assessing a patient for surgery, such as spinal fusion in muscular dystrophy. The results are not very reliable until the age of 5–7 years.

For both the PEFR and the FEV_1/FVC readings, a table of predicted values is available corrected for height (Table 17.6).

Exercise tolerance

This can be difficult to assess in the young child. Observation of the child at play may give a useful guide to the child's exercise tolerance but the very breathless child may select more sedentary play activities rather than push himself into an uncomfortable and often frightening breathless state by exertion beyond his limits. The older child (around 9 or 10 years) can generally be relied upon to perform more technical exercise tests, e.g. on a bicycle ergometer or treadmill.

Exercise is sometimes deliberately used to induce airway narrowing.

A peak flow recording is taken prior to a vigorous run in an enclosed corridor, walking on a treadmill or cycling on a bicycle ergometer. This activity is then followed by serial peak flow readings, which will often unmask exercise-induced asthma.

Auscultation

Using a stethoscope

Listening to a chest through a stethoscope is a necessary skill when treating acutely ill children and the skill can only be acquired by practice.

Paediatric stethoscopes are available and are recommended for listening to the neonate and small baby.

The most obvious sounds heard on first applying the stethoscope are often the heart sounds, because of the relatively large size of heart in comparison to lungs in the infant. The breath sounds are similar in character to those of adults, e.g. normal (vesicular) sounds and added sounds such as wheezes and crackles (formerly rhonchi or râles) etc.

Table 17.6 Normal lung function values for FVC, FEV$_1$ and PEFR in healthy boys and girls of European descent derived from the regression equations of Cotes (1975) Gas volumes in BTPS

Height (cm)	FEV$_1$ (litres)		FVC (litres)		PEFR (1/min)
	Boys	Girls	Boys	Girls	Boys and Girls
100	0.81	0.79	1.00	0.95	124
105	0.93	0.90	1.15	1.07	146
110	1.06	1.02	1.30	1.21	169
115	1.19	1.15	1.47	1.36	191
120	1.35	1.30	1.65	1.52	215
125	1.51	1.45	1.84	1.69	237
130	1.68	1.61	2.05	1.88	260
135	1.86	1.79	2.27	2.07	283
140	2.06	1.97	2.50	2.28	305
145	2.27	2.17	2.76	2.49	328
150	2.49	2.38	3.02	2.72	351
155	2.73	2.61	3.31	2.97	374
160	2.98	2.84	3.60	3.22	397
165	3.25	3.09	3.92	3.49	420
170	3.53	3.35	4.25	3.78	442
175	3.83	3.63	4.60	4.07	465
180	4.14	3.92	4.97	4.39	487
SD	10%	10%	11%	10%	13%

FEV$_1$, forced expiratory volume in 1 second; FVC, forced vital capacity; PEFR, peak expiratory flow rate; SD, standard deviation; BTPS, body temperature and ambient pressure saturated with water vapour.

Cooperation from children

Young children are often unable to cooperate with taking deep breaths on request and babies frequently cry during auscultation. Crying can, however, be advantageous as the child will take in a large breath after a lusty cry.

Stridor

A harsh, rasping inspiratory wheeze, called stridor, may be heard in infants and is caused by obstruction around the epiglottis or upper trachea. The noise is audible without the stethoscope, and on auscultation is heard throughout the chest. It will mask any other added sounds.

Chest X-ray

Chest X-rays are difficult to perform on children as the child must lie or sit still and the young child is not able to control his breathing when asked.

Child–adult differences

Noticeable differences between a child's and an adult's chest X-ray are the rib positions, which are much more horizontal in the child, and the presence of the thymic shadow, which is shaped like a sail and may be confused with upper lobe collapse in the child (Fig. 17.13). Generally speaking, upper lobe abnormalities are more commonly seen in the infant than in the adult. This is due to the more horizontal posture of the child and the anatomical differences of airway sizes between the child and adult.

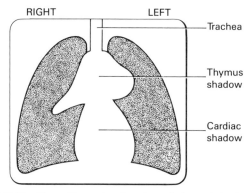

Fig. 17.13 Chest X-ray showing the sail-shaped shadow of the thymus gland.

Fractures

It is rare for young children to fracture ribs because of the cartilaginous nature of their bones. However, they do occur after severe trauma or if there is underlying pathology. Chest X-rays should therefore be checked for fractures.

CONCLUSION

The elements of assessment described above are intertwined in a complex way. No one element can be taken in isolation. In the assessment of gait the need to take into account both the child's stage of development and any respiratory disorders is stressed. Similarly, breathing patterns are discussed in the section on muscle tone.

It is hoped that by combining the four modalities the paediatric physiotherapist will be enabled to draw up a comprehensive picture of the skills and difficulties of the individual child, and hence to plan effective intervention strategies.

REFERENCES

Atkinson H W 1986 Principles of assessment. In: Downie P A (ed) Cash's textbook of neurology for physiotherapists. Faber & Faber, London

Best C H, Taylor N B T 1973 In: Brobeck J R (ed) Physiological basis of medical practice. Williams & Wilkins, Baltimore, ch 5, p 9–89

Bobath B 1983 (reprint) Adult hemiplegia: evaluation and treatment, 2nd edn. W. Heinemann, London

Butler P, Engelbrecht M, Major R E, Tait J H, Stallard J, Patrick J H 1984 Physiological cost index of walking for normal children and its use as an indicator of physical handicap. Developmental Medicine and Child Neurology 26: 607–612

Cotes J E 1975 Lung function — assessment and application in medicine, 3rd edn. Blackwell Scientific Publications, London

DeSouza L H, Musa I M 1987 The measurement and assessment of spasticity. Clinical Rehabilitation 1: 89–96

Drillien C M, Drummond M B 1977 Neurodevelopmental problems in early childhood. Blackwell, Oxford

Grimley A M D, McKinlay I A 1977 The clumsy child. The Association of Paediatric Chartered Physiotherapists Publications, Crawley

Hare N 1984 Ideas developed at the Cheyne Centre, Regeena Printing, Nottingham

Inman V T, Ralston H J, Todd F 1981 Human walking. Williams and Wilkins, Baltimore

King H A, Staheli L T 1984 Torsional problems in cerebral palsy. Foot and Ankle 4(4): 180–184

Lance J W 1980 Pathophysiology of spasticity and clinical experience with baclofen. In: Feldman R G, Young R R, Koella W P (eds) Spasticity: disordered motor control. Year Book Medical Publications, Chicago, p 485–494

Milner A D, Martin R J 1985 Neonatal and paediatric respiratory medicine. Butterworths, London

Young R R, Delwaide P J 1981 Drug therapy: spasticity. The New England Journal of Medicine 304(1)

FURTHER READING

Basmajian 1978 Muscles alive. Williams and Wilkins, Baltimore

Burus R B 1986 Child development. Croom Helm, Beckenham

Craik R L, Oatis C A 1985 Gait assessment in the clinic: issues and approaches. Measurement in Physical Therapy. Churchill Livingstone, Edinburgh

Downie P A (ed) 1987 Cash's textbook of chest, heart and vascular disorders, 4th edn. Faber and Faber, London

Godfrey S, Kamburoff P L, Nairn J R et al 1970 Spirometry, lung volumes and airway resistance in normal children aged 5–18 years. British Journal of Diseases of the Chest 64(1): 15–24

Gregory G A (ed) 1982 Respiratory failure in the child. Churchill Livingstone, Edinburgh

Griffiths M, Russell P 1985 Working together with handicapped children. Souvenir Press. London

Illingworth R S 1983 The development of the infant and young child. Churchill Livingstone, Edinburgh

Laughman R K, Askew L J, Bleimeyer R R, Chao E Y 1984 Objective clinical evaluation of function: gait analysis. Physical Therapy 64(12): 1839–1845

Law H T, Minns R A 1989 Measurement of the spatial and temporal parameters of gait. Physiotherapy 75(2): 81–84

Medeiros J 1984 Automated measurement systems for clinical motion analysis. Physical Therapy 64(12): 1846–1850

Rose G K, Butler P, Stallard J 1982 Gait. Principles, biomechanics and assessment. Orlau Publishing, Oswestry

Sharrard W J W 1979 Paediatric orthopaedics and fractures. Blackwell Scientific Publications, London

Sheridan M D 1977 Children's developmental progress. NFER Publishing, Windsor

West J B (ed) 1985 Best and Taylor's physiological basis of medical practice, 11th edn. Williams and Wilkins, Baltimore

Yack H J 1984 Techniques for clinical assessment of human movement. Physical Therapy 64(12): 1821–1830

18

Treatment systems

P. Eckersley   L. King

PRINCIPLES OF TREATMENT

Numerous philosophies can be adapted for use in the treatment of both neurological and non-neurological disorders of childhood. The concepts and objectives are wide-ranging. Some are common and complementary to each other, whilst others appear to conflict. This is particularly so in the area of early independence of mobility versus the attainment of 'correct' motor patterns.

The need to increase the number of clients and patients seen and to reduce waiting lists may lead to a policy of encouraging early functional independence. This may be to the detriment of fully establishing more 'normal' motor patterns, automatic balance responses, etc. Early mobility is also believed to help diminish the feelings of frustration in children, to motivate them, and to aid their learning.

It is essential, therefore, that great care is taken in order to:

1. Establish effective working relationships with others, both parents and professionals.
2. Develop clear guidelines and explanatory information.
3. Cooperate with alternative needs and objectives.
4. Minimise the damaging effects caused by team conflicts and confusion.

There is little empirical evidence to suggest

whether an integrative and eclectic approach or a specific concept approach is the most effective when working with children. This is a difficult question to answer. However, it is probably more helpful for the newcomer to paediatrics to work with one philosophy initially, in order to gain a measure of expertise and confidence. The therapist should always be prepared to examine and use other ideas as and when appropriate so that the therapeutic approach becomes broad based and capable of adaptation to the needs and circumstances of individual children and their families. Although 'dabbling' in concepts without any real skill or thought can invite confusion or misunderstanding, it is only by keeping minds open to new ideas and challenging older and possibly more accepted ones that the therapy approaches to the management of childhood disorders can continue to develop.

In this chapter the concepts of management are given in outline only. The choice of emphasis is personal to the authors' ideas and experiences.

A simple comparative overview follows, based upon and developed from the excellent work of Levitt (1982).

COMMON DENOMINATORS OF TREATMENT PRINCIPLES
General principles

1. Careful *assessment* and *recording* should be an *ongoing* process, not an isolated event.
2. *Realistically* planned therapeutic measures should be derived from the assessment.
3. *Early* 'treatment' should be incorporated into the daily *management* of the child.
4. *Repetition* and *reinforcement* are essential for learning and for the establishment of modified motor patterns.
5. *Maximise* sensorimotor experience (Fig. 18.1).
6. *Involvement* of the child as an active participant.
7. *Motivation* of the child is essential.
8. *Teamwork*. The multidisciplinary approach is invaluable and must include the child

and his or her family. Conflicts and confusions should be minimised by discussion and demonstration.

Specific principles

1. A consideration of *developmental training*. Philosophies differ as to whether sequences should be strictly followed or modified. (Compare Rood, Fay, Doman, Bobath, Vojta, for example.)
2. A *modification* of abnormal tone. Some schools of thought give much less emphasis to this aspect and more to functional independence.
3. The use of *afferent stimuli*.
4. The facilitation of *purposeful, active* movement (although some use passive movement also).
5. *Minimising* and *preventing* deformity.
6. *Functional independence*. The levels at which the use of compensatory movements and aids are introduced vary greatly between the philosophies.

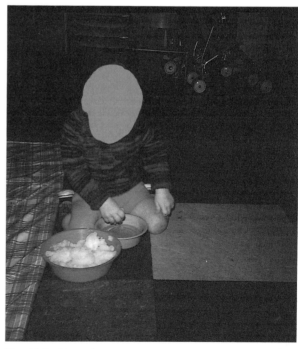

Fig. 18.1 Sensorimotor experience: the sensation of cold snow and warm water.

OUTLINES OF SELECTED MANAGEMENT SYSTEMS

Selected systems of management available to therapists are outlined below. Further reading, training and practical experience are recommended.

Phelps

Phelps was an American orthopaedic surgeon who pioneered the treatment of children with cerebral palsy and encouraged therapists to form habilitation teams. Specific treatment techniques were applied to his diagnostic classification of cerebral palsy and included muscle education and bracing. He described 15 'modalities', or phases of treatment, which were used in various combinations within his classification. The five modalities described below are central to his approach to treatment:

1. Massage, which was used for hypotonia but contraindicated for spasticity and athetosis.
2. Passive motion (movements) for joint mobilisation, maintaining soft tissue length and for demonstrating the movement required.
3. Active assisted movements, active movements, and resisted movement according to the individual's ability and needs.
4. Conditioned motion and synergistic motion involving resistance to one muscle group in order to facilitate contraction of an inactive muscle group in the same synergy, a familiar concept in proprioceptive neuromuscular facilitation (see p. 326).
5. Periods of rest were also included and their beneficial effect should not be forgotten in more recent approaches.

Braces and calipers

The use of braces and calipers was also included as a modality in Phelps' approach (Egel 1948). These were used to correct deformity, obtain the upright position and control athetosis. Their use was extensive and they were worn for many years. As the child progressed, the support was gradually removed until, finally, where possible the child used only below-knee irons and boots. More recently, this extensive bracing was considered by some to be detrimental to the child and the use of all types of bracing and splinting in the management of children is now very carefully assessed and monitored. Many authorities would now consider the use of bracing and splintage, providing it has been carefully designed for a particular purpose and for a specific individual (Fig. 18.2).

Physical principles, as well as the neurophysiological standpoint (balance reactions) suggest that, if the base is unstable, the rest of the body will have difficulty in gaining segmental balance and control (i.e. in standing: head on trunk, on pelvis, on feet). In this situation the body segments must make a compensatory adaptation to accommodate the unstable base. This compensation can be seen when observing the standing position of a child with hemiplegia or diplegia. The child stands on one leg with the foot of the weight bearing leg held flat, and the other ankle held plantar flexed with the ball of the foot on the floor and the hip inwardly rotated. Correction of the posture so that pelvic and shoulder girdles are level and the head is in midline cannot occur easily or naturally from such a base. In these circum-

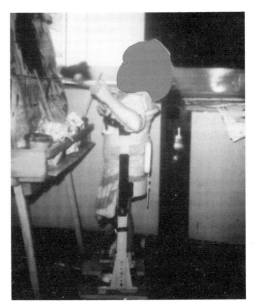

Fig. 18.2 Use of a standing frame during painting.

stances the use of an ankle foot orthosis (see Chapter 21 Aids and Appliances) or serial splinting (see Chapter 19 Treatment Methods) would be relevant to Phelps' philosophy.

Proprioceptive neuromuscular facilitation (PNF)

This technique of facilitation was devised by Kabat, Knott and Voss, in America, between 1946 and 1951 in response to the need to rehabilitate patients following poliomyelitis (Knott & Voss 1972). The majority of British-trained physiotherapists will be familiar with at least the basic premises of the technique.

There are eight basic components of PNF technique:

- patterns of movement
- stretch
- manual contact
- joint position
- verbal stimulus
- timing
- reinforcement
- maximal resistance.

Patterns of movement. Muscle action is more efficient when working in patterns. These patterns are three-fold:

1. Movements are diagonal and rotational.
2. Movements in distal joints follow those of proximal joints.
3. Movement commences with the rotatory component.

Stretch. By putting skeletal muscles on the stretch, the actions produced by the vast majority of muscles are in a diagonal direction and involve rotation (Waddington 1984). This stretch stimulus results in a more efficient and dynamic action. The movement in pattern starts with the muscle at the limit of its extensibility and is completed when the muscle is fully shortened.

Manual contact. The therapist's hands are placed on the limb to be moved in a position allowing him or her to lead the movement and to provide an appropriate level of resistance. Firm, comfortable contact through the palm of the hand is used.

Joint position. Traction is used to facilitate flexion, i.e. lifting, and joint approximation is used to facilitate extension, i.e. pushing.

Verbal stimulus. The therapist provides verbal encouragement by talking the patient through the movement pattern and motivating each degree of success.

Timing. All components of the movement pattern are carried out with a rhythmic flow.

Reinforcement. The action of the weaker muscles is facilitated by using patterns involving stronger muscle groups. The action of the stronger muscle leads to overflow into the weaker.

Maximal resistance. In order to gain the potential of a muscle it must be exercised maximally in all parts of its range (Waddington 1984). The level of resistance must be such that the patient can move in a smooth coordinated way. This can be achieved by using high resistance over a low number of repetitions or minimal resistance over a high number of repetitions.

PNF techniques

These eight components can be applied to a number of PNF techniques of which the three described below have been used by the author (P.E.).

- repeated contraction
- slow reversals
- hold–relax.

Repeated contractions. A muscle works more strongly after a slight stretch. In this way abduction of the shoulder using the deltoid muscle could be encouraged in order to develop a child's saving reaction through arm propping. Deltoid could be worked in a pattern of flexion/abduction/lateral rotation. The instructions would be:

- pull up
- hold (slight stretch by therapist)
- pull up (cycle of instructions repeated as necessary).

This movement would be repeated over the range of the pattern.

Slow reversals. A muscle works more strongly

after its antagonist has worked hard and in this situation the pattern of the stronger muscle group is used first. Weak finger and wrist extensors can be strengthened by first working wrist and finger flexors, and the movements would then alternate without relaxation between the patterns of flexion and extension. This technique can be helpful in preparing a child for the activities of grasping and releasing a toy, or for constructional activities.

Hold–relax. A muscle relaxes maximally following maximal resistance. Where a child has tight adductors relaxation can be enabled by:

- taking the legs to the limit of abduction
- actively resisting static adduction
- allowing supported relaxation to take place in this position
- passively abducting the hips to the new limit.

This process is repeated a number of times.

Application

A major obstacle in the use of PNF techniques has been that the use of maximal resistance in patterns of adduction and internal rotation may reinforce patterns of spasticity in the child with a neurological deficit. However, therapists are now taking a fresh look at the technique and its possibilities. The author (P.E.) has found that progress may be achieved using PNF techniques with children with spina bifida, and may also help some children with athetosis. As with all treatment systems the physiotherapist must be guided by continuous assessment and an awareness of the desired outcomes. Thorough training in the method makes it more effective and also increases the therapist's confidence and ability to adapt the techniques into play and exercise activities.

Brunnstrom

Most of Signe Brunnstrom's work has been with adult hemiplegia, but her views are included here in summary. Her work has been thoroughly documented over many years (Brunnstrom 1956, 1962, 1970).

In this system, movement is produced by provoking primitive motor patterns on synergistic movement patterns and later by training conscious volition of movement. Control of the head, neck and trunk is promoted by stimulating the tonic neck, labyrinthine and lumbar reflexes with the facilitation of righting reflexes and balance training being encouraged later.

Brunnstrom also uses associated reactions and hand reactions, e.g. extension of the thumb reduces flexor hypertension of the fingers.

Much emphasis is placed upon the use of sensory stimulation including proprioception.

The Rood approach

This approach is based upon the work of Margaret Rood, an American physiotherapist and occupational therapist.

Rood's basic premise is that motor patterns are developed from fundamental reflex patterns, which are present at birth. These are used and modified through sensory stimuli until the highest control is gained at the conscious cortical level. If the correct sensory stimulus is applied using the appropriate sensory receptor (as it is used in normal sequential development), it should be possible to elicit motor responses reflexly and, by repetition, gain correct movement patterns.

Theoretical components

The five major components of the theory are:

1. Normalisation of tone and stimulation of normal motor responses, achieved reflexly by using appropriate sensory stimuli.
2. Sensorimotor control is developmentally based and thus therapy begins at the child's current level of development and progresses in sequence to higher levels.
3. The movements should be purposeful, with the child's attention being directed towards the end goal (not the pattern of movement).
4. Repetition of sensorimotor responses is essential for learning.
5. Facilitatory and inhibitory techniques are carried out within the movement sequences.

This method has been underused in the United Kingdom in recent years although Goff (1969,

1972) advocates its adoption as a valuable treatment.

Treatment sequence

There are four phases to the treatment sequence:

- skin stimulation
- weight bearing
- movement
- developmental sequence.

The facilitation of wrist and finger extension is used as an ongoing example in the sequence described below.

Skin stimulation. Techniques of skin stimulation facilitate muscle action through the relationship between dermatomes and myotomes. The afferent stimuli from a sensory input prepares the muscle for contraction by raising receptivity. The sensory techniques described by Rood must be carried out in a well-defined manner and are frequently applied by fast brushing using the hand or soft bristles:

- the stimulus must change rapidly
- a period of stimulus should be limited to 3 seconds in any one place
- each period of stimulus should only be repeated two to three times in any one place
- there is a delay of 30 seconds before any effect is seen (Goff 1969).

The use of skin stimulation alone can be useful in working with children with spasticity. Slow stroking over the back has a central inhibitory effect, and stroking over the lateral outer third of the forehead can inhibit a Moro response. Stroking not only raises the receptivity of the prime mover, but also relaxes the antagonistic muscle group. This can be particularly helpful when working with children with tightly fisted hands. Stroking the dorsum of the hand and extensor surface of the forearm encourages flexor relaxation and is a useful preparation for fine motor activities, self-help skills and play.

Ice can be used briefly immediately before other stimuli. It is particularly successful for extension and for skilled movements, particularly those of the lips and tongue. Considerable care should be taken when using ice as many children find it both uncomfortable and distressing. It should never be used behind the ear, on the sole of the foot, on the back, or on the left shoulder.

Weight bearing. Deep pressure is given along the long axis of the limb using counter-pressure at each end. This stimulates the mechanisms of weight bearing both by facilitating deep postural muscles and inhibiting spastic muscles.

Pressure at the heel of the hand and counter-pressure at the elbow would be used following the stroking of the dorsum of the hand and forearm described above (see Fig. 18.3).

Weight bearing can be modified by:

1. Pressure through tapping may be given — tapping the lateral malleolus activates the everters (Goff 1969).
2. Compression can be given by squeezing the child's hand whilst a cone is grasped in the hand with the wide end towards the medial palm (little finger).

Movement. Weight bearing and pressure is followed by a simple movement that takes place with the distal extremity of the limb fixed. Compression through the forearm would therefore be followed by a game of pushing or by using a toy activated by pressure or squashing. The child's hand remains in one position whilst the trunk and shoulder move over and around the hand.

Developmental sequence. The final phase of the sequence is a purposeful activity appropriate

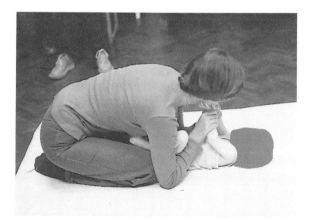

Fig. 18.3 Encouraging a child to push with arms using pressure at the heel of the hand with support and counterpressure at the elbow.

to the developmental level of the child such as grasping a toy, painting or feeling textures and shapes. It takes place using compression throughout, and the position of the therapist's hands is instrumental in guiding and enabling movements to take place. Counter-pressure would continue to be given between the elbow and heel of the hand whilst encouraging the child to reach and carry out the activity, for example, drawing.

Application

The use of sensory afferent stimuli is a component of a number of treatment systems and methods (see page 324 and Chapter 19 Treatment Methods). The author (P.E.) has found the Rood treatment sequence described above particularly helpful when working with children with cerebral palsy, both for achieving hand use and, in an adapted form based on bench-sitting, for encouraging dorsiflexion and standing. It can be used in conjunction with an exercise programme following serial splinting of the foot (see Chapter 19 Treatment Methods). Compression and joint approximation are possible in a number of body positions to which Rood techniques can be applied. Pelvic girdle stability can be developed in crook lying and that of the shoulder girdle in prone forearm support.

Temple Fay

In Temple Fay's philosophy, the child is taught to move according to evolutionary development and Fay suggests that human ontogenic development is based on phylogenetic development in the evolution of the species. Thus, he contended that movement sequences should be built up from reptilian squirming and amphibian creeping, through mammalian quadripedal reciprocal movement (reciprocal movement on all fours), to the erect walking of the primates. He believed that as lower order animals with simple nervous systems could carry out squirming and creeping movements, so the human who has an abnormal cerebral cortex should be able to perform the same patterns.

These creeping movements are taught initially with passive movements known as patterning. The child is later encouraged to perform them alone. The movement patterns are developmental and Fay suggested that they should be followed in strict sequence of:

- prone lying — head and trunk rotation
- primitive homolateral creeping
- contralateral creeping (Fig. 18.4)
- crawling
- elephant walk on hands and feet
- walking pattern.

Another aspect of this system used extensively with young people with severe head injuries by the author (L.K.), is the use of unlocking reflexes to reduce hypertonus.

Doman–Delacato

The system described by Glen Doman and Carl Delacato includes the basic tenets postulated by Fay and described above, but adds other factors

Position 1

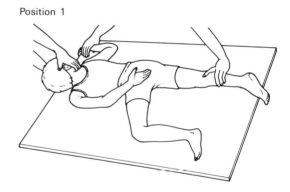

Position 2

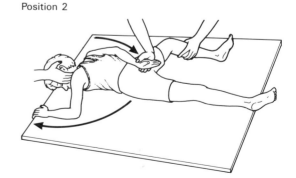

Fig. 18.4 Contralateral creeping pattern: pattern alternates rhythmically between positions 1 and 2.

such as restriction of fluid intake, the development of cerebral hemispheric dominance and the encouragement of deep breathing and breathing control using periods of CO_2 inhalations (by rebreathing).

This system has caused concern to some because it is costly both financially and in terms of numbers of people. It may also appear to place added stress upon family units and their helpers. However, many parents find the techniques helpful and welcome the positive belief that there is always something they can do to help. The authors feel that physiotherapists should keep an open mind so that parents feel supported and encouraged in their choice of method.

Doman and Delacato consider that damage occurring in the brain results in disorganisation of sensory experience and of motor function. They believe that by highly systematic movement and sensory input the undamaged brain cells can be stimulated, resulting in sensory and motor integration (Doman & Doman 1960).

The motor and sensory modalities of input are:

- motor
  — mobility
  — manual skill
  — language
- sensory
  — tactile competence
  — understanding of sound
  — visual competence.

Treatment techniques

The programme established would contain a sequence of activities for each of the above modalities, the predominance of any one modality being dependent on individual assessment. It is usually recommended that the programme sequence is repeated every 2 hours and frequently volunteers as well as family are needed to carry out this sequence. Temple Fay patterns form a central component of the mobility modality and, as with all passive movements, great care must be taken in assessing levels of spasticity, possible pain or discomfort, safety during head movements and the condition of hip, knee and shoulder joints.

Brachiation is used in developing manual skills and is a form of ladder-walking, with the child hanging by the arms from a horizontal ladder above head height. One author (P.E.) has found this both helpful and motivating when working with older boys with hemiplegia and diplegia. Considerable trunk rotation is required for brachiation which results in reduction of central spasticity.

Flash cards are used from an early age in the development of visual competence. These flash cards progress from dot patterns to familiar shapes such as animals, and to letters and words.

The Vojta approach

An approach that is not well known in the United Kingdom, but which merits consideration, is that developed by Vaslav Vojta, based on the work of Fay and Kabat (Vojta 1974). The main features of this concept are:

1. Reflex creeping and rolling.
2. The use of afferent sensory stimulation through touch, stretch and pressure for facilitation of movement.
3. 'Triggering' — the use of resistance to provoke either a tonic or a phasic muscle action and rising reactions.

Collis

A British pioneer, Eirene Collis, postulated a number of practical and constructive tenets (Collis 1953):

1. Early treatment was advocated, in the belief that this would aid a more beneficial outcome.
2. The physiotherapist should conduct a scheme of management of the child throughout the day, rather than sessional 'treatments'.
3. Dressing, feeding, toileting and washing should be included in the treatment programme.

Collis also considered that the child should follow a strict developmental sequence and should not be permitted to perform motor skills beyond his or her developmental level. This would be challenged today on the following basis:

1. Although a general sequence can be helpful, children rarely develop at precisely the same rate or in the same sequence (e.g. some children crawl, but others bottom-shuffle).
2. In order to achieve one level of development the child needs to have progressed to a higher level (e.g. balance in sitting is not fully established until standing is attained, and so on).
3. Children may become frustrated when their experiments with movement are curtailed or their participation is not sought, and lack of motivation may ensue.

Collis established the idea of a 'cerebral palsy therapist'. This was further developed, especially in recent work such as that of the conductor in conductive education, and the idea of amalgamating occupational therapy and physiotherapy.

Conductive education

This concept was developed in Hungary by Professor Peto from 1945 onwards, and the work now continues in Budapest at the Institute for the Motor Disabled which he established in 1952. The philosophy was introduced into the United Kingdom in the late 1960s and early 1970s by Cotton (1970).

The system of conductive education is one of total integration. Peto did not view children with cerebral dysfunction as merely having a motor disability, but rather that they also have resulting changes in personality and reduced ability for spontaneous adaptation, and thus problems of learning. The concept which has evolved is essentially educational rather than medical.

Children work in groups selected according to their age, needs and ability. It is hoped that these groups will increase motivation and socialisation and provide an optimal environment for learning. The operators of these groups are called the conductors, who in Hungary have become a unique new professional group whose task it is to stimulate learning.

The child learns how to function through movement. Careful task analyses of each functional activity are made and the child then works through task-series (built up from task parts) until the end goal is reached. The task and task parts are taught by the use of facilitation — rhythmical intention. This term is used to describe how language is used to plan, intend and carry out a movement by starting it in words. The intention does not vary, although how it is achieved by the child may. When the movements become automatic, new intention for a new movement is introduced (see p. 333).

Philosophical background

Conductive education is an educational approach aimed at teaching children with motor disorders how to overcome their problems of movement and control and live with a degree of independence. The process of progress towards these goals is known as orthofunction (Read 1991). Orthofunction is the determination to succeed which equips the person with the physical and mental capacity to live and adapt into home, school and the working environment. It is not what is learned, but how it is learned (Todd 1990).

Professor Peto developed a system which integrated all aspects of a child's day into a unified approach which combines treatment, education, self-help skills and social skills. In order to ensure this unified approach a child's whole day is planned, guided and monitored by a single professional, the conductor, who has the responsibility for all aspects of development.

Active participation of the child. Although the day is planned by the conductor the active participation and initiative of the child is central to Peto's philosophy. He believed that all movement starts with the intention of the person who is to perform that movement, and that this intention in turn stems from a desired goal. Conductive education aims to promote and expand the goals which individual children have and hence to develop their individual intention to move and to learn. It is an active system which increases a child's own spontaneity and involvement in the day, which links all treatment and learning to purposeful functional activity. In this way the child always has an understanding both of what he or she is doing, and why it is necessary to do it. It is a system which seeks to change intention rather than performance and which describes intention as a general animation of our personal organisation (Hari 1988).

There are three central components to the conductive education system:

- task series
- rhythmical intention
- daily routines through group activity.

Task series

The activities of daily life and of learning form a sequence of events for the child from waking to sleeping. It is one of the roles of the conductor to analyse this sequence of events and break it down into its component parts.

The child is then guided individually, or in a group, to the successful completion of each component. The whole pattern of life through the day becomes an opportunity both to learn and to practise motor skills. Each functional activity is analysed and broken down into its individual elements or stages known as a task series.

There would therefore be a task series for activities such as:

- rolling over in bed
- sitting on a potty
- rising from sitting to standing (Fig. 18.5)
- putting a coat on (Fig. 18.6)
- holding a pencil
- drinking from a cup.

The challenge for the conductor is to identify those skills which are useful in the greatest number of ways or the greatest number of times (Kinsman et al 1988). In this way sitting on the potty can be generalised to independent box-sitting, sitting listening to a story, sitting to have a meal and sitting as preparation to standing. The child becomes motivated to succeed because each task series has an immediate relevance and significance to the child and to a practical situation.

A task series for sitting at a table holding on is given in Table 18.1.

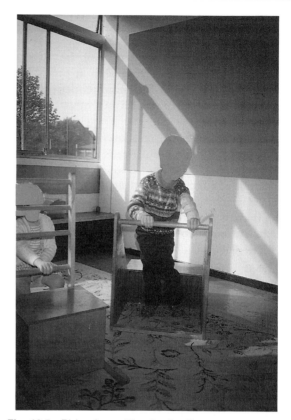

Fig. 18.5 Rising from sitting to standing.

The process is not a passive one but one in which the child shares the process of problem-solving to develop the task series and is

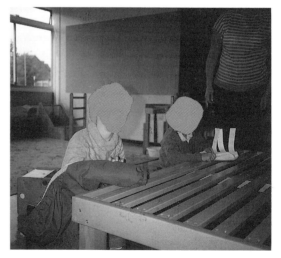

Fig. 18.6 Putting a coat on.

Table 18.1 Task series for sitting at a table

Child's bottom at back of chair

Thighs in contact with chair

Knees at right angles

Feet flat on floor

Back held upright

Head aligned with shoulders

Eyes looking straight ahead

Hands on the table

Hands holding on to the table slats

encouraged to initiate the activity for him or herself. The child learns to organise and plan his or her own movements.

Rhythmical intention

Rhythmical intention is the guidance of speech or inner speech which is used to direct conscious action. Each specific goal or activity is always reached through the same task series and verbal intention so that repetition reinforces the learning process (Todd 1990). The conductor designs a phrase or instruction for each part of the task series. The following sequence of events then takes place:

1. The conductor speaks the first phrase of the task series.
2. The conductor and child or group repeat the phrase.
3. The conductor and child or group repeat the phrase a second time.
4. The action is performed whilst the action word is repeated.

In conductive education it is considered that the repetition of the action in words before the action takes place prepares the motor set for that movement and also that by performing the movement *only* during the action word spastic patterns are inhibited. In the early years all activities are regulated by adult speech, but as the child gets older and skills develop this verbal reinforcement is taken over completely by the child. In this way the child's understanding of the motor plan develops as well as his or her motor memory and personal autonomy. Once a task is learned the

counting can be discarded (Cotton & Kinsman 1983).

The rhythmical intention for the first stage of the task series shown in Table 18.1 is given in Table 18.2.

Daily routines for group activity

Each part of the day is used as a learning situation and complex programmes of activity are developed which shape the group's daily routines. Conductive education uses a group setting as its means of teaching, of motivation, and of developing social skills. The essential feature of the group is the ability of the group members to develop effective interpersonal relationships (Todd 1990). Each small item in the task series must have a context in group activity or it will become an arid exercise or an empty session (Hari 1988).

The activities of the group bring the task series to life and each child is given the time and opportunity to show his or her skills to the group (Fig. 18.7). Activities are designed for success. It is in the group that play and learning take place. A task series for pressing and turning may become a session on collage in art; a task series for pushing a ball might develop into objects which roll and a lesson on circles and shapes; and one for grasp and release can be a stage in progression to building, counting bricks and number work.

The conductor, who combines the multiprofessional roles of physiotherapist, speech therapist and teacher, would select activities appropriate for the group which build into a daily programme which incorporates all aspects of child learning and development.

Table 18.2 Rhythmical intention for task element 'Child's bottom at back of chair'

Speaker	Verbal intention
Conductor	My bottom is on the chair
Conductor and Group	My bottom is on the chair
Conductor	I push my bottom back
Conductor and Group	I push my bottom back
Conductor and Group	I push my bottom back back *BACK**

* The movement only takes place when the word *BACK* is spoken

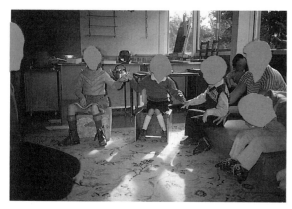

Fig. 18.7 Activities in a group.

Equipment

Conductive education does not advocate the use of wheelchairs, calipers or equipment unless essential. Children are encouraged to perform appropriate activities as independently as possible or with the help and guidance of one or more conductors. They are given as much time as they need to complete each task for themselves. Two types of equipment have, however, become known as Peto equipment: the ladder-back chair and the slatted bench (see Fig. 18.5). These are used on the basis that, both to move in lying and to support the trunk and shoulder girdle in sitting, a child will need many points of support to grasp, push, reach for and pull up to in order to move independently. The Peto bench and chair provide these numerous pivots and points of reference. The ladder-back chair is also used as a walking aid.

Conductive education is a holistic approach to the disabled child in which a motor disorder is seen as a learning difficulty to overcome rather than a condition to be treated (Hari 1988).

The Bobath concept

The Bobath concept is arguably the most familiar and widely used approach known to British physiotherapists working with children with neurological disorders. It originated in the 1940s and early 1950s and has subsequently been developed and modified by herself, Dr K. Bobath and the staff of the Bobath Centre.

Philosophy

The approach was originally based on neurodevelopmental principles which view development as:

- dynamic
- sequential
- cephalocaudal
- proximal to distal
- automatic before conscious
- responsive and adaptive.

The basic premise is that a child in the first few months of life undergoes a maturation of the central nervous system. At first the child is dominated by reflex, unconscious movement patterns, but gradually these involuntary movements become part of conscious experience; they become controlled, rhythmical and coordinated. Once the child is able to control movement at a particular level of maturation, the developmental process then moves on to the next level.

For the child with a neurological disorder, however, the maturation of his or her central nervous system has been arrested at a particular level and the child is unable to progress beyond it. This means that stereotypical primitive reactions and responses become obligatory and the adaptive coordinated development of more skilled movements does not take place.

Basic principles

The Bobaths outlined a number of basic principles which should be incorporated into any treatment approach intended to overcome the above problems. These are:

- patterns of movement
- use of handling
- prerequisites for movement.

Patterns of movement. Movements work in patterns, and it is patterns which are represented at cortical level rather than isolated muscle activity. It is therefore essential that all activities designed to increase movement skills should be based on developmentally appropriate movement patterns. The child with cerebral palsy may acquire movement patterns in a number of ways:

- by retaining primitive reflexes and reactions
- by developing abnormal patterns of movement because of restricted movement possibilities
- by compensating or adapting to abnormal movements.

These restricted movement patterns may themselves become limiting and prevent the aquisition of more skilled, responsive movements. The more the child uses an abnormal pattern the more it becomes part of the child's movement vocabulary. In this way a pattern of walking on the toes with inwardly rotated hips and flexed knees becomes the only way of walking which feels right to the child. Correct walking is therefore not just a matter of learning a new way, but of also unlearning the incorrect way. When using the Bobath approach the physiotherapist would aim to ensure that all movement patterns are learned in a more normal manner. The quality of the movement is as important as its performance.

As movement is created in patterns the action of any one muscle group will result in an adaptive response from all other muscle groups in the body. In this way the act of opening the mouth to speak may result in a loss of control over the pelvic girdle; reaching for a toy may cause plantar flexion in the ankle of the opposite leg. The greater the effort required to perform any individual movement the greater these responses will be.

It is therefore important that abnormal inappropriate movement patterns are recognised and that therapy programmes are designed to overcome them. Normal responsive and effective patterns are then encouraged and developed.

Use of handling. These responsive and effective patterns of movement are developed through the use of special handling techniques. During treatment sessions the physiotherapist becomes part of the sensory input system of the child, and handling is a constant interplay between the therapist and the reactions of the child. The Bobath concept of handling aims to normalise tone, improve co-ordination of posture and movement, and develop skilled, adaptive responses.

In this way the child is helped and guided to improve the quality of movement rather than being left to struggle on his or her own. Automatic movements are the basis of all motor sequences and are therefore facilitated in the first instance, the child responding to skilled handling more easily than to spoken requests.

Prerequisites for movement. The Bobaths listed three factors, or prerequisites, for efficient movement (Table 18.3) (Bobath 1971).

1. Normal postural tone is necessary to resist gravity whilst at the same time allowing movement to take place.
2. Reciprocal innervation to muscle groups enables the action of agonists and antagonists to be coordinated and balanced.
3. Postural fixation is necessary so that central muscle groups can give stability whilst dynamic movement takes place in more distal parts of the body.

Bobath concepts

A dynamic management concept has been developed from these basic principles in which the responses of the child are guided through handling towards the achievement of consistent sensorimotor goals. These special techniques of handling also counteract the abnormal patterns of tonic reflex activity (Bobath 1983).

The cyclical pattern described below could be incorporated into any therapy session (Fig. 18.8).

Inhibition. Reflex inhibiting patterns (RIPs) are used to reduce abnormal reflex activity and associated reactions and to overcome abnormal tone. By passively rotating or rocking the body

Table 18.3 Prerequisites for movement: handwriting

Prerequisite	Resultant skill
Normal postural tone	Independent upright sitting balance
Reciprocal innervation	Finger flexors and extensors enable movement of pencil to form letters or shapes Shoulder abductors and adductors enable movement of pencil across page
Postural fixation	Shoulder girdle stability Wrist and elbow stability

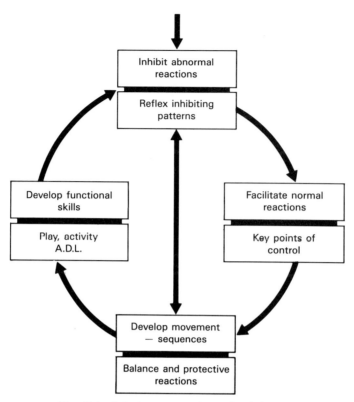

Fig. 18.8 Bobath concepts: the cycle of therapy.

in a range of sequences the normalisation of tone is promoted. These sequences are constantly evolving through therapy practice and frequently:

- the least affected part is worked on first
- handling begins proximally.

Thus, the reduction of spasticity in the hand might first be encouraged by working on the movements of the shoulder girdle.

It is neither necessary nor desirable for therapists to use static reflex inhibiting postures by passively reversing the abnormal patterns and controlling and holding every part of the patient's body. Though this reduces spasticity, it makes active and more normal movements impossible (Bobath 1983). Instead the RIP is used throughout the performance of an activity to inhibit an inappropriate return of altered muscle tone associated reactions and abnormal movement patterns. In this way RIPs are incorporated into therapy both as a preparation for active movement and as a support for control of its

performance. Examples of RIPs are shown in Table 18.4 and Figure 18.9.

Table 18.4 Examples of RIPs

Pattern of increased tone	RIP	Supplementary RIP
Flexor spasticity shoulder and arm	Neck extension Spinal extension External rotation shoulder Extended elbow	Wrist extension Supination Abduction thumb
Extensor spasticity trunk and neck (see Fig. 18.9)	Hip flexion Protraction shoulder girdle Hip abduction	Internal rotation shoulder Trunk flexion Neck flexion Jaw retraction
Extensor spasticity trunk and legs	Retraction shoulder girdle Hip flexion Hip abduction	External rotation hip Flexion trunk Flexion knees Dorsiflexion toes and ankles

All of the above patterns can usefully be combined with rotation of the shoulder girdle against the pelvic girdle

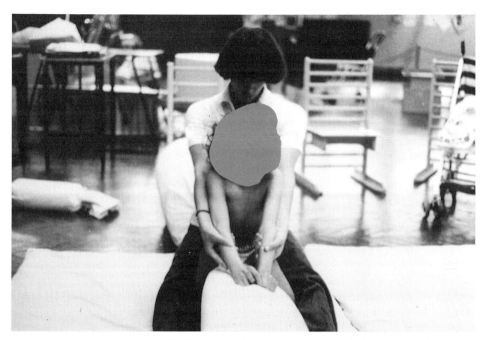

Fig. 18.9 One reflex inhibiting pattern for extensor spasticity in trunk and neck.

Key points of control. Key points of control are those parts of the body at which handling by the therapist normalises tone and guides normal active movement. As with RIPs the key points of control are frequently proximal (Fig. 18.10).

Facilitation. Facilitation is used to enable the child to:

1. Achieve a more normal postural background for movement.

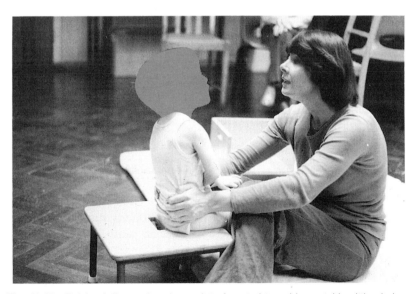

Fig. 18.10 Pelvic girdle used as key point of control to achieve stable sitting balance.

2. Develop righting and equilibrium reactions (Fig. 18.11).
3. Develop fundamental movement patterns on which more skilled activities can be built.
4. Adapt to movement during its performance.

The input from the therapist is carefully graded and is based on a careful and detailed assessment of the motor responses of the child. Treatment becomes an ongoing and reciprocal interchange between the actions of the therapist and the response of the child. The therapist must be guided by the child's reaction (Bobath & Bobath 1964). This assessment will have led to a choice of RIP and appropriate key points of control for the performance of movement. The motor support and sensory stimuli given by the therapist must be sufficient to gain a response but must not prevent the child's active participation in the movement. They must also take into account:

1. The child's developmental level (without adhering rigidly to it, e.g. early standing may be promoted to encourage back extension and head control).
2. The way in which a child without a disability would perform that movement.

A sound knowledge of normal movement is paramount to the therapist. The action of moving from lying to sitting has been chosen as an example of the facilitation of movement.

> **CASE HISTORY**
>
> Example of one approach to developing a child's ability to move from lying to sitting.
>
> Two factors must be taken into account when planning to facilitate this action.
>
> Developmentally a child will achieve sitting by rotating to one side and *not* by performing a 'sit-up'. It is easier for a child with any disability to start a movement from a position of most control over gravity.
>
> Therefore:
> * the movement may first be facilitated from sitting to lying
> * the movement may be facilitated through rotation.
>
> The position of the therapist in relation to the child must also be considered. Whilst facilitating the movement from sitting to lying it is important that extensor spasticity does not occur and therefore that head control is not lost. As eye contact with the child is important throughout the movement the therapist must be positioned in such a way that his or her eyes and those of the child are on the same level. Any extensor spasticity can also be controlled by ensuring that the hips are flexed and abducted and by using the shoulders as a key point of control. As the child develops control of the movement the key point can move to the elbows and subsequently to wrists. At each stage the therapist must stop and wait for the child's motor response and must facilitate the child's return to upright sitting before any loss of control takes place. Only when the movement from sitting to lying has been achieved with control throughout the range can lying be used as a starting position, with chin retraction, shoulder protraction together with shoulder girdle rotation continuing to be achieved through the key points of control.

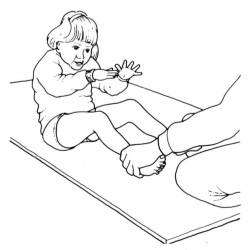

Fig. 18.11 Developing righting and equilibrium reactions.

Proprioceptive stimulation. Proprioceptive stimulation can be used as an adjunct to facilitation where the child has low muscle tone, where weak muscles underly spasticity, or where the child has a lack of sensorimotor experience. The techniques of pressure and/or tapping can be used in combination with the techniques of facilitation.

In the example given above, pressure through the pelvic girdle in sitting can be used to achieve postural stability prior to and during movement (see Fig. 18.10). In the final stages of the facilitation it may also be used, for example, to encourage the child to push him or herself into sitting with one hand on the floor. The key point of the shoulder is used to give pressure through the long axis of the arm to promote weight bearing.

Tapping is used to give intermittent input to enable the child to maintain a position. By tapping the posterior aspect of the shoulder and the triceps muscle the child may be stimulated to maintain weight-bearing on the supporting arm. The stimulus is given at a speed which is rapid enough to prevent loss of control, but slow enough to allow the child to react. As control increases the stimulus can decrease in frequency. As with all techniques of facilitation the balance between support and independence must be achieved.

Movement sequences and functional skills. All techniques of inhibition and facilitation are used to develop purposeful movement sequences and functional skills. Movement sequences are varied and flexible and should not be followed rigidly. However, the following form a basis for consideration:

• rolling
• lying to sitting
• prone lying to forearm support to all fours
• all fours to high kneel
• high kneel to stand
• sitting to standing.

Balance and protective reactions:

• transfer of weight on all fours
• arm support in sitting
• trunk balance in sitting
• transfer of weight in high kneel
• transfer of weight in standing
• protective leg extension in standing.

As with all activities the child must understand the reason for achieving these basic skills and be motivated through play and purposeful activity.

Discussions with parents and carers can lead to practical and relevant objectives being included where inhibitory and facilitatory techniques have a direct impact on dressing,

undressing and toileting. It is essential that children are 'managed' throughout the day and everyone involved should ideally be taught appropriate handling for each child.

Equipment

The Bobath approach is one which first and foremost uses direct handling of the child. However, some items of equipment may on occasion be used as additional tools to achieve movement skills, for example:

• the large therapy ball (Fig. 18.12)
• the 'sausage' roll (see Fig. 18.9)
• the hoop.

The equipment is only used as an adjunct to handling, for example, as a means of maintaining central stability so that more skilled distal movements can take place, or to promote automatic balance reactions.

AN ECLECTIC APPROACH

As stated at the beginning of the chapter there is little empirical evidence as to whether an integrative and eclectic approach or a specific concept approach is the most effective when working with children. Whilst the choice is one for the paediatric therapist to make it should

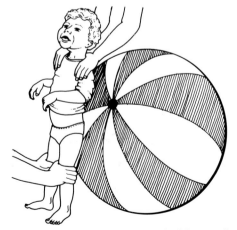

Fig. 18.12 Use of large therapy ball for standing. Note the legs held in abduction and lateral rotation with support of knee joints. Trunk and pelvis aligned through contact with therapy ball.

always be based on the needs of each individual child and his or her circumstances.

There is a danger that an overview of the various approaches to and philosophies of paediatric physiotherapy serves to emphasise those aspects which differentiate rather than those which are shared. It appears to the authors that there are a number of common factors to all approaches and philosophies, even where their implementation and emphasis may differ. They are:

- assessment and planning is necessary at all stages
- early treatment is essential
- team work is important
- the child must be motivated and involved
- parents should be involved and supported.

During treatment:

1. Neurodevelopmental sequences should be considered but not followed rigidly.
2. Postural mechanisms and normal postural tone should be developed involving
   — postural fixation
   — antigravity mechanisms
   — righting reactions
   — equilibrium reactions.
3. Deformity should be prevented.
4. Afferent stimuli can be used
   — touch
   — temperature
   — vision
   — pressure
   — stretch
   — hearing.
5. Sensorimotor experiences should be encouraged
   — voluntary skilled movement
   — cognition
   — perception
   — function.
6. Gross motor activities generally precede fine motor movements.
7. Repetition and reinforcement are necessary.
8. The development of movement should lead to purposeful activity and independent function.

CONCLUSION

Physiotherapists interested in paediatrics should strive to keep informed of new advances in techniques and neurophysiological understanding. Equally, they should continue to develop their own ideas, and be prepared to question and challenge and to be questioned and challenged.

In this chapter we have attempted to identify and introduce a few of the main concepts of treatment. In the final analysis the approaches which are adopted will inevitably be influenced by the personal views, experiences and training of the individual therapist. One concept has not been recommended as being superior to another, nor has every available treatment approach been covered. This chapter is essentially, a starting point for the therapist to explore different concepts and philosophies and thereby identify effective treatment strategies for individual children.

AUTHORS' COMMENTS

The authors have given their own perspective on and interpretation of these methods. Any misinterpretations of any method or concept are the responsibility of the authors and in all circumstances the reader is encouraged to gain further information from source material and relevant practitioners.

REFERENCES

Bobath B 1983 Adult hemiplegia: evaluation and treatment. Heinemann Medical, London
Bobath K 1971 The normal postural reflex mechanism and its deviation in children with cerebral palsy. Physiotherapy: Reprint
Bobath B, Bobath K 1964 The facilitation of normal postural reactions and movements in the treatment of cerebral palsy. Physiotherapy 50(8): 246
Brunnstrom S 1956 Methods used to elicit, reinforce and coordinate muscular response — upper motor neurone lesions. American Physical Therapy Association, New York: APTA-OVR Papers

Brunnstrom S 1962 Training the adult hemiplegic patient: orientation of techniques to patient's motor behaviour. In: Approaches to the treatment of patients with neuromuscular dysfunction (Third International Congress: World Federation of Occupational Therapists)

Brunnstrom S 1970 Movement therapy in hemiplegia: a neurophysiological approach. Harper & Row, New York

Collis E 1953 A way of life for the handicapped child. Faber & Faber, London

Cotton E 1970 Integration of treatment and education in cerebral palsy. Physiotherapy 65(4): 143

Cotton E, Kinsman R 1983 Conductive education in adult hemiplegia. Churchill Livingstone, Edinburgh

Doman G, Doman R 1960 Children with severe brain injuries: neurological organisation in terms of mobility. Journal of the American Medical Association 174: 257

Egel P 1948 Techniques of treatment for the cerebral palsy child. Henry Kimpton, London

Goff B 1969 Appropriate afferent stimulation. Physiotherapy 55(1): 9–17

Goff B 1972 The application of recent advances in neurophysiology to Miss Rood's concept of neuromuscular facilitation. Physiotherapy 62(11): 358–361

Hari M 1988 The human principle in conductive education. In: Going to Budapest information pack 1991. The Foundation for Conductive Education, University of Birmingham

Kinsman R et al 1988 A conductive education approach for adults with neurological dysfunction. Physiotherapy 74(5): 227–230

Knott M, Voss D E 1972 Proprioceptive neuromuscular facilitation: patterns and techniques, 2nd edn. Harper & Row, New York

Levitt S 1982 Treatment of cerebral palsy and motor delay, 2nd edn. Blackwell Scientific Publications, Oxford

Read J 1991 Conductive education? In: Going to Budapest information pack. The Foundation for Conductive Education, University of Birmingham

Todd J E 1990 Conductive education: the continuing challenge. Physiotherapy 76(1): 13–16

Vojta V 1974 Die cerebralen Bewegangstomingen im Sauglingsalter. Verlag, Stuttgart

Waddington P 1984 Proprioceptive neuromuscular facilitation techniques and plasticity. Physiotherapy 70(8)

FURTHER READING

Aubrey C, Sutton A 1986 Handwriting: one measure of orthofunction in conductive education. British Journal of Special Education 13(3): 110–114

Bobath B, Bobath K 1975 Motor development in the different types of cerebral palsy. Heinemann Medical, London

Bryce J 1976 The management of spasticity in children. Physiotherapy 62(11): 353–357

Cash J E 1986 Textbook of neurology for physiotherapists, 4th edn. Faber & Faber, London

Campbell S K 1984 Pediatric neurologic physical therapy. Churchill Livingstone, Edinburgh

Cottam P J, Sutton A (eds) 1985 Conductive education: a system for overcoming motor disorder. Croom Helm, Kent

Cotton E 1980 The basic motor pattern. The Spastics Society, London

Fay T 1954a Rehabilitation of patients with spastic paralysis. Journal of the International College of Surgeons 22: 220

Fay T 1954b Use of pathological and unlocking reflexes in the rehabilitation of spastics. Americal Journal of Physical Medicine 33(6): 347

Finnie N R 1974 Handling the young cerebral palsied child at home. Heinemann Medical, London

Gillette H E 1969 Systems of therapy in cerebral palsy. C C Thomas, Springfield, Illinois

Hari M, Akos K 1988 Conductive education. Transl. Smith N H, Stevens J. Routledge, London

Kabat H, McLeod M, Holt C 1959 The practical application of proprioceptive neuromuscular facilitation. Physiotherapy

Levitt S 1984 Paediatric developmental therapy. Blackwell Scientific, Oxford

Stockmeyer S A 1967 The Rood approach. American Journal of Physical Medicine 46(1): 900

Voss D E 1959 Proprioceptive neuromuscular facilitation. American Journal of Occupational Therapy XIII (4 part 2)

19

Treatment methods

*E. Bell   P. Eckersley   V. Bastow
M. Jones   S. Steel*

INTRODUCTION

Children with physical disabilities or chronic sickness may have their movement restricted in a number of ways. These restrictions may result from poor muscle control, delayed or inappropriate movement patterns, lack of strength and stamina, pain, reduced opportunity, or a lack of awareness of what movement is about.

Physiotherapists have access to a variety of treatment methods to address these issues. A major challenge when planning physiotherapy programmes for children is to devise varied activities which are purposeful, enjoyable, energetic and challenging. In this way some of the physical and emotional frustrations felt by many children can be reduced.

In this chapter a range of methods is discussed, all of which offer increased opportunity to develop movement skills and to encourage that self-confidence, enjoyment and motivation which enables all children to exert physical control over their own immediate environment.

The chapter begins with two sections which look at the physical activities involved in exercise and hydrotherapy. Methods which help overcome physical restriction are then covered in sections on respiratory therapy, vibration therapy and serial splinting and strapping. The chapter ends by looking at the way in which the physiotherapy programme can be incorporated into the overall individual learning programme of the child and hence be established as an important part of the daily routine.

EXERCISE AND ACTIVITY
P. Eckersley

INTRODUCTION

Movement is as natural and essential to young children's lives as loving care, rest and nutrition. Movement provides children with an outlet for expression, creativity and discovery. Through movement children learn about themselves, their environment and others. Movement is a stimulus for physical growth and development. Children enjoy moving for its own sake (Curtis 1982).

The concept of movement through exercise and activity is central to much of the work of the paediatric physiotherapist.

Development of movement

The development of gross and fine motor skills has already been described in Chapter 4. Exercise and activities are gradually developed by children and adults together as the child gets older. Opportunities to practise and repeat activities consolidate skills. Physical maturation can gradually help to broaden the range of skills and heighten levels of performance.

The first five years of life form the basis for all activity and Curtis (1982) describes the changes in movement which take place during this period (Table 19.1).

The movement patterns of the disabled child follow the same maturational pattern. However, the impact of the majority of disabling conditions and illnesses will mean that this pattern is delayed or restricted in varying degrees. The games and exercises devised should always work towards the next stage in movement, allow time for skills to be achieved and plan imaginatively for the child to experience the more adventurous activities even when they cannot be performed without considerable assistance. They should also be enjoyable and build in self-motivation and reward.

Table 19.1 Changes in movement skills

Year	Changes in movement skills
1st	Master gravity Increasing control of hands
2nd	Run, climb, jump Rudimentary ball skills
3rd	Language and socialisation Concepts and labels Playmates
4th–5th	Complex movement patterns Increasing speed and strength Basis of later sports skills
7th	Throw and catch
11th	Swim Follow a map
14th	Tackle high jump
16th	Technical skills in gymnastics Ice skating

Adapted and developed from Curtis (1982)

AIMS OF EXERCISE AND ACTIVITY

Increasing evidence points to the value of exercise in a wide variety of areas related to fitness and health (Kerr 1988). Exercise also has an important part to play in the development of self-concept, creativity and socialisation. The aims of exercise and activity can be divided into five components:

1. Health-related
   a. motor fitness
      — strength
      — speed and power
      — agility
   b. cardiorespiratory fitness
   c. weight control
   d. posture, flexibility.
2. Skill-related
   a. use of objects, equipment and texture
   b. rhythm, balance and coordination
   c. laterality
   d. spatial awareness
   e. body and movement potential
   f. learning and concept formation.
3. Individual-related
   a. enjoyment and self-expression
   b. self-confidence and self-esteem
   c. stress reduction and relaxation

d. purposeful use of time

e. adventure and challenge.

4. Social aspects

   a. sharing and taking turns

   b. cooperative skills

   c. comradeship and interaction

   d. rules, planning and problem solving

   e. leadership.

5. Creative aspects

   a. quality of movement

      — heavy/light

      — fast/slow

   b. imagination and experimentation

   c. dance and music

   d. expanding the environment.

All of the above components can be built into therapy programmes using exercise and activity regardless of the nature of the disability. All are as relevant for the disabled as for the non-disabled child.

When considering the appropriate plans for working with an individual child, consideration should not be restricted to what appears to be the primary disorder experienced by that child. Cardiorespiratory fitness is as important for the child with diplegia who is learning to walk as it is for the child with cystic fibrosis.

The child with profound and multiple disabilities needs an opportunity to develop cooperative and interactive skills as well as the child with spina bifida who is in the school basketball team. Nothing is more expressive of ourselves than our body movements and the language of the body can be used to communicate feelings; physical activity is an important creative outlet (Bracegirdle 1990).

TYPES OF EXERCISE AND ACTIVITY

All types of exercise and activity incorporate the five components described above in various degrees.

Games and sport

Games and sport focus on particular events which have a beginning, a middle and an end. They take place in a context which requires co-operative skills and an understanding of rules and regulations. Simple games develop from childhood play and may also require a basic understanding of action–response, e.g. skittles. Others require the generalisation of skills and forward planning, e.g. the tactics of wheelchair hockey.

Many sports have a community relevance and even where activities such as archery require individual performances there is usually a team with which to share triumphs and disasters. Where the purpose of the activity is purely recreational, confidence and self-esteem can functionally increase.

A wide range of games and sports is available to disabled children:

- archery
- bowling
- badminton
- fencing
- table tennis
- hockey
- swimming
- basketball
- football.

A variety of handles, grips, velcro supports, tripods and wheelchair attachments make the majority of sports accessible to disabled children (see Appendix: Voluntary and Statutory Resources).

Physical education

PE is vigorous and physically demanding (Price 1980). It provides children with an opportunity to explore their own body potential, to handle a variety of objects in different ways, to move on different surfaces in different ways and to make demands of their own abilities in a safe environment. Imagination in movement can be explored in PE sessions to music; this can be an invaluable means of developing a sense of rhythm and timing. It can also create an enjoyment of movement and a sense of achievement.

Whilst planning the instructions for a PE session beforehand is essential with mixed ability classes, it is particularly important where a disabled child is integrated into a mainstream school. A simple instruction such as 'This half of the class lie on the floor and make wide and narrow shapes; the rest of you stand up' means that the child who usually spends time in a wheelchair or who can only walk with a walking aid can join in without being individually identified.

PE incorporates a wide variety of activities:

- object manipulation — balls, beanbags, hoops
- projectile skills — throwing, catching, kicking
- movement through space — running, jumping, hopping, rolling, sliding, climbing, swinging
- rebound skills — height and length, take off and landing
- stamina and endurance — distance, repetition, weight.

In many instances PE activities are used as training for sport, wheelchair athletics and outdoor activities. Programmes of circuit training, weight training and rhythmic activity can form part of group and individual sessions.

Outdoor activity

Access to the outdoors can be limited for many disabled children, and opportunities need to be deliberately created to extend disabled children's experiences. The 'outdoors' is a natural form of exercise, it has a recreational value and therefore a motivating force (Price 1980).

Recent years have seen the growth of outdoor resources for disabled children and adults, and as a result the use of outdoor activities to promote self-confidence and enjoyment alongside balance, coordination and stamina, is being encouraged.

Local and national outdoor centres now have many facilities available:

- riding
- sailing and canoeing
- fishing
- adventure playgrounds
- orienteering
- rock climbing
- cross-country running.

Facilities and adaptations are wide-ranging, from sailing techniques for visually handicapped young people to wheelchair abseiling.

Play and relaxation

All children experience times of stress and tension. These experiences can range from the loss of a parent, a new baby at home, to being bullied at school and not being picked for the school team (Madders 1987). Disabled children may also experience the additional stress of feeling ill, being in hospital away from home, a sense of physical isolation, pain or the frustration in teenage years of realising the restrictions of disability. Play and relaxation have a therapeutic value by providing outlets for stress and ways of managing aggression and frustration.

Play is self-initiated and is carried out for its own sake. It can give the child an opportunity to act out experiences through 'let's pretend' or to let-off steam through rough and tumble. Tugs of war and coconut shies give directed means to defuse aggression. Dances which incorporate jumping for joy or freezing with terror can give outlets for imagination and emotion and for the child's own thoughts and feelings.

Teaching relaxation should be considered for all children, particularly where possible stress has been highlighted, and should be incorporated into individual therapy programmes.

Passive exercise

For many children, passive exercise is essential if range of movement is to be maintained and movement skills increased. However, although the child is being moved by an adult it should not be a purely passive activity. It is an opportunity to talk to each child about what is taking place, to engage their interest, to use words such as 'up' and 'down', 'bent' and 'straight' and to work with music to develop rhythmical body movements. We must involve the children in what is being done (Eckersley 1990), and show they are valued by seeking their views and opinions.

Alternatives

The use of imagination is as important for the therapist as for the child. Creativity, independence and a valued use of time can also be developed through less demanding activities. In this way the sense of rhythm and timing, direction and planning, which are all important for sport and exercise, are promoted at other times.

Alternatives can include:

- listening to records and the radio
- creative work — design, printing, sewing or cooking
- construction games — modelling
- reading and debating
- visiting — museums and theme parks
- collecting — stamps, records.

USE IN CHILDHOOD CONDITIONS

It should be stressed that all the components of exercise described above are important for all children, regardless of disability. The description of those components of particular relevance to particular conditions should not be seen as totally exclusive. Some examples of the types of activity which can be used to reinforce the various components of exercise are given in Table 19.2.

Cardiorespiratory conditions

- breath control
- relaxation
- cardiovascular efficiency
- stamina, strength and endurance.

It can be helpful for the therapist to know the distances involved in moving around school, whether books and equipment will need to be carried around and whether pupils are expected to go outside at break and lunch times. This information can aid planning discussions with mainstream school staff and means that breath control and stamina can be developed in a practical and relevant way.

Spina bifida

- sitting balance
- manual dexterity

Table 19.2 The components of exercise

Component	Examples
Relaxation	Breathing exercises, Tension/release Robot and rag doll
Stamina and endurance	Obstacle courses: ball games Wheelchair slalom
Sitting balance	Simon says: large stacking toys Nursery rhymes, i.e. Jack and Jill, Incy Wincy Spider
Manual dexterity	Posting, threading Construction
Arm strength	Wheelbarrows, pushups, Weighted arm bands, Push/pull toys
Coordination	Hand-clapping games, Windmills Angels in the snow, rocker boards
Movement experience	Soft play areas, trampolines, swings, hammocks, slides, rolls
Imagination	Music and movement, Pretend games Making body shapes
Concept formation	Matching, sorting Directional movement — up, under, over
Planning and problem-solving	Choosing own exercises, Keeping own timetable, Cleaning own wheelchair
Aggression management	Large apparatus play, dance, Mime, tug of war

- arm strength
- coordination.

Particular care should be taken with the management of incontinence, fragile bone structures and consideration of valves for hydrocephalus.

Cerebral palsy

- movement experience and imagination
- fine motor skills
- coordination and timing
- balance
- motor fitness and flexibility.

The child with cerebral palsy has limited movement experiences and a limited understanding of movement possibilities. These experiences can be extended by talking about activities and then developing these creatively. For example, facilitating rolling from supine to prone can be followed by a discussion on how the child would plan to do this unaided, and could subsequently lead to rolling being incorporated into a movement-to-music session on the seashore (rolling waves) or on an autumn day (blown leaves).

The therapist should be aware that the effort and excitement generated by many activities increase spasticity. Whilst their effects should be noted and mediated using positioning, inhibition and relaxation, the feelings themselves are a natural part of childhood.

Cognitive problems

- concept formation — what, where, how, up, down, over
- concentration
- games as prerequisites for skills, i.e. prewriting.

Children who experience learning difficulties will not be able to acquire experiences in a way and at a rate which is appropriate to their age. A child may have all the necessary motor responses available but be unable to decide what is appropriate (Price 1980).

Clumsy children

- all skill-related activities
- relaxation
- aggression management
- roles, planning and problem-solving
- motor fitness.

ORGANISING AN EXERCISE SESSION

The following factors should be taken into consideration when developing group or individual activity sessions:

- planning
- safety.

Planning

Session structure

An exercise and activity session should have:

- A beginning, which includes a warm-up.
- A middle, which is planned around a central theme or concept.
- An end, which includes relaxation and a cooling down period.

All children, however young, should be involved in the skills they are working on and given an opportunity to share the planning process.

Clothing and footwear

Consideration should be given to clothing and footwear. The ability to observe the effects of exercise on a particular body part can be important to the therapist. The effect of an energetic basketball session on body temperature may mean the clothing becomes damp, with implications for the skin condition of the wheelchair player, personal comfort and social acceptability after the game.

Choosing activities

It will be necessary to decide whether dressing and undressing form part of the session. Thought must also be given to:

- group size
- range of difficulties experienced
- equipment available
- venue available
- activities included — short activities/long games
- method of instruction
  - spoken details throughout
  - explanation which is then carried out
  - asking 'How can you . . .?'
  - children working it out in pairs or groups.

Practice

The importance of practice and repetition cannot be overemphasised and opportunities for this will need to be planned into sessions on an ongoing basis. A child's persistence can be surprising, for example, a 9- or 10-year-old seeing an older sibling kick a ball during a football match will continue to practise the same skill until he has mastered it, even if exhausted (Hoole 1981). The element of practice may be particularly difficult for the disabled child unless opportunities are deliberately created and structured.

Safety

Safety is important for all children. All games and sport carry risks and when planning activities for disabled children the risks should be neither unacceptable nor unreasonable. However, the risks resulting from inactivity need to be balanced against risks resulting from activity and can only be assessed on an individual basis. Discussion with, and the agreement of, parents will be necessary:

Particular consideration must be paid to:

- exposure to sun and weather
- presence of sores and infections
- ear conditions
- brittle bones
- haemophilia
- cardiovascular and respiratory problems
- presence of valves for hydrocephalus
- atlantoaxial instability in children with Down's syndrome.

CONCLUSION

PE, sport and games are as much a part of the childhood of the disabled child as they are of able-bodied children. If well planned they can motivate the child to practise the more difficult aspects of the therapy programme and give a reason to keep up exercise on leaving school. They can also be a powerful source of enjoyment and achievement.

Children are different; not only because of their physical condition but also because they think differently, have different likes and dislikes, and different strengths and weaknesses. Recognising and valuing this individuality is central to the improvement of the motor skills of young children with disabilities. Although they may need equipment adaptations, their greatest need is to be

challenged, motivated, engaged and rewarded for their achievements.

It is not enough to maintain that since archery is good for paraplegics, it is therefore an appropriate activity for all paraplegics (Price 1980).

Physiotherapists should begin with the assumption that for each child there is an activity which is enjoyable. The challenge is to establish what that activity is for each individual, and to plan it in a way which develops self-confidence and self-esteem.

HYDROTHERAPY: THE HALLIWICK METHOD
E. Bell

HISTORY AND PHILOSOPHY

The Halliwick method of teaching swimming was developed by James McMillan MBE, an engineer by profession, and is named after the school at which he was working at the time. He founded the Association of Swimming Therapy (AST) in 1952 to promote the Halliwick method and ensure its continuation in its pure form.

Hydrodynamic principles and the scientific understanding of the human body in water form the basis of the method, which stresses ability instead of the disability that is apparent on land (Table 19.3). The instructor and swimmer work together as a pair and minimal, but constant, sensitive and flexible support is given to the swimmer. This allows each person to learn to appreciate the upthrust of water and to find his own balance. The main objective is learning to be safe and competent in water, rather than learning to swim.

The Halliwick method has the tripartite aims of breath-control, relaxation and balance, which are interdependent and interrelated. A swimmer who is truly adjusted to the water will have mastered all three aspects.

HYDRODYNAMIC PRINCIPLES

Awareness of the hydrodynamic principles affecting the behaviour of the human body in water will ensure the maximum potential benefits of hydrotherapy for the child. The physiotherapist

Table 19.3 The Halliwick philosophy

- Stresses ability not disability
- Incorporates adjustment to water
- Develops the individual's understanding of being in water
- Teaches movement in water on a one-to-one basis
- Stresses the importance of breath control
- Uses balance and positions of safety rather than flotation equipment
- Promotes relaxation and the enjoyment of being in water
- Develops confidence in water
- Uses group dynamics and games for motivation.

must be able to teach the physically handicapped child how to utilise or counteract these dynamic effects. The principal hydrodynamic factors affecting the handicapped swimmer are described below.

Buoyancy

The relative density of water is 1 and any body with a relative density of less than 1 will float. The average relative density of the human body is 0.95, therefore it will float with approximately 5% of that body above the surface of the water. Body weight, muscle bulk, presence of spasticity and deformity will all affect the relative density of the child's body. This can be seen, for example, when the child with spina bifida has difficulty in keeping his legs, which have a low relative density, down in the water and preventing his bottom from sinking. The skilled physiotherapist will be able to assess whether the swimmer is a 'sinker' or a 'floater'. Halliwick requires that as great a proportion of the body as possible should be kept beneath the surface of the water, whilst keeping the face above it.

Pressure

Water exerts an equal horizontal pressure which provides support; to maximise this the body should be kept well down in the water. The vertical pressure, or upthrust, increases with depth and the child will feel more support when the body is low down in the water.

Metacentre

Each swimmer has a metacentre around which body rotation occurs. One of the most important features of Halliwick is that the swimmer learns to control this rotation and is able to maintain a safe, balanced position in the water.

Impedance

The physiotherapist must be aware that a greater amount of energy is required to move through water than to move on land. However, this impedance to movement can also have beneficial effects by constraining any unwanted involuntary movements.

Turbulence

The physically disabled swimmer must be taught how to make himself as streamlined as possible, to eliminate unwanted turbulence and facilitate movement through the water.

Turbulence causes low pressure areas, which have a suction effect that can aid movement through water. It can also be used, as the child gains confidence, to develop balance and co-ordination skills.

There is less turbulence at the edge of a pool than in the centre, although irregularly shaped pools can cause unexpected turbulence currents.

USE OF FLOTATION EQUIPMENT

The disabled child will experience a number of restrictions to movement. Flotation equipment will make it more difficult for the child to overcome the effects of water pressure and will therefore restrict his movement further. This equipment may also give a false sense of balance, therefore making it more difficult for the child to learn to compensate for his lack of motor ability and asymmetry of body posture. In some situations the equipment may hold the child in a dangerous position: for example, a child with cerebral palsy may be turned face down in the water and be unable either to right himself or to lift his head to breathe. The child will gain more from the support of an adult than from the use of flotation equipment.

THE TEN-POINT PROGRAMME

The Halliwick method is built around the principles described above, using a programme consisting of ten separate points, which divide into four phases (Table 19.4). These ten points form a sequence on which any individual or group programme is based.

Mental adjustment

A child's adjustment to water has both physical and mental implications and is a continuous process, working through the entire hydrotherapy programme. The initial, and most vital, point of support and contact is through the eyes.

Adjustment to water

The hydrotherapy pool is a strange and exciting environment for many children. Sounds are altered and echoes are present; smells are different and suddenly being placed in a warm, wet and unusual environment can be frightening (Eckersley 1990). Many children prefer to be introduced to the pool slowly and a number of sessions can be spent constructively, watching other children in the pool or sitting on the edge and having feet splashed. Many children become frightened when water comes near to their chins or ears, and for some the very activity of undressing can be distressing.

Talking to parents about a child's responses to being bathed at home or to having his or her face washed can be helpful. Sand and water play in the classroom can also be a useful introduction to play in the pool. Even familiar songs can be used to prepare the child and the song 'Here we go round the mulberry bush' can be changed to 'Here we go round the swimming pool.'

Young children often prefer the security of a smaller space to play in. Introductory games facing into the corner of the pool rather than facing out across the whole expanse of water can add to this sense of security (Fig. 19.1).

Disengagement

The Halliwick method is based on a one to one adult to child relationship. This allows the child's confidence to grow as skills develop, so that they progressively disengage from the adult. The sense of security described above is an essential pre-requisite to this disengagement.

Disengagement can be seen in a number of ways:

1. In the increasing independence when a child gets into the pool.
2. When a child standing in water and supported at the waist is gradually able to stand alone whilst the physiotherapist creates turbulence at waist level.
3. When a child who has achieved a point of balance in supine floating with support under the shoulder blades progresses to

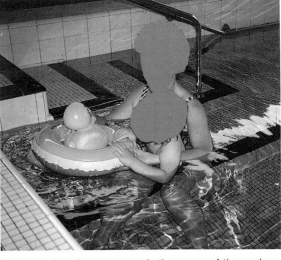

Fig. 19.1 Introductory games in the corner of the pool.

Table 19.4 The ten-point Halliwick programme

Phases	Points
Mental adjustment	Adjustment to water Disengagement
Balance restoration	Vertical rotation Lateral rotation Combined rotation
Movement inhibition	Upthrust Balance in stillness
Movement facilitation	Turbulent gliding Progression to swimming Movement in water

achieving this same balance without support.

The first step to becoming disengaged is when eye contact with the helper is dropped, of the swimmer's own volition. Disengagement has also taken place when the child can lift his feet from the floor of the pool and therefore loses all the points of reference he has on dry land. This can be a difficult progression. Physiotherapists working with children out of their depth should be very aware of the different patterns of movement on land and in water. The instructor has a very important role in encouraging complete disengagement, so that the swimmer can eventually swim safely on his own.

All such progressions take place in a relaxed environment and all support is given with flat hands and a steady, firm pressure; grasping and holding should be avoided.

Balance restoration

Vertical rotation

Vertical rotation occurs around the transverse axis of the body. The first aim is to achieve head control in lying, as the position of the head determines the position of the body in water. The head should therefore never be held when using the Halliwick method. The swimmer will first be asked to put his head forward or backwards, in order to learn how he can bring his body under control. Vertical rotation is used to enable the swimmer to move easily between vertical and horizontal positions, the movement always being head-initiated. To achieve supine lying the head is taken slowly backwards and as the action takes place the feet move forwards and upwards to the surface (Campion 1985). The culmination of vertical rotation is the ability to execute a forward or backward somersault, through 360°, with postural and breathing control. This is to ensure that the swimmer will always be able to regain a safe breathing position, should he be submerged and put off balance. He must be able to control his exhalation throughout so that his breathing is not compromised. 'Blow' should be the most common word heard in the pool area (Campion 1985).

Lateral rotation

This can occur when the child is both vertical or horizontal in the water. Learning about rotation should start in the upright position, until the swimmer is sufficiently adjusted to lying back in the water. Lateral rotation takes place around the longitudinal axis of the spine and, like vertical rotation, is initiated by the head. Children will learn to turn, perhaps from one instructor to another, looking in the direction in which they are travelling. This encourages lateral rotation of the head, which will trigger the rotation of the body.

Once this has been mastered, the swimmer should adopt a supine position in the water, supported by the instructor, who will first show him how he can counteract any unwanted roll by using his head. Physically disabled children will roll in the water because of their asymmetrical shape, and it is important that they learn to control this unwanted rotation. Once this control is achieved, the child can be taught to use his head movements to turn over in the water, and to use arm movements to assist this. Complete rotation in the horizontal, through 360°, is the ultimate aim.

Combined rotation

The placing of combined rotation after vertical and lateral rotation does not necessarily imply that it will be taught later. It is the combination of the two previous rotations, and its mastery which means that the swimmer is able to be in complete charge of his position in the water. He will be able to adopt a safe breathing position when he chooses, and also be able to move easily from the upright to the horizontal, from supine to prone, and vice versa, at will.

Movement inhibition

Upthrust

The swimmer gradually learns to appreciate the buoyancy of water. An understanding of this effect reassures the swimmer and a change in attitude develops when it is clearly understood that water acts as an upward force rather than a downward one (Campion 1985). An advanced level of breath control is required for this, as the swimmer must be able to exhale against the pressure of water while submerged. Changes in shape will influence the body's buoyancy. The swimmer discovers that he is unable to remain submerged, and that upthrust will always be the dominant force. Body type predetermines whether the swimmer will have a tendency towards floating or sinking, and a great deal of patience and skill will be required to assess the most appropriate movements of head and limbs to achieve balance for each individual child.

Games can be used to increase a child's understanding of this property of water. A floating toy can be pushed under the water so that the child can watch it rise to the surface like a pop-up toy. Splashing and pushing the water can create waves which will move toy boats or animals across the water in a race. Waterfalls and showers can be created using colourful plastic colanders.

The physiotherapist should also be aware that the thrust of water can have an unwanted effect on movement. Where children have diplegia or hemiplegia, walking forwards against the pressure of water can result in an increased plantar flexion and increased adductor spasticity through effort. Walking backwards or sideways can counteract this; and is frequently more fun.

The thrust of water may also damp down the athetoid movement of many children and the sudden removal of this stabilising action may result in increased athetoid movements. It is important that children are removed from the pool, or leave the pool independently, in a relaxed and calm frame of mind. The final exciting and active game should be followed by a period of relaxation.

Balance is stillness

The seventh Halliwick point means an ability to balance against the turbulence present in any pool. Contrarotation will be required as the swimmer is tilted by the moving water, and the head must be used to achieve balance. The swimmer will first attempt to keep his balance while in the vertical. He can passively resist turbulence

set up, or actively create his own, by moving through the water before coming to an abrupt halt, so that he has to work against the momentum built up. The second stage of *balance is stillness* is to maintain balance while in the horizontal plane. This is harder, as there is no solid surface to react against.

Movement facilitation

Turbulent gliding

This phase involves using turbulent force to tow the swimmer through the water. The swimmer adopts a back float position and makes only small, contrarotationary movements with the hands, in order to maintain his balance. Meanwhile, the instructor moves backwards, thus creating a low pressure area into which the swimmer will be pulled. The strength of tow can be increased by adding turbulence beneath the level of the swimmer's scapulae, by means of circular movements of the instructor's hands. The area in which turbulence is placed will be of significance, as will the speed of movement through the water, and the physiotherapist must ascertain the correct placement and generation of turbulence. The swimmer remains still, maintaining as streamlined a shape as possible, and is able to appreciate the sensation of moving through the water without physical support. His balance will not be upset by having to make any large movements to assist his locomotion.

Gliding can also be used to reduce spasticity and increase the range of trunk movements. The instructor gently moves the shoulder girdle from side to side whilst towing the child through the water. A rotatory contramovement is created between shoulder and pelvic girdle, which reduces spasticity and allows freer and more rhythmic arm and leg movements to take place. This activity can be linked to imaginative games when the child moves through the water whilst pretending to be, for example, a tug boat, a sailing ship or a small boat in a storm. This type of activity will result in a variety of creative and expressive movements which the child may find impossible on dry land.

Progression to swimming

Confidence by this stage, and full balance control, will enable the swimmer to propel himself through the water independently. He adopts the back float position he used during the turbulent gliding phase, then provides his own power by performing a small sculling action at hip level with his hands. The movement remains small so that balance is not greatly affected. Halliwick introduces swimming on the back as in this position the child will have fewer problems with breathing. Where head control in prone lying is difficult for the child, swimming on his back will be a preferred position.

Movement in water

The physiotherapist must assess the relative strengths of the swimmer in order to decide which stroke best suits that individual. For many children it will be a backstroke, with the arms used either alternately or together and the legs kicking. There are many variations, however, and frequently an adjustment must be made by the swimmer to compensate for weaker limbs, deformities and restricted movement.

Side stroke is often a good choice, particularly for children with hemiplegia. Front crawl is a suitable early prone stroke, provided that breathing can be controlled, and adapted breast stroke is more advanced.

SAFETY

Safety is of paramount importance and the physiotherapist is responsible for ensuring not only their own safety but that of their swimmers and instructors. All aspects of safety must be considered and rules rigorously observed. Medical and parental permission to swim must be obtained in writing. A number of additional safety factors must be borne in mind at all times:

Incontinence

This should not be a barrier to a child's going in the pool. All children should go to the toilet before entering the pool. If a spina bifida child is being trained by expression of urine this must be attended to prior to entering the pool (Campion 1985). Any urinary bag should be emptied and the tap closed. Plastic pants give added security.

Infection

Many children may be prone to ear infections or to pressure sores. It is helpful to have advice from nursing or medical staff in these situations.

Environmental safety

Toys and equipment can easily be pushed off the side of the pool and care must be taken that pool sides remain uncluttered, with ease of access to all areas. A member of staff experienced in life-saving techniques should be present at all times.

Rest period

Hydrotherapy pools are warm and therefore tiring, although they present a contrast to the temperature of the outside world. All children will require a short period of rest after activity and where children have travelled to the pool care must be taken that hair is dry before the return journey. Where possible a drink should be available.

Lifting and handling techniques

The physiotherapist must be certain that correct lifting and handling techniques are taught and adhered to, both on land and in the pool.

Halliwick demands human support, therefore it is vital that holds are scrupulously taught to potential instructors. Gripping and being gripped is discouraged, instructors' hands being held flat and supinated (Fig. 19.2).

Halliwick has specific holds for facing towards and away from the instructor, in addition to holds used in circle and line formations. Minimum support is emphasised, and holds will generally be at the centre of gravity of the body, between thoracic vertebra II and sacral vertebra 2. The physiotherapist must be certain that they are

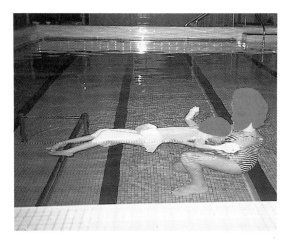

Fig. 19.2 Support with flat hands.

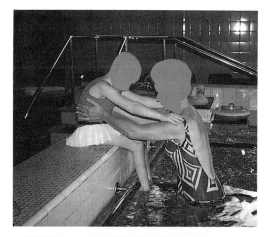

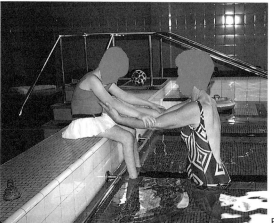

Fig. 19.3 Progression of holds for entry to water.

stable in the water at all times, as the swimmer relies on them totally for support.

Holds for entry and exit

There is a graduated scale of holds for entry to the water, with support being withdrawn as disengagement progresses. At first the physiotherapist places her arms around the swimmer, who is sitting on the poolside, hands over the scapulae (Fig. 19.3A); they graduate to using forearm and hand support (Fig. 19.3B); and finally the swimmer makes an independent, head-first entry from the side. There is also a rotating entry within the Halliwick scheme. Swimmers using the Halliwick method are strongly encouraged to exit over the side of the pool, if at all possible. The physiotherapist will assist the exit, using the upthrust of water to take the weight of the swimmer.

GROUPS AND GAMES

Halliwick is frequently used by a physiotherapist working with only one child. However, as the accepted method of using Halliwick is through the use of games and activities, working in a group is advantageous. The ideal number to have in a therapeutic group is between four and six children. Both individual and group programmes, based on the ten-point programme, will need to be devised which incorporate both therapeutic aims and the use of games.

Games as a teaching medium have a number of advantages. A game is an enjoyable and successful method of teaching skills. Language development, social development, problem-solving, memory, discrimination and competition are just a few of the positive aspects. Play is, after all, a child's learning tool. Games may include a variety of toys, but the majority are singing games, which bring rhythm into play. The songs used may be well-known nursery rhymes, adaptations of popular songs or specially formulated songs. Games must have a structure, so that formation, engagement with the swimmer, action and teaching points are understood. Most games will incorporate elements of several of the

Halliwick points. Practically every game will aid the development of mental adjustment and disengagement.

Fishes in the net

Formation. A circle, with joined hands to form a 'net'.

Engagement. Each swimmer is on the right of his instructor; long arm hold.

Action. One swimmer, the 'fish' (and instructor), starts in the centre of the circle. The circle rotates, and the individual swimmer (and instructor) must try to escape from the 'net' by going over the joined hands, rotating onto his back and standing up (combined rotation). The group sings the relevant song. The circle changes direction, while the swimmer then has to go underneath the hands in order to return to the centre. Where the child has not achieved good breath control the 'net' can lift arms up or down as appropriate to make the movement easier for the swimmer.

The swimmers take turns to be the 'fish'.

Teaching points. Mental adjustment, disengagement, combined rotation, upthrust and balance in stillness.

Entry songs

A number of songs are used on entry to the pool so that the child cues into the precise moment that he will be coming into the water. The advantage of this is that he is fully prepared and can cooperate by bringing his head forward at the right time.

One suitable entry song is an adaptation of 'Ten Green Bottles', using the appropriate number of 'dry swimmers sitting on the wall'. The swimmers may all make their entries together, or by number. Most games can be progressed, so that the task is made more demanding in various ways and the degree of support diminished.

Other suitable songs for adaptation are 'Here we go round the mulberry bush (swimming pool)' when the words are changed to 'This is the way we get into the pool', and 'Johnny Green, where are you?'.

THERAPEUTIC ASPECTS OF HYDROTHERAPY

Independence in water without the use of artificial flotation aids, and the rotational elements link the Halliwick method of working in water to the important features of physiotherapy intervention in the treatment of cerebral palsied children on land:

1. Emphasis on using the head to initiate and control movement in water relates directly to the importance of head control on land.

2. Halliwick requires eye-to-eye contact between the swimmer and physiotherapist, and it is the visual system that cues in the motor system.

3. Smell plays a large part in introducing a deaf or blind child to an alien environment, such as a swimming pool, and the olfactory nerve is the first of the cranial nerves to develop.

4. Games entail repetition, a necessary element in teaching a skill, particularly with the mentally handicapped, and this repetition can be achieved without boredom.

5. The confidence built up as the child progresses through the ten-point programme is not confined to the time spent in the water.

6. Working in neutral gravity, in water, helps to create a better body image.

7. Although most work done in Halliwick, in the horizontal, is done in the supine, the prone position can be used as long as natural breathing is not impeded, as spontaneous reflex lower limb movements will appear in children who have been released from cortical control.

8. Structured work in water increases the range of management procedures that can be constructed by the parents of a child with a mental or physical disability. This increases their ability to handle their child with confidence.

The therapeutic effects of exercise in water are considerable and include:

- the relief of pain and muscle spasm
- the maintenance or increase in range of motion of joints

- strengthening
- re-education
- improvement
- encouragement
- maintenance.

In addition, the ability to be independent in water, to achieve skills that may be difficult or impossible on land, can only have favourable and lasting psychological effects which boosts confidence and morale, and which may well be carried over into life on land (Campion 1985).

RESPIRATORY THERAPY
V. Bastow

INTRODUCTION

The techniques used in the treatment of respiratory problems in children may vary from child to child and from age group to age group. A degree of imagination is required to obtain co-operation from children and familiarity with a child's favourite toys and games will often help ease the problem of winning his confidence. Children feel the same fear and pain as adults but are less able to understand why they are in pain and the reasons for hospital admissions and physiotherapy treatments.

CHEST PHYSIOTHERAPY IN CHILDREN

They are many differences between the anatomy and physiology of a child's respiratory system and that of an adult (Kendall 1987) and these must be considered when planning treatments.

Timing of treatment

Whatever the age of the child, treatment is best avoided immediately following food or drinks. In a young baby it is advisable to treat in the half-hour prior to a feed, and in the toddler and older child to leave at least an hour after a meal before treatment to avoid vomiting. If the child is being fed via a continuous nasogastric infusion it may be advisable to arrange for the feed to be stopped prior to and during treatment, unless it is a very slow and small volume infusion.

Postural drainage

The young baby is often the least difficult to treat as they generally enjoy the proximity of another person, find chest percussion a soothing procedure, and may fall asleep with the steady rhythm. Where possible the baby should be treated on the parent's or physiotherapist's knee. Wrapping the baby in a towel or small blanket induces a feeling of security and also prevents flailing arms and kicking legs in the more active baby. Between 18 months and 4 years, treatment can be more difficult with the added problem of catching your patient if he or she is mobile! However, by approaching slowly and calmly, explaining to the parents where possible what has to be done and perhaps demonstrating on teddy first, the child's confidence can usually be won over. Letting the child pat teddy whilst you are treating the child may also be helpful. Singing 'pat-a-cake' and other familiar nursery rhymes may help, and if the child will join in, an element of deep breathing may be achieved. Initially it may be necessary to treat in the position the child chooses rather than the optimal postural drainage position. When the trust of the child is assured the position can be changed to that of your choice.

Over about 5 years of age, the child may not need as much play or distraction to obtain co-operation and will usually be able to understand why treatment is necessary. The very ill child, however, often regresses in behaviour, and toys and comforters can still be important to an older, apparently 'grown-up', child. Displaying an interest in the child, his family, friends, school and personal belongings will help the child to trust you.

Duration of treatment

In the very ill child — as in the very ill adult — length of treatment may well be dictated by the heart rate and blood pressure of the patient. A 'little and often' is the maxim best observed, with treatments being as short as 2 or 3 minutes.

As the child improves longer treatments should be possible, although a compromise often has to be made between the child's tolerance and cooperation and achieving optimal effective treatment. Leaving the nurses and parents with some 'fun' exercises, such as blowing bubbles, can be beneficial in between formal treatment sessions.

Percussion

No matter what the age of the child percussion can be performed, although non-cooperation may require the use of other techniques. It is also worth noting that the physically abused child may perceive this to be a further abuse and so be very frightened and uncooperative.

Percussion should not be performed over bare skin as this can be painful: a folded towel, terry napkin or flannelette sheet should be placed over the child's chest. In a small baby a face mask may be used or the technique of 'tenting', where three or four fingers are used with the middle one raised (Parker 1987). Single-handed percussion is the preferred technique because of the small size of the child's chest and it is often more comfortable, less frightening and the child is better able to maintain a steady respiratory rate. A cough will often be produced during percussion of a baby's chest.

It is desirable in the older child (around 3–4 years and upwards) to encourage deep breathing during percussion, interspersed with quiet, relaxed breathing. This way the arterial oxygen level will be better maintained during treatment and the collateral ventilatory channels may open up atelectatic areas and help increase the ventilation of areas blocked by mucus plugging and so dislodge secretions.

Shakings and vibrations

These may be performed on a child but the method of application will vary depending on the size of the child's chest. Finger tips only should be used on the small baby, progressing via whole fingers to one and then two hands with the bigger child. In a baby with a high respiratory rate it is often easier for the therapist to vibrate the chest wall on every second or third breath with the phase of vibration being kept very short — to the length of each expiration. In a very young child, where the chest wall is very compliant, it is possible to impair cardiac venous return and therefore cardiac output by performing simultaneous bilateral chest wall compressions; hence it is advisable with these patients to keep to unilateral techniques.

Expansion exercises

From the age of about 18 months the child can be taught to take deep breaths, although it is easier initially to get them to 'make big blows' using paper, windmills, bubbles, etc. Performing a deep expiration will usually be preceded by a large inspiratory effort. Such activities also help to make treatment more enjoyable and they are games that parents and nurses can also enjoy playing with the child. Inspiration may be actively achieved around 3 years and 'tummy', diaphragmatic or relaxed breathing can be easily taught to most children around this age.

Where there is persistent segmental or lobar atelectasis, a positive expiratory pressure (PEP) bottle may be useful (Campbell et al 1986). Most children enjoy blowing through straws into their drinks and so to be actively encouraged in this activity can be quite exciting. A plastic bottle, part filled with water, is fitted with a short length of wide bore (2 cm) tubing. A second hole is made in the top to allow for air escape and the tube adjusted so that the open end sits approximately 5 cm below the water level (Fig. 19.4). The child is encouraged to blow into the bottle and to 'make bubbles'. The PEP may be increased or decreased by altering the tube immersion depth. Some caution must be exercised with this technique if there is risk of pneumothorax, e.g. if the child has undergone thoracic surgery or has a history of pneumothorax.

Incentive spirometry is another useful and enjoyable tool and may be used to achieve a deep and sustained inspiration (Fig. 19.5). When the child is unable to inhale voluntarily, the device may be upturned and expiration used to produce ball movement.

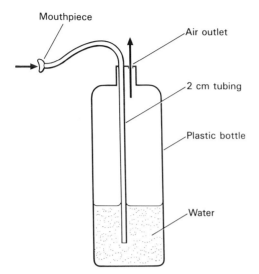

Fig. 19.4 Positive expiratory pressure bottle.

Suction

The indications for suction in children are similar to those in adults — chiefly the inability to cough effectively when secretions are present in the airways. It may also be necessary in children to obtain a specimen of secretions from the upper

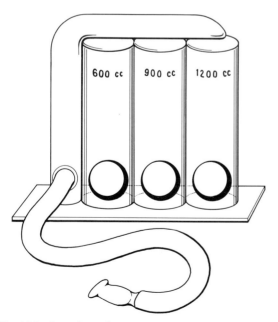

Fig. 19.5 Incentive spirometer.

airways as expectoration is often difficult under the age of about 5 years. However, this should not be undertaken lightly in these youngsters as it can be a very distressing procedure and is best avoided unless essential.

Intubated patients

In an intubated patient, regular suction may be necessary as the natural upward movement of mucus from the airways to the pharynx (the mucociliary escalator) is inhibited by the presence of the tube. Mucus from the nasopharynx may track downwards past the endotracheal tube into the large airways, particularly when an uncuffed tube is used (as is common paediatric practice). The frequency with which suction is needed must be assessed for each individual patient.

Non-intubated patients

In a non-intubated, spontaneously breathing patient, suction may be needed to remove secretions from the airways when the child cannot cough effectively, although an effective cough can sometimes be stimulated in these patients by percussion and shakings or by tracheal compression whereby finger pressure is applied either side of the trachea below the thyroid cartilage. This technique will often stimulate the cough reflex in a baby, but it may also produce a bradycardia and so should be used with great care.

Nasal suction

Nasal suction is frequently carried out in the physiotherapy and nursing care of babies with respiratory and upper respiratory problems, and its use prior to feeding may often facilitate sucking and swallowing. However, the procedure is not without problems as it may induce hypoxia, bradycardia, bronchospasm and cause mucosal damage. It should therefore be used with caution and with careful heart and oxygen monitoring in the very sick child. Once over the age of about 9 months, the procedure is needed less often because the increase in airway calibre allows mucus to be more easily dislodged by other manoeuvres such as shakings and coughing. Also, it is rather distressing for the older child and more likely to cause trauma if the child struggles. The procedure has been well researched by Young (1984a, 1984b, 1988) and her recommendations for a safe, sterile and comfortable technique should be adhered to: using sterile catheters — size 5 or, more usually, size 6 FG in the premature and small baby and size 6 or 8 FG in the child up to 5 years. The catheter should have a control valve or be attached to the main suction tubing by way of a 'Y' connector in order to control the suction pressure and prevent the development of high pressures which may cause mucosal damage. A sterile glove should be worn when handling the catheter and, if the nasal route is used, the catheter should be lubricated with suitable sterile jelly — unless the child has a particularly moist nasal passage, when lubrication may not be necessary. Each catheter should be used once only and then discarded safely.

Teaching suction methods

It is often the role of the physiotherapist to teach the procedure to parents and carers when a child requires suction at home or school. The procedure must be carefully taught and those under instruction observed to carry out the technique a number of times prior to the child's discharge. A review of the technique and a regular check on equipment should be maintained.

Forced expiration technique

The forced expiration technique (FET) is a help in moving secretions within the airways to a point where they may be expectorated. The technique consists of performing one or two forced expirations (or huffs) from a midlung volume to a low-lung volume followed by a period of relaxed (diaphragmatic or tummy) breathing. The latter is necessary to allow the airways to return to their resting calibre as they will narrow following any forced expiratory manoeuvre, be it a 'huff', cough or laugh. The period of time needed to be spent in the relaxed phase will depend on the lability of each child's airways and can only be gauged by observation.

Active cycle of breathing techniques

These techniques are learnt gradually with relaxed breathing being the first component. Next, deep breathing is taught with emphasis on full expansion and quiet expiration. This deep breathing encourages airflow through the collateral ventilatory system (pores of Kohn and canals of Lambert) and so increases the airflow in the smaller bronchi, helping to mobilise secretions. This is followed by the 'huff', or forced expiration technique, which itself needs accurate teaching to ensure that the child is forcing the air out without narrowing his glottis and using midlung to low-lung volumes in order to effectively remove peripheral secretions. It is sometimes helpful to keep the child's lips open during the 'huff' by using a cardboard disposable peak flow tube (Gaskell & Webber 1987).

The forced expiration technique is described by Pryor & Webber (1979) who emphasise its application in asthma and cystic fibrosis and show a reduction in the time needed for the removal of secretions when compared with conventional postural drainage. It also brings independence for the older child, as many no longer need to rely on others during their postural drainage.

Preferential ventilation

The positioning of the very ill child requires careful consideration. Heaf et al (1983) have demonstrated, in a study of ten infants, that oxygenation improves when the good lung is uppermost — the reverse of the situation in adults. This postural effect persists in young children up to 27 months old (Davies et al 1985) and possibly in much older children too. This observation must be considered in the management of critically ill infants and young children with unilateral lung disease. Monitoring of oxygen saturation is desirable when treating these patients, particularly when employing postural drainage, as the position required for optimal drainage may compromise the ventilation and oxygenation. As yet the age at which this pattern of preferential ventilation changes to that seen in the adult is unknown.

VIBRATION THERAPY
E. Bell

INTRODUCTION

Vibration therapy is relatively new as a method of treatment, being comparatively unknown until twenty years ago. In 1965 research was initiated to look at the neurophysiological changes produced when vibration was applied to skeletal muscle (Eklund & Hagbarth 1965).

TYPES OF VIBRATION

There are two kinds of mechanically produced vibration:

- linear
- multidirectional

Linear vibration is produced along a single plane and is usually, but not necessarily, of fixed frequency. The effect is a percussion action which has only a surface application. Multidirectional vibration projects along three planes — longitudinal, lateral and vertical. It produces a cycloidal action of a type used in therapy.

Frequency of vibration

The parameters of vibration considered safe for therapeutic use range from 15 Hz (cycles per second) to 150 Hz (Table 19.5).

NEUROPHYSIOLOGICAL EFFECTS OF VIBRATION

Nearly all muscles contain sensory endings known as muscle spindles. They play a major role in the control of posture and movement. Primary endings are sensitive not only to the length of the muscle but also to the rate at which the length changes, and therefore to a combination of stretch and the rate of stretch.

They are particularly sensitive to vibration in the range of 100–200 Hz (cycles per second) Through this route the tonic vibration reflex (TVR) is set up. This reflex is not very powerful in normal muscle and may take several seconds to develop. Where brain damage is present, the stretch reflex in muscle is often exaggerated, giving rise to the clinical condition of spasticity. In many patients with this exaggerated stretch reflex the tonic vibration reflex is also brisk, and tone is increased.

However, the effect of other lower frequencies of vibration may induce an inhibitory phenomenon.

INDICATIONS FOR USE
Cerebral palsy

There are a number of possibilities for using vibration in the treatment of children with cerebral palsy. By using low frequency vibration in the treatment of spasticity the following effects may be achieved or encouraged:

- reduction of muscle tone
- increase in range of movement
- motivation in developing patterns of movement
- ease in handling and positioning for dressing and feeding
- prevention of postural deformity.

Where mild contractures are present, high frequency vibration can be applied to the antagonist group of muscles whilst gently moving the limb in order to regain range of movement.

Circulatory and respiratory problems

The effect of vibration can assist in the improvement of circulation and the dispersal of tissue fluids. It can also be used as a useful adjunct to postural drainage, especially where a child finds percussion techniques uncomfortable or distressing.

Table 19.5 Frequencies of vibration and their neurophysiological effects

Cycles per second (Hz)	Effects
20–50	Inhibition of spastic motor patterns
80–120	Stimulation of tonic vibratory reflex
100–250	Postvibratory facilitation

Reward and reinforcement

Vibration is a pleasant tactile stimulus and can be an alternative means of reward and reinforcement. This can be especially useful when working with children with profound and multiple disabilities (see Chapter 10 Profound and Multiple Disability). Vibration can be a most effective stimulation for those whose mental and sensory abilities are limited, enabling us to encourage a group who have previously been very difficult to motivate (Rushfirth 1984). Vibrating pads have frequencies which can be altered and this may enable children to experiment with the use of their own voices in the production of sounds (Eckersley 1990). It is important that in any such situation vibration equipment is introduced slowly and calmly, and that the child does not become apprehensive.

TREATMENT METHODS AND EQUIPMENT

Hand unit vibrator

These hand-held machines operate at a frequency of 20–100 Hz. They are most often used in their higher range to increase muscle tone by producing the tonic vibratory reflex. Muscles which are warm and relaxed, or when muscle relaxant drugs have been administered, will respond more slowly. The following methods can be used:

1. Vibration along the triceps muscle to encourage arm support.
2. Vibration on either side (not across) of the spinal column to encourage back support.
3. Vibration along the anterolateral aspect of the lower leg to encourage dorsiflexion.

Many children find touching the hand-held vibrator a motivation to movement and this can be used to develop actions such as reaching for a toy, rolling over and turning the head.

Cyclopad vibrator

The cyclopad is a soft pad measuring approximately 20 inches by 14 inches. It has a frequency range of 20–60 Hz and is useful in the treatment of babies and young children. Young children can lie on the pad or, with older children, an arm, leg or the trunk can be supported on the pad. The low frequency vibrations can be both relaxing and comfortable. They can also be a means of introducing gentle movement and sensory experience to a child who is distressed by touching and handling.

Where spasticity is present the cyclopad can be used as an additional technique for reducing adductor spasticity of the legs and retraction of the shoulder girdle.

Base units (platforms)

Base units operate at a frequency of 15–60 Hz. These sturdy platforms come in a range of sizes and are fitted with a vibration molar. They are useful for promoting whole body movements since their effect is transmitted throughout the entire body. Although the frequency is one which is relaxing, experience has shown that this effect is temporary and develops into a facilitation of more normal postural tone. This effect is particularly helpful when, for example, a chair or a standing frame is placed on the vibrating platform. The child is encouraged to achieve a more upright position, and in some instances is encouraged to rise from sitting to standing and to retain an independent standing position.

SAFETY ASPECTS

As with all therapy techniques, a child should never be left alone whilst resting on a vibrating pad. This is not only essential for safety reasons but also so that the response of the child can be noted and built on in subsequent physiotherapy sessions. In view of the close contact between child and equipment it is suggested that a circuit-breaker is used.

SERIAL SPLINTING AND STRAPPING
M. Jones

INTRODUCTION

Serial splinting and strapping are two methods of

applying gradual stretch to soft tissues to bring about the correct anatomical alignment of muscles and joints in order to improve their function. The objective is to fix temporarily the position so gained, before repeating the process until the desired tissue lengthening or realignment has been achieved. A particular example of the use of serial splinting is with hemiplegic cerebral palsy patients, where the aim is to develop a correct heel strike pattern during walking. This process may attain the required correction or it may have to be repeated on a number of occasions over a number of years as the child continues to grow. The methods may be used as an end in themselves but they are generally used as an adjunct to other forms of treatment and offer in some cases an alternative to surgical intervention (Jones 1992). In babies too small or too ill to withstand operative procedures, treatment of this nature can often be safely considered, and corrective intervention initiated.

CONDITIONS IN WHICH THE TECHNIQUES MAY BE EMPLOYED

Adaptive shortening may occur in a number of disorders such as:

* orthopaedic conditions — talipes, chronic juvenile rheumatism
* trauma
* neuromuscular disease
* central nervous system disorders.

Orthopaedic conditions

Talipes

A combination of splinting and strapping may be used successfully, but the presence of a short tendon or skeletal abnormality, for example, in congenital vertical talus, may necessitate other forms of treatment, such as surgery, or fixed splinting for an extended period.

Chronic juvenile rheumatism

In the joints of the upper and lower limbs, where pain and spasm have led to abnormal positioning, serial splinting can be used to realign the joints. Once this is achieved a resting splint is used to maintain the desired position and permit the joints to be rested. The treatment is designed to promote the return to a full range of movement.

Trauma — burns and nerve damage

Where there are contractures of soft tissue due to scarring and adaptive shortening, serial splinting of various forms may be used, for example a picture frame splint (Fig. 19.6). The simple design and construction of this splint facilitates inspection of the traumatised area as the stretching proceeds.

Neuromuscular disease

The process of adaptive shortening associated with the development of muscular dystrophies can be delayed by treatment with an aggressive programme of serial splinting and the use of appropriate orthoses, such as polypropylene splints and standing frames.

The deformities created by arthrogryposis can be helped by prompt intervention at an early stage before growth adds to the problem.

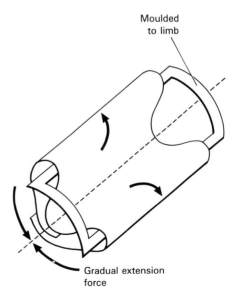

Moulded to limb

Gradual extension force

Fig. 19.6 Picture frame splint.

Central nervous system disorders

Imbalanced muscle activity resulting from hypo/hypertonia in spina bifida and cerebral palsy leads to deformity and a treatment programme of serial splinting may be appropriate.

SERIAL SPLINTING IN HEMIPLEGIC CEREBRAL PALSY

Serial splinting can make a valuable contribution to the attainment of improved gait in the hemiplegic cerebral palsied child. Success can be achieved in both the early treatment of the condition and in the treatment of the child with an established poor gait pattern. An examination of this specific use of the technique will illustrate the general principles of the method.

The technique can be used in all cases where there is evidence of a poor gait pattern. There is still no clear understanding of the underlying neurological processes involved. The procedure is effective, but more evidence is needed of why this is so. It has been suggested that: 'the clinical problem solving process involves not only the analysis of motor behaviour and consequent intervention, but also the ability to extrapolate relevant information from current scientific knowledge and use this information to develop clinical strategies for the motor disabled' (Shepherd 1987).

Indications for use

The technique is appropriate for very young children referred with hemiplegic cerebral palsy, prior to the developmental stage of 'pull to standing', where it is considered that the paucity of spontaneous foot movement and the tendency to a plantarflexed and valgus foot posture will eventually lead to a 'toe–heel' pattern of walking.

The application of the technique is not, of course, limited to children with this condition. Beneficial results can be obtained from the use of the method with patients suffering from the more complex bilateral problems associated with diplegia, both ataxic and athetoid.

Gait pattern

In the treatment of established poor gait patterns the time needed for the serial correction from plantarflexion towards dorsiflexion is variable and depends on age, the type and degree of spasticity and the frequency of application. In the early treatment of the condition the aim is to ensure that the developmental stages of standing and coasting around furniture are established in as normal a manner as possible, enabling movement to be as effective (and consequently physiologically efficient) as possible.

Where possible, treatment should take place at an early stage in the child's development, when it is possible to establish a good motor pattern. Once over-correction has been achieved a heel strike gait pattern can be facilitated. As the child grows a subsequent deterioration in the gait pattern may make it necessary to repeat the procedure.

Parental involvement

Parental involvement in the decision to adopt this procedure, the application of casts and the subsequent regime of home exercise programmes is a major advantage of the method. There is likely to be a greater understanding on the part of the parents of the responsibility for the child's well-being because of the interactive nature of the procedure than would be the case with surgery.

There may also be considerable parental influence on the interval between episodes of casting, related to their degree of diligence in ensuring treatment exercise programmes are adhered to. The parents will need extra encouragement during the child's growth spurts and at times when the patient's motivation is low.

Decreased associated spasticity and improved circulation in the splinted limb are observed as a bonus in most patients and in this context good results can be obtained from serial casts of elbows and hands. This is particularly evident in older children being serially splinted for the first time. The presence of the cast draws attention to the limb and this is beneficial to patients with parietal inattention.

If the foot requires further support after casting, ankle–foot orthoses have been found to be helpful or they may themselves be used serially.

Non-invasive

Perhaps the most significant advantage over surgery is the non-invasive nature of the treatment.

Planned timescale

In a majority of cases treatment cycles can be arranged to avoid interrupting schooling, socialisation processes or play activities. By planning periods of splinting to coincide with times convenient to parents, the disruption of normal family life is minimised. Once treatment has commenced it is normally very soon accepted as being a painless process and the consequent psychological comfort to both child and parent cannot be undervalued. Indeed, making the cast decorative, with stick-on pictures or using bright colours, transforms a visible sign of disability into a status symbol in peer group evaluations.

Both early and late intervention must be accompanied by a specific exercise programme which is carefully monitored to ensure that it is diligently completed, particularly during growth phases and in periods of low patient motivation.

Procedures

The cast is applied with care in a series of gradual stretches, at approximately weekly intervals, from plantarflexion to overcorrected dorsiflexion. As previously indicated, the number of casts required varies greatly depending on the condition, the severity of any spasticity and the degree of any contractures present.

There are many casting materials now available and choice will be influenced by factors such as cost, availability and ease of application or removal. Commercially made products are now available which are easily removed by plaster shears and, if necessary, have the added advantage of being easily removed at home with strong scissors.

The technique described below is Deltacast® specific.

The basic equipment

- stockinette
- felt
- orthopaedic bandage — Soflex® or Softban®
- splinting material — two bandages and one splint (Deltacast® or other similar materials)
- adhesive tape
- heel — where appropriate
- bowl to hold water at room temperature
- plaster shears and scissors
- crepe bandage
- rubber gloves.

Preparation for splinting

Before starting to apply the splint, it is essential to make an initial examination to ensure that the skin is free from abrasions, athlete's foot, etc. The patient is then positioned prone with the knee flexed so that gravity will assist the holder.

The required position for splinting will be determined by such factors as:

- the patient's age
- the type and degree of tone
- presence and degree of soft tissue contractures
- the degree of deformity
- emotional factors — patient and parent.

It is very important to stretch and fix the ankle in a position that holds the calcaneum vertical without valgus or varus. Only then can the forefoot be corrected using enough pressure to keep the toes dorsiflexed, tightening the plantar ligament and maintaining a good arch. It is essential to maintain this position until the cast is set, and the holder must be able successfully to anticipate clonus, and to counteract impatient wriggling, etc. whilst the bandaging takes place.

Application procedure

Inner protective layers. The first step is to cut and fit a length of stockinette to extend from above the knee to beyond the toes. A piece of adhesive felt is then cut as shown in Fig. 19.7 and attached from the back of the heel and around the ankle, the felt being smoothed towards the toes so as to prevent wrinkles forming. For children with sensitive skin it is wise to use non-adhesive felt or acrylic-type adhesive felt. This serves to protect the bony prominences. Alternatively, the felt can be applied directly on to the skin before putting on the stockinette.

The orthopaedic bandage is then applied in the conventional manner of covering half the previous turn, from the toes to just below the knee, the process starting and ending with a double turn. Care in the application of the felt, the orthopaedic bandage and the casting material is vital to the comfort of the patient, as pressure is, of necessity, applied to gain the required position.

Corrective bandaging and casting. A suitably sized Deltacast® bandage is selected and, after removal of the foil, is immersed in water at room temperature for between 5 and 10 seconds. The bandage is squeezed several times during the immersion to ensure thorough wetting. After removal from the water the bandage is allowed to drain before being applied firmly and evenly to the limb, pleating where necessary to conform to contours. The polymer-impregnated bandage reacts rapidly with the water and sets hard in 5–7 minutes, being completely cured in 30 minutes. The slab splint is next removed from its foil pack,

placed over the limb and cut to a length which is slightly less than the area covered. The splint is immersed in water for 5 to 10 seconds and then placed over the calf and sole of the foot, prior to bandaging in position.

The whole cast is then firmly covered in a crepe bandage for 3 to 4 minutes to allow the layers to bond together; the crepe bandage is then removed. If required, the heel is fixed in place using elastoplast strapping. As more dorsiflexion is introduced, a wedge of slab material can be positioned under the forefoot to encourage weight to be taken at the heel.

Finishing the splint. The splint is finished off by turning the stockinette back over the top edges of the cast and ensuring that the edges are smooth. Any excess material covering the toes is cut away whilst leaving a platform below the toes to ensure that they are dorsiflexed. The turned-back stockinette is covered and secured by elastoplast tape. This finish is designed to allow parents to investigate any areas which may cause minor irritation and trim off the problem areas.

Activity after splinting

Although the cast is cured in 30 minutes, it is normal practice to ask the parents to ensure that the limb is non-weight-bearing and kept as still as possible overnight, to facilitate accommodation to the new position. After this the child is encouraged to be as active as possible, so as to avoid any perception of being an invalid. Because the splinting materials described are light, strong and waterproof there should be little interference with the child's normal play and social activities.

Changing the splint

The serial process of splinting involves changing the splint on a weekly basis (or sooner) to increase gradually the degree of stretch. After removal of the splint using plaster shears, the limb is carefully checked for pressure sores or abrasions, and washed prior to the beginning of the next cycle.

The limb is remanipulated into a position of further correction, and resplinted. The amount of manipulation possible will vary with the

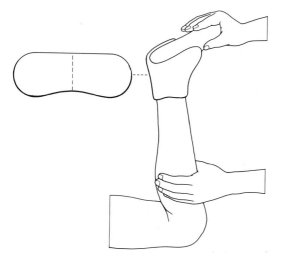

Fig. 19.7 Felt protection for bony prominences.

tightness of the tendon/soft tissue resistance but gradually each child's requirements become clear. During the period between removal of the original splint and a resplinting process taking place, it is advisable to prevent weight-bearing and thus unwanted stimulation of the plantar thrust. When a significant degree of dorsiflexion has been obtained it is worth considering the removal of part of the cast under the heel to allow it to make contact with the ground when standing and walking, and thus to stimulate proprioception.

The exercise programme

Parents are encouraged to continue to give daily therapy to their child by various methods of sensory motor stimulation. All aspects of daily life are geared to involve the hemiplegic side of the body.

During leg-splinting periods parents are expected to give extra active extension exercises to combat an initial overflow of flexor activity into hip and knee. Parents are also made aware of the necessity to check the circulation of the splinted limb.

In the event of the cast's becoming wet, it has to be dried and checked to ensure that it is still comfortable for the patient.

Most parents help on treatment days by removing the splint with shears and assisting with the casting process.

The exercise/night splint

Once the desired degree of overcorrection has been achieved by the serial splinting programme, a removable fibreglass-reinforced plaster of Paris exercise splint is used to maintain the limb in the attained position of overcorrection (Fig. 19.8). It is possible, as with the serial splint, to remove part of the cast under the heel to facilitate direct ground contact. This is used both during the day for normal activities and special exercise therapy and can be used as a night splint. The exercise splint is normally made on the penultimate resplinting day, so that it is ready as the child's serial casting programme is completed.

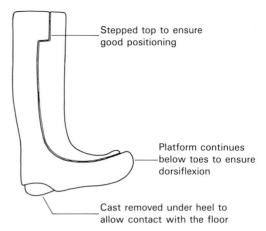

Stepped top to ensure good positioning

Platform continues below toes to ensure dorsiflexion

Cast removed under heel to allow contact with the floor

Fig. 19.8   The exercise/night splint.

Making the exercise splint

1. With the child prone, lying with the affected limb flexed at the knee, the lower leg is wrapped in an orthopaedic bandage and covered with stockinette, care being taken to avoid wrinkles forming.

2. The child's foot is held in the overcorrected position, which is maintained until the plaster cast is set. The lower limb is then bandaged using only two layers, so as to keep the final cast as light as possible. The bandage is smoothed and moulded to the contours of the limb.

3. The intended line of separation of the two halves of the splint is marked into the plaster while it is still soft, this indentation subsequently serving as a guide and weak point along which the scalpel blade can penetrate. It will be noted from Fig. 19.8 that:
   a. separation is not on the midline but off-set to leave a deep 'base' section and shallow 'lid';
   b. a step section at the top has been incorporated to help keep the splint halves in register.

4. While the cast is setting, and before full hardening occurs, the scalpel blade tip only is used at right angles to the cast in a reciprocating motion to cut along the previously marked line. Care must be taken to avoid any slicing action or contact with the patient's skin.

5. Final separation of the two halves is completed by cutting through the stockinette and any thin layer of plaster that remains uncut with scissors.

6. The lid is removed from the limb and then the deeper base is eased off, care being taken not to distort the two halves.

7. The stockinette lining is removed from inside the shell halves and all edges are trimmed with thin strips of plaster of Paris moulded to give a smooth edge finish. The inside is similarly finished by 'creaming' with plaster of Paris.

8. The shell is then fibreglassed to give added strength.

9. Micropore tape is used to edge the splint. The splint is then lined with felt.

Fitting the splint. Final adjustments are made to ensure a comfortable fit for the splint by adding or removing felt. It is suggested that a thin sock is worn for the first fitting as the skin may be tender after the serial splinting. Keeping the patient prone provides a good position from which to manipulate and hold the foot prior to application. Alternatively, if supine, the foot should first be plantarflexed then inverted before dorsiflexing.

SERIAL TREATMENT — OTHER APPLICATIONS

As previously mentioned, good results may be obtained from serial casting programmes used in the treatment of, for example, adaptive tissue shortening at the elbow, or deformities due to inflammatory conditions of the hand. Over-correction of the elbow is not possible due to the joint configuration.

Congenital talipes equinovarus

Serial strapping can be effective in the treatment of congenital talipes equinovarus (CTEV). The foot is progressively manipulated and then immobilised, using felt and adhesive strapping (Fig. 19.9), until an over-corrected position is achieved or operative procedures become necessary.

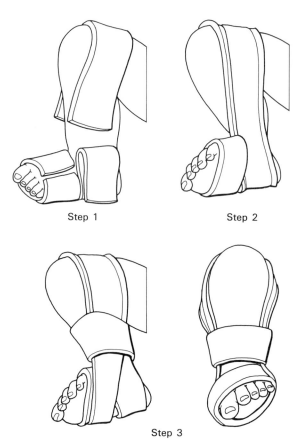

Step 1   Step 2

Step 3

Fig. 19.9 Strapping for congenital talipes equinovarus.

Splinting the hand

It is essential to identify clearly whether rest or function is the aim when splinting, particularly splinting of the hand. Extension at the wrist for a hand in resting position is 12 to 20 degrees compared with 25 to 35 degrees for a functional position splint (Fig. 19.10).

The ultimate overcorrection is the totally extended pattern indicated for the serial casting of a spastic wrist, thumb and fingers (Fig. 19.11).

GENERAL CONSIDERATIONS IN SERIAL TREATMENT

As with the use of orthoses, physiotherapists must carefully consider the following factors when applying strapping or splinting:

• correct alignment of the joint

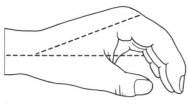

Position of rest (12 — 20°)

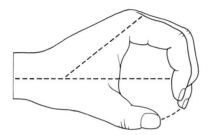

Position of function (20 — 35°)

Fig. 19.10 The wrist: positions of rest and of function.

- the loading forces applied to growing bones
- any sensory impairment which may lead to undetected problems of pressure points or abrasion
- protection of pressure points or bony prominences
- care of the circulation.

The physiotherapist must be aware of the forces involved, evaluate the need for splinting or strapping and be aware that, particularly when dealing with a very young baby, a stretched pos-

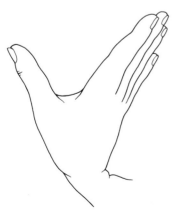

Fig. 19.11 Overcorrection of the hand.

ition may be achieved beyond which point further force may be contraindicated. Surgery then becomes the most appropriate treatment. For example, in some patients with CTEV, 'to persevere with stretching in these cases results in a rocker-bottom deformity and flat-topped talus' (Shaw 1977).

Nevertheless, in some conditions, the need for non-invasive corrective procedures at the earliest possible time after diagnosis is desirable, if fixed deformities are to be prevented, even though it may subsequently become necessary for surgery to take place.

INDIVIDUAL LEARNING PROGRAMMES
S. Steel

Introduction

The 1981 Education Act, formally implemented in April 1983, laid a duty on local education authorities to define the needs of individual children and show how and where those needs would best be met (see Chapter 25 Legal Aspects in Paediatric Physiotherapy). The Act abolished the traditional categories of handicap in favour of the wider concept of special educational needs proposed in the Warnock Report (Department of Education and Science 1978), with the child becoming the centre of focus, rather than his or her disability. Emphasis is placed on looking at the whole child and, on the basis of a multidisciplinary assessment, the local education authority may prepare a 'statement of special needs'. This must specify the child's special needs and the provision required to meet those needs, including non-educational provision. The 1981 Education Act requires that any statement is subject to annual review, but ongoing assessment of a child's special educational needs can also be provided according to the school's perceptions of the child's needs.

Although many schools have had a written curriculum document stating the philosophy and aims of the school and the core areas of curriculum, it is only within the last 10 years that there has been increasing focus on planning individual learning programmes for children through the use of behavioural objectives. This approach is in contrast to a medical or traditional remedial style of intervention. Both these approaches are curative, as the expert is called in to diagnose the problem once it has developed and then prescribe appropriate treatment. This allows children to fail before any action is taken and is then preoccupied with fitting them to a descriptive label or category of handicap. The behavioural objectives approach concentrates on factors within the professional's control and advocates immediate action as soon as it is seen that a child is having difficulty. The focus is on the content of the teaching programme and its management. It forces professionals to ask fundamental questions about what they are doing and how they are doing it, thus ensuring that work is set for individual children at an appropriate level (Ainscow & Tweddle 1979).

HOW TO PLAN FOR INDIVIDUALS

Planning individual learning programmes using a behavioural objectives approach involves setting clear and precise behavioural objectives, analysing tasks into appropriately sized steps and developing appropriate teaching strategies. Implementation of the programme will then lend itself to a continuous cycle of assessment, choice of objectives, teaching method and record keeping (Ainscow & Tweddle 1979).

The major planning steps in this cycle will include setting up:

- profiles
- priorities
- behavioural objectives
- programme content
- assessment of achievement.

Profiles

The first step towards devising an individual learning programme is for the teacher to draw up a profile of the child. This is an assessment of what the child can do based on advice from all professionals involved. It should produce a picture of the whole child rather than looking at aspects of his or her development in isolation.

Depending on the needs of the child, contributions may come from physiotherapists, occupational therapists or speech therapists amongst others, as the following profile illustrates:

Profile 19.1   Simon.
Simon is 3 years old and is in the nursery class. He is a very social little boy and enjoys the company of other children, but he tends to flit from activity to activity. He likes listening to stories and looking at books when he has the undivided attention of an adult, but again his concentration span is limited. He enjoys singing and action games. He eats messily with a spoon and drinks from a feeder cup. He needs to be reminded to go to the toilet and has to be held on the seat because his sitting balance is poor. He can pull himself along the floor in the classroom. He uses a wheelchair to move around school and can wheel himself, but has to be lifted out.

Priorities

Once a profile of the child has been drawn up, priority curriculum areas which reflect the child's special educational needs are selected, and behavioural objectives are set based on staff perceptions of the level of improvement possible over a specified period of time, for example, 6 weeks. The teacher should take advice from all professionals working with the child, whether contributing a specific objective or giving advice on implementation of an objective.

The following priority areas of curriculum might be selected for Simon: social skills, language and motor skills.

Programme content

Once the behavioural objectives have been set, the content of the learning programme can be decided. In the example shown, implementation of the language objective for Simon could incorporate the priority areas highlighted in his profile. Although Simon enjoys stories when he has an adult's undivided attention, he will now be expected to work as part of a small group. The group activity could have a specified time limit, perhaps 5 minutes initially, during which time Simon would be expected to stay with the group and not move to another activity. The motor objective, specified by the physiotherapist, could be linked with an activity Simon enjoys so that he has a purpose for getting out of his wheelchair.

Behavioural objectives

Behavioural objectives would then be devised for each of these areas and could be as follows:

Social skills

Will ask to go to toilet (advice on suitable seat from occupational therapist).
Will drink from a two-handed cup, no lid (advice on suitable cup from occupational therapist).

Language

Will 'read' a storybook with an adult in group of three children.

Motor skills

Will get out of wheelchair independently (objective from physiotherapist).

Assessment of achievement

At the end of the specified period of time, 6 weeks for the examples shown, the objectives achieved can be recorded and new objectives set. A sequence of these profiles will give a long-term picture of the achievements of the child. The following example shows what Simon might have achieved:

Social skills

Can ask to go to the toilet.
Can sit independently on toilet seat (following both advice and practical intervention from the occupational therapist).
Can drink from a two-handled cup, no lid.

Language

Can 'read' a storybook with adult in group of three children for 5 minutes.

Motor skills

Can get out of wheelchair with verbal prompts.

ADVANTAGES OF BEHAVIOURAL OBJECTIVES

There are many advantages to using a behavioural objectives approach to learning, but in particular, as Ainscow & Tweddle (1979) indicated:

- the child is viewed in a positive prescriptive way
- objectives are written in terms that are clearly understood
- record-keeping provides a system of ongoing assessment.

Opponents of this approach argue that it is impersonal and stifles creativity by staff and demands too much paperwork. Perhaps their real objection is that they become accountable because progress is measurable — this approach does not allow for vague statements such as 'her social skills show some improvement'!

It is possible to train all staff, for example, teachers, classroom assistants and paramedical staff, in behavioural techniques, and thus all staff have the opportunity to participate in devising individual learning programmes. One such package is the EDY Project (Foxen & McBrien 1981). Although this was designed particularly for professionals working with children with severe learning difficulties and profound and multiple handicaps, the teaching methodology can be adapted and applied in any setting. If professionals work in isolation it is possible not only to slow down a child's progress but to stop it. Teacher and therapist working together using a behavioural objectives approach creates a common language and suggests a sharing of expertise and a cooperation which will ensure that the child is looked at as a whole and not as separate parts.

IMPLEMENTING INDIVIDUAL LEARNING PROGRAMMES

Planning a programme which is individually tailored to a child's special educational needs involves:

- assessment of need
- concentrated individual attention daily

- the opportunity to generalise the specific skills and concepts learnt
- a coordinated consistent approach.

It is becoming increasingly apparent that effective responses to the initiative of the 1981 Education Act will have to be based on maximising and managing resources, time and personnel within the classroom, so that providing individual help is feasible (Thomas 1986). The notion that teacher expertise should be focused on the content of the learning programme, the teaching process and the management of resources is in sharp contrast to the traditional diagnosis/treatment model, which owed more to medicine than education. As Thomas (1986) indicated, teachers are increasingly fulfilling the role of managers in the classroom.

The high pupil:teacher ratio in special schools, and the increasing trend for support staff to work alongside teachers in mainstream schools as more children are integrated, is not automatically advantageous. When adults work together in one room, various management systems exist:

- all 'muck in' together approach!
- one person leads, the others follow
- class split into groups doing either similar or different things
- individual and group work going on at the same time.

However, such ratios can be used to improve both the quality and quantity of education for the children. What is needed is an approach in which:

- everyone knows what he is doing and why he is doing it
- planning takes place before the teaching sessions
- adults do not spend unnecessary time talking to each other in teaching sessions
- interruptions are dealt with efficiently and effectively.

CLASSROOM MANAGEMENT

One such organisational approach is Room Management. This system of organising staff arose out of the work of Hart & Risley (1976),

in the United States, and was taken up in this country by Porterfield et al (1977), who used the system in institutions for people with a mental handicap. Since then Room Management has been implemented in both special and mainstream schools.

Staff roles

Room Management aims to increase the amount of individual teaching time possible in a busy classroom by organising specific periods of time, usually 1 hour, when the minimum number of staff usefully occupy groups of children and so free others to conduct the individual teaching sessions (Thomas 1985). Staff take on three specific roles:

- individual helper
- activity manager
- mover.

The individual helper works with individual children on a rota basis for short specified periods of time. The work for these children will have been planned beforehand.

The activity manager supervises the rest of the class who are consolidating and generalising tasks already learnt. Most attention is given to children who are working appropriately, while those who are not are prompted with minimal attention, such as a gesture.

The mover maintains the flow in the classroom by dealing with distractions and interruptions and moving equipment.

This system of organisation can be adapted to any setting and the precise arrangement will depend on the needs of the class. In a school for children with physical disabilities Room Management has been adapted and developed from the system used during the Anson House Preschool Project (Gunstone et al 1982), into a model which incorporates two specific roles:

- individual worker
- coordinator.

The individual worker works with individual children, for a specified length of time, on specific objectives from the child's individual educational programme, uninterrupted.

The coordinator ensures the smooth running of the class and consequently deals with all interruptions and the positioning of children, as well as supervising children working independently to consolidate skills and concepts previously mastered in individual sessions.

The class teacher has overall responsibility for what happens in the classroom in terms of teaching content and management, but roles within Room Management are interchangeable. Staff may wish to change roles weekly or take specific roles on specific days. Where classroom teams consist of more than two staff, the number of individual workers is increased.

Timetable

Room Management in this setting lasts for half-day blocks, and in order for the system to be implemented smoothly the class teacher is responsible for drawing up a daily Room Management timetable, which the coordinator uses as a basis for directing staff during the session. The session is divided into 15-minute blocks of time to ensure that each child has an individual teaching session daily as well as the opportunity to work independently. Teaching sessions with other professionals, such as speech, occupational or physiotherapists, are also timetabled to ensure that sessions do not clash. Figure 19.12 shows a Room Management timetable for

Time	Co-ordinator	Individual worker		Children out
	Nursery nurse	Teacher	Child care attendant	
9.30	Supervision of class	Kate	Michael	Stephen (physiotherapy)
9.45	Ian into standing frame	Tracy	Mark	
10.00		John		Nicola (speech therapy)
10.15		Stephen	Ian	
10.30	Coffee break	Supervise children's break	Supervise children's break	Jacqueline and Mark (physiotherapy)
10.45	Ian out of standing frame	Coffee break	Jennifer	
11.00		Carl	Coffee break	Tracy (physiotherapy)
11.15	Nancy on to prone board		Nicola	Kate (occupational therapy)
11.30	John to walk to individual worker using rollator	Nancy	Jacqueline	Michael (speech therapy)
11.45				Ian (physiotherapy)
12.00	Tidy classroom	John	Kate	

Fig. 19.12 A Room Management timetable.

a class of 12 children with a team of three staff: two individual workers and a coordinator.

Although the fourth column specifies 'children out' it may well be that a therapist chooses to work with the child in the classroom.

Advantages and disadvantages

The advantage of a Room Management approach is that all members of staff know what they are doing and why they are doing it, and therapists are included as part of the classroom team. An obvious disadvantage is that all the planning must take place before the Room Management session begins and it therefore demands a great deal of initial preparation by the class teacher. Once the organisation and content has been decided upon, it still needs to be continually monitored and modified as necessary.

CONCLUSION

In recent years schools have been required to look in detail at the kind of educational programme they offer children and how effective they are in helping children to learn. There is no doubt that children need to have a balanced school day with opportunities for both individual and other kinds of learning. At the same time schools have a responsibility to meet children's individual special educational needs. It is suggested, in conclusion, that one of the most successful ways of doing this is through devising individual learning programmes, and the most effective way of implementing these programmes is by well-planned Room Management.

ACKNOWLEDGEMENTS

The author (E. B.) wishes to acknowledge the advice of Jocelyn Ness, Scottish Council for Spastics, on the hydrotherapy section and the advice of Dr G. E. Walsh, Department of Physiology, University of Edinburgh, in the preparation of Vibration Therapy.

REFERENCES

Ainscow M, Tweddle D A 1979 Preventing classroom failure — an objectives approach. Wiley, Chichester

Bracegirdle H 1990 Developing physical fitness to promote mental health. In: Creek J (ed) Occupational therapy and mental health. Churchill Livingstone, Edinburgh

Campbell T, Ferguson N, McKinlay R G 1986 The use of a simple self-administered method of positive expiratory pressure in chest physiotherapy after abdominal surgery. Physiotherapy 72: 498–500

Campion R M 1985 Hydrotherapy in paediatrics. Heinemann Medical, London

Curtis S R 1982 The joy of movement in early childhood. Teachers College Press, New York

Davies H, Kitchman R, Gordon I, Helms P 1985 Regional ventilation in infancy. New England Journal of Medicine 313: 1626–1628

Department of Education and Science 1978 Special educational needs (Warnock Report). Her Majesty's Stationery Office, London

Eckersley P M 1990 Cerebral palsy and profound retardation. In: Hogg J et al (eds) Profound retardation and multiple impairment. Chapman and Hall, London

Education Act 1981 Her Majesty's Stationery Office, London

Eklund G, Hagbarth K E 1965 Motor effects of vibratory stimuli in man. Electroencephalography and Clinical Neurophysiology 19: 619

Foxen T, McBrien J 1981 Training staff in behavioural methods — the EDY in-service course for mental handicap practitioners. Manchester University Press, Manchester

Gaskell D, Webber B 1987 The physical treatment of cystic fibrosis. Cystic Fibrosis Research Trust Publication, Bromley, December 1987

Gunstone C, Hogg J, Sebba J, Warner J, Almond S 1982 Classroom provision and organisation for integrated preschool children — Anson House preschool project papers 2. Dr Barnardo's, Hertford

Hart B, Risley T R 1976 Environmental reprogramming: implications for the severely handicapped (unpublished paper). Center for Applied Behavior Analysis, Kansas

Heaf D, Helms P, Gordon I, Turner H 1983 Postural effects on gas exchange in infants. New England Journal of Medicine 308: 1505–1508

Hogg J et al (eds) Profound retardation and multiple impairment. Chapman & Hall, London

Hoole B 1981 Motor development in children. Blackwell Scientific Publications, Oxford

Jones M 1992 Serial splinting in hemiplegic cerebral palsy. APCP publications (reprint)

Kendall L 1987 A comparison between adult and paediatric intensive care. Physiotherapy 73: 495–499

Kerr K M 1988 Exercise and health related fitness. Physiotherapy 74(8): 411–420

Madders J 1987 Relax and be happy. Unwin Paperbacks, London

Parker A 1987 Paediatric and neonatal intensive therapy. In: Downie P (ed) Cash's textbook of chest, heart and vascular disorders for physiotherapists, 4th edn. Faber & Faber, London

Porterfield J, Blunden R, Blewitt E 1977 Improving environments for profoundly handicapped adults: establishing staff routines for high client engagement. Mental Handicap in Wales Applied Research Unit, University of South Wales, Cardiff

Price R J 1980 Physical education and the physically handicapped child. Lepus Books, London

Pryor J A, Webber B A 1979 An evaluation of the forced expiration technique as an adjunct to postural drainage. Physiotherapy 65: 304

Rushfirth S 1984 Physiotherapy for severely mentally handicapped children. In: Levitt S (ed) Paediatric developmental therapy. Blackwell, Oxford

Shaw N E 1977 Treatment and prognosis in clubfoot. British Medical Journal 1: 219–222

Shepherd R B 1987 Movement science and physiotherapy — deriving implications for the clinic. Proceedings of the Tenth International Congress of the World Confederation for Physical Therapy.

Thomas G 1985 Room management in mainstream education. Educational Research 27(3): 168–193

Thomas G 1986 Integrating personnel in order to integrate children. Support for Learning 1(1): 19–26

Young C S 1984a A review of the adverse effects of airway suction. Physiotherapy 70: 104–106

Young C S 1984b Recommended guidelines for suction. Physiotherapy 70: 106–108

Young C S 1988 Airway suctioning: a study of paediatric physiotherapy practice. Physiotherapy 74: 13–15

FURTHER READING

Association of Swimming Therapy 1981 Swimming for the disabled. EP Publishing Ltd, Wakefield

Cotton M 1981 Out of doors with handicapped people. Human Horizons Series. Souvenir Press, London

Eklund G, Hagbarth K E 1966 Normal variability of tonic vibration reflexes in man. Experimental Neurology 16: 80–92

George S J, Hart B 1983 Physical education for handicapped children. Human Horizons Series, Souvenir Press, London

Gregory G A (ed) 1982 Respiratory failure in the child. Management of respiratory failure of cardiac origin. Churchill Livingstone, London, ch 6

Levitt S (1982) Movement training. In: Norris D (ed) Profound mental handicap. Costello, Tunbridge Wells

Skinner A T, Thomson A M 1983 Duffield's exercise in water, 3rd edn. Baillière Tindall, London

Sutherland A, Soames P 1984 Adventure play with handicapped children. Human Horizons Series. Souvenir Press, London

20

Living skills and the environment

*R. Bates G. Hall K. Newton
P. Pott*

INTRODUCTION

As children grow they develop increasing control over both themselves and their environment (Table 20.1). The disabled child is more dependent on parents and carers for those self-help activities which are increasingly taken for granted by the non-disabled child. In this chapter the skills of feeding, toileting and dressing are discussed not only from a practical perspective but also for the contribution their acquisition makes to a child's involvement in the wider social community and to the development of choice, self-determination and independence. The chapter ends with a section on the ways technology is used to enhance the disabled child's access to decision-making, communication and learning.

FEEDING
K. Newton and P. Pott

INTRODUCTION

There are many occasions in life when eating and drinking form an opportunity for social interaction. This can occur in different contexts, such as close family contacts on a daily basis; less frequent but regular meetings with friends, relatives or peer groups; and special celebrations (parties, weddings and religious festivals). Food and drink are also used to break down barriers

Table 20.1 The development of functional skills

Age	Functional skill
6 months	Feeds self biscuit
9 months	Holds own cup Puts arm out for dressing
12 months	Finger feeds
15 months	Takes spoon to mouth but upside down Very interested in going to the toilet
18 months	Takes off shoes, socks, hat
2 years	Drinks without spilling Uses spoon well Undoes zip Understands going to the toilet but has no control
$2\frac{1}{2}$ years	May use fork Pulls pants down but not up Puts on hat and shoes Toileting — may remain clean during the day — controls bladder for up to 2 hours
3 years	Washes hands, may need help drying
$3\frac{1}{2}$–4 years	Brushes teeth Can do buttons but not laces Toileting — child clean day and night
5 years	Dresses and undresses Uses knife and fork

and uncertainties between people who are getting to know each other.

However, many children with disabilities have difficulty in developing efficient eating and drinking skills. This may impede their development of social skills and hence their ability to establish a range of social contacts.

At a more basic level, feeding is an essential activity, because food sustains life. It is therefore vitally important that a child should be offered a balanced diet to ensure maximal benefit from eating, and that the child chews the food as well as possible to assist digestion. Feeding problems need to be dealt with as soon as possible and appropriate, bearing in mind that skill in this aspect of development is acquired and refined over many years in any child. The development of feeding patterns reflects neurological maturation and the change from reflex behaviour to that which is under voluntary control.

Physiotherapists, speech therapists and occupational therapists may all be involved, in collaboration with parents and others, in improving feeding patterns in children. All, too, may take others' roles in developing the child's sensory awareness of the process of feeding, in reinforcing motor skill, in paying attention to the social aspects of mealtimes and encouraging as much independence as possible.

PROBLEMS ENCOUNTERED WHEN FEEDING

The development of satisfactory eating and drinking behaviours may be impeded by the presence of one or more of the following difficulties, which will be discussed under Remediation:

- poor trunk position and head control
- poor grasp
- poor coordination
- persistence of infantile reflexes, such as extensor thrust and ATNR
- altered reflexes involving the oral musculature
- hypersensitivity to different textures and flavours of food; this is sometimes associated with exaggerated reflexes
- hyposensitivity, with lack of awareness of the presence of food in the mouth
- drooling
- abnormal or limited movements of the tongue, jaw, lips and soft palate
- respiration.

Where several of these difficulties co-occur, careful consideration should be given to determining priorities for assisting the child to overcome or modify them.

Postural stability, grasp and controlled movements of the tongue, jaw and lips are important in feeding. They are also necessary for the acquisition of other skills, e.g. writing and speech, and are therefore significant for cognitive development and emotional maturation.

The anatomical structures involved in speech production (thorax, larynx, pharynx, tongue, soft palate, mandible, teeth, lips) are primarily used for the life-sustaining functions of respiration and taking nourishment. Utilisation of these structures for speech requires extensive adaptation of motor control. The exact nature of the relationship between them is not clearly understood but it is widely held that abnormal development of the earlier occurring feeding patterns negatively influences speech development/acquisition (Treharne 1980).

In normal development, much of the motor activity of eating and speech becomes automatic, but proprioceptive feedback has a monitoring function which ensures that the behaviours can be quickly brought back under voluntary control if required. Neurophysiological dysfunction, as in cerebral palsy, for example, may cause impairment in proprioceptive feedback and this must not be overlooked in planning remediation.

REMEDIATION

In order to develop an appropriate feeding programme, very careful observation and assessment are necessary to highlight the child's particular problems (Coupe et al 1987).

The problem areas identified earlier as contributing to the impairment of eating and drinking will now be considered in some detail. Although these difficulties are primarily viewed as sensorimotor problems, all are closely related to the child's level of cognitive development and before embarking on a self-feeding programme it is important that the child has attained the cognitive level that makes self-feeding a realistic aim. Although these aspects are discussed below in the context of a feeding programme, the improvement of function is likely to be a goal of other parts of the child's developmental programme. So, for example, attaining and maintaining sitting balance will be included in the toileting programme, as well as the feeding programme. Similarly, controlled and differentiated oral movements will be a goal in the speech therapist's programme for a child with sensorimotor impairment leading to dysarthria and dyspraxia of speech.

Poor trunk position and head control

The child should be as near as possible to an upright sitting position with head and shoulders in the midline and slightly forwards. A child who has only recently achieved stability in unsupported sitting may need support when eating, to enable competent hand–mouth coordination and oral control to be achieved.

A hypotonic child may be helped by being seated at a high table giving arm support at shoulder level. This fixation facilitates head control. Occasionally, a minimal reclining position may be necessary to eliminate the effect of gravity on the head, but great care will be required to avoid choking.

Poor grasp

Adequate grasp may be facilitated by the use of padded utensil handles. Waiting until the child can consistently maintain grasp independently may unnecessarily delay the acquisition of self-feeding skills and the use of strapping/splinting may reduce frustration arising from the continual dropping of the utensil.

A child who has limited pronation and supination will have difficulty in loading a spoon, and may be helped by the use of specialised cutlery. Consultation with an occupational therapist is recommended.

Poor coordination

The more difficulty the child has with coordination, the more important it is to stabilise the trunk. If further help is required, fixation of the non-active arm by splinting or by holding a grab bar will enable more efficient use of the active arm (Fig. 20.1). It may also be necessary to rest the elbow of the arm being used on a non-slip mat on the table to facilitate spoon loading and controlled hand–mouth coordination.

When a severely athetoid child is being fed, he will be able to control his oral movements better if both arms and trunk are stabilised.

Persistence of infantile reflexes

A child with extensor thrust needs increased flexion at hips and knees. The foot support may have to be removed to prevent the possibility of pushing down and thus initiating this extension.

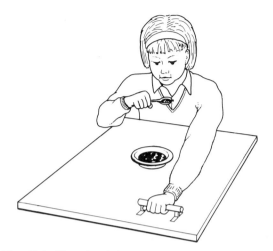

Fig. 20.1 Use of grab bar.

Asymmetrical tonic neck reflex will also interfere with feeding. The hands must be fixed in the midline to allow the head to face forwards.

Altered reflexes involving the oral musculature

Initially feeding is dependent on the oral reflexes:

- sucking
- biting
- chewing
- swallowing.

Sucking reflex

This is normally present at or soon after birth. The jaw moves up and down with accompanying rhythmical tongue movements, which enable the baby to squeeze the nipple or teat to gain nourishment. However, in some babies the sucking reflex is not present or well-enough developed and attempts may be made to facilitate it. For example, gentle upwards, downwards and sideways movements of a teat which has a sweetened liquid on the outside may help. If sweetened substances must be used, then care must be taken with dental hygiene afterwards.

Larger holes on the teat do not necessarily help as more liquid flows into the mouth without the child's making any effort. This may lead to choking. It is preferable to use a plastic bottle which can be squeezed rhythmically to force out the liquid, simulating the result of pumping action of the tongue. Alternately applying and releasing pressure under the chin to help the tongue press the teat against the gums may also be useful, as may stroking the cheeks downwards.

Some babies never achieve a sucking response so may be fed from a spoon instead.

Biting reflex

This is also found in very young babies, occurring when something is placed into or near the mouth. It usually begins to disappear around 4–5 months, although voluntary biting continues.

However, if the reflex persists there will be problems with drinking and chewing. If the baby clamps gums or teeth on to anything between them, he cannot make the necessary rotatory movements.

Applying upward pressure below the chin can help because the child resists and so releases the jaw.

Chewing

This requires the tongue to move independently from the jaw and as chewing develops the sucking reflex gradually disappears. However, chewing will only be acquired if there is something to chew on, so the child must be introduced to thicker consistency and coarse textures. This must at first be easily chewed and digested, e.g. rusks, ripe bananas, etc., in case the child swallows the food before it has been properly chewed. He may be helped by having small pieces placed directly between the back gums or molars and the cheeks manipulated in a circular movement to encourage chewing.

If the jaws are held closed when a piece of food has been placed between the teeth, this may result in the child's resisting the jaw closure, leading to a chewing movement.

Swallowing reflex

Although problems with the actual swallow mechanism do occur, difficulties attributed to this are often incorrectly diagnosed. They may be due to poor tongue control, leading to problems in directing food towards the back of the mouth so that swallowing can be initiated. A sensory deficit may make the child unaware, either that the food is in a state suitable for swallowing, or that there is an accumulation of fluid, e.g. saliva, which needs swallowing. This is discussed further under Hyposensitivity.

It is important to remember that swallowing is extremely difficult and, for some people, impossible, if the mouth is open or the head is thrown back. Hence, a flexed position with the head and shoulders slightly forwards is a prerequisite for efficient swallowing once the child no longer needs to be fed in a nursing position. So, too, is mouth closure. Normally the top and bottom lips are brought together, but alternatively top teeth and bottom lip (or occasionally top teeth and tongue) make contact in cases of limited oral movement.

For those children with specific swallowing difficulties, an effective procedure can be stroking the upper neck gently and then pressing upwards under the chin. If the child's mouth is open, gentle downward pressure towards the back of the tongue with a polythene spoon, which should then be quickly removed, may also stimulate a swallow.

Hypersensitivity

Some children, especially those with increased muscle tone, may be hypersensitive around the face and mouth. This makes it very difficult for them to tolerate a helper's touch or assistance with movements of the mandible, tongue or lips. The child's experience of the more normal movements required for eating and drinking will be reduced.

In some cases, hypersensitivity may also be associated with a heightened gag reflex. While this is a normal reflex which prevents choking, when exaggerated it may lead to the rejection of some foods and inability to tolerate certain utensils.

Procedures for reducing hypersensitivity may include stroking, brushing and tapping the child's face starting at the forehead, ears and chin and gradually working towards the oral region. These will help build up the child's tolerance of touch.

Careful consideration must be given to systematically developing the child's tolerance of an increasing variety of food textures and flavours. The child may tolerate smoother texture and more bland flavours at first. For detailed guidance on desensitisation, refer to Warner (1981).

Acceptance of more adult food types may take longer for a child with disabilities, but is an important aspect of emotional and social maturation.

Hyposensitivity

Conversely, reduced oral sensitivity may mean that the child swallows food before it has been adequately masticated, leading to choking. The child may also be unaware when there is enough food inside the mouth — too much is taken in to be satisfactorily dealt with — and so meal times can be excessively messy, with food spilling out. There may also be reduced awareness of temperature and burning may occur.

In all cases, attention should be paid to helping the child to become more aware first of large differences in texture, flavour or temperature and then gradually of finer differences. Kinaesthetic discrimination, initially, may need to be augmented by visual discrimination.

Drooling

A commonly encountered problem, with or without associated eating problems, is drooling. While problems in swallowing may be responsible for this, there are other reasons why persistent dribbling of saliva may occur.

Insensitivity to the accumulation of saliva inside the mouth may result in its spilling forward out of the mouth. If it spills backwards down the throat, without the swallow reflex being initiated, then choking may occur as the saliva will enter the trachea rather than the oesophagus. In a child who has great difficulty in coughing, it is potentially dangerous if saliva, fluids from drinks or food, enter the lungs, and suction may have to be carried out.

In cases where the child is unaware of the build-up of saliva, then it may be helpful to develop his awareness externally first, by drawing attention to the difference between wet and dry lips and chin. This may be achieved visually using a mirror as well as kinaesthetically. From external recognition, the child may then be helped to build up awareness of saliva within the oral cavity and the need to swallow before it dribbles out.

Problems in closing the mouth to assist swallowing (see p. 380) and prevent drooling may arise because of tooth alignment, spastic muscles or poor muscle tone in the oral region, or a habitual open-mouth posture. Since these problems have considerable implications for speech, liaison with the speech therapist is important.

Abnormal or limited movements of the tongue, jaw, lips and soft palate

Food is normally moved around the mouth by action of the oral musculature. Where difficulties occur, the speech therapist should be approached for appropriate intervention.

A child who is unable to direct food around the mouth will be helped by the food's being placed laterally between his teeth rather than centrally. It is important to check that food does not become compacted in the roof of the mouth and that the mouth is cleaned after meals.

Respiration

In order to develop an adequate sucking and swallowing pattern in early infancy, the baby must be able to maintain nasal breathing during the stage of rhythmic oral sucking movements, with temporary suspension of breathing during the swallow stage of feeding. If breathing is not synchronised with sucking and swallowing, choking will occur.

While the nasal pattern of breathing is normally maintained throughout life, including while eating and drinking, it is not impossible to chew during oral inspiration and expiration (e.g. if talking while eating, even though this may be considered undesirable in some societies). However, breathing continues to be suspended during the swallowing stage.

WIDER CONSIDERATIONS

There are also wider considerations to be made as part of overall remediation. These include:

- the meal
- utensil use
- linguistic, social and emotional aspects.

The meal

The food should be placed where the child is able to see it. The consistency should be appropriate for the competence of the child, but helpers should be aware of the need to promote developmental skills. Items should be chopped separately so that the child can experience a variety of flavours and textures. The child will be more confident about taking food if he sees the helper test the temperature.

Children will vary as to the quantity of food they can manage to take from the spoon and the speed at which it will be consumed. If choking has previously occurred, some children will be afraid of the foods which caused the problem, e.g. skins of peas and beans, dried fruit, minced beef, cabbage.

Children's personal preferences should be respected and where possible choices given. Allowing the child to select the order and/or combinations of food to be eaten, e.g. carrot plus potato or alone, and whether or not he would like seasoning or sauces to be added, may make a difference to the acceptability of the meal. This enables the child to have some control over the meal, as does allowing him to say when he is ready for the next spoonful. Even a non-speaking child can indicate that he wants more, e.g. by eye-pointing. The child should be encouraged to cooperate fully with the removal of food from the spoon.

The importance of adequate fluid intake should not be overlooked and a drink should be offered at mealtimes.

Utensil use

The provision of suitable utensils will aid efficient eating and drinking. In some cases specially designed cutlery, plates and cups will be required;

in others, simple modification of conventional utensils may be needed, e.g. angled spoons, padded handles and lightweight cutlery (Burnett & Greenfield 1983).

Particular points to consider in the early stages of cup use are:

1. Use a cup with a piece cut out of the upper rim so that it can be tilted further without the child's needing to push his head back (Fig. 20.2).
2. Present the cup from below to reduce the possibility of an extensor thrust.
3. Where there is a persisting bite reflex, place the rim on the lower lip rather than between the teeth.

The use of a straw may be considered as an alternative means of drinking independently. Collaboration with the speech therapist is recommended here.

Spoon feeding is an acceptable option for presenting liquid to a child who cannot suck, but is also a normal stage in the acquisition of eating skills. Non-breakable spoons of the appropriate size with shallow bowl and a rounded end, are best.

If the child has an exaggerated bite reflex or tongue thrust, present the spoon from the side, although eventually the aim should be to present it from the midline. Applying firm pressure with the spoon to the middle of the tongue helps eliminate a tongue thrust. If attempting to remove the spoon from the mouth precipitates a bite reflex, applying pressure under the chin around the base of the tongue usually releases the bite.

When the spoon is removed, mouth closure should be obtained with the helper providing manual assistance if necessary (Fig. 20.3). A more detailed discussion of techniques than is possible here may be found in Warner (1981) and Blockley & Miller (1971).

Where progression to self-feeding is taking place, some initial deterioration in oral competence may be encountered until the child has mastered manipulative skills, e.g. a child who has managed to control a tongue thrust may lose this ability when concentrating on holding a spoon and directing it to the mouth. Some subsequent attention to the coordination and refinement of manual and oral feeding skills may be necessary.

To facilitate a consistent approach between all involved in helping an individual child with feeding, a feeding profile chart may be useful in ensuring that all are aware of his needs (Fig. 20.4).

Linguistic, social and emotional aspects

All who are involved in helping children to increase competence in eating and drinking should take care not to confine themselves to the mechanical aspects.

It is important that the person helping with the

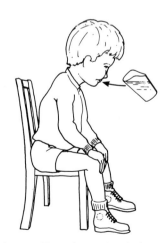

Fig. 20.2 A cup with a piece cut out of upper rim.

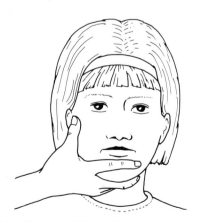

Fig. 20.3 Manual assistance for mouth closure.

Feeding profile Name .... Date			
	Yes	No	Describe

1. What does the child sit in?
    e.g. box, arm chair, etc.
    Does child need assistance to
    maintain optimum posture?			

2. Does child need :
    apron/bib
    arm fixation
    non-slip mat			

3. Does child use :
    spoon (normal, padded, angled,
    fork   lightweight)
    knife
    special plate (e.g. lipped, plateguard)
    special cup (e.g. shallow, shaped)			

4. What textures can child manage :
    liquidised
    mashed
    chopped
    normal			

5. Is child on special diet :
    medical
    religious
    has child any particular preferences?			

6. Does child need help?
    Where does helper sit?
    Is help needed with loading spoon?
    Is help needed taking food from spoon?
    If fed, where in mouth is food placed?			

7. Are there oral problems :
    bite reflex
    sucking
    gag reflex
    hypersensitivty, intolerance
      or lack of awareness
    difficulty in closing mouth
    difficulty in using tongue
      to manoeuvre food			

8. How does child communicate :
    verbally
    eye pointing
    signing			

9. Will child accept a new feeder?			

10. Is child easily distracted :
    by noise
    by activity			

Fig. 20.4 Feeding profile.

meal sits in a position where the child's face is in good view and preferably at the same level so that eye contact is facilitated. For visually handicapped children, verbal or tactile prompts should be given so that they are not surprised by food being suddenly thrust into the mouth. It is essential that the helper can see and is sensitive to the various signals given by the child, particularly if he is non-speaking. The helper should have a relaxed and attentive manner and, if possible, not be restricted by a time limit. Tension and anxiety impede feeding.

If the child is reluctant to take food, other possible reasons for this may be: a sore mouth because of ulcers or toothache, threatening illness, apprehension about a new helper, general distractions in the environment.

Mealtimes are important in developing a child's social skills, which are closely related to emotional maturation. They provide a context in which cognitive development may be enhanced, not only in relation to motor skill development, but one in which language can be learned. Labelling, e.g. categories of food, utensils, mouth parts, the vocabulary of action, e.g. open, close, chew, swallow; descriptive vocabulary, e.g. sweet, tart, salty, soft, smooth, lumpy, cold, full, hungry and colours, may all be extended at mealtime.

Language as a social activity is enjoyed at mealtimes and pauses to enable the disabled child to participate are important. The desirability of the child's eating at the same time as the rest of the family is acknowledged from the point of view that he should not be made to feel different. However, it is also pertinent to consider the practical difficulties for a child who cannot feed himself and has great difficulty in dealing with the food in his mouth, or for a child who is easily distracted by noise and activity around him. It may be easier for the child to participate in the social aspects of a mealtime if he has already had his food and can then more easily listen to and take part in the conversation. The person helping the child can then give full attention to him and to promoting the goal of independence without being distracted by others. The needs of the individual must be as carefully evaluated with respect to the social aspects of a mealtime as it is to other aspects.

TOILETING
G. Hall

INTRODUCTION

Toileting is one of the most intimate and personal of self-help activities. It cannot be assumed that nappies are only worn by the disabled baby, nor that toilet training is only necessary for the under 5-year-old. Great sensitivity is needed when changing the nappy of an older profoundly disabled child, or when embarking on a toilet training/self-continence regime with an older child with spina bifida. In the examples of activities described below it will be necessary to develop the suggestions to encompass the needs of a wider age range.

NAPPY CHANGING

Nappy-changing time should be a routine enjoyed by mother and child, a time when many kinds of learning can take place. Babies love the freedom of being without a nappy. It is an opportunity to kick, babble and smile, and the mother spontaneously talks, tickles, pats and smiles back. Eye contact is made and the child listens. With the disabled baby who cannot kick spontaneously it can be a time of correct passive movement when the baby can learn that his feet and toes are a part of him.

Sensory experiences

Putting the baby on his tummy, over his mother's knee, on a towel or rug on the floor or on a wedge, increases body awareness and tactile input. Using cream and talc can help to develop both olfactory and tactile awareness.

Activities to develop listening skills can be continued during nappy changes. Water running, bin lids banging and the sound of cubicle curtains being drawn can extend the sensory input included in the classroom programme. However, whilst this is appropriate for younger children it may not be so for older disabled children who wear nappies. In these situations changing must be dealt with in a calm, friendly manner which retains a sense of respect and the need for privacy.

Profoundly disabled children

Very physically disabled and profoundly disabled children often dislike being touched and handled by people who are strange to them but they learn to accept the care and handling of school staff quite quickly. The one-to-one situation existing during the changing routine is ideal for developing eye contact, communication and bonding at whatever level the child needs.

POTTY TRAINING

Potty training for the young disabled child needs very sensitive handling. Correct and comfortable positioning is essential.

Support

Potties with good back and front support should be used (Fig. 20.5). Without good support the child will feel insecure and be unable to relax. Training will seem impossible to the mother and her anxiety will transfer to the child, making the task the harder. An adult can sit behind the child to give additional support where necessary and perhaps prevent a child going into extension. The proximity of a familiar adult will also give emotional security.

Many children will manage on an ordinary potty facing the wall with a fixed hand rail to hold onto for sitting balance. For children needing a lot of physical support, potty chairs with a good grab bar are useful, they are quite easy for patients to make in hospital workshops and should ideally be tailor-made for each child (Fig. 20.6).

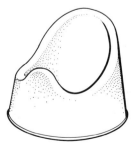

Fig. 20.5 Potty with good back and front support.

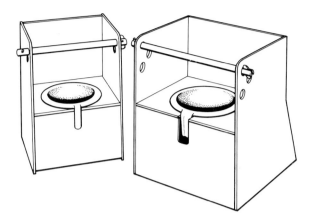

Fig. 20.6 Potty chair with grab bar.

The feet must be firmly on the floor with the exception of some athetoid children who achieve a relaxed position more easily if the feet are unsupported, as tactile input to the soles of the feet increases involuntary movement. Such children should be individually assessed for toilet seating.

Positive reinforcement

Musical potties can help by giving positive reinforcement. Whatever potty is used positive results should be rewarded with praise.

TOILETING
Seats

Many disabled children manage well on a toilet and a toddler's seat from a baby store can prevent them from falling in. Others needing more support should be assessed thoroughly. A wide range of toilet aids is available from firms catering specifically for the needs of disabled children and many are sensitively designed to fit in with family bathroom design. It is often easier to suit the needs of the individual than to cater for the needs of many in the school setting.

Frames and rails

Ambulant children needing only support in balancing will be helped by grab bars at the side of the toilet or by toilet frames. The walls should be sufficiently well constructed for the fixtures to be firm.

The toilet is often too far from the wall for the grab bars to be effective and toilet frames that look ideal may not fit because pipes are in the way. Detailed measurements should be taken before fitting frames.

Hinged bars at either side of the toilet can be used by many children, but the water cistern is frequently the wrong shape or size to allow for these to be correctly placed. As a final resort a rail can be fixed to the floor, although this can cause problems if the toilet is to be used by children in wheelchairs.

Plinths

While babies and small children can usefully be changed on the carer's lap, it is necessary for changing areas in schools to have plinths for older children in nappies. These should have a simple height-adjustment mechanism so that children can be transferred from wheelchairs with ease, and then the plinth height adjusted to suit the carer. For safety, plinths should have side pieces that can be let down while transferring the child, then easily put up again, so that the child cannot fall off if the carer's back is turned.

WHEELCHAIR USERS

Access to the school cloakroom is often through narrow doors and round sharp corners, so access routes should be checked. Can the child manage the door into the wheelchair users' toilet? Sliding doors take up the least space and are the easiest to operate. Doors opening in the normal way need a great deal more space, because the wheelchair user needs to go through and then be able to turn in order to close the door behind them. They are also more complicated to open and shut from a wheelchair. There must be sufficient room on either side of the toilet so that wheelchair users have space to transfer from either side. Raised toilet seats, making wheelchair and toilet seat a similar height, make the transfer easier (Fig. 20.7).

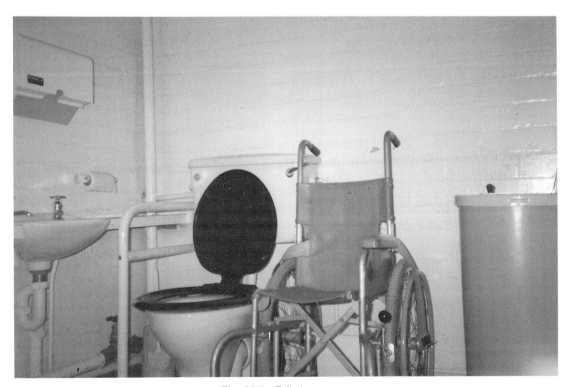

Fig. 20.7 Toileting area.

Independence

For those coping independently with problems of incontinence a wash-hand basin adjacent to the toilet is indicated, unless a toilet which also washes and dries the user is installed. There also needs to be a full length mirror both for self-catheterisation and for checking clothing before leaving the toilet area.

Design of changing areas

Changing areas need careful planning so that cupboards containing nappy pads, powder and creams are near to the plinth, and the sink is easily accessible. This will both encourage independence and ensure that, if the child needs washing, the sponge or flannel does not get cold in transit. Confidence, comfort and the reduction of tension are necessary if this most personal activity is to be dealt with sensitively.

Design of toilet areas

At home people like to furnish their own bathrooms with care and to decorate them pleasantly. Careful thought should likewise be given to the furnishing and design of school toileting areas.

Toilet areas easily become cluttered with equipment which has been individually prescribed and is no longer used, so the more multiply adjustable toilet aids are, the more likely they are to be used long-term.

CONCLUSION

Children need to become independent of adult help as soon as possible, and their dignity and need for privacy must always be respected.

DRESSING
G. Hall

POSITIONS FOR DRESSING
Parent's knee

A plastic changing mat is commonly used to change and dress even the tiniest baby. This may have the advantage of convenience but, for the disabled child the mother's lap can be the best position for correction and support.

Parents and carers can be shown how to seat the child appropriately on the lap in order to dress him. For example, for a spastic child who inwardly rotates from the hips it usually helps to sit him with his legs abducted over the mother's knee. The mother must also be sitting comfortably (Fig. 20.8).

Floor

The parent can sit on the floor with the child in front — supporting him from behind, to give him the balance he needs, keeping his head in midline and shoulders forward.

At the same time the child can be helped to use both hands to assist with his own dressing. The parent's hands come round the child from behind and model and assist the child's own movements.

Sitting in the corner of a room can also help the child to balance in order to dress independently.

However, in a child's home, classroom or

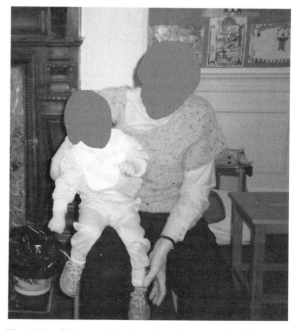

Fig. 20.8   Sitting position for dressing on mother's lap.

cloakroom, corners often have pipes going up or round them, or are obstructed by furniture, so a floor level corner seat is probably the best substitute. If firmly positioned, this is all the support many children need.

Chair

Some children need only a chair of the correct dimensions, or a stool that is at the correct height so that their feet are firmly on the floor, with the knees and hips flexed at right angles. The stool or bench should be sufficiently deep and wide for them to balance with weight going through one or both arms, either laterally or behind, depending on individual needs (Fig. 20.9).

Side-lying

There are children who find it simpler to dress and undress while side-lying, when knees and

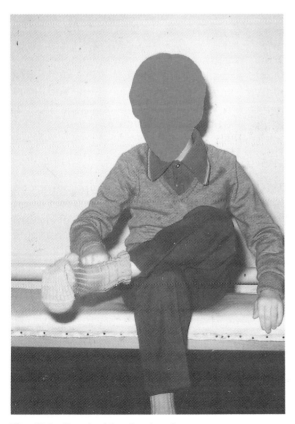

Fig. 20.9 Bench sitting for dressing.

hips may bend more easily. For this reason changing areas must have space for a therapy mat or should, at least, be carpeted.

BONDING AND SELF-AWARENESS
Bonding

Parents of disabled babies will often share their feelings with therapists or carers they have come to trust and tell them that bonding has not been spontaneous, and that they have had to learn to love their children. In these circumstances direct individual contact with the parent and the close handling and involvement with the child can be beneficial and supportive.

Self-awareness

If parents talk to and laugh with their baby during dressing or changing, he will begin to establish a positive image and feel he is special. He can also be helped to develop his spatial perception through being moved from lying to sitting, sitting to standing or at least to an upright position if the mother tells him what is happening. The baby will feel secure because of the parental closeness and familiar handling and may explore by pulling his mother's hair, playing with a necklace or poking her nose, eyes and mouth. She may play with his nose, mouth, hands and feet, giving the opportunity to learn about body parts.

THERAPY
Positioning

By carefully positioning the clothes, midline positioning of the head can be encouraged, as well as reaching and visual tracking, if indicated. This can be particularly helpful with hemiplegic children.

If handling and therapeutic positioning can be used during daily routines, parents will often find therapy easier to understand and this understanding can then be expanded.

The parent can be shown how to position the child to further his therapy programme; for example, a child lying prone across his mother's lap with his arms forward will be encouraged towards improved head control and any hyperextension will be discouraged (Fig. 20.10).

Self-help dressing skills

Clothes should always be placed near to hand and the child encouraged to look at named clothing, to relate clothes to body parts and to help with dressing as appropriate to his ability. Allowing him to achieve or help achieve the final task, at least, helps him to feel successful and able.

Where a child has right–left confusion, a red mark on the right sleeve, shoulder, leg or shoe is often very helpful, but for children with spatial–perceptual problems greater difficulties arise; 'top', 'bottom', 'back', 'front', etc. have little or no meaning.

While the child is learning to dress, clothes should be placed on a chair in the order in which they are to be put on and the right way round. Many will need this sort of help for a very long time.

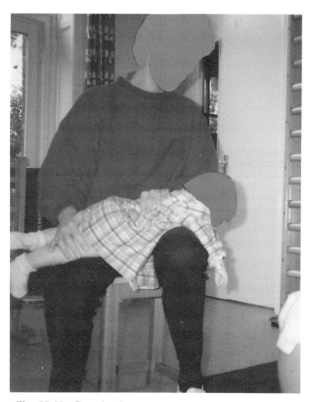

Fig. 20.10 Dressing in prone.

It also helps if the child always puts on each item in the same way, for example, arms into the jumper sleeves first, leaving just one hole to put over the head. If the head goes in first the child has to try to find armholes that cannot be seen, resulting in frustration and in the jumper's being pulled and stretched.

Aids and equipment

Mirrors can help both mother and child to monitor what is happening but children need to be individually assessed, as the mirrored image can confuse directionality, although this happens surprisingly seldom.

Mirrors

A full length mirror should be provided, so that the child can check that all is well before returning to class, rather than be teased if clothes are back to front, inside out or caught up at the back.

Pegs

Clothes pegs should be at a suitable height, of a suitable size and firmly fixed to the wall, so that children with poor hand function and poor balance can safely manage during busy periods such as playtime and hometime.

Bars

Many children need only a bar at an appropriate height for them to hold on to. In schools where a number of children need this kind of facility, Peto chairs are invaluable because the bars give firm support at the correct height for many children, either standing or high kneeling. The latter gives the child a more stable base (Fig. 20.11).

Dressing sticks

Methods of dressing to suit most children can be found, so aids are seldom needed. Dressing sticks with a rubber thimble at one end and a hook at the other can help children with poor reaching ability, as can long-handled shoe horns and stock-

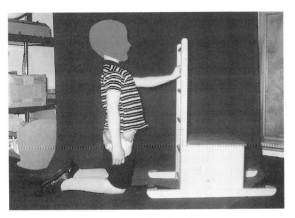

Fig. 20.11 Peto chair used for dressing.

ing aids, but these dressing aids are individually rather than generally needed.

GENERAL CONSIDERATIONS

Cloakroom areas

School cloakrooms often lack suitable facilities, particularly those not used to providing for handicapped children in these settings.

School cloakrooms are often the draughtiest, coldest rooms in the building, but it is essential that changing areas for disabled children are adequately heated, as they take longer to dress and change than their able-bodied peers.

Clothing

A thick winter coat may make it impossible for a child to fit correctly into a moulded seat. Thin, equally warm, coats are available and avoid many problems. For wheelchair-bound and incontinent children, fabric that does not slip on the wheelchair seat surface and does not retain odour is of the greatest importance.

Fitting

When greater independence is indicated, it should be remembered that undressing is a lot easier than dressing. Tight clothes are very difficult to manage, particularly tight-necked sweaters and fine nylon socks. Bearing in mind how expensive children's clothes are, parents should be encouraged to buy loose fitting clothes for their children. However, loose fitting clothes are not always fashionable, so clothes, and particularly fastenings, may need to be adapted.

Fastenings

Velcro or large buttons can replace small ones, cuffs can be joined with elastic making it unnecessary to do up buttons. Even zips can be difficult if hand function is limited; attaching a ring or bobble can be helpful. Shoes with velcro fastenings are easy to put on.

Fabrics

It is only recently that detailed attention has been given to the fabric used in clothes for handicapped people and research is ongoing. Natural fibres may be comfortable and absorbent, but may be hard to care for and crease easily.

If waterproof material is indicated, unless very carefully chosen, it can result in the child's becoming very hot and sweaty.

Dressing is fun

There are various ways of making the learning of skills more enjoyable for young children, and those who have a long-term dressing problem. Appliqued trains, for example, can have zips for the railway lines, different fastenings to join the carriages, which can be in pocket form with small dolls to put inside. Handkerchiefs can be attached to their hands with poppers. Colour matching can also be incorporated, with dolls dressed in the colours of the carriages. Similarly, trees with fruit, birds and animals in the branches are fun.

Toy shops now have dolls that are specifically designed to help children learn dressing skills, although some handicapped children need more detail, so home-made devices using buttons of different shapes and sizes and toggles are often more suitable.

CONCLUSION

The clothes children wear are of great importance

within their peer group. Their dignity and social acceptance is largely dependent on their appearance, and almost equally on their skills of independence. The environment in which these skills are learned should be as conducive as possible towards meeting the individual needs of every child receiving help.

COMPUTERS AND TECHNOLOGY
R. Bates

INTRODUCTION

Physical disability imposes restrictions on how an individual is able to interact with the environment. Depending on the degree and type of handicap, modern technology can be used to help overcome this restriction and to enable the individual to function more fully. For many years various aids have been designed to help the disabled person control his environment more effectively. These have used various technologies and materials in their design and manufacture.

Microtechnology plays an important part in present day living, making many everyday tasks easier and life more comfortable. Much everyday equipment now incorporates micro-electronics; making it increasingly accessible to disabled people. In some cases very slight adaptation, such as extending or enlarging a switch or a control knob may allow easier operation. Improving access to standard commercial equipment has many advantages for the disabled. The cost of designing, manufacturing and servicing specialised equipment for a small market is avoided and the user is not made to feel different.

The computer represents one of the most dramatic manifestations of the new technology of micro-electronics. Today a computer can fit into a briefcase, or even a pocket. Only a few years ago it would have taken an air-conditioned room to hold a machine with the same power. The computer can carry out many different tasks, if suitable instructions are presented to it in the form of a program. This versatility is one reason why computers are becoming of so much importance for disabled children and adults. The same

computer can be used for playing or for writing a book, by using different software. A young child can begin by using a switch connected to the computer. Pressure on the switch can produce sound and a picture on the screen as a reward and a motivation for this activity. The same computer and switch can later be used with other software to become a word-processor.

CHOOSING TECHNOLOGY FOR COMMUNICATION AND LEARNING

Electronic devices have become very important in the lives of many disabled people. Electronic aids and computers are used to help in learning, communication, both written and face to face, and environmental control. Most professionals working with disabled people gain their first experience of such technology on the job. Its very newness has meant that few have encountered such technology in their training.

Team approach

The choice and provision of electronic equipment has created new problems for all concerned. A team approach is essential to ensure that all aspects of the child's situation are considered in making the choice. The team can include:

- parents
- physiotherapist
- teacher
- speech therapist
- occupational therapist.

Each person involved has a part to play in deciding how best to meet the child's needs, bringing to the discussion their professional skills and knowledge of the child.

The decision-making process can be broken into six stages:

- identification
- referral
- assessment of needs
- provision of equipment
- training
- monitoring.

Identification

There must be an initial decision to consider the use of some technological aid with the child. A number of factors can lead to this decision. The child may be:

- having problems communicating
- not making satisfactory progress in the classroom
- having difficulties with writing
- having problems interacting with their environment.

Referral

If a decision is made to investigate the use of technology, further support may have to be called upon. A number of sources are available, including Communication Aids Centres, ACE Centres, local education Information Technology support centres, etc.

Assessment of need

This involves having available a range of equipment and expertise to help choose appropriate technology. The child will be given the opportunity to try various pieces of equipment, ideally in a familiar setting. The results observed can then give a basis for further discussion. A longer term loan of equipment may be needed to evaluate possible strategies fully.

Provision of equipment

Funding can be very difficult and may involve charity as well as statutory provision. Equipment for use in school may be provided as a result of a child having a statement of special educational needs (see Chapter 25 Legal Aspects in Paediatric Physiotherapy). This is drawn up from reports and discussions involving parents and professionals and sets down the educational provision needed for that individual. Communication aids may be funded from local health authority provision. Provision of funding varies considerably from region to region and no clear structure of statutory provision is apparent.

Training

Not only will the child need time to learn how to use the equipment, but all those involved with the child will need to understand the day to day operation of equipment and why it is being used. When a communication aid is being introduced considerable time is needed to build up the vocabulary stored and to make it suitable for the individual using it.

Monitoring

Regular review of the effectiveness and appropriateness of any equipment used must be carried out. Equipment and strategies can fail or become unsuitable for many reasons, including:

- inappropriate choice of equipment
- insufficient training for user
- insufficient support for parents and staff
- improvements in technology could provide a better aid
- access method becomes inappropriate due to improvement or deterioration in the child's physical condition.

ACCESSING EQUIPMENT — DIRECT ACCESS

To obtain maximum benefit from any piece of equipment, the child needs to be able to control it effectively. The degree of control possible depends on the child's physical and cognitive abilities.

Access methods can range from the full keyboard of a computer to a single switch. It is desirable, where possible, to provide the physically handicapped child with a way of using the machine via the standard keyboard so that he can access the full range of software available. Many trial modifications can be made to the keyboard before deciding whether this is an effective way of using the computer or whether switch operation would be more appropriate.

Keyboard modifications

Position, posture and seating

The aim should be to obtain the best possible

relationship between the user, the keyboard and the screen. This should allow a clear view of the screen and keyboard as well as encouraging good posture. For most classroom situations where the computer is shared this can only be done by providing an adjustable table or trolley. Computers that have separate keyboard units can help further by allowing the keyboard to be easily placed in the best position for each pupil. Provision of wrist or arm supports can help to overcome problems presented by pupils who have difficulty reaching because of muscular weakness.

Keyguards

Guards are now made for many types of keyboard. These protect against unintentional key presses, and allow the hand to be rested on the keyboard. The keys are operated by poking a finger through the holes (Fig. 20.12).

Sticky keys

The user who can only press one key at a time may have problems using some programs. Special modifications can be made to many computers to allow them to 'remember' key presses until the user has completed a sequence. Thus, programs that require simultaneous key presses can be used. Similar modifications to the software or hardware used can allow the repeat and accept delays of the keyboard to be altered. This can help those who because of difficulty in timing their key presses produce unwanted letters.

Alternative keyboards

Because of the way that a computer is constructed, it is often fairly easy to connect a different type of keyboard to it. Alternative keyboards are available that can be larger, smaller, or with a different layout to the standard one, providing access to the computer for children and adults with a wide range of handicaps. Very small keyboards are ideal for those who have a limited range of movements. Larger keyboards with recessed keys may help those who have erratic and less well coordinated movements.

Concept keyboard

The concept keyboard has been developed as an alternative way of accessing computer software. When used with suitable software it allows the computer to be operated by the child pressing on a simple flat board. This can be covered by a paper overlay showing pictures, words, sentences etc. (Fig. 20.13). This presents a much simpler input method than the full keyboard for children with learning and physical handicaps.

Switch operation of computers

Children with severe physical disabilities are often unable to interact with or influence their environ-

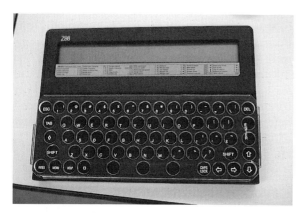

Fig. 20.12 Lap-top computer fitted with keyguard (reproduced with permission from the Northern ACE centre).

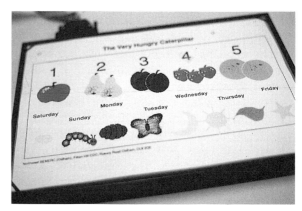

Fig. 20.13 Concept keyboard overlay (reproduced with permission from the Northern ACE centre).

ment. The use of switches to provide a simplified method of controlling toys and computers has given many of these children a way of controlling their surroundings. They can press a switch, make a sound or touch the screen to cause a reaction. This can be immediate, stimulating and consistent and take many forms, a tune, bright graphics or a combination of these.

For these children the keyboard will not provide satisfactory access to the computer. They may be unable to make the precise finger and arm movements to operate the keys, even with the range of modifications already discussed. Alternative methods of controlling the equipment will then have to be considered.

If the child has already had experience with switch operation of toys then the same switching may be used to operate the computer. Early training with toys and simple computer software will already have established the prerequisites of switch control. The awareness of cause and effect is essential; that is when the child clearly understands the relationship between his operation of the switch and the resulting operation of the toy or computer. It is also important to be sure that the child can clearly see the screen of the computer being used. In some cases it may be necessary to begin by using bright and stimulating pictures on the computer screen to encourage visual perception and awareness of the screen.

Early experience of switch operation is very important for the severely disabled child as it may be his key to spoken and written communication, as well as environmental control, in later life. It is important that they begin to control and operate switches as soon as possible, and that the task to be carried out is kept simple yet interesting. Such a switch can also be used to carry out simple environmental control tasks, such as switching on a torch or, with a suitable adapter, switching on and off a mains-operated appliance.

Factors influencing the choice of switch

Range of movement

The identification of the best movement to use to operate a switch can depend on many factors.

The child may already have been using toys and be familiar with switch operation. The movement chosen should be repeatable, consistent, not too tiring, acceptable, practical and appropriate to the type of task being attempted. The most obvious way of switch operation is by using hand or finger movements. Head movements are often found to be suitable; for many children the use of head switches is found to encourage a much better posture, enabling them to maintain good eye-contact with the screen. Much trial and error may be required to establish the best position for the switch and then to arrange for its firm mounting. Switches that will respond to the slightest movement, or even to electrical signals generated by eye movement, are available. The range of movement will also govern the number of switches to be used. Two or more switches may potentially give more control over the software. This is not always of benefit as the effort and concentration required to move between switches may take more time than can be saved by using a multiple switch.

Switch position

This is obviously governed by the movement the child uses to operate the switch. The final positioning can often be quite difficult, as it also depends on the mounting method available.

A number of clamping and mounting systems is available to attach switches and other equipment to wheelchairs (Fig. 20.14). These are not always very pleasant to look at and can in some cases be replaced by a purpose-built mounting when the exact position is settled on.

Care has to be taken to ensure that switches are not mounted in such a way as to obstruct other movements, for example, getting in and out of a wheelchair. Where a computer is being controlled by a switch the child must be able to look at the screen whilst operating the switch. Some children find that they have to look at the switch in order to press it. If this is so the switch would need to be carefully positioned for computer use or an alternative switching method may have to be adopted. A considerable period of learning may be needed before a child becomes a competent switch user. Sufficient time for practice

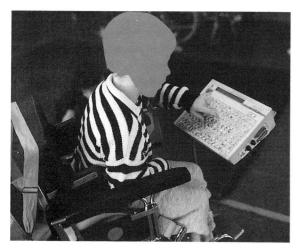

Fig. 20.14 Portable computer mounted on wheelchair (reproduced with permission from the Northern ACE centre).

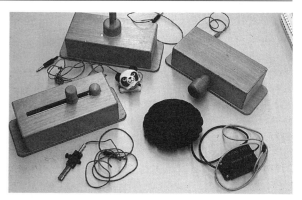

Fig. 20.15 A variety of switch types (reproduced with permission from the Northern ACE centre).

should be allowed before trying alternative switches and positions.

Switch type

Switches can take many forms, but are basically a means of completing an electrical circuit. The computer can detect that a switch is on and then carry out some action.

The simplest switches are just boxes with hinged lids. When the top is pressed a small microswitch inside is closed. Touch-sensitive switches are more complex and respond to the proximity of a hand or any part of a person. Pressure is not required. There is often a feeling that the more complicated electronic switches will somehow be better for many children. However, experience has shown that simpler switches that give a definite 'click' when operated are often more effective than those that do not provide any form of tactile feedback. The choice of movement for switch operation and the careful positioning of the switch can often make the largest contribution to successful switch operation (Fig. 20.15).

Switch method

Devices and computer software that have been designed to work with switches can often be tailored to suit individual users. Some will be able to hold a switch down while others will only be able to make momentary contact.

Other input methods

A variety of alternative inputs has been developed for computers, usually to provide quicker or more direct access for particular applications. The mouse or tracker ball are frequently used to control graphics software, and these can also enhance access for disabled children.

The touch screen can provide a very immediate form of control as the child can use this to interact directly with the screen display. This has proved very useful for children with severe learning difficulties.

Speech and sound input systems are being developed but they are not yet sufficiently consistent and accurate to be an effective long-term input method for children. Simple sound activation of computers and toys has proved to be of benefit for younger and less able children to encourage vocalisation and develop awareness of cause and effect.

Software used

The mere connection of a switch to a computer will not in itself provide access for the disabled user. The machine also has to have suitable software designed to be controlled by switches. Initially this would be of the simple 'cause and effect' variety. Each time a switch is pressed a result is observed on the screen; for example, a picture is built up step by step.

To enable different activities to be carried out using a switch the software must offers choices, to be made by pressing the switch at an appropriate time. This requires a much greater degree of switch control and awareness than the cause and effect software. Choices are often offered by a process of scanning. The computer displays a selection of choices in the form of a grid, for example, the letters of the alphabet. Switch presses are used to select which line of the grid contains the desired choice, the final choice then being made as the items in that line are offered in turn. This process makes considerable demands on the user, who may also be struggling with the spelling of a word as well.

Control of the computer

The flexibility and design of computer systems can confer other advantages on the disabled child. It is possible to carry out many operations from the keyboard or switches using suitable systems. With word-processors the user can store and retrieve written work, print it out, or even send it to another place using electronic mail. Previous material can be recalled and edited or referred to again. Computers can be linked to environmental control systems, providing a greater degree of independence.

Software that can 'learn' from the user is becoming available. It will learn the words he uses and the likely context and will offer intelligent guesses as he types. If a single switch is being used for writing, three presses are needed for each letter, if the computer can guess one word in ten, a significant reduction in time and effort results.

TECHNOLOGY AND PLAY

Play is an essential part of all children's education. It is by playing that children form many of the concepts that will be necessary in later life. Play with bricks helps form spatial concepts; play with sand and water develops concepts of properties of materials.

Play opportunities for young physically disabled children can be restricted and limited. In many cases they can only play through obser-

vation: it is by watching their parents and others play with toys that they gain some of these concepts. Battery-operated toys can be adapted by using a simple lead to work from easy-to-operate single switches. This can allow a severely physically disabled child to experience controlling something outside himself. This can be an important part of learning and will help the child become ready for more complicated tasks in the future. The ability to control toys can also be used to develop simple interactive games which can be used to encourage communication with other children and adults.

TECHNOLOGY AND COMMUNICATION

The speech of many disabled children is difficult to understand, and they can benefit from electronic communication aids which can 'speak'. Electronic aids have many advantages over traditional charts:

Voice output

Audible output can more readily attract attention, can be understood by other children and is more appropriate to many situations.

Message store

A much larger store of messages can be held electronically than on a chart; in some cases hundreds are available.

Switch input

The aids can be controlled by the same variety of input switches that are used to operate computers.

Versatility

Output from some models can be spoken, printed on paper or displayed on a screen, which allows messages to be prepared in advance. Models based on portable computers are also available combining the functions of a communication aid and word-processor.

The choice of aid and its introduction requires a great deal of support for the user and others involved. A communication aid should be available at all times, which can take considerable organisation and planning. Not only does the user have to be trained but listeners have to be introduced to the idea of listening and acting on what the child is trying to say. The introduction of a communication aid is perhaps the most difficult of all the new technologies to implement successfully.

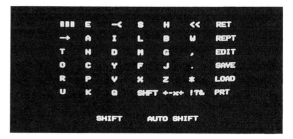

Fig. 20.16 Screen display for scanning word-processor (reproduced with permission from the Northern ACE centre).

COMPUTERS AND LEARNING

Although computers are now seen in all classrooms it is in the field of special needs that they have had their greatest impact. The computer has been found to be an ideal tool for motivating and enabling children to produce a much higher standard of work.

This has resulted from the development of software that provides a framework on which teachers can build materials to suit the individual needs of their pupils. The flexibility of the computer has given the physically disabled pupil access to much of this material. Developments in software design and computers are resulting in there being fewer but more powerful computer programs.

This range of software makes use of the computer as a tool rather than a teaching machine. The development of software for 'drill and practice' learning was a feature of some early educational software, particularly that from America. These programs often involved the computer presenting problems such as sums for the child to answer; the computer would then reward correct answers. This use of the computer was felt to be unsatisfactory and a waste of the potential of the equipment.

The development of software for English schools concentrated on using the computer as a tool, in many ways echoing its use in the real world outside schools.

Perhaps the most successful use of computers in the classroom is as a word-processing tool (Fig. 20.16). This has given many children the opportunity to produce for the first time acceptable written work. They have been able to become familiar with the way that computers are used in the business world. It is now a requirement of the National Curriculum that all children become familiar with this application of the computer and also are given the opportunity to develop keyboard skills. An additional benefit for many children with physical disabilities is that they are able to produce work of identical quality to that of other children. Additional features, including prediction and spelling checkers, can help the handicapped user speed up his output and improve its quality.

Many of the framework packages that have been developed make use of the concept keyboard and programs such as Touch Explorer can be adapted by teachers to meet a range of curriculum needs. This flexibility allows the same piece of software to be used by pupils of all ages and abilities.

Although in many cases standard software can be made accessible to children with physical disabilities it has been found necessary to develop a selection of specially written switch software. This material will not only provide the child with learning experiences such as colour matching, but can also be used for providing practice in switch control. Just as children need to practise the skills needed for pencil control, the disabled child will need time to practise and develop switch skills.

CONCLUSIONS

The use of new technology has opened many opportunities for learning, leisure, play and eventually employment for handicapped people. It is also, however, presenting many extra problems for parents, carers and everyone concerned and involved with the handicapped child.

The variety of the issues surrounding the introduction and use of technology with the handicapped child makes it essential that a team approach is adopted.

REFERENCES

Blockley J, Miller G 1971 Feeding techniques with cerebral palsied children. Physiotherapy 57(7): 300–308

Burnett A, Greenfield E 1983 Summary report on an assessment of feeding aids for handicapped children (spoons, beakers and handstraps). DHSS Aids Assessment Programme. Her Majesty's Stationery Office, London

Coupe J, Aherne P, Crawford N, et al 1987 Assessment of early feeding and drinking skills. Manchester Education Committee, Manchester

Treharne D A 1980 Feeding patterns and speech development. In: Jones F M (ed) Language disability in children. MTP Press, Lancaster

Warner J 1981 Helping the handicapped child with early feeding. Winslow Press, Winslow

FURTHER READING

Clothing for the handicapped child. The Disabled Living Foundation, London

Finnie N 1974 Handling the young cerebral palsied child at home, 2nd edn. William Heinemann Medical Books, London

Goldsmith S 1977 Designing for the disabled, 3rd edn. RIBA Publications Ltd, London

Harpin P (undated) With a little help. The Muscular Dystrophy Group of Great Britain

Jenkins G, Lamb J 1987 Fabric wise. Disabled Living Foundation

Penso D E 1987 Occupational therapy for children with disabilities. Croom Helm, London

COMPUTERS AND TECHNOLOGY

The rapid rate of change in technology can make most books out of date before they are written. The most useful information can be obtained from the following annual publications and information sheets.

Mary Marlborough Lodge
Nuffield Orthopaedic Centre
Headington
Oxford OX3 7LD
Publish an excellent series of annual publications including 'Communication' which deals with all aspects of aids to communication and daily living.

ACE Centre
Ormerod School
Waynflete Road
Headington
Oxford OX3 8DD (0865 63508)

and

Northern ACE Centre
Park Dean School

St Martins Road
Fitton Hill
Oldham OL8 2PY (061 627 1358)
Provide information, assessments and advice on all aspects of communication technology for handicapped children. A series of publications and information sheets are available. Those dealing with equipment and software are updated on a regular basis.

Northwest SEMERC
Fitton Hill CDC
Rosary Road
Oldham OL8 2QL (061 627 4469)
Provides a comprehensive catalogue of computer software for pupils with special educational needs.

The Advisory Unit for Microelectronics in Education
Endymion Road
Hatfield AL10 8AU (0707 265443)
Publishes factsheets on technology in support of the national curriculum for students with severe learning difficulties.

21

Aids and appliances

D. G. I. Bardsley   M. Jones

ORTHOSES AND FOOTWEAR
M. Jones

ORTHOSIS

Physiotherapists are faced with a daunting array of devices, frequently known as surgical appliances. These were traditionally made from metal and leather with straps, buckles and laces, and were frequently named after their designers. The advent of thermoplastics introduced a wider choice of design materials and the range of available appliances has been further extended as designs incorporating the use of electronics have been developed.

The situation is confused by a lack of precision in the use of nomenclature. The use of calipers (irons), for example, is frequently termed 'bracing' and a surgical appliance can be a harness, a splint or an iron. An orthosis has been defined as 'an external appliance designed to apply forces in the body in a controlled manner, to control motion and/or cause alteration in the shape of body tissues' (Rose 1977). The use of orthoses in their various forms to correct by force, for example, the results of muscular imbalance or skeletal deformities, has been described as 'closed' or 'bloodless' surgery.

Current practice acknowledges the potentially dysfunctional aspects of this treatment and therapists must be aware of the dangers of the use of excess or wrongly directed force. It has been suggested that 'physiotherapists, surgeons and orthotists usually have only an informal introduction in the clinical situation' to the use of orthotic devices (Rose 1977).

In the use of orthoses, an understanding of basic and applied mechanics is essential (Bowker 1987a and b).

CONVENTIONS FOR APPLIANCE SPECIFICATION

The approach to the prescription of orthoses is based on a number of principles:

1. An orthosis is 'any medical device applied to, or around, a bodily segment in the case of physical impairment or disability' (Stedman's Medical Dictionary).
2. The body comprises three major anatomical divisions: the spine, upper limbs and lower limbs.
3. Each orthosis is described by the joints it will surround.

It is therefore useful to consider orthoses in relation to the function required and the anatomical area (the joint(s) and the body segment(s) involved) in the format and convention described by Harris (1973). The function required may be:

- prevention of movement
- movement correction
- stabilisation at a joint
- a combination of these effects.

For purposes of description, complex joint systems such as the hand, wrist or foot are considered to be units but these may need to be further subdivided:

1. The spine is considered to comprise four non-divisible sections — cervical, thoracic, lumbar and sacroiliac.
2. A device involving only one joint, for example, a shoe insert, would become simply a 'foot orthosis'.
3. An orthosis which involves the hip, knee, ankle and foot, which would formerly have been referred to as a 'long leg caliper' or 'long leg brace' is prescribed under this system as a 'hip-knee-ankle-foot orthosis' (HKAFO).

4. The action which the orthosis is designed to create in relation to the affected joint is categorised as one of the following:
   — flex/extend
   — abduct/adduct
   — rotate.

Current terminology is then directed at a clear description of the body segment involved, e.g. ankle-foot orthosis (AFO) followed by a description of the function required. In the case of an AFO this could have several possibilities:

- to limit plantarflexion (weakness of dorsiflexors or overactive plantarflexors)
- to limit dorsiflexion (no plantarflexion power)
- to correct angular deviation of the foot, either valgus or varus.

Control exerted by orthoses

The control which is exerted by the orthosis is specified for the five joint motions required:

1. Free — movement allowed in any direction.
2. Assist — the application of external force (e.g. spring) to assist the correct movement.
3. Resist — the application of external force to decrease or resist the unwanted movement.
4. Stop — the use of a fixed device to prevent unwanted movement.
5. Hold — the prevention of all movement in a specified direction.

COMMON ORTHOSIS FUNCTIONS

An understanding of the use of orthoses can be developed by considering some of the common functions served by the conventional orthoses from which have developed more complex contemporary designs.

The body brace

An example is the Milwaukee brace (Fig. 21.1). This consists of a metal-reinforced moulded plastic or leather pelvic pad from which three metal bars are arranged vertically (one anterior and two posterior). These terminate in a mandibulo-

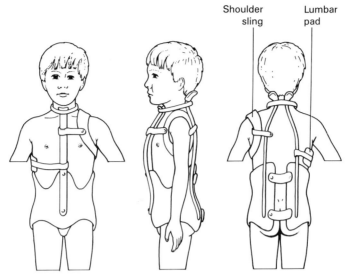

Shoulder sling   Lumbar pad

Fig. 21.1 The Milwaukee brace (adapted with permission from Physiotherapy 63(3)).

occipital support. The brace thus combines three-point pressure and traction and is used in the treatment of scoliosis, in an attempt to constrain the abnormal curvature of the spine, compensate for asymmetrical muscle activity and counteract the force of gravity. These correcting forces are illustrated in Figure 21.2. It is worn continuously apart from bathing and is used in conjunction with trunk strengthening exercises. Contact sport and vigorous gymnastics are contraindicated but other vigorous activities are positively encouraged. The design is complex, and accurate prescription and fabrication is critical.

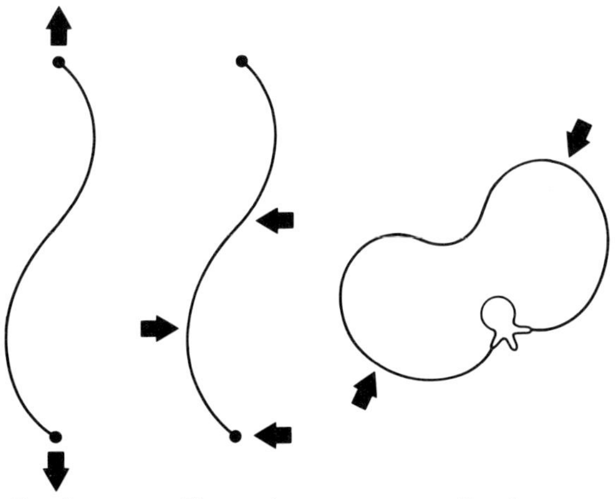

Calipers

Long-leg caliper

A long-leg caliper or knee-ankle-foot orthosis (KAFO) would conventionally consist of either a leather-covered ring top or a moulded leather corset top with a posterior metal supporting band; adjustable metal side pieces; bands of leather behind the thigh and calf or a calf-band with posterior metal insert; a narrow leather buckled ankle-strap and a broad leather buckled knee-strap (Fig. 21.3). In the treatment of valgus or varus, or hyperextension of the knee, an additional strap may be incorporated. Designs may or may not incorporate knee-hinges. A leather covered metal pelvic band with a free joint may be added to control hip motion. Where this addition is used to link two calipers, the appliance is known as a 'full set', or double calipers. This configuration can be used with trunk support in the treatment of spina bifida or paraplegic patients. Major factors to be considered in prescribing this design are its weight and its tendency to break under high load.

Traction   Three-point   Couple

Fig. 21.2 Milwaukee brace: the correcting forces (adapted with permission from Physiotherapy 63(3)).

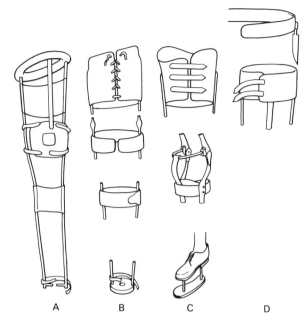

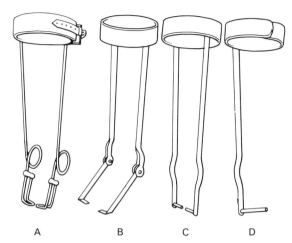

A   B   C   D

Fig. 21.4 Below knee calipers. (A) Coiled spring toe raising. (B) Double iron with ankle joint. (C) Double iron unjointed with shoe attachment. (D) Single iron with shoe attachment. (Adapted with permission from Physiotherapy 73(8).)

A   B   C   D

Fig. 21.3 Long leg calipers. (A) Ring top, unjointed with thigh and calf-bands, knee-cap and ankle-strap. (B) Corset top, ring joints with calf-band and paten. (C) Weight-bearing thigh corset, Barlock joints and shoe with paten. (D) Pelvic band with free joint and cuff top.

Below knee caliper

A below knee caliper or ankle-foot orthosis (AFO) can be used in the treatment of total loss of muscle function or imbalanced muscular activity (Fig. 21.4). This can comprise either a single or double iron with foot attachment. Designs can incorporate coil spring or hinge modifications strategically placed to assist, resist or stabilise ankle movement. A 'T' strap attached to the footwear can be used to correct varus or valgus conditions of the hindfoot (see Fig. 21.13).

Force transmission orthoses

All orthoses transmit or react to force in some form, but in some designs this function is the predominant feature. The simplest and most common illustration of this is the crutch, which is used to extend the length of the arms and together with the feet, to provide a stable four-point base, thus giving a large area of support within which the line of gravity of the trunk may be centred.

A second function may be to act as an aid to propulsion, in the manner of ski sticks, with the effect of transferring the motor function from the legs to the arms and shoulders. The crutch may also be used as a pivot or prop upon which downward pressure may be exerted to facilitate the lifting clear of the ground of one leg in the process of reciprocal walking.

Finally, this relatively simple orthosis may be used to divert the weight from, for example, a sprained ankle and thus relieve pain resulting from compressive forces on the joint.

Protective orthoses

For children who fall excessively or who are otherwise at risk because of, for example, epilepsy, small-scale adaptations of the standard construction worker's protective helmet have been produced. Alternatives which may be more acceptable to the child or the parents include American football-style helmets, leather cycling headgear or riding hats.

The Von Rosen splint

This is used in the treatment of congenital dislocation of the hip in infants, to facilitate the correct positioning of the femoral head in the acetabulum. The orthosis comprises a lightweight rubber covered dorsal aluminium splint which is used to keep the hip joints in the reduced position.

Contemporary developments of this design are the Pavlik harness and the Cambridge CDH orthosis (Fig. 21.5).

ASSESSMENT

When deciding on a treatment regime which includes the use of an orthosis, it is essential for physiotherapists to be familiar with the mechanical forces involved and their relationship to the child's pathological condition, the prescribed appliance and the resultant interaction.

Place in treatment plan

The use of the aid should be carefully incorporated into the overall treatment plan for that individual patient. Thought must be given to the child in his family situation and any problems discussed stage-by-stage in view of the possible psychological problems, such as acceptance and cosmetic features, and the physical difficulties, including ease of putting on and taking off the orthosis.

Child development

Careful consideration should be given to the physical and neurological development of the patient, and where appropriate to his/her cardiovascular system, in order to establish the presence of any limiting factors or contraindications for use of the proposed appliance. Factors to be considered include the presence of areas of diminished sensation, for example, with spina bifida patients, or problems of point-loading on the patient due to the presence of a bony prominence or possible skin sensitivity.

Functional requirement

A precise definition of the problem is essential to establish what functions the orthosis will be required to fulfil. This may include one, some, or all of the following:

- the prevention of unwanted movement
- the correction of movement
- the stabilisation of movement
- the assistance of movement.

Having defined the required function(s), a choice of orthosis can be made from the basic range available, with condition-specific modifications being developed in conjunction with the prescribing consultant and the orthotist.

Initial fitting

The initial fitting should be planned so as to

Von Rosen splint

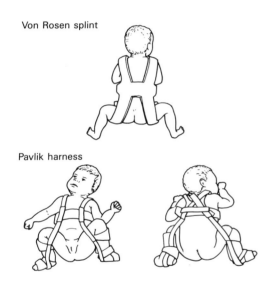

Pavlik harness

The Cambridge CDH orthosis

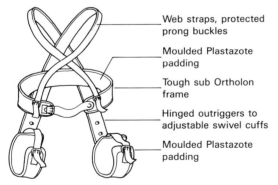

Web straps, protected prong buckles

Moulded Plastazote padding

Tough sub Ortholon frame

Hinged outriggers to adjustable swivel cuffs

Moulded Plastazote padding

Fig. 21.5 The Von Rosen splint, Pavlik harness and Cambridge CDH orthosis (adapted with permission from Physiotherapy 71(9)).

allow sufficient time to ensure that the orthosis meets the required specification, and in the case of a complex appliance to teach the correct use. The patient should be encouraged to exercise for a period of time sufficient to allow any pressure or friction areas to become evident. This will enable any necessary remedial action to be taken immediately, thus avoiding problems which might otherwise arise. These may be due to a negative attitude developing towards using the appliance, or as a result of initial discomfort or pain experienced after leaving the treatment centre.

Evaluation

Subsequently, careful evaluation of the patient is essential so as to identify progress, stability or deterioration in the condition. Children grow, and care must be taken to ensure that either adjustments are made to accommodate this growth, or a new appliance is prescribed. With infants, consideration must be given to the possible inhibition of activities which are asociated with normal development; for example, the use of calipers may inhibit crawling.

CONTEMPORARY ORTHOSES

A wide range of thermoplastic and thermosetting materials is now available for use in the construction of orthopaedic rehabilitation appliances. Two main categories of materials are used.

Low temperature direct forming plastics

These materials include:

1. Plastazote.* When preheated in a hot air oven to 140°F, Plastazote is self-adhesive and can be shaped. Used for cervical support collars, spinal jackets and foot orthoses (insoles).
2. Hexcelite.* A matt mesh structure moulded in hot water. Used for fracture bracing, spinal supports, hand splints and seating.

_____
* Trade name.

High temperature thermosetting materials

These materials include:

1. Polypropylene. Moulded from a positive plaster cast using vacuum or other pressure techniques.
2. Polyester and acrylic liquid resins. Used in conjunction with fibre reinforcement.
   Forms a laminate which can be smoothed, drilled and riveted.

Aluminium

Lightweight aluminium appliances have further extended the range of orthoses.

The ankle-foot orthosis (AFO)

Based on a plaster of Paris (POP) cast, these splints are made of polypropylene and can be used serially if required, to allow the controlled lengthening of shortened tissues with no inhibition of function.

The production of the AFO begins with the normal POP bandage technique, with the limb held in the desired position. Particular care should be taken to identify and mark bony prominences prior to casting. The cast is removed and filled with plaster to form a positive mould from which the polypropylene AFO is produced using vacuum or other pressure techniques. The orthosis can be worn inside normal footwear and is secured by velcro fastenings. The main advantages over the conventional lower limb caliper are the splint's lightness and cosmetic appearance.

The physiotherapist, more than any other member of the team, should have assessed the appropriate muscle activity, studied the child's gait and thought through the effects of the proposed prescription, which could read:

Ankle-foot orthosis (AFO) with plantarflexion resist and valgus support

This could be an orthosis prescribed for a child with hemiplegic cerebral palsy, walking with a toe-heel gait. A physiotherapist should ask for the trimline of the foot piece to extend just past the toes; by so doing it is thought that the plantar grasp will not be stimulated (Fig. 21.6). The conventional alternative would be a below knee caliper with posterior stop and valgus 'T' strap.

Ankle-foot orthosis (AFO) with plantarflexion assist

This represents the prescription for a spina bifida child with weak/absent plantarflexors. In this case the physiotherapist could ask for the trim line of the foot piece to be proximal to the metatarsal heads, based on the converse of the preceding example. The intention would be to try to ensure that the plantar grasp reflex would be stimulated (Fig. 21.7). The conventional alternative would be a below knee caliper with an anterior stop.

Either of these two examples of orthoses could be used to improve the gait pattern. By dispensing with their use for increasing periods of time, the physiotherapist can evaluate the progress towards a more normal pattern of walking. An important aspect of the above examples is the close liaison between the physiotherapist and the orthotist, both in drawing up the prescription and in making the cast.

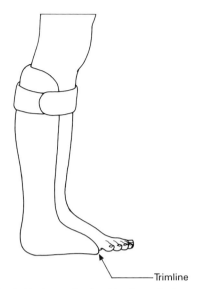

Fig. 21.7   Ankle-foot orthosis with plantarflexion assist.

The swivel walker: hip-knee-ankle-foot orthosis (HKAFO)

For children with a considerable degree of disability who have great difficulty in maintaining the upright position, for example, the severe athetoid cerebral palsy patient, there are significant psychological and developmental advantages associated with the use of a standing frame. The Orlau swivel walker, developed originally for spina bifida patients, is a rigid stable frame which terminates in a base plate mounted on swivelling footplates (Fig. 21.8).

Simply by rocking from side to side using upper body and head movements, the child causes the device to swivel forward on alternate footplates. This is achieved by a careful adjustment of the line of gravity of the child and the walker, so that it falls just in front of the bearing centres of the footplates. Paraplegic children can be taught a wide range of activities of daily living, from getting into and out of the appliance and transferring to a wheelchair, to learning a swing-through gait with crutches (Rocca & Hopkins 1978).

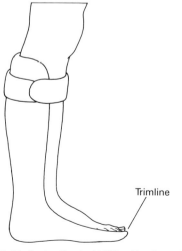

Fig. 21.6   Ankle-foot orthosis (AFO) with plantarflexion resist and valgus support.

The parawalker (PW)

The parawalker (PW) was formerly known as the

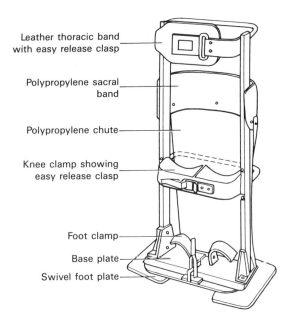

Leather thoracic band with easy release clasp

Polypropylene sacral band

Polypropylene chute

Knee clamp showing easy release clasp

Foot clamp

Base plate

Swivel foot plate

Fig. 21.8 The Orlau swivel walker (HKAFO) (adapted with permission from Physiotherapy 68(10)).

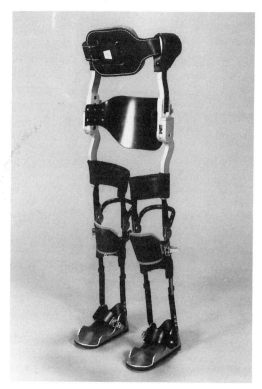

Fig. 21.9 The Parawalker (PW) (reproduced by permission of Orlau Publishing).

hip guidance orthosis (HGO). The high energy demand of the conventional 'full set' previously described stimulated considerable research to analyse the ground reaction force involved when patients were walking with the aid of crutches. As a result the PW was developed to allow the patient to walk with a reciprocal gait. The body weight is supported by the stance leg and the swing leg held clear of the ground by the brace, resulting in significant reduction in energy expenditure. This is achieved by the design of the HGO, which incorporates a body brace with low friction hip joints which limit the range of flexion and extension. The knee and ankle functions are stabilised and there is a shoe plate with rocker sole. The orthosis is provided with simple fastenings to facilitate donning and doffing. The construction is lightweight aluminium, with a moulded polypropylene buttock support (see Fig. 21.9). Applications are for paraplegic and spina bifida conditions, and the HGO is used in conjunction with crutches.

Current developments centre on the use of functional electronic stimulation (FES) used in conjunction with the PW to further reduce the physiological cost of walking. This represents the so-called 'hybrid' orthosis.

Reciprocating gait orthosis (RGO)

The Louisiana State University (LSU) RGO is one example of this type of lightweight thoraco-hip-knee-ankle-foot orthosis (THKAFO). It is made from polypropylene, carbon fibre inserts and aluminium tubing. The reciprocating element in the model is provided by a Bowden cable coupling system which links both left and right orthoses. Thus the action of hip flexion on one side promotes hip extension in the other joint. The cable can be disconnected at each hip joint to allow both sides to flex simultaneously for sitting (Fig. 21.10). The design allows adjustment for growth for approximately 3 years. The original model was for spina bifida children, but subsequent developments have made it suitable for use by both children and adults suffering from lower trunk and lower limb neuromuscular disorders, for example, cerebral palsy, muscular dystrophy and multiple sclerosis. A recent development has been to combine the RGO with

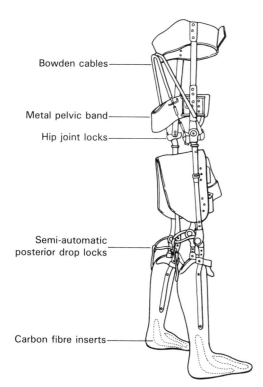

Fig. 21.10 Reciprocating gait orthosis (adapted with permission from Physiotherapy 73(8)).

Labels on figure:
- Bowden cables
- Metal pelvic band
- Hip joint locks
- Semi-automatic posterior drop locks
- Carbon fibre inserts

an FES system (Bajd et al 1985) and prior to this, investigation was made into computer-controlled walking using the RGO for patients with complete spinal injuries (Petrofsky & Phillips 1983).

Cast bracing

Using chemically reactive low-temperature thermo-setting materials such as Hexcelite* or Dynacast*, a lightweight brace can be made which is a cheap, easy to use alternative to the conventional Thomas splint (long-leg caliper). The energy cost to the patient is much reduced and again there is a cosmetic appearance value, but above all the patient becomes ambulatory more quickly which, together with early discharge from hospital, is psychologically better for the patient (Thomas & Meggitt 1981).

---

* Trade name.

Orthoses incorporating FES

There are also FES applications in the design and development of brace appliances. The functional electronic peroneal brace (FEPB) attempts to correct a plantarflexed and inverted foot during the swing phase of hemiplegic gait. The FEPB consists of an electrode strapped to the skin just behind the fibular head, powered by a small 9-volt battery and triggered by a heel switch. As the patient walks, the ankle dorsiflexors are stimulated to contract at the correct point in the swing phase. As the heel comes off the ground the switch is activated in the heel of the shoe. The device is considered suitable only for a relatively small number of patients, in the main adults with upper motor neurone lesions who are able to cooperate and are relatively physically fit and able to walk with or without some assistance.

Other areas of development in FES include:

1. Multichannel systems (MCS) where work has been done to improve dynamic support of the paralysed limb during the stance phase.
2. Implanted systems (IS) which are not widely commercially available, but offer advantages over surface electrode systems for everyday use.
3. Nerve blocking systems (NBS) which are concerned with the peripheral blockage of motor activity by stimulation. The advantage is that there exists the possibility to regulate contraction strength compared with the on/off facility of simple FES designs.

Summary

The aim of this section is to present an overview of what is an extremely wide-ranging area of treatment. Whilst reference has been made to well-established designs and their applications, it must be remembered that the physiotherapist should be aware of the principles involved so as to use this knowledge in the prescription of treatment regimes. For each individual patient, using this knowledge of the forces involved where appropriate, opportunities to design aids which are unique, or modifications/adaptations of standard models, may be considered, thus providing the most specific assistance in the most appropriate manner. The patient's need may be for educative assistance, where inappropriate phasic action is the problem, or effort reduction assistance by the use of force transmission devices, or cosmetic/protective help with the orthosis fulfilling a dual role of both physical and psychological support.

FOOTWEAR

A valuable confirmation of gait abnormalities can be obtained by observation of the child's usual footwear. Normal wear can be observed on the outer edge of the heel and sole. Any wear to the inner side of the midline can be considered abnormal (Sharrard 1979).

Where appropriate, AFOs can normally be accommodated in the child's standard boot or shoe, including fashion wear and 'trainers'. This is an important psychological advantage over conventional calipers, particularly with the young adolescent. In general terms, a well-fitted boot or shoe should comfortably enclose the contours of the foot with a half-inch growing space available at the toe.

Special footwear

Some special shoes and boots can be obtained as 'off-the-shelf' items, for example, Piedro* boots (Fig. 21.11) made with ski hooks as fastenings to facilitate fitting and to observe the position of the child's toes before fastening the boot. This is particularly important where there is a sensory deficit.

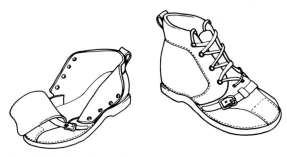

Fig. 21.11 The Piedro boot.

* Trade name.

Made-to-measure surgical footwear

Where there is a need to protect swollen or painful joints or to accommodate bony prominences or deformities, footwear can be specially prescribed. In these cases a last, which is a model of the weight-bearing foot, is made.

Footwear adaptations

These may be made to suitable normal boots or shoes, either as temporary or permanent modifications, again with both cost and cosmetic considerations. These adaptations can include:

1. A raise. This can include the whole foot area where there is a leg length discrepancy, and can be achieved by the addition of material to the sole and heel in the form of a pad, or in extreme cases the deficiency can be compensated for by the provision of a paten.
2. Heel raise. Where there is a fixed deformity and a need to redistribute weight. This can take the form of either an internal (soft) wedge or an external wear-resistant addition to the normal heel.
3. Metatarsal bar. This can be either an internal or external device positioned under the metatarsal heads and is used in Pes cavus in an attempt to stretch the high arch of the foot (Fig. 21.12A)
4. Valgus support. Foot orthosis (FO). This is an insole made from either cork, rubber or sponge and is prescribed in the treatment of flat feet (Fig. 21.12B)
5. Attachments. Where the child needs conventional components, these can be incorporated into a strong shoe or boot (Fig. 21.13)

Footwear adaptations can fulfil a number of functions: they can offer support to the foot to improve the patient's balance, both in standing and in walking; they can be used in the accommodation, treatment or correction of deformities; with additions, footwear can be used to compen-

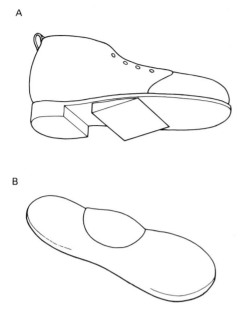

Fig. 21.12 Footwear adaptations. (A) The metatarsal bar. (B) Valgus support.

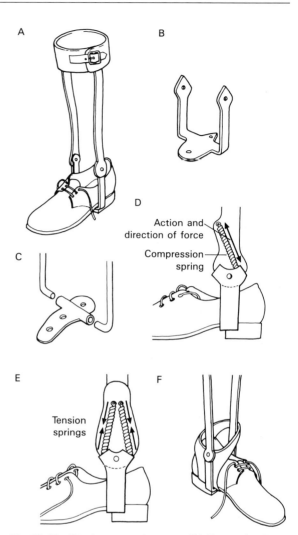

Fig. 21.13 Attachments to footwear. (A) Conventional components attached to a shoe. (B) Stirrup method of attachment. (C) Caliper attachment. (D) Spring-loaded dorsiflexion assist. (E) A double action assist. (F) Varus/valgus correction straps.

sate for unequal leg lengths. Additional boot stability can be used to limit motion or provide stability for unstable joints. The physiotherapist should consider carefully the degree of severity of the deformity and the attitude and tolerance of the child, when considering the prescription of special footwear. The use of foot orthoses may be appropriate in a wide range of mid- and hind-foot conditions, including Pes planovalgus, Pes equinus and Pes cavus.

As with all types of orthoses, it is essential that the progress of the patient is closely monitored to ensure that the original diagnosis was accurate and that any change in the deformity is quickly accommodated by a revision of the prescription followed by careful checks for accuracy of fit and designed corrective features.

Parental understanding and cooperation is vital in achieving the therapeutic goals for which devices are introduced to their children. In addition, the physiotherapist must be aware of how much they may be expecting from carers in constantly checking the fitting, comfort and safety of devices and in alerting the appropriate agencies if they detect anything of concern.

SEATING
D. G. I. Bardsley

INTRODUCTION

In general, the purpose of a seat is to help stabilise the body in desired postures which facilitate the individual's chosen activity with maximum comfort. At the same time, seating for disabled children must be consistent with constraints imposed by their medical and physical status, promoting the process of development and preventing any deterioration. Inevitably conflicting requirements are involved. The 'art' of seating involves determining compromises which satisfy the majority of requirements.

POSTURAL OBJECTIVES

Ideally the posture shown in Figures 21.14 and 21.15 should be achieved. Of primary importance is the pelvis, 'the keystone' of the body. This should be upright and balanced over the ischial tuberosities, which should be directly under the centre of gravity of the trunk. The spine should follow its natural curvature, particularly at the lumbar region where the highest loads are transmitted. Hips and knees should be flexed to approximately 90 degrees and the feet supported flat in a plantigrade position. Arm and head position are largely dictated by the individual's activity. When viewed in the frontal plane, the body should be symmetrical about its midline.

Compromises immediately arise in postural considerations. For example, a forward trunk position can help to improve hand/eye function

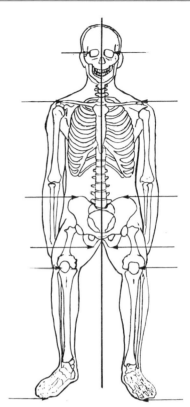

Fig. 21.15 Ideal posture — frontal view. Arrows show symmetry about midline.

but may require more effort to maintain and is therefore less comfortable. Higher comfort levels may be achieved by reclining the trunk but this is at the expense of function.

Fixed skeletal deformities of spine, pelvis and femurs inevitably limit the achievement of this 'ideal' posture. Similarly, postural instability may reduce the range of stable postures which can be used.

Comfort (or lack of discomfort) is a priority requirement of any seat. Lack of comfort probably accounts for the large majority of rejected seats as a seat will not be tolerated if it does not meet the comfort requirements of the occupant.

Comfort is difficult to define but may involve a wide number of factors. Impeding functional desires either by obstruction or by inappropriate posture may be perceived as discomfort. Restriction of movement by too much postural support is often perceived as discomfort because of sustained loading of soft tissues and because the body has an inherent habit of movement. On

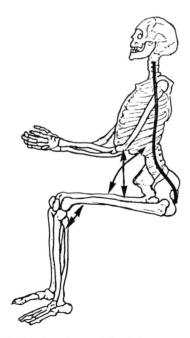

Fig. 21.14 Ideal posture — lateral view.

the other hand, inadequate support requires more muscle action and associated effort to maintain a desired posture. This may contribute to discomfort.

Conditions of pressure, temperature and humidity at the supporting surfaces also play a major part in comfort. Pressure sustained over certain threshold values for prolonged periods of time prevents the circulation to soft tissues. This may be perceived as discomfort and, if maintained sufficiently, results in tissue necrosis and formation of a pressure sore. Elevated temperature and humidity levels reduce the resistance of tissues to this form of damage and may also be perceived as discomfort (Barbenel et al 1983).

Finally, disabled children and their parents or attendants are often extremely sensitive to the appearance of their seating. It is important that aesthetic comfort is not disturbed by any obtrusive or ugly seat, however well it performs.

SEATING ELEMENTS

A wide range of support elements can be incorporated in a seat to achieve the postural objective described above. Depending upon the needs of the child, they may vary in complexity from the simple flat surface of a stool, to the total support provided by a whole body mould.

Figure 21.16 illustrates most of the possible seating elements which may be incorporated in a seat. Detailed knowledge of how a seat supports the human body is lacking. However, useful information may be obtained from Zacharkow (1988).

TYPES OF SEATING

Over recent years, a wide range of seating systems have been developed for the disabled, particularly for children. Consequently there are many options available to meet the seating requirements of children.

In general, the simplest solution should be chosen to avoid unnecessary complexity and cost. However, increasing problems and requirements of seating often lead to the need for more complex solutions.

The following is a summary of the different types, commencing with the simplest and finishing with the more complex designs. Some indications of the applications of the different types of seating are included.

Fixed format

An enormous range of fixed formats of seating is available in a wide variety of sizes. These may meet the needs of a large proportion of disabled children who simply require an accurately fitting chair. The majority provide a horizontal seat with upright backrest. Armrests are sometimes included and may be useful as reminders to maintain an upright posture but usually give little lateral support (Fig. 21.17).

The majority of these designs are intended primarily for the able-bodied but can be applicable to the disabled. Mass-produced plastic shell seats are widely used for normal babies before they are capable of sitting and can be highly appropriate for the first few years of disabled children (Fig. 21.18). Similarly, school furniture is produced in incremental sizes for normal children and consequently may permit the accurate matching of size required by the disabled.

The majority of wheelchairs have fixed formats of seating and are designed in incremental sizes to give the necessary dimensional matching. However, wheelchair seating, particularly of the buggy type, suffers from the use of sling-types of material (Fig. 21.19). This is helpful for folding but gives rather poor support as it sags and hammocks to encourage flexed postures.

Recent developments in children's pushchairs have resulted in considerable improvements in their seating. The sling seats have been stiffened by wooden inserts and additionally give further support as required. Their major drawback is that these pushchairs tend to be very expensive.

The intimacy of support provided by fixed designs is inherently limited by their mass production. However, simple modifications can extend their applicability considerably and solve mild instability problems. Layers of foam may be added to adjust dimensions to provide lateral support where required (Fig. 21.20). This may be achieved rapidly with few more resources than a knife and pot of glue.

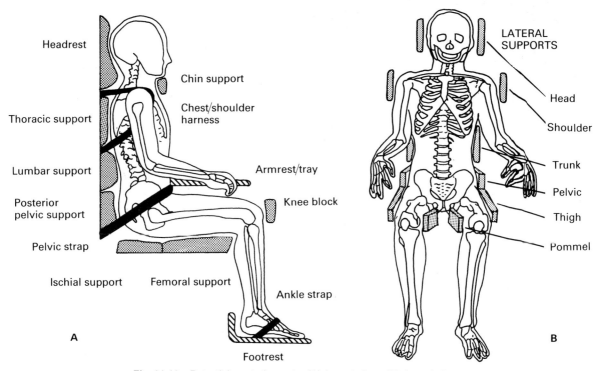

Fig. 21.16   Potential seat elements. (A) lateral view; (B) frontal view.

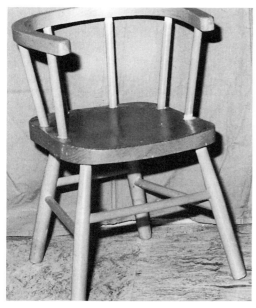

Fig. 21.17   Fixed format nursery seat.

A 'sticky' mat (e.g. dycem) may be placed under the buttocks using friction to discourage sliding forwards. A simple pelvic strap can be added, again to prevent forward sliding. Care should be taken to locate such straps to pull down over the iliac crests of the pelvis, bisecting the angle between the seat and backrest (see Fig. 21.16).

Cushions with firm bases may be added to sling seats to give a horizontal surface which helps maintain the pelvis horizontally in the midline (see Fig. 21.16). Ramping may be added under the cushion to help maintain horizontal femurs and to inhibit forward sliding (see Fig. 21.16).

The approach of using simple modifications often suffers from poor appearance as the modifications are often glaringly obvious. Also these modifications are limited in the extent of problems they can handle.

Adjustable seating

A number of seating designs incorporate adjustable features which permit more matching to

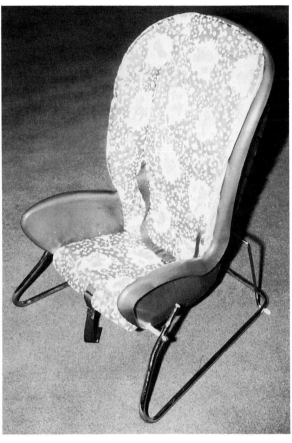

Fig. 21.18 Plastic shell seat.

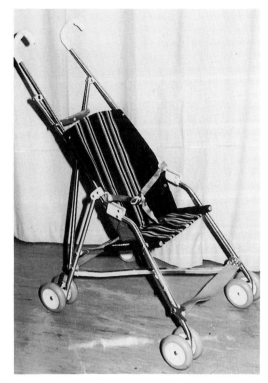

Fig. 21.19 Buggy with sling seat (reproduced by permission of Maclaren Ltd).

individuals' requirements than is possible with a fixed format. This adjustability may permit changes to match the changing needs of the child either in the short term during the day or in the longer term as their sitting abilities develop. Angle of recline is the most common adjustable feature and may affect the whole seat or the backrest alone. Further features such as lateral supports, leg supports, armrests and head supports may be incorporated to give variability (Fig. 21.21). Nearly all wheelchairs incorporate adjustable footrests to accommodate the inevitable variations in leg lengths.

Clearly there are benefits of adjustable types of seating systems but usually the extent of adjustability and hence the severity of problems they can accommodate is limited. Some highly adjustable systems have been developed for this reason but these tend to suffer from excessive com-

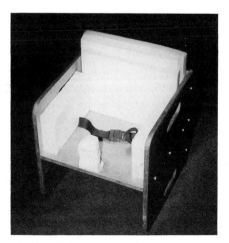

Fig. 21.20 Modified nursery seat.

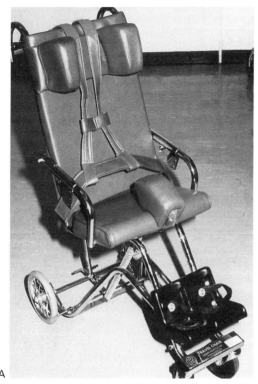 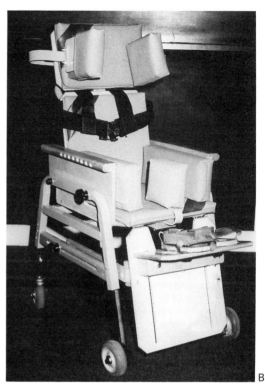

A   B

Fig. 21.21 (A) Adjustable seat (reproduced by permission of Ortho-kinetics (UK) Ltd); (B) Highly adjustable seat (reproduced by permission of James Leckey Design Ltd).

plexity, weight and a less attractive appearance (Fig. 21.21B).

Modular seating

Recent developments have concentrated on a modular approach to seating design (Fig. 21.22). This involves assembling a seat from a standard kit of components to give the desired size and configuration. Usually some adjustability is retained in the assembled seat which consequently can accommodate changing needs. The advantages of this approach is that it provides a wide range of adjustability without excessive complexity and avoids expensive fabrication involved in customised seating. The versatility of this approach can be appreciated through the ability to combine different types of 'module' in one seat. For example, individually contoured elements and special pressure distribution cushions can be combined with standard components to produce a hybrid seat.

Customised seating

Customised seating involves fabrication of a seat specifically for the individual. It is used only for the most difficult seating problems as it is usually expensive, has a limited life and tends to 'lock' the occupant into one posture. However, it is sometimes the only applicable solution, particularly for children with no sitting ability and severe skeletal deformities. A wide variety of different types is available as follows:

Foam and wood

This is probably the most versatile type of customised seating and requires a minimum of special equipment. It involves production of a wooden structure which is approximately the shape of the desired seat. This is padded with foam to give the required precision of support and then upholstered (Fig. 21.23).

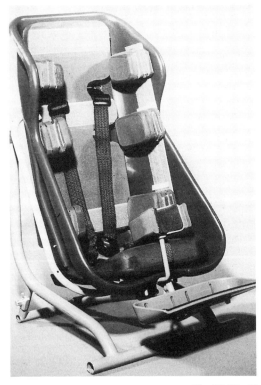 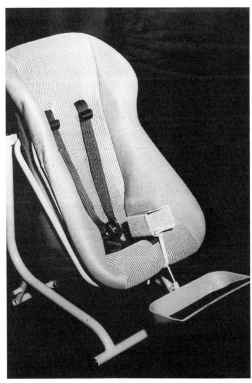

Fig. 21.22 Modular seats.

The technique suffers from being time-consuming and requiring highly skilled technicians to achieve an acceptable quality of finish. Also, errors in configuration easily occur and it is difficult to modify the seat once it has been completed. The use of a simulator greatly assists in producing an accurate seat.

Despite its problems, this approach is often required as a 'last-resort' solution for some people because of the comfort and the freedom of movement it can provide.

Matrix systems

These systems rely on a series of small interlocking components which can be released to produce a flexible surface (Fig. 21.24). This may be shaped to follow body contours and subsequently can be locked into the desired shape. It has considerable advantages of versatility and adjustability but can be rather heavy and difficult to manipulate.

Moulded foam

Polyurethane foam may be obtained in two liquid components which, when mixed together, form the foam which sets in the shape of the containing mould. Customised seats can be made using this technique by foaming around the individual in a sitting posture. This can produce a comfortable customised seat very rapidly but difficulties may be experienced in maintaining the required posture during the foaming process. Also, it cannot be adjusted. The technique can be improved by using a bead bag system to determine the seat shape and then foaming around the cast of the bags.

Bead bag vacuum consolidation

This technique relies on the use of plastic bags filled with small polystyrene beads. These conform to the shape of the individual. When vacuum is applied to the bag, it consolidates in a rigid form which follows the shape of the in-

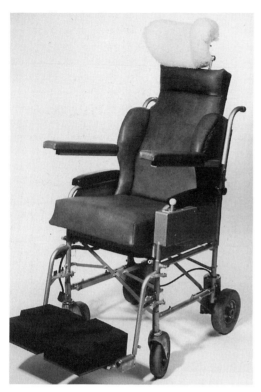

Fig. 21.23 Foam and wood seat.

dividual. Some systems use this approach as the final seat for day-to-day use by the individual. It requires to be reshaped as required or when vacuum is lost through the inevitable leaks. This is particularly attractive as an adjustable customised seat but requires skilled operators on hand at all times.

Other systems introduce adhesive at the time of moulding. This sets to hold the seat in a fixed form without the need for a vacuum.

The most elaborate development of the vacuum consolidation technique involves copying the seat shape in plaster which subsequently forms the mould for a vacuum formed plastic shell lined with foam (Fig. 21.25). Skilled staff are essential to determine the optimum seating configuration and to manipulate the bead bags.

The process can be greatly assisted by the use of separate bead bags to support different areas of the body and by an adjustable simulator type of chair to support the bags.

Associated devices

A number of devices can be used in association with a seat to improve its supporting characteristic and to extend its usefulness as follows:

Wheelchairs

Many disabled children require a wheelchair to provide mobility whilst seated. This article does not attempt to cover the wide subject of wheelchairs. However, several seating systems are designed to fit into wheelchairs which were not designed for this purpose. This need arises most frequently for the customised forms of seating. Special care is required to ensure that the configuration of seat, wheelchair and occupant is stable over the likely range of slopes, and that the occupant is positioned within easy reach of the propelling wheels if necessary. These objectives can often be difficult to achieve.

Orthoses

Orthoses sometimes present the only solution to problems of supporting parts of the body. The spinal orthosis in the form of a rigid jacket worn close to the skin is the most effective spinal support but is not tolerated by many people. Neck orthoses of a sheet or tubular form may be the only solution to the collapse into flexion of the cervical spine. Ankle-foot orthoses are essential to control foot position accurately and also may be used in dorsiflexion to reduce extensor patterns.

Cushions

A wide variety of cushions is available to control pressure distributions under the buttocks. They are intended to improve comfort and prevent or help treat pressure sores. Normally, high quality foam with an appropriate stretch cover is sufficient for most people.

The use of a firm base or convex shape of bottom surface to the cushion is beneficial to negate the effects of the inevitable sagging wheelchair canvas.

More vulnerable buttocks require the use of

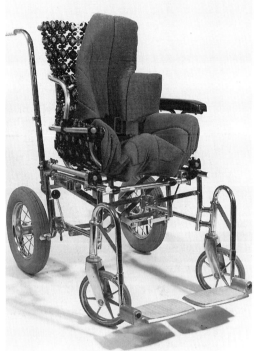

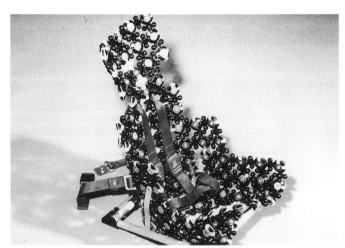

Fig. 21.24 Matrix seats.

gel or air-filled cushions to achieve the required pressure distribution. Expert advice should be sought in these cases.

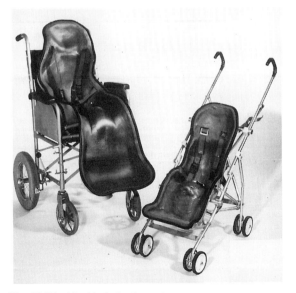

Fig. 21.25 Moulded plastic seats.

Straps/harnesses

Ideally these should be avoided as far as possible in view of the restraint they impose on the individual. However, they may be required as a simple safety precaution in a wheelchair or where forward flexion or sliding is a problem. Lap straps may hold the pelvis back at the desired upright position but must be located low over the iliac crests and should bisect the angle between the seat and the backrest. More extensive support can be achieved for the upper body by chest harnesses which are located by shoulder and chest straps. Walking reins for controlling errant toddlers are similar and may be used as seating straps.

Foot straps may provide the necessary location for wayward feet and can have surprising effects in stabilising the lower part of the body. Alternatively they can aggravate instability by converting foot movement to whole body movement and consequently should be used with caution.

Trays/tables

Nearly all seats are intended to facilitate function. This consideration often extends to incorporate table-top types of activities such as feeding, writing, play, etc. It is essential that this surface is in an optimum position relative to the individual to ensure maximum function. Trays can usually be fitted to wheelchairs for this purpose without too many problems. Trays may fulfil a dual function for some individuals by providing arm support to inhibit flexion at the trunk.

Tables often present difficulties in compatibility with seating systems and associated wheelchairs. These should be selected with care to ensure accessibility by the wheelchair and optimum height relative to the seat.

PROVISION OF SEATING

A 'system' of provision is required to ensure that each individual receives the seat which is most appropriate for their needs. The system involves the following sequence of events:

Assessment

The characteristics and the needs of the child are determined at this important stage. Seating can be involved in many aspects of the lives of the disabled and assessment has to be correspondingly wide-ranging. Ideally it should be multidisciplinary, including medical, physical, functional and associated elements. Where possible it should be a quantified process as shown by Mulcahy et al (1988) but this is not always practical for all elements. The assessment should end with a clear specification of the objectives which the seat should fulfil.

Prescription

The type of seat is selected at this stage. Correct selection of the type is dependent upon knowledge of the available range of seats, their indications and contraindications. Some guidance can be obtained from literature and catalogues but at present experience is the primary source of knowledge.

Positioning

Selection of the appropriate configuration of seat requires positioning the child in his optimum posture (or range of postures) and determining the support required from the seat to maintain that posture. This is a critical part of provision. In particular, 'positioning the disabled child' is a subject in its own right and beyond the scope of this article (Ward 1984). A trial and error approach is often adopted by trying out different configurations to determine the best.

This process is helped considerably by 'simulators', which simulate different seating configurations in a highly adjustable format (Bardsley & Taylor 1982) (Fig. 21.26). The required seat is then selected or manufactured to provide this optimum configuration. Some seating systems are sufficiently adjustable to be considered as incorporating their own simulator.

Fabrication

Ideally, all seats should be provided instantly on an off-the-shelf basis. This avoids delays in provision and minimises costs. The more customised seats, however, inevitably need

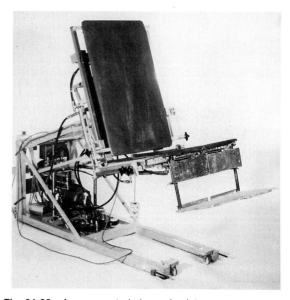

Fig. 21.26 Assessment chair — simulator.

fabrication. An intermediate fitting stage is often necessary as part of this process. This has the benefit of allowing fine tuning of the seat and is a useful check that it is an appropriate prescription.

Delivery

The definitive seat requires to be handed over to the child at the delivery stage. It is important to check that the seat fulfils the objectives set out at the assessment. In addition, instruction should be provided on how to use and care for the seat.

Review

Children in particular require regular review of their seating to ensure that it continues to be appropriate and that it continues to function satisfactorily. Consequently, a delivery system must ensure that the appropriate reviews occur at regular intervals.

REFERENCES

Bajd T, Andrews B J, Kralj A, Katakis J 1985 Restoration of walking in patients with incomplete spinal cord injuries by use of surface electrical stimulation — preliminary results. Prosthetics and Orthotics International 9: 109–111

Bardsley G I, Taylor P M 1982 The development of an assessment chair. Prosthetics and Orthotics International 6: 75–78

Bowker P 1987a Basic mechanics: forces and their effects. Physiotherapy 73(6): 264–270

Bowker P 1987b Applied mechanics: biomechanics of orthoses. Physiotherapy 73(6): 270–275

Harris E E 1973 A new orthotics terminology: a guide to its use for prescription and fee schedules. Orthotics and Prosthetics 27(2): 50–63

Petrofsky J S, Phillips C A 1983 Computer controlled walking in the paralysed individual. Journal of Neurological and Orthopaedic Surgery 4(2): 156–164

Rocca L, Hopkins P 1978 Swivel walkers. Physiotherapy 64(1): 14–18

Rose G K 1977 Total functional assessment of orthoses. Physiotherapy 63(3): 78–83

Sharrard W J W 1979 Paediatric orthopaedics and fractures Vol 1. Blackwell Scientific Publications, Oxford, p 507

Thomas T L, Meggitt B F 1981 Comparative study of the methods for treating fractures of the distal half of the femur. Journal of Bone and Joint Surgery 63b(1): 3–6

Ward D E 1984 Positioning the handicapped child for function. Phoenix Press, Missouri

Zacharkow D 1988 Posture, sitting, standing, chair design and exercise. Thomas, Illinois

FURTHER READING

Barbenel J C, Forbes C D, Lowe G D O 1983 Pressure Sores. Pitman, London

Butler P B, Major R 1987 The Parawalker: a rational approach to the provision of reciprocal ambulation for paraplegic patients. Physiotherapy 73(8): 393–397

Condie D N 1987 Long leg braces. Physiotherapy 73(6): 275–279

McHugh B, Campbell J 1987 Below knee orthoses. Physiotherapy 73(8): 380–385

Major R E, Stallard J 1985 Structures and materials — an introduction based on orthotics. Orlau Publishing, Oswestry

Mulcahy C M et al 1988 Adaptive seating for motor handicap. British Journal of Occupational Therapy. October 51(10): 347–352.

22

Planning for progress

P. Eckersley

INTRODUCTION

As children grow their development is characterised by an increasing control over their own movement. All overt behaviour is expressed through movement. This is true whether the child is interacting with the physical environment or involved in social communication (Laszlo & Bairstow 1985). When working with those children who are disabled or ill the paediatric physiotherapist should be seeking to guide and promote those aspects of development which are usually learned through self-directed movement and exploration.

As children develop a skill they use it to explore, to play, to eat, to learn and even to get into trouble. Movement is used as a response to instruction, sensation, conversation and the child's own plans and ideas. All movement becomes a basis for learning.

The physically disabled or ill child may be denied many or all of these experiences and it is central to the work of the physiotherapist that an individual programme should be based on a sound assessment of responses, problems and skills. If this programme is truly to reflect fully the needs of the child the total context of the child's experiences must be brought to bear on the planning process. In this way the ability to plan for progress becomes a valid expectation, not only for families and therapists, but more importantly for the child himself.

In this chapter assessment strategies, treatment systems and methodologies are discussed as tools in the planning process. Choices and decisions on their use are informed by:

- an understanding of the purpose of movement
- knowledge of the relationship between movement, learning and general education
- awareness of the barriers to movement
- choices in approach to physiotherapy
- the views and concerns of parents
- the needs and rights of the child
- involvement with colleagues from all agencies
- individual attitudes and expectations (Fig. 22.1).

THE PURPOSE OF MOVEMENT

It is necessary to spend only a short time with a child or group of children to realise that every activity is carried out for a reason and with a purpose in mind. The child's purpose does not necessarily coincide with that of the adult.

However, part of the process of growing up is reconciling what may be these very different purposes.

Purpose and motivation are complex subjects and have been explored by a number of authors, with varied conclusions. However, all agree that curiosity and intrinsic motivation seem to be inextricably linked and must therefore be looked at closely when children are taught how to learn (Curtis 1989). Piaget (1930) proposed that children respond to situations which are new and complex and generate intrinsic motivation to explore, whereas Miller & Dyer (in Curtis 1989) found that well-planned experiences and interaction with adults and peers were more likely to stimulate curiosity. Zimmerman & Rosenthal (Curtis 1989) stressed the importance of the presence of, and reinforcement from, trusted adults to encourage exploration and activity.

These senses of purpose, motivation and curiosity must be harnessed and developed by the physiotherapist working with children. All paediatric physiotherapists will be aware that working on a skill, task or problem as an isolated

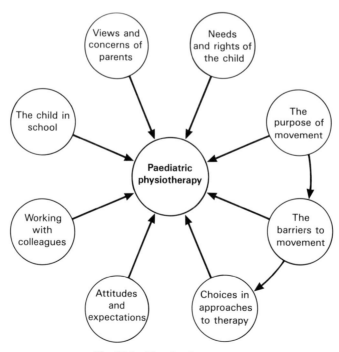

Fig. 22.1 Planning for progress.

movement activity will meet with little success. All movement activities which are taught or learned must answer the question 'Why is this activity necessary; what is its purpose?'

In order to understand the purpose of movement a number of factors should be analysed and subsequently incorporated into the planning cycle:

* developmental progress
  — sequential
  — age-related
* components of movement
* stimulus to movement.

Developmental progress

Chapter 4 The Developing Child states that most children follow a fairly predictable sequence of development, but that there is a wide variation in the age at which children reach milestones and emphasises that from the infant's earliest days new positions and movements are experienced. Chapter 17 Common Assessment Procedures also emphasises the need for a flexible approach when considering milestones as indicators of developmental progress. Many experienced developmental physiotherapists find lists of milestones unacceptable and have made their own individual adaptations of these checklists according to the child and his or her particular paediatric condition. However, such developmental charts do help to convey the important message that there is a sequence in the development of motor capacity (Levitt 1984). In order to plan appropriate intervention programmes this sequence must be understood, adapted and applied.

Two parameters can be considered in any discussion of developmental progress:

* sequential development
* age-related clusters of skills.

Sequential development

The sequences of motor development have already been described in Chapter 4 The Developing Child and it can readily be seen that the sequence forms a progression from simple to complex coordinated movement. Those developmental skills of particular relevance to any assessment leading to programme planning are:

* communication
  — by eye movements
  — with sounds
  — with bodily responses
* eye contact
  — with people
  — with toys
* head control
  — to lift and turn
  — in lying and in sitting
* mouth and tongue control
  — for sounds
  — for feeding
  — for mouth closure
* arm support
  — for propping in prone
  — to crawl
  — to balance in sitting
* hand use
  — to reach and grasp
  — to pass objects from hand to hand
  — to manipulate
* trunk control
  — as a base for movement
  — to balance and respond to outside faces
* stable sitting
  — supported
  — independent
* mobility
  — rolling and crawling
  — lying and sitting
  — sitting to standing
  — walking
  — running, jumping, hopping (from Eckersley 1990).

Age-related clusters of skills

The outline given in the previous paragraph gives a broad picture of progression in the development of a range of motor skills and emphasises that, for example, head control is achieved before stable sitting and arm propping in prone before standing and walking. However, skills are not developed in isolation. There is an interrelationship between the various movements and activities a child is beginning to perform, is learning through repetition, or has perfected at any particular age. In clinical practice the author (P.E.) found that the cluster of skills achieved by a 6-month baby to be a particularly useful foundation on which to build treatment programmes (Table 22.1).

Any analysis of developmental progress must therefore take account of both the sequence of development of any particular skill and the interplay and reinforcement which occurs with the parallel development of additional skills. A therapy session which has the objective of promoting independent sitting could therefore include arm support in prone, pulling to sitting and rolling. It could also be useful to use a mirror as reinforcement when working on independent sitting, since both are similar age-related skills. However, it is equally important to realise that for many older children this method may be inappropriate unless the mirror is used as a tool for the self-correction of position rather than as a game.

Components of movement

Movement and the ability to be still from choice, form the basis of most daily activities (Eckersley 1990). Movement can be assessed and enabled by considering the components which underpin developmental skills. Those components which can be applied to all gross and fine motor activities are:

- selectivity
- coordination
- strength and stamina
- understanding
- imagination
- consolidation.

Selectivity

The acquisition of higher movement skills demands an increasing selectivity of movement and is shown in a number of ways:

1. Isolation of movement within a limb:
   — pointing with one finger alone
   — grasping an object whilst the arm remains extended.
2. Separation of one half of the body from the other:
   — moving legs independently of the arms and vice versa
   — moving the right side independently of the left.
3. Combination of dynamic and stable muscle work:
   — writing: where shoulder and elbow remain stable but wrist and finger movements are dynamic
   — eating: where shoulder and neck remain stable but tongue, lips and jaw movements are dynamic.
4. Changing and alternating movements:
   — wide and narrow jumps
   — changing direction when running
   — colouring within a shape
   — playing 'statues'.

Coordination

There is an optimal way to carry out each movement. As children grow they practise a skill continuously until it can be achieved in a way which is satisfactory to them. A coordinated movement has, for example, appropriate:

Table 22.1 Child development at 6 months

Developmental area	Skill
Prone	Extended arm support One arm reach
Supine	Reach with both arms Pulls to sitting (legs extended)
Sitting — independent	Forward arm support (approximately 1 minute) One arm reach
Hand use (supported sitting)	Transfers objects hand-to-hand Reaches and grasps in pronation Feels feet and body Plays with toes

Movement	Rolls prone to supine
	Jumps on tiptoes when held
	  upright in standing
	Takes some weight when held
	  in standing

Vision	Fixates and reaches
Social	Drinks from a cup Smiles at mirror image

1. Rhythm — marching in time to music.
2. Timing — bringing hands together at the right moment to catch a ball.
3. Balance — reaching for a toy without falling over.
4. Force — turning a handle and pulling a door shut.
5. Direction — running around a room without bumping into everything.
6. Spatial organisation — arranging toys and objects in patterns around themselves.

Strength and stamina

Children frequently appear to have endless energy and continuous movement. At first the force and strength required is judged in a very arbitrary way. Large or small, and heavy or light objects are all approached in the same way. Short and long distance walks are begun with the same vigour and enthusiasm and being told to 'save your energy' rarely has any effect. However, children gradually learn through experience that an object of a particular size is likely to need a certain amount of force to lift or to push; or that a walk to the shops requires a particular degree of effort. This anticipation of effort extends to the pacing and timing required for sport, athletics and swimming.

Understanding movement

As young children play and experience movement they develop an understanding of the consequences of their actions. Action/response games, pop-up toys, switch toys, sand and water play all give children an opportunity to learn that their actions have a purpose and a consequence and that similar environments have similar possibilities. Young children can use this developing skill to considerable effect to explore the possibilities of puddles, closed doors, stairs and ornaments on shelves. They gradually understand what their bodies are capable of, and become able to repeat activities in many different situations. They can also increasingly anticipate appropriate contexts in which particular actions and activities are relevant.

Imagination

Once a child has developed and understood a movement skill it is further refined by choice, imagination and enjoyment. At the highest level of skill they become dance, mime or skating, but they are equally important for responses to nursery rhymes, for 'pretend to be' games and playground competitions.

Consolidation

A child will move through the stage of repeated practice of a skill, considerable concentration on working out what to do next, and effective performance to a point at which all the basic movements are consolidated. It then becomes possible to:

- carry a cup *and* open a door
- draw a picture *and* talk to a friend
- kick a football *and* direct it at the goal.

Concentration is directed towards, or away from, any particular movement as appropriate.

Stimulus to movement

All movement has a purpose, and is a response to motivating factors which may come from within the child or from external influences. The various stimuli to movement are:

- touch
  - turn to look
  - respond to tickling
  - guide direction of walking or action
  - calm, relax and comfort
  - exploring own body
- smell
  - move away
  - come in for a meal
  - investigate the unknown
  - make a face, hold breath, breathe deeply
- hearing
  - investigate sounds and voices
  - respond to music
  - put hands over ears
  - run to a recognised voice
- vision
  - copy a TV character

— walk around to investigate

— go to get food or drink

- comfort
  — put a jumper on if cold
  — cry if distressed
  — move to a softer chair
  — blow nose
  — go to the toilet
  — change position
- outside forces
  — balance on an escalator or moving bus
  — keep upright in a crowd
  — go down a slide
  — respond to being pushed
  — passive* movement
- wish to impose movement
  — pedal a tricycle
  — move a swing
  — push a toy
  — pull an adult
- instruction
  — respond to request
  — follow verbal, written and demonstrated directions
  — give instructions
- pleasure
  — move for its own sake
  — enjoy messy play, e.g. sand, water and clay
  — expression, e.g. dancing
  — keeping fit, e.g. sport, hobbies
  — play with a toy
- necessity
  — move from danger
  — open a door
  — make a meal
  — self-help skills
  — getting up
- experimentation
  — trial, error and self-correction
  — practice
  — turning and pressing all knobs, buttons and switches
  — begin a new skill
  — construction and building
- communication
  — gesture
  — demonstration

— attract attention

— self-expression.

MOVEMENT, LEARNING AND EDUCATION

Physiotherapists working with children use language to direct and guide movement, to explain what is required, to motivate, to praise and to encourage independence and understanding. It is therefore essential to have an understanding of the development of language skills, learning and the formation of concepts. The words we use must at all times have a meaning and relevance to the child.

All physiotherapy programmes must be informed both by:

1. A knowledge of the relationship between movement and learning.
2. An awareness of children learning in an educational context.

Movement and learning

The development of movement influences intellectual, social and emotional development. Exploration leads to knowledge about the environment which, in turn, leads to concept formation (Laszlo & Bairstow 1985). A well-planned physiotherapy programme is also an ideal opportunity for the child to develop learning skills and understanding through movement (Table 22.2).

Play

Learning begins with play and each stage of development is accompanied by a different kind of play. As children grow and develop their play reflects their own level of competence (Sylva & Lunt 1988). Play is frequently used by physiotherapists as a means of encouraging and promoting movement through enjoyment. The use of movement through play is analysed below in terms of a programme to develop hand–eye coordination. Many types of play might be used and could include the use of:

- jigsaws

Table 22.2 Movement skills and concept formation

Movement	Concept
Movement by progression	Space, distance, perspective Direction
Moving through manipulation	Shape, weight, texture, size
Coordinated movement	Time, rhythm, flow
Moving during games	Position, direction Planning, anticipation cooperation Rules and routines

- bricks
- toys
- songs.

Jigsaws. The size and thickness of pieces should be chosen with care and suitable pegs should be available as handles if this is necessary. There are other equally important factors to consider:

1. Does the child have a concept of colour required to match the pieces?
2. Is the background and foreground clearly divided to allow for any figure ground problems in perception?
3. Does the jigsaw have a picture with a meaning or is it purely for learning colour and size?
4. Has the child developed the concept of symbolic representation? A 2-year-old child recognises miniature toys and pictures but at 3 years is not able to complete a jigsaw of a man. At 6 years a jigsaw man may be correct but there may still be problems with the direction of the feet.

Bricks. Bricks may be used for building or to create patterns and shapes. Size and weight must be chosen with care and the words used to direct their use and motivate the child must also be relevant to each child:

1. Does the number of bricks used relate to the child's developmental level?
2. Does the child have an understanding of the concepts of colour and position necessary to give meaning to the statement 'the red brick is on top'?

3. If bricks are used in container play has the child developed concepts of:
   — ends and means?
   — container and content?
   — object permanence?
4. Where different-shaped bricks are used in a posting-box, is the box chosen relevant to the child's concept of shape, rotation and position?

Toys. Activities such as dressing a doll, feeding teddy or driving a car are not only enjoyable, they also demand skills relevant to fine motor control and eye–hand coordination. The ways in which these toys are used can also reinforce learning if they are linked to the stages in development of play:

1. Sensorimotor play uses only the physical properties of an object and many physiotherapists might feel it inappropriate for a teddy, or even a toy car, to be thrown, hit or pulled. However, stroking fur, moving toy arms and legs, or patting and feeling a hard surface are valid experiences.
2. Representational play — objects are used in context. A doll is put to bed, teddy is bathed, a car is driven.
3. Imaginary play — situations are acted out. The doll is taken to the seaside, teddy rides an imaginary horse, the car breaks down and is repaired.
4. Double knowledge — the type of toy is generalised and used for a number of purposes. The doll becomes a television character, teddy is the doctor who saw a child in hospital, the car miraculously changes into an ambulance or tractor.

Each stage in play requires increasing understanding and imagination. The use of toys must reflect the ability and understanding of the individual child.

Songs. Nursery rhymes and songs have always been central to the concept formation of preschool children. Where they are built into therapy programmes their language content should be considered so that they can be used effectively. Children are particularly fascinated by nursery rhymes and musical toys from the age of 18 months and as well as developing rhythm and timing, they also develop concepts of:

- direction
  - Jack and Jill went *up* the hill
  - *Down* came the rain and washed the spider out
  - Here we go *round* the mulberry bush.
- body parts
  - *Fingers* like to wiggle waggle
  - *Heads* and *shoulders*, *knees* and *toes*
  - This is the way we clap our *hands*.
- movement
  - The people on the bus *bounce* up and down
  - He *marched* them up to the top of the hill
  - *Wind* the bobbin up, *pull, pull, clap, clap, clap*
  - *Point* to the ceiling.

Learning in an educational context

Childhood is a time of exploration and learning through movement, sensory experiences and the routines of daily life. It is also a time when more formal learning takes place and the child learns:

- to read, write and work with numbers
- concepts of time, size and weight
- to use money
- about the environment: history, geography
- to follow a timetable and use time effectively
- to follow rules and routines
- to behave appropriately
- to be responsible for him/herself
- to cooperate with others.

All these aspects of learning can be supported during the time the physiotherapist spends with the child and can complement the work of the classroom teacher.

Reading, writing and number

For many physically disabled children, perceptual difficulties, poor manipulative skills and restricted concrete experiences can adversely influence learning. Restricted life experiences, as a result of illness and hospitalisation can have a similar effect. Children who have intellectual disabilities will experience both a slower rate of progress in learning and considerable difficulties in coping with the abstract and symbolic nature of concepts such as number, time and money as well as language itself (Westwood 1987). It is essential that the paediatric physiotherapist has an opportunity to discuss both the child's level of understanding with the classroom teacher and whether this understanding is concrete, symbolic or generalised. For example, counting to ten by rote, counting ten bricks, knowing ten is more than eight, waiting until someone counts to ten, and doing something ten times requires increasingly complex levels of understanding. Teachers should welcome such a dialogue and the opportunity it presents to extend 'classroom based' learning.

It is unrealistic to expect a child to be excited at having stood for a count of ten if there is no understanding of the 'ten-ed-ness' of ten, or its relationship to the numbers which come before it.

If a child is asked to do a reciprocal arm movement three times, this is the equivalent of multiplying 2 by 3. 'Give me three red bricks' requires not only an understanding of three but the ability to recognise two concepts in the instruction, number and colour, in addition to the motor instruction. When planning the language to be used with the child, the physiotherapist should be clear whether the objective is the learning of the concept or the reinforcement and motivation of the movement.

Reading and writing skills are developed through fine motor activity and spatial awareness sessions, including advice on seating, positioning of books and paper and use of pencil grips and typewriter guards. They can also be progressed through a knowledge of classroom themes for project work, topic webs, and practical science activities. Classroom themes are many and varied, for example:

1. The colours around us — could be developed using particular pens, crayons and chalk when working on fine motor skills.
2. Materials which keep us dry — could be

linked to swimming hats in hydrotherapy, wearing gloves when practising wheelchair use along wet pavements.

As children mature and consolidate their skills the use of writing and reading as practical skills can be emphasised by writing the instructions for an activity rather than speaking them, by having a written appointment card system for which the child is responsible, and by using a diary record of activities and progress which is kept by the child. Effective planning must try to link all of the activities in a child's day into a coordinated whole. Therapy activities and classroom programmes are interrelated and both complement and reinforce each other. Without coordination and planning the effectiveness of each is reduced and the overall impact diminished.

Planning and independence

The progression through nursery, primary, junior and secondary schooling makes increasing demands on the planning skills of children. There is a general expectation that higher levels of independence should and will be achieved, although this may not be explicitly acknowledged. Paediatric physiotherapists are increasingly faced with the dilemma of having to choose between the more time-effective and resource-efficient system of seeing children in clinics, and the more child-centred and effective system of seeing children at home and in school. Physiotherapists have to resolve these conflicts in the light of the existing resources and policies within each District Health Authority or Hospital Trust. There can be little doubt that seeing children in the relevant context leads to the development of activities which are more constructive, appropriate and above all developmentally relevant than those developed in a clinical setting.

Whatever the circumstances faced by the physiotherapist a number of questions should be considered:

1. How much time can be given to discussing 'why' and 'how' with children?
2. Is it possible to have timetabled sessions where the child is responsible for keeping the appointment?
3. Can systems be developed with class teachers whereby the information that the class is, for example, 'out on a visit next Tuesday' is given by the child?
4. Can discussions be held with child and class teacher to plan which lesson will be missed? — this should not be the most enjoyable, or always the end of the day.
5. How much time is to be allowed for the child to choose
   — which mat to go to?
   — where to park a wheelchair?
   — which games to play before breathing exercises?
   — whether a jumper is inside out or upside down?
6. How long can we wait whilst he/she works out how to fasten a caliper strap?
7. How do we plan choice into activities for children with severe learning difficulties?
8. Is it possible to let something go wrong without stepping in and correcting it?
9. Do we remind the child of the time of the next appointment or expect him/her to take responsibility for knowing the next lesson after the therapy session?

These questions are central to the use which a child will make of the motor skills practised during the 'hands on' therapy session. Motor learning does not take place in a vacuum but in the context of the child's understanding of their relevance both in the school and the home setting.

Patterns of learning

Children's progress in physiotherapy is not only linked to movement but also to development of formal learning. Such learning follows a pattern which can usefully be extended to all aspects of daily life and can be incorporated into the planning process. Haring & Eaton (1978) outlined an instructional hierarchy of five stages:

1. Aquisition — children are shown a new skill and learn to perform it.
2. Fluency — the skill is performed with fluency and accuracy.

3. Maintenance — the skill is retained even when no longer being taught.
4. Generalisation — the skill can be used in different contexts.
5. Adaptation — the skill can be applied to solve problems or applied in novel ways.

CHOICES IN APPROACH TO PHYSIOTHERAPY

The third stage in the planning of a therapy programme is to decide on the content of that programme. This decision should be informed by an understanding of the purpose of movement and its relationship to learning as described earlier in this chapter. It also results from accurate assessments and observation of the skills and problems experienced by the child. Planning the objectives for the programme has four stages:

1. Analysis of the barriers to movement.
2. Selecting the aims of the therapy.
3. Choice of systems and methods.
4. Recording and evaluation.

Barriers to movement

All children referred to a paediatric physiotherapist experience some barrier to their movement skills. Barriers can range from breathlessness during sports and games to a degree of disability which means that movement only occurs with adult intervention. Levitt (1982) detailed three different barriers:

1. Psychological — inability to concentrate, level of mental and perceptual function, lack of understanding;
2. Medical — spasticity, paralysis, lack of sensation, poor vision, poor general health;
3. Environmental — reduced opportunities given by people, access to buildings, furniture and equipment.

These categories can be extended to include:
— lack of opportunity and time
— pain and discomfort as a result of constipation, hunger, hyperspasticity or cold
— distress — at a recent family event
— at being taken out of story-time or an enjoyable activity
— fear of the unknown
— being taken away from parents
— a new physiotherapist.

It is also helpful to remember that all children behave as children and sometimes simply do not want to do something for reasons which are meaningful but personal to them, but may also appear idiosyncratic, arbitrary or as a result of awkwardness to adults.

Aims of therapy

The aims of therapy relate to:

- fine and gross motor function
- social skills
- communication
- perception and self-awareness
- self-help skills
- experience
- learning.

There will be a unique combination for each individual child. The general areas from which aims should be drawn are summarised in Table 22.3.

Choice of systems and methods

The various systems and methods available to paediatric physiotherapists have been described in detail in Chapters 18 to 21. In this chapter the choice is described from three perspectives:

- the components of therapy
- choice of method
- achieving progress.

Components of therapy

Levitt (1982) described five aspects of movement as being for:

- function
- fun
- fitness
- treatment
- learning.

Table 22.3 Aims of therapy

Establishing a relationship of trust

Involving children in all activities at all stages

Encouraging development of normal movement sequences

Developing symmetry and choice of movement

Normalising tone

Preventing deformity

Improving exercise tolerance

Improving fitness and strength

Improving circulation

Achieving a stable, safe and independently maintained position

Finding a comfortable and secure means of support

Developing balance and coordination

Finding a means of movement across space

Encouraging enjoyment and self-expression in movement

Developing creative activity

Enabling self-help skills

Developing understanding, awareness and planning skills

Training for sporting activities

Learning spatial concepts and perceptual skills

Widening choices and experiences

Linking activities and learning

Supporting and reinforcing classroom activities

Table 22.4 Components of therapy

Component	Considerations and examples
Position	In lying, sitting, kneeling or standing — order and progression Relevant position of therapist for eye contact
Equipment	Use of roll — for forearm-supported long sitting — for arm support in prone — as horse for balance Use of hoops, beanbags, balls Choice of standing frames, splints, seating Choice of electric or manually operated wheelchair
Exploration of self	Hands to parts of body Touching, stroking, patting self Hands to mouth, feet to mouth
Movement	Rough and tumble Rolling, pushing, swinging Balancing
Environment	Indoors or outdoors Hydrotherapy, riding, athletics
Sensory awareness	Use of texture, music, crinkle paper, light stimulation Links between, e.g. music and movement
Treatment	Vibration and intermittent positive pressure Postural drainage and breathing exercises Passive movement
Play	Use of toys and games Songs and nursery rhymes
Reaction to others	Group or individual Concentration and behaviour Social responses
Purpose	Relevance of activity, i.e. why sit up if only to lie down again? why lift my head if there is nothing to see?

This is not to suggest that an activity can be linked to only one aspect of movement (e.g. hydrotherapy can be fun, will develop fitness and can be used to reduce spasticity), but that where possible the whole range of movement experiences should be incorporated into a therapy plan. These five aspects lead the physiotherapist into making choices about those components of therapy which are relevant to the aims drawn up for each child. These components are summarised in Table 22.4.

Choice of therapy

A point will be reached when the paediatric physiotherapist has to choose between the various systems of working with children, such as Conductive education, Bobath, Doman–Delacato. At this point it will be necessary to identify an appropriate philosophical starting point on which to base assessment, planning and intervention. It is not the intention of the author (P.E.) to either advocate or deter the use of any particular approach. However, the following guidelines should be considered:

1. It is impossible to choose between systems unless they have been studied and practical experience gained. They need to be understood in functional terms.
2. All systems are effective with some

children and choices should be made which fit systems to children and not children to systems.

3. No system should be advocated or discounted on the basis of publicity or rhetoric.

4. All systems are related to particular aspects which underpin child development.

5. Each physiotherapist will be more comfortable with some philosophical approaches than with others.

6. The experience and opinions of colleagues and parents must be respected.

7. Most paediatric departments have established parameters of professional practice and the most effective have processes to evaluate progress and modify approaches.

8. The response of the child is the most effective feedback in monitoring appropriate choices.

9. Different systems and approaches to working with children are not mutually exclusive.

10. How well does a particular system relate to the child's other experiences — formal (e.g. school, speech therapy) and informal (e.g. family life, interests)?

Children learn from all the experiences available to them, whether the experiences are sensory, motor or cognitive, and no adult would attempt to limit experience to one modality. This is equally true of work with disabled children. The facilitation techniques of a Bobath approach can be used to great effect to enable and guide movement during a conductive education group. A conductive education task series can be incorporated into a hydrotherapy session. Vibration can be used to relax spasticity prior to breathing exercises with a child who has cerebral palsy and a respiratory infection. As long as therapists assess the child's problems from observation and not from mere assertion or second-hand opinions, then appropriate techniques can be chosen from any system (Levitt 1984).

Achieving progress

Physiotherapy intervention is a dynamic process

which should lead to the achievement of planned objectives (Fig. 22.2). As the child progresses these objectives will increase in complexity even within the same overall aim. This increasing complexity can be described with regard to arm reach/eye–hand coordination as described on page 328. A planned progression would be:

- preparation through vibration, intermittent positive pressure or inhibition
- passive movement for arm reach
- passive movement for arm reach with use of tapping or approximation to maintain
- supported active arm reach using placing
- arm reach in response to supported balance in sitting using trunk as key point
- using rhythmic intention and self-directed movement through language
- reach in response to request with no verbal self-direction
- reach to grasp a toy using internal self-direction and choice
- reach arm out for protection and balance
- gesture or point as communication
- copy a person or picture of someone reaching
- describe reaching to another person
- read an instruction to reach and grasp and understand it
- alter the speed and timing of reaching
- reach with one arm or with both
- reach against resistance
- incorporate reaching into dressing, feeding, etc.
- reach to throw or grasp
- do two things at once
  —reach and balance
  —reach and talk.

Progress must also reflect the generalisation of a skill so that it can be used in other relevant contexts. Physiotherapists working with children will be familiar with the words 'He did do it so well at home yesterday', 'She did this in physio last week', 'Come on, the doctor would love to see you do it.' Children frequently make choices about how, when and for whom they will 'perform'.

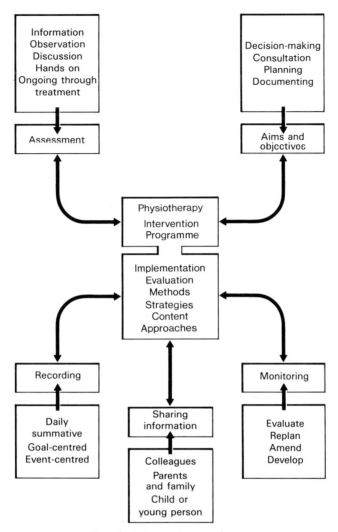

Fig. 22.2 The physiotherapy intervention programme.

The timescale of progress and the size of the individual steps along the way will vary considerably for all children. Expectations must be both adjusted accordingly and based on accurate assessment. All achievements, however small, must be looked on as praiseworthy. Motivation is vital.

Progress should incorporate the consolidation of behavioural skills. Disability and illness are no excuse for naughtiness and inappropriate behaviour, and it is important to distinguish between unnecessary bad behaviour and that which results from immaturity, stress or hyperactivity which the child cannot control.

Recording and evaluation

Recording systems support the identification of problems, progression of skills and evaluation of outcome. As well as being important to the planning of a therapy programme they also ensure that information is retained giving both a baseline picture of the child at initial assessment and of the key events over the period of intervention. Effective records also ensure that information is available for a smooth transfer between therapists in the same department or when a child moves to a different part of the country. They are also necessary in the event of legal action, for health and safety matters, and as statistical information. Not least, they are relevant to the individual therapist's effectiveness and development as a practitioner.

Seven types of record can be considered:

- checklists
- aims and objectives
- use of equipment and aids
- specific records
- narrative
- permission slips
- confidential.

Checklists. Checklists usually record the developmental stages of fine and gross motor skills, communication, social skills, self-help skills and perception and are charted on an age-related basis. Many are individually designed or adapted. They are most effective when they give an instant visual picture of initial assessment and the course of progress. Most physiotherapists will have a preference for columns which can be ticked and dated, or a matrix which can be colour-coded with a felt-tipped pen. However, whilst they list the skills which have been achieved they do not record the manner in which the skill is performed (see p. 70).

Aims and objectives. It is good practice to draw up aims and objectives for all courses of intervention however short. Where therapy is long-term they should be revised and updated on a quarterly basis as a minimum.

Use of equipment. Records should be kept of the type of equipment chosen, the date it was first used, the length of time the child used it and its effect. This is important not only to record and monitor the use of vibration or IPP but also to indicate progress in the length of time spent at a standing frame, the distance of independent walking with calipers or of independent wheelchair use.

Specific records. These files will include relevant specific charts such as:

- referral forms and general information
- initial assessment forms
- centile charts
- charts of range of movement
- sensory distribution charts

- peak flow readings
- letters from parents, consultants.

Narrative records. Narrative records give a consecutive daily or periodic picture of events and incidents as they occur. They can be used to give a picture of the responses and emotional state of the child, discussions with parents and colleagues, and as a working document on which to plan future sessions. They are helpful in recording information for use as a quarterly summative record which can be used as a basis for future aims and objectives.

Permission slips. Permission slips from parents for activities such as hydrotherapy, riding and outdoor mobility should be available.

Confidential records. These will be necessary in a few situations. Departmental guidelines on the recording systems for sensitive and personal family information, accidents and injury and incidents of non-accidental injury and child abuse should be available.

VIEWS AND CONCERNS OF PARENTS

Partnership between parents and professionals involves a full sharing of knowledge, skills and experiences in helping children with special educational needs to develop as individuals. Mittler & Mittler (1982) describe this partnership as a two-way process of joint assessment and decision-making and identify a number of ways in which parental involvement can fall short of a true partnership:

1. Where professionals assess and decide the intervention required and then show parents how to implement activities at home.
2. Where parents are shown how to keep records which show whether progress is made at home with skills taught at school.
3. Where parents are shown what to do without explanation about why certain exercises are necessary.
4. When home programmes are set up without consultation on the needs of the

family as a whole and the resources available to it.

5. When assumptions are made that all parents of disabled children have characteristics in common.

There are many ways in which parents and physiotherapists can collaborate in planning therapy priorities and objectives. These include:

• making information available to parents
• incorporating information from parents into planning
• planning priorities and objectives jointly with parents
• involving parents as therapists
• providing support for parents
• respecting parents' wishes on the extent of their involvement.

Information for parents

The first stage in any working relationship with parents is to establish how information can be shared. Each different setting in which paediatric physiotherapists work contains its own barriers to effective parental contact. Hospital departments and clinic settings may give little opportunity for privacy, and appointment systems need to be carefully arranged if there is to be an opportunity for more than a cursory discussion on 'how things are going'. Special school settings mean that whilst the physiotherapist is available during the day children often travel from a distance by special transport and therefore contact with parents does not readily occur. When children attend mainstream schools the physiotherapist may only visit for the therapy session and, in the majority of cases, may not be present at the beginning and end of the day to see parents. Opportunities must be deliberately created for information and contact to be shared at all levels. They will rarely arise spontaneously.

Decisions should be made as to whether:

1. Parents will be seen individually or also have an opportunity to meet as a group.
2. All information will be shared in the 'work' setting or home visits will be offered as routine.

3. Information will be given directly in discussion or whether termly reports or reports to parents at the end of a course of treatment will be given.
4. A general departmental newsletter will be sent to parents on general issues relating to work with children, e.g. how the department responds to requests for advice under the 1981 Education Act; the implications of the National Curriculum and PE with children; project work.
5. Information sheets will be made available on subjects such as breathing exercises, footwear, lifting and carrying, games and songs to promote developmental experiences.
6. Parents are to be invited to join a departmental steering group.

The need for information does not diminish with the passing years, but rather changes its focus (Marks 1985). The need for information on child development and welfare benefits in the early years later changes to a need for information on teenage behaviour and responses, after-school issues, leisure activities, employment and concerns about the future.

Levels of involvement

Having created opportunities for parental involvement it must be recognised that parents will make use of the opportunities to different degrees. It is easy to group all parents of a disabled or ill child together and discuss them as if they were a unique and homogeneous population. Parents have individual needs and preferences for counselling, support and other involvement. Parental preferences must be taken into consideration, including parents' expressed confidence in special educators' skills (Rodger 1986). This can only be achieved if physiotherapists listen to what parents have to say. All professionals communicate not only *to* parents but *with* them. We have to give information but also to take steps to enable parents to express their viewpoints, ask questions and make comments. We have to create a situation in which dialogue between listeners can take place (Atkin et al 1988).

A number of levels of involvement have been described by Pugh (1989) as:

- Active non-participant — active parental decision not to participate.
- Passive non-participant — a parent who feels unable to participate.
- Support — through practical general help which supports the school or department.
- Participation — physical involvement in the work of the department, i.e. running the toy library, going on outings, attending school assemblies.
- Partnership — involved in a working relationship with joint planning, shared decision-making, shared skills.
- Control — parents determine and implement decisions.

Whatever the levels of involvement it is essential that it is welcomed and supported by all members of staff and that processes are set up to ensure that decisions are representative of the whole group of parents on whom they will have an impact.

Parents as therapists

Most parents will wish to be actively involved in working with their child to overcome problems, to develop skills and widen experiences. It is essential that their partnership with physiotherapists answers the question 'What can I do to help?' In order to achieve this:

1. Assessments must be shared and information on outcomes given in a way which deals sensitively with issues of severe illness and profound developmental delay. In the author's experience most parents know the extent of their child's needs and are only hoping that someone will give time to discuss them openly.
2. Aims and objectives should be planned jointly and decisions achieved by negotiation. Parents and professionals may not have the same goals and it is important to provide opportunities for a free discussion to identify expectations (Mittler & Mittler 1982).

3. Time should be available to enable parents to learn how to carry out a physiotherapy programme and to feel confident in their own skills and choices.

Parents can also have a direct impact on the planning of a therapy programme with information on a child's likes and dislikes, i.e. 'He dislikes red bricks', 'She loves playing with cars', 'We learned a new nursery rhyme this weekend'.

Support for parents

Each child and family has a different range of experiences, needs and expectations and should therefore be supported by a range of options and flexibility of approach. There may also be a range of needs and expectations within the family to take into account and the different views between two parents, or between parents and grandparents can require careful handling.

The pressures and personal distress experienced by parents of a disabled or ill child are considerable. Physiotherapists should be aware that situations can arise where too much information or expectations of a high level of practical involvement will simply overburden the family. There must be a range of parental involvement options. The type of home programme advocated by Parcella (1980) which is likely to succeed is:

- easy to run
- fits in with the daily routine
- is not too time-consuming
- can involve all family members
- has been clearly modelled and practised by parents
- has been suggested by parents so they are motivated to carry it through
- is reinforced by other professional staff who have contact with the family
- is constantly monitored.

NEEDS AND RIGHTS OF THE CHILD

If given freedom of choice a child will select activities which he or she judges can be performed successfully and this further strengthens self-concept (Laszlo & Bairstow 1985). Children have both a need and a right to experience success and to have a positive self-image of themselves. The cooperation, involvement and enjoyment of the child is essential if physiotherapy intervention is to result in progress and achievement. There are three major factors to consider when planning activities:

- the development of a sense of self
- family and culture
- involvement in planning.

Development of a sense of self

Normal growth and development do not necessarily mean a trouble-free progress from early infancy to healthy adulthood. In each developmental phase distressing features of a physical, social, environmental, emotional or psychological nature may occur. For instance, psychological distress can result from physical problems such as pain and discomfort; while mental excitation such as frustration or laughing may disturb sleep, food intake or elimination.

Erikson (1950) described how the needs and abilities of children change as they pass through the various stages of development:

- sense of trust
- sense of autonomy
- sense of initiative
- sense of industry
- sense of identity.

Sense of trust

The basic feeling of trust usually develops during the first year of life, although it can be strengthened or undermined in later years. The child develops a basic view of the world as either a dependable and satisfying place or a place of pain and uncertainty. The ways in which people respond to a baby's physical and emotional needs influence the development of a sense of trust or mistrust.

Sense of autonomy

During the second and third years of life, the child concentrates on developing a mind and will of his own. Self-awareness develops as the child wants to do things for himself. With the growth of physical and mental abilities children test out for themselves how much they can do things independently. Given encouragement and opportunities they will develop a sense of confidence in their own abilities. If they are denied these opportunities they develop doubt about their ability to trust themselves.

Sense of initiative

Between the ages of 3–6 years children are usually willing to try things out and develop the self-confidence to take risks. At this stage the child's curiosity, imagination and need to experiment have a great influence on what he does. This is the time when the child understands more clearly what people expect from him and at the same time invents fantasies. Both conscience and imagination develop. A sense of initiative grows when the child is encouraged to make plans and given opportunities to express his fantasies. Too much retribution or reprimanding can lead to excessive guilt.

Sense of industry

This stage begins around 6 years of age and expands over the next five or six years. The child wants to be engaged in real tasks that he or she can complete. Adults can help by providing interesting ideas for work, both in school and at home, and by helping him to learn how to do things. Feeling successful encourages a child's sense of self-worth and eagerness to learn more. If a child is denied opportunities and encouragement the resulting feeling of defeat may lead to a sense of inferiority and can adversely influence the motivation towards future learning.

Sense of identity

Adolescence is a complex phase of life when problems of identity can be overwhelming. The young person's mind swings between that of a child and an adult. Patience and understanding are needed as an adolescent struggles to find appropriate roles, values and sexual behaviour. Peer group support or disapproval can be of great significance to an adolescent.

Family and culture

The developmental phase within childhood is influenced by cultural aspects. What is frequently described depicts Western culture where the nuclear family of mother, father, child and siblings provides the fundamental unit for the early development of a child. 'In other cultures, and in some circumstances in Britain today, other forms of family pattern networks involving grandparents, uncles and cousins may be as important a background to a child as his mother and father.' (Raynor 1973).

Strong religious values coupled with a sense of how to be a member of the family is nurtured within the developmental process. Cultural identity becomes a very important issue for a child from another culture growing up in Britain.

Health and social care staff, the majority of whom are trained in Western traditions, may find it difficult to assess normality and abnormality in a culture which is different from their own. Misdiagnosis both of a child's growth development and of family relationships is likely to take place.

Involvement in planning

Recommendations in the European Charter on the Rights of the Child contained the general principles that children must no longer be considered as parents' property but must be recognised as individuals with their own rights and needs; that policies and programmes must take into account the importance for children of love and affection as much as their need for material assistance; and that education and upbringing should aim at cooperation and equality of rights.

Physiotherapists can contribute by involving children and young people in the planning of their physiotherapy sessions. This is especially important where adolescents have been receiving physiotherapy for as many as 19 years. There are a number of areas in which discussions with, and the concerns of, young people can provide important information:

- comfort and security
- new experiences

- independence and responsibility
- recognition and achievement.

> CASE STUDY: Ayesha, aged 6 years
>
> Ayesha, a mentally handicapped girl of 6 whose parents came from Pakistan, was admitted to a hospital ward for 6 weeks. The medical, nursing and paramedical staff felt concerned about her mother not visiting her, although Ayesha's father and her aunt visited her regularly. The issue of 'child neglect' and lack of bonding between mother and daughter was raised. The social worker was asked to make an assessment of the home situation and found Ayesha's mother to be very concerned and loving towards her daughter. Her inability to speak English prevented her from visiting Ayesha, but she was happy for Ayesha to be visited by her husband and sister. This demonstrates how easy it is to make inaccurate cross-cultural assessments. (Bhaduri 1981.)

Comfort and security

Comfort. Discomfort is perhaps the most immediate factor in any decision to change position and as adults we curl up, sit sideways, slide down in a chair, rest our heads sideways or cross our legs. Children react in the same way. Yet there is a strong belief that the disabled child must be contained in an anatomically correct position for a major part of the day in order to prevent or correct deformity. This is not an easy issue to resolve and deformity can ultimately prevent freedom of movement and cause pain and illness. However, unrestrained movement is important and children do have a right to have the need for calipers, splints and supportive seating explained to them. Young people are also giving strong views about their preference to stay in a wheelchair rather than stand in calipers and find decisions based solely on medical grounds unacceptable. The London marathon has highlighted the fact that hip, knee and ankle flexion may be more important for wheelchair sporting activities than extension is for standing.

Comfort is also intimately related to self-help skills and can influence self-image. The child should never feel that blowing noses, changing nappies, being taken to the toilet and clearing up if food is knocked over is something the physiotherapist would not take part in.

Security. Security stems from being accepted as a child with a disability which is acknowledged, but which does not limit experiences or ignore concerns and above all, does not place a lesser value on the child as a human being. A child needs to know that nothing untoward will happen. This can extend to considering:

1. How objectives are discussed with parents in front of the child.
2. How a new therapist or a student observer is introduced to the child.
3. How the child is prepared for the first visit to the hydrotherapy pool or to go horse-riding.
4. How more distressing techniques, such as passive movements, postural drainage and suction, removing plaster of Paris splints, are approached.
5. How confidence is developed for that first step alone or to sit unaided; to know either that someone will catch you if you fall *or* that you have been taught to fall.
6. How a child might react to joining a group when previous treatment has been individual.
7. How a period of hospitalisation is discussed.

New experiences

All children grow wanting to explore new possibilities and experiences. It is part of the work of the paediatric physiotherapist to find ways of incorporating exploration, questioning, discovery, adventure and experiment into therapy activities.

Independence and responsibility

Planning and independence skills have already been discussed in this chapter (p. 431). This independence must be supported alongside the development of responsibility by channelling discipline, initiative, self-control and cooperation. Independence can be achieved in mobility, self-help skills, toileting and hobbies. It can also be supported by involving young people in the choices they make:

- when working in a group
- in involving adolescents with younger children
- in waiting for decisions about the order and combination of food when being fed
- by asking for their views on building adaptations for access
- by discussing their own priorities during physiotherapy sessions
- by recognising that contracts may need to be drawn up with older students
- by recognising that young people may have different views to those of their parents
- by acknowledging any practising or work they have done at home
- by trusting them to work unsupervised.

Some decisions are not easy, and many will also be the concern of parents and teachers. Joint discussion, sound professional judgements based on knowledge, assessment of individual circumstances and well-documented reasons are important.

Recognition and achievement

Children respond to encouragement, praise, realistic challenge and the opportunity to influence the activities of others. All children, however disabled, are able to do something well and have a right to have this acknowledged. The role of the physiotherapist is to recognise that skill, identify how to motivate it and develop ways of building it into additional more complex activities. Achievement can take many forms from a child turning his or her head to sound, to blowing bubbles in the hydrotherapy pool, holding a cup for the first time, painting a picture, climbing to the top of the wall bars or being a member of a basketball team.

Whilst for the ill or disabled child these skills may not be directly related to the age of the child, they must be recognised and progressed in a way which reflects a respect and understanding for the age the child or young person actually is.

INVOLVEMENT WITH COLLEAGUES

The importance of planning alongside class

teachers has already been stressed earlier in this chapter (p. 430) and issues of cooperation between team workers are developed in Chapter 24 Team Workers. This section considers the involvement with colleagues in the process of planning objectives.

Cotton (1984) identified a number of factors which result in a linear intervention of the various professional and voluntary agencies involved in supporting child and family. She expresses concern that the child may move from one operator to another at prescribed times whilst each individual deals with the symptom or function which comes under his or her particular jurisdiction. This mechanistic approach leads to the separation of education, treatment and care and results in each being episodes of intervention which are outside daily routines. They become isolated events rather than parts of a planned process.

Partnership and cooperation with the various agencies begins with a knowledge and understanding of the work they do and a willingness to share information. Each individual should also accept that they will have a different perspective on the priorities and methods of working with children and families. Even when these perspectives are recognised there will be a need for discussion, liaison and negotiation if the individual decisions made are to complement rather than conflict with each other. Each multidisciplinary team will need to identify whether joint working practice is one of:

1. Friendly cooperation — where the role and priorities of other services are acknowledged.
2. Goal planning — where a common objective is identified and each member works in an individual way to achieve the common goals.
3. Expertise sharing — where the methods and strategies for achieving common objectives are shared and implemented across the agencies.

In this way behavioural objectives established by a clinical or educational psychologist would be implemented in clinic, school and departmental environments and systems would be established to record outcomes in all settings.

Independent dressing skills would be monitored by the occupational therapist during PE in school, after hydrotherapy and during physiotherapy sessions. Toileting and feeding would be the responsibility of all agencies, and strategies devised by the speech therapist to encourage vocalisation would be incorporated into work in all settings.

Real partnership is difficult to achieve and sustain. Working in isolation is invariably less demanding on the professional. It is easier for one service to ask for help and support from others in fulfilling its responsibility, than for services to share responsibility or to carry out jointly agreed decisions (Sayer 1987). Recognition, joint networks of support, shared knowledge and information and cross-disciplinary opportunities for planning and training are increasingly being established in many authorities and it is hoped that current legislation will provide the impetus to enable these initiatives to be progressed (see Chapter 25 Legal Aspects in Paediatric Physiotherapy)

ATTITUDES AND EXPECTATIONS

In the final analysis it is the attitudes and expectations of the individual paediatric physiotherapist which have the most impact on the way in which intervention is planned and implemented. The most important attitude is one of realisation that the child is more than the disability or illness which is presented; that physiotherapy is more than the clinical implementation of a treatment programme to overcome disability. It is an opportunity to increase the child's experiences of the physical environment and of himself or herself by planning sessions so that:

1. A child's sense of humour is harnessed. Children love to fall down on purpose, walk backwards, upend toys, run away or say 'no'.
2. Activities have a definite conclusion. Children enjoy closing doors, giving a toy, closing a book, being caught.
3. The need for tireless exploration is harnessed. Children love to upend

containers, look in cupboards, climb up every step when outside, look through windows.

Children demand constant attention and frequently get angry when things do not go their way. The child who is ill or disabled has the same feelings, emotions and ambitions. The conviction that these childhood experiences are valid and important and that it is possible to incorporate them into therapy programmes should precede the planning of the activities themselves.

Physiotherapists working with older children will be well aware that teenagers work cooperatively when they are consulted as young adults, when their views are sought and when activities planned relate to leisure activities, independence and pre-employment activity skills. It is important to hold the expectation that for all young people it will be possible to find a valued and fulfilling use of time after leaving school.

Involvement with colleagues and parents has already been discussed. A key attitude to be considered is that of the paediatric physiotherapist as advice giver. The present and hopefully the future moves towards integration, resource constraints within health authorities and the need to spend increasing time in documenting and recording activities mean that less time is spent with the individual child. Paediatric physiotherapists are already involved in planning their work on an advisory basis, where assessment, training and monitoring are carried out by the therapist but programmes are implemented on a day-to-day basis by physiotherapy aides, classroom assistants, parents and teachers. This requires a belief that skills can and should be shared and that there are therapy routines and activities which can be competently carried out by people other than physiotherapists.

It also means that the advice which is given and the activities recommended must be practical and relevant and that the responsibility for their effectiveness rests more with the physiotherapist than with the implementer.

ACKNOWLEDGEMENT

The author (P.E.) wishes to acknowledge the assistance of Mrs R. Bhaduri in the preparation of the section on the Needs and Rights of the Child.

REFERENCES

Atkin J, Bastiani J, Goode J 1988 Listening to parents. Croom Helm, London
Bhaduri R 1981 Contact with children in distress is not all grey and gloomy. Community Care Journal (April 28)
Cotton E 1984 Integration of disciplines in the treatment and education of children with cerebral palsy. In: Levitt S (ed) Paediatric developmental therapy. Blackwell, Oxford
Curtis A M 1989 A curriculum for the preschool child. NFER-Nelson, Windsor
Eckersley P 1990 Cerebral palsy and profound retardation. In: Hogg J et al (eds) Profound retardation and multiple impairment. Chapman & Hall, London
Erikson E 1950 Children and society. Penguin, London
Haring N G, Eaton M D 1978 Systemic instructional procedures. In: Haring N G et al (eds) Research in the classroom. Charles E Merrill, Ohio
Laszlo J, Bairstow P J 1985 Perceptual motor behaviour. Holt, Rinehart & Winston, Eastbourne, Sussex
Levitt S 1982 Movement training. In: Norris D (ed) Profound mental handicap. Costello, Tunbridge Wells
Levitt S 1984 Paediatric development therapy. Blackwell, Oxford
Mittler P, Mittler H 1982 Partnership with parents. National Council for Special Education, Stratford upon Avon
Parcella A 1980 Increasing parent involvement. Education and Training of the Mentally Retarded 15
Pugh G 1989 Parents and professionals in pre-school services. In: Wolfendale S (ed) Parental involvement. Cassell Educational, London
Raynor E 1973 Human development. Allen & Unwin, London
Rodger 1986 Parents as therapists. In: The Exceptional Child, Vol 33, No 1, Queensland
Sayer J 1987 Secondary schools for all. Cassell Educational, London
Sylva K, Lunt I 1988 (reprint) Child development: a first course. Basil Blackwell, Oxford
Westwood P 1987 Common sense methods for children with special needs. Croom Helm, Kent

This section explores the concept of the paediatric physiotherapist as a member of a team. It highlights the importance of joint planning, communication, advisory networks and effective partnership with parents. Chapter 23 describes the impact on family relationships of the birth of a disabled child or of a developing illness. Chapter 25 concludes the section with information both on the legal implications of working with children and on current legislation in the fields of children's health, education and social services.

SECTION 5
Allies in the provision of services

23

Parents and children

P. Hartley

INTRODUCTION

In any therapeutic interaction, certain key factors exert considerable influence on the therapist's perception of the patient's needs and consequently on the quality of care provided. Initial evaluation of these factors will contribute to patient motivation and to recovery rate, where this is relevant. Such factors include:

1. The age or developmental level of the child (particularly relevant in paediatric care, Platt 1959).

2. The interrelationships of the patient. No one is sick in isolation. Illness for children has implications for parents, siblings, grandparents, teachers and even friends. These relationships should be acknowledged in the provision of services and the importance of effective communication within a wide radius of the child's contacts stressed.

3. Effective communication was emphasised in the Platt report (1959) for a variety of reasons. Appropriate information can reduce tension and anxiety (Hayward 1975) and may also serve to involve the relatives more actively in the process of recovery. This is particularly important in the care of children, whose compliance rate depends to some extent on the motivation and attitudes of their parents.

4. The impact of the parent–child relationship on the child's experience of

hospital will be explored in more detail
(see p. 451).

5. For children with chronic disability or a
terminal condition, the experience of illness is
further complicated by the sense of loss
involved. Parents of disabled or terminally ill
children will grieve over the loss of the healthy
child they knew or expected, or the impending
loss of the sick member of the family. To
provide adequate care of the patient and
family some knowledge of the grieving process
is invaluable for the therapist.

HOSPITALISATION

Preparation

Much of the distress associated with the experience of hospital is due to the suddenness with
which admission often occurs. A positive attitude
to hospitalisation and medical care in particular
could be encouraged by various means, for example, children's books featuring hospital, with
emphasis on the nurse or doctor. Television
programmes can demystify hospital procedures
for children by featuring popular animal charac-
ters in hospital mingling with real human
patients. Where possible, pre-admission visits
may be arranged, similar to the immediate preschool visits, which are fairly standard procedures
intended to familiarise children about to enter
reception classes.

Admission

The Platt Committee emphasised the importance
of the initial impression for both child and
parents and stated that admission is the time
when children are most vulnerable and apprehensive. It was recommended that the admissions
procedures should be carried out in the ward by
experienced staff, who should reassure the child
and ask parents for information relating to the
child's specific likes and dislikes. This should include diet as well as family expressions for
toileting and hygiene, to help to reduce the gap
between home and hospital. In addition, whenever possible, a favourite toy and the child's own
day and night clothes help to maintain a link with
the outside world.

Stacey et al (1970) found that in a group of
95 preschool children admitted to hospital, most
parents felt that reception arrangements were
inadequate, with very limited information being
given.

The Fassler Study (1980)

The effect of information and emotional support
on children's experience of hospital was studied
by Fassler (1980) using three groups: A, B and
C. All children used in the study were admitted
on a planned, not an emergency, basis. Group
A, acting as controls, were not given any
information or emotional support during their stay.

Group B were given 'emotional support' only.
The experimenter read stories, provided a set of
toys and talked informally about general
interests, school and family. There was little
reference to hospital.

Group C were given the same support as
Group B but in addition they were given
information about the hospital. Toys for Group C
included an operating table, which focused
discussion on treatment. The children were
shown a film about a child going into hospital
and concerns about their own stay were
discussed.

Each child was tested for degree of anxiety.
Group A, the non-informed, were found to be
the most anxious, with Group C showing
significantly less anxiety than Group A or B.

Psychological reactions

Illness is the most common form of stress affecting the developing child according to Lewis
(1982). Findings suggest that some degree of
psychological reaction is inevitable and may be
classified as:

• general
• specific to the illness.

Coping mechanism

Removal from a normally safe and familiar environment such as the family home to a new and
potentially distressing environment is a major
stress (Kent & Dalgleish 1986). They suggest
that hospitalised children may exhibit a three-
stage coping mechanism involving:

• distress and protest

- misery and apathy
- detachment and loss of interest in the parents.

These features can be recognised in grieving adults but may be more serious in young children whose life experience has not equipped them with the necessary concepts or skills appropriate for dealing with crises such as sickness.

Developmental level

The child's developmental level is crucial. A child whose verbal skills and understanding of time are reasonably developed is easier to reassure and more likely to benefit from information about his situation and the immediate future. For young infants, much can be achieved through frequent, gentle handling and a soothing tone of voice. Gentle handling, cuddling and verbal reassurance of the infant may also be beneficial to the therapist who may feel inadequate in dealing with small children whose level of intellectual development makes feedback somewhat limited.

The child's developmental age, both cognitive and emotional, has an important bearing on adjustment. Anxiety and distress may result in regression to patterns of behaviour more typical of an earlier developmental level. Repeated hospital admissions are associated with a slight increase in enuresis, especially in children undergoing surgery (Douglas 1975). Douglas postulates that family background may also be an important factor, suggesting that frequent hospitalisation in early infancy is more likely to occur in large families. Where social class and reasons for hospitalisation were taken into account, repeated admissions appear to be related to later disturbances.

The focus of anxiety also changes with the age of the patient:

- pre-5-year-olds were most afraid of separation and hospitalisation.
- The 5–7-year group most feared hospitalisation and the operation.
- The 7–10-year group feared the anaesthetic and the operation.
- From 10 years upwards the focus of

anxiety was anaesthesia and associated loss of self-control and consciousness.

The progression in focus here from the immediate and observable (e.g. separation, change in environment) to the possible and only hitherto imagined, reflects the sequence of cognitive development outlined by Piaget (1950) (see Chapter 4 The Developing Child). Some knowledge of major developmental theories may thus help therapists to understand the patient's anxiety at different life stages.

Personality

Some children may be more vulnerable to the traumatic effects of hospitalisation than others and some knowledge of patterns of interaction between the ages of 3 and 6 years might help to predict those children at risk. Brown (1979) found that those children who stayed in close proximity to the family at home showed high distress in hospital. Those who were less 'clingy' at home and more independent in their activities were more likely to become involved with other children in the ward and less likely to remain in bed.

To some extent the child's reaction to hospitalisation will be determined by existing personality factors. Regardless of the theoretical perspective used, some personality features will have been apparent prior to admission. It will therefore be possible to predict at some level the child's general mode of coping with stress. This pattern will of course be modified by the anxiety, discomfort and pain involved in the specific situation. An early study found that children with previous neurotic tendencies showed the most disturbance on hospitalisation.

Loneliness. Children may feel profoundly lonely in hospital. Not only are patients isolated from their parents and family but also from their friends and normal society network. The presence of other children in the ward does not necessarily reduce this loneliness. When adults are sick they make less effort to make social contact. In children, where some regression to a more egocentric level is likely, it is possibly even more difficult. The professional may help to reduce this isolation by involving a small group of children of similar ages in treatment wherever possible.

Play. Where appropriate, play is an important treatment medium and may also serve the social needs of hospitalised children.

Privacy. Young patients also have a need for privacy. They too need 'personal space'. Even quite young children may be distressed by being examined or treated in full view of other patients in the ward. Self-consciousness reaches a peak during adolescence but many prepubertal children may privately object to displaying their bodies to the rest of the ward. Working through a heavy case-load may sometimes result in carelessness but if such embarrassment can be avoided the rapport between patient and therapist is more likely to be positive and consequently a higher degree of cooperation is achieved.

Professional awareness

Greater attention should be paid to the emotional and mental needs of the child in hospital (Platt 1959), bringing about change:

- in attitudes towards children
- in the hospital's place in the community
- in medical and surgical practice.

The authority and responsibility of parents, the individuality of the child and the importance of mitigating the effects of the break with home should all be more fully recognised.

Attitudes

Hospitalisation can be traumatic for some children and the break with home and separation from parents is particularly distressing. Discrepancies in attitudes to children occur between general staff and those with paediatric training in the same hospital (*Which* 1980). This report stressed the acute need for some paediatric orientation among staff not specifically trained for children's care.

Effective hospitalisation depends on:

- hospital facilities
- the age of the child
- the attitudes of the parents to the disease

- the quality of the relationship between the family and the doctor
- the course of the specific disease.

Staff should have considerable knowledge of child development so that the environment and resources could encourage a more positive adjustment to hospital. Individual children have different levels of anxiety which may not be related to the complexity or degree of any individual procedure.

There is also a need for more specialist units in local general hospitals and for nursing children in peer groups (Platt 1959).

The patient's perception of the hospital environment is of course very different from that of the therapist. Uniforms, high technology, medical and surgical procedures are all commonplace to the professional, not to the sick child. Complex machinery and some therapeutic procedures are often frightening and frequently involve discomfort at best and pain at worst.

Expectations

Parsons (1958) clearly defined the 'part' the patient plays. Being ill involves both rights and expectations (see Chapter 9 Developmental Delay). These rights and expectations are conferred on the sick individual by society as part of the socialisation process. The sick person knows, through learning, that he/she has certain rights: to be cared for, to be treated and to be helped to adjust. Patients expect professionals to furnish these needs. At the same time professionals have certain expectations of patients: that they accept the credibility of the medical team and comply with instructions and treatment. Any infringement of these rights and expectations may result in problems for both patient and therapist. If the patient does not receive satisfaction of his/her needs he may demonstrate dissatisfaction in a variety of ways, e.g. verbal abuse, uncooperative behaviour and unpleasantness. The therapist may see such patients as 'difficult' and awkward. The popular patient is one who does not complain, who shows a high degree of compliance and who often requires little from the professional.

In dealing with children it is particularly easy to slip into an authoritarian role. Highly dependent children may to some extent welcome this, but more independent adolescents may find this approach an additional source of stress. In families where children have learnt to play one parent off against the other, the same tactics may be used with different members of the professional team.

Parental involvement

The parents' anxiety, and particularly the mother's, also affects patterns of adjustment to hospital. Children who have poor relationships with adults and other children, and who are so-cially inhibited, aggressive or uncommunicative before entering hospital, are more likely to be disturbed by the experience (Stacey et al 1970). Certain types of pleasant separation, e.g. good babysitters or staying overnight with relatives, may lead to good adaptation in hospital. Children from a secure home base are less likely to be disturbed by hospitalisation (Harlow 1959, Bowlby 1971, Rutter 1979).

Parental involvement may do much to reduce the traumatic effects demonstrated by a large proportion of young patients. In spite of this, *Which* (1980) found that some hospitals restrict and discourage parents from staying in with their children. They found also that visiting restrictions still exist and that hospitals need to be more flexible about allowing parents to be present during treatment of their children.

Many health professionals maintain that a parent's presence during the child's treatment increases the level of distress shown by the child, but this theory has not been fully tested. Most research shows that where parents are involved they themselves experience less anxiety as they feel more in control over what is happening to their own child. In turn, they transmit less anxiety to the child. A parent with whom a therapist has established a good relationship can be an invaluable extra pair of hands, leaving the professional to carry out the highly skilled treatments for which he/she has been trained. Often some treatment is required when the child is back home with his/her family. Initial involvement of the parent during hospital treatment will greatly

increase the likelihood of continued treatment when the child returns home.

The physical presence of the child's mother has been shown to be of enormous importance. All children interviewed in the *Which* (1980) survey wanted to have their mothers with them and were particularly distressed at night when the mothers had to leave. This feeling was not confined to the youngest children. Not only are mothers a valuable emotional support but they are also a vital link with the child's life outside hospital. The parent may also be seen by the child as his/her representative in the adult world of the hospital, and a useful mediator.

The adolescent

Adolescence is frequently described as that period of life in which the major developmental task is the establishment of a stable identity, leading to the formation of an individual in his or her own right (Erikson 1963). This phase often has negative associations, for example, with regression and rebelliousness, involving defiance and rejection of parental and societal values. These responses may be more positively viewed as important 'self-statements'. There may be the assumption of new responsibilities and newly found independence. Illness during this period of profound change may well have radical implications and hospitalisation may occasion disquieting and profound psychiatric situations (Hoffman et al 1976).

Coping strategies

In common with other age groups, adolescent responses to illness and disability will be idiosyncratic. The coping strategies used will vary according to:

- the nature of the illness
- the prognosis
- the medical or surgical techniques involved
- the patient's premorbid personality
- present developmental level.

Fear and anxiety may be expressed through aggression or apathy, both difficult responses for the therapist. Aggression, however, may be utilised to motivate the patient if the appropriate channel can be found (see Chapter 22 Planning for Progress). The apathetic patient may prove a greater challenge.

Self-concept

Such reactions to illness may be understood in the context of the patient's life situation. The young person may be faced with many and sometimes painful investigations, with the possibility of impaired function and future disability. Surgical disfigurement may result in body-image and self-concept problems. Self-worth is to some extent in our society measured in terms of body integrity and conformity to certain physical norms. Children are particularly vulnerable in this respect and many health problems, both physical and mental, occurring during adolescence, focus on issues relating to body and self-evaluation. Adler (1927) demonstrated that even a minor bodily imperfection can be generalised to the self as a whole. Deaf adolescents, for example, judge their disability to be far more extensive than just hearing loss (McDaniel 1976). In eating disorders the body is the target for the patient's personal sense of inadequacy and low esteem.

Anxiety

The sick or disabled adolescent may experience a resurgence of old anxieties previously mastered. Struggles for freedom may reappear as the patient recognises his/her dependence on health professionals. Uncomfortable and unpleasant symptoms and painful procedures involve reasonable fears and discontent, which may inevitably be discharged on professionals. In some patients the anger and aggression may be internalised, resulting in withdrawal and depression. The closeness of the relationship between physiotherapist and patient provides a vital opportunity for the child to talk about these feelings. As touch is so important in physiotherapy, massage and relaxation training may facilitate the expression of these fears within the therapeutic interaction.

Cooperation and motivation

The adolescent patient faced with a very different future as a result of a permanently disabling illness or accident, may need considerable help in feeling motivated to cooperate with treatment. Professionals sometimes hold unrealistic expectations of patients, assuming that disabled people will adjust to their impaired function. Later in this chapter the stages in the grieving process will be outlined. At this point it is sufficient to state that this process also applies to loss of function or body part. Just as parents would mourn the untimely death of an adolescent son or daughter, a disabled adolescent may mourn the future for which he had been preparing but will not now experience as he had expected. Career and even partnership prospects may need radical revision.

CHRONIC ILLNESS

As many of the acute childhood illnesses which formerly led to the development of paediatrics have largely been overcome, chronic disease may now be seen as the major health problem. For these patients, many of whom will not get well, small progress in improved function is all that can be achieved. Parents of such children are often under tremendous strain, with the knowledge that the situation will not improve and will, in many cases, deteriorate. For the health professional the philosophy must be to improve function wherever possible, but always to support and care.

Professional attitudes

The present incidence of chronic illness or disability reflects between 5 and 10% of the population below the age of 16 (Pless & Pinkerton 1975).

These children and their families are often burdened by social and behavioural difficulties, frequently involving intervention by social workers and psychologists. Many such difficulties are related to adjustment both by the sick child and the family.

One problem is that adjustment is itself difficult to define. One possible definition reflects the extent to which the patient has accepted the reality of his condition and has learned the best way of adapting to it. This would necessitate making optimal use of remaining skills and abilities, as well as coming to terms with the level of impairment and the inevitable treatment.

Another definition of adjustment involves the concept of psychological balance of freedom from abnormality in the face of pathological circumstances. In some respects, psychological wellbeing may be best achieved by refusing to accept the reality of the illness and the disability it imposes (Pless & Pinkerton 1975).

Concept of normality

The concept of normality is even more difficult to define. A useful working baseline would be that normality is a process, the end result of interacting systems which change over time. These systems involve normality in physical, mental and social terms, not merely the absence of disease and illness. In addition, normality equates with the average, the middle range of the distribution of traits and characteristics in which both extremes are equally deviant. In any adjustment response it is likely that both positive and negative patterns will occur.

Looking at the sick or disabled child in a more global way resulted in the self-concept model suggested by Barker et al (1953). Within the timescale of the illness, intrinsic attributes (temperament, personality, intelligence, age and sex) forming the pre-illness self-concept, were seen in interaction with the stress of the illness itself. Included under this concept of stress were factors such as the effect on the patient's body image, the response of family and other people of significance to the child and his or her altered self-concept as a result of the illness experience.

According to the nature of this interaction, the response to illness or disability will involve modified behaviour, both positive and negative (Fig. 23.1).

Patterns of reaction

Three patterns of reaction to chronic sickness or disability are often described:

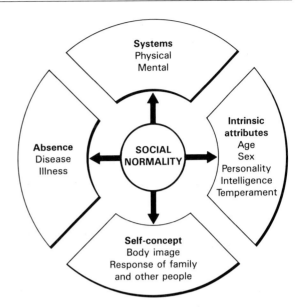

Fig. 23.1 Social normality: an interactive process.

- withdrawal
- rejection (denial)
- acceptance.

It is usually assumed that the first two are unhealthy and that acceptance is the most desirable, but this is a value judgement for which there is little supporting evidence. If the sick child is genuinely happier and functions more effectively having withdrawn from a challenging situation or denying the limitations of his illness, he could be said to be in harmony with the real world, coping by using those methods which are most suited to his personality.

Symptoms such as strong self-centredness, emotional instability, intensive worrying and anxiety are cited by many health workers as signs of maladjustment, but these traits can also be seen as a normal and understandable reaction to genuine trauma. It is more realistic to look at the period of time over which such responses are maintained. The task of the therapist is to help the patient to use existing strengths and minimise negative coping strategies in the period of adjustment. It is useful for the therapist to remember that coping patterns will tend to reflect genetic, familial, environmental and social factors. In this respect each child's reaction to sickness or disability will be unique.

PARENTAL REACTIONS

The reactions of parents to sickness and disability vary according to a number of factors (Lewis 1982). Many of these have already been discussed in this chapter, but it is helpful to focus on specific examples.

Types of childhood disorder

Birth defects

The delivery of a baby with congenital defects may result in initial rejection by one or both parents. Feelings of revulsion, anger, anxiety and low self-esteem are experienced. Mothers in particular feel guilty and inadequate. This is similar to the sense of bereavement following the death of a child, in that the birth of a less than normal child is just as much of a 'loss'. The prospect of caring for such children is daunting, as defects tend to progress and change with time (Lewis 1982).

Acute illness

When children regress under the stress of acute illness, it is obviously difficult for many parents to understand and cope with behaviour which may seem inappropriate for someone of the child's actual age. Bed-wetting, thumb-sucking, food refusal and temper tantrums have been observed by paediatric staff. The nature of the illness itself, coupled with the anxiety surrounding the strange hospital environment, may lead to outbursts of anger towards parents and staff. Parents themselves may feel that their child is rejecting them and in turn direct these feelings towards the professional health carers. This may be particularly so should the child respond more favourably to the nurses or other hospital staff. Mothers may feel redundant in these circumstances, describing hospital visits as 'distressing' or 'a waste of time'.

The burns patient

Children with burns may manifest severe emotional reactions. Studies suggest that the patient may feel guilty about the cause of the burn (play-ing with fire or matches) and afraid of the consequences of the disobedience sometimes involved. It may be that some children perceive the burns themselves as punishment. The period of acute care is traumatic, involving hospitalisation, separation, frequent and painful procedures and immobilisation (see Chapter 13 Infection and Trauma). The child must also cope with the reactions of parents, who may feel both anger and guilt, frustration and distress. Professional staff will sometimes be the target for these feelings.

The pain of severe burns may in itself lead to anger, aggression and depression. Studies reviewed in Lewis (1982) suggest various interesting features relating to burns. For example, children lacking pain sensation below the waist showed less adverse reaction to burns and more cooperation with staff. Other workers in the field found that in some cases emotional difficulties existed prior to the burns injury and that a major proportion of the families concerned had serious psychosocial problems before the accident occurred. The patients themselves may have long-term fears in relation to disfigurement and social isolation.

Parental attitude

Several studies of childhood illness and disability have suggested that children have to contend not only with the illness but also with parental attitudes (McDaniel 1976). Other studies suggest that chronic conditions such as cystic fibrosis or haemophilia may trigger negative attitudes towards the sufferer. Mothers may feel guilty and inadequate at their own inability to care for their sick child. The mother of a child with haemophilia may feel particularly guilty for handing on the defect. Fathers of such sons have sometimes lost interest in their boys, who were discouraged from participating in family pursuits and games like football. Studies of epilepsy indicate that the child with this affliction is frequently the victim of his environment, with well-meaning family and friends being over-protective (see Chapter 8 Disorders of the Central Nervous System).

Stress

There is little doubt that families with a chronically sick or disabled child are under considerable stress, and it is likely that some of the related anxiety will be transmitted to the child. Should the patient feel that the parent is reacting negatively towards him, his own sense of worth will be diminished. Many professional carers believe that if the patient's self-esteem has been strong prior to disease or injury there may be fewer problems in self-evaluation following the trauma. We should bury the belief that mothers are neurotic, and recognise their prolonged stress (Roskies 1972).

Rejection

Rejection by family members, particularly a brother or sister, may lead to poor self-esteem, which may, in turn, be expressed through hostility to the family. Rejection is sometimes perceived in spite of evidence to the contrary. When the patient himself feels worthless, there is often the expectation that others will find him equally so. This 'set' or expectation may lead to behaviour by the patient which triggers off the response expected from those involved: the 'self-fulfilling prophecy'.

Positive attitudes

Despite the lack of credible evidence to support such ideas, people frequently associate certain physical attributes to certain personality characteristics. Increasing emphasis on physique and appearance during adolescence has an important effect on personality development, particularly for the physically disabled adolescent (Bansavage 1986). Health professionals may help to counteract any problems by adopting positive attitudes towards the patient's body, stressing the patient's strengths and abilities and minimising any negative qualities within realistic limits.

DEATH IN CHILDHOOD

There are still some childhood illnesses for which

there is no known cure. At best, these children have to be supported and treated with confidence by professional staff who will inevitably experience some anxieties themselves throughout the treatment programme. The physiotherapist may have feelings of failure and inadequacy. There may be problems dealing with parental anxieties, anger, resentment, depression and even denial. Most importantly, the professional may bear the impact of the child's loneliness, sense of insecurity and feelings of being abandoned.

Talking to the child

This is a particularly difficult area and one in which parental wishes should always be respected. Parents should be asked how they would respond if their child asked them about death. It is said by many health professionals that children can usually cope with such stresses when a trusting relationship gives them the opportunity to discuss these matters openly and honestly (Kubler-Ross 1982). Once a decision has been made, the child should be engaged in a dialogue about his future, perhaps being given information over several gradual stages but not in the form of an announcement. The child must still be given hope in the knowledge that professionals will continue to fight on his/her behalf. It is important that the child is enabled to express concerns and anxieties through play and other media (Kubler-Ross 1982). Where the child is using denial of the illness as a defence, this must be respected. Any idea that death is a punishment should be removed, and regressive behaviour should be dealt with as, although both responses are understandable, they are counterproductive.

The child's concept of death

In general, a child's understanding of death is linked with the level of cognitive and emotional development attained. A 4-year-old child may see death as 'disappearance' and a slightly older child may feel guilty and wonder 'Was it my fault?'. If not dealt with early enough, such thoughts may trigger serious psychological problems. For example, a 16-year-old anorexic girl remembers thinking that she did not deserve to eat as she had failed to summon an ambulance for her dying brother. She was 6 at the time of his death and the telephones in the neighbourhood had been vandalised.

Older children may understand the implications of death but will nevertheless have emotional difficulties. If a long illness and hospitalisation are involved, then all the psychological defences related to illness may be present. The child's own coping strategies will to some extent be determined by the parents' reactions.

Parental grief and mourning

Engel (1962) described the grieving process as 'work'. It is an inevitable part of everyone's life, not only following the loss of a valued person but also following the loss of function or body part. Engel maintains that this working through involves four important stages.

Disbelief and shock. This may last for a few days, while refusal to accept what has happened may dominate the mind. The concept can apply in the case of sudden death or the diagnosis of a terminal condition. Exceptionally, such denial may persist for many months.

Developing awareness. Sometimes this is accompanied by guilt and bitterness. 'If only I had . . .'. 'Why my child . . .?'

Apathy and exhaustion. These may also be seen at this stage, and parents are in need of someone willing to listen and accept the expression of these feelings. This is an important stage in the grieving process.

Resolution. The work of mourning is complete with the establishment of a new identity, acceptance of what has happened and a new adaptation to the environment. For example, a child may have adapted positively to a newly acquired disability or a mother may realise that there are some pleasures in caring for a handicapped baby.

Reactions to death and loss

Specific reactions to death or impending loss do vary according to the precise nature of the situation and the personality characteristics of the people involved. For example, the stillborn child is just as much a loss as the death of an older child may be. Stillbirth is frequently associated with guilt and feelings of inadequacy in the mother, as miscarriage may also be. Parental grief needs careful handling. Some dying children, for instance, are 'over-idealised' by parents trying to deal with the loss of expectations they may have had for their child. It is not uncommon for parents to overprotect remaining siblings or to try to fill the void with another pregnancy. Occasionally, their grief forces them to withdraw, sometimes from the dying child himself. Although professionals may feel anger in such situations, their role is to support the patient and his/her relatives without being in any way judgemental.

Where the process of dying is prolonged, the mourning process will involve anticipatory grief (Burns 1980). Parents may be troubled by unacceptable thoughts, wishing this child dead, thus relieving the emotional and financial burden. Such thoughts will lead to guilt and anxiety, which may be expressed to hospital staff. After the child has died, relief may be mixed with guilt and remorse.

Unfortunately, most paediatric therapists will encounter such children in their caseload and it is necessary to understand the reasons for parental insistence that their child should be kept alive and intervention continued. All the features of bereavement are present, however, but initially parents cannot accept that there is no hope. They need time to come to terms with the reality of the situation and staff must acknowledge the responsibility of the parents in the decision-making about continued intervention. The sense of guilt could be very great if parents were pressured into making any decision before they had reached the appropriate stage in the grieving process. When such a child dies in the absence of the parents the ensuing guilt is sometimes the trigger of serious psychosocial problems.

CONCLUSION

From the studies carried out it is reasonable to suggest that illness and hospitalisation may be traumatic not only for the child but also for the parents and other family members. Some understanding of child development, the emotional needs of the child and the family, should improve the nature of the therapeutic interaction for both patient and therapist. With greater implementation of the recommendations of Platt (1959), and increased understanding of behaviour in sickness and bereavement, it should be possible to reduce the fears and anxieties of patients, parents and therapist.

Although it must be accepted that a cure is not always possible, that progress may be very limited, and that sometimes death is the only outcome, a sensitive awareness of the global needs of sick children and their families should improve the quality of the illness experience for patients and therapists alike.

REFERENCES

Adler A 1927 The practice and theory of individual psychology. Harcourt Brace, New York

Bansavage T 1986 Social acceptance in a group of orthopaedically impaired adolescents. APA Proceedings

Barker R G, Wright B A, Myerson L, Gonick M R 1953 Adjustment to physical handicap and illness: a survey of the social psychology of physique and disability. Social Science Research Council, New York

Bowlby J 1971 Attachment and loss, vol I. Attachment. Penguin Books, Harmondsworth, Middlesex

Brown B 1979 Beyond separation: some new evidence on the impact of brief hospitalisation on young children. In: Hall D, Stacey M (eds) Beyond separation. Routledge and Kegan Paul, London

Burns R B 1980 Essential psychology. MTP Press, Lancaster

Douglas J W B 1975 Early hospital admissions and later disturbances of behaviour and learning. Developmental Medicine and Child Neurology 17: 456–480

Engel G, 1962 Psychological development in health and disease, Saunders, Philadelphia

Erikson E H 1963 Childhood and society. Norton, New York

Fassler D 1980 Reducing pre-operative anxiety in children. Patient Counselling and Health Education 2: 130–134

Harlow H F 1959 Love in infant monkeys. The nature and nurture of behaviour. Readings from Scientific American 1973. Freeman, San Francisco

Hayward J 1975 Information: a prescription against pain. Royal College of Nursing, London

Hoffman A D, Becker R D, Gabriel H P 1976 The hospitalised adolescent. Psychological and Cognitive Aspects of Medical Management. The Free Press, Macmillan, New York

Kent G, Dalgleish M 1986 Psychology and medical care. Bailliere Tindall, London

Kubler-Ross E 1982 On death and dying. Tavistock, London

Lewis M 1982 Clinical aspects of child development. Lea and Febinger, Philadelphia

McDaniel J W 1976 Physical disability and human behaviour, 2nd edn. Pergamon, Press, London

Parsons T 1958 Definitions of health and illness in the light of American values and social structure. In: Jaco E G (ed) Patients, physicians and illness. Free Press 1958, Glencose, Illinois

Piaget J, 1950 The psychology of intelligence. Routledge, London

Platt Committee Report 1959 The welfare of children in hospital. HMSO, London

Pless I B, Pinkerton P 1975 Chronic childhood disorder. Promoting patterns of adjustment. Henry Kimpton, London

Roskies E 1972 Abnormality and normality. The mothering of thalidomide children. Cornell University Press, Ithaca

Rutter M 1979 Parent–child separation. In: Clarke A, Clarke A. Early experience. Open Books. London

Stacey M, Dearden R, Pill R, Robinson D 1970 Hospitals, children and their families. Routledge and Kegan Paul, London

Which? Campaign Report 1980 Children in hospital. Consumers' Association, London

24

Team workers

A. M. D. Grimley

INTRODUCTION

The needs of sick and disabled children are designed to be met through the provision of a range of services through different agents, for example, health and local authorities. In the UK, for example, the purpose of a Joint Children's Service in a District is to provide a comprehensive service for children and young adults from conception up to 19 years of age.

If a child with special needs is to receive maximum benefit from family, health, education, social and voluntary services, it is essential that there is a managed team approach to assessment, sharing of findings, agreement on hypotheses, on setting objectives and in the active management of the identified problems (Bauer 1989a).

Joint planning coordinates the resources of social services, health, education and voluntary bodies to create a range of closely integrated services. Such services should be organised and delivered in a way that is appropriate to meet individual needs in order to:

- safeguard and promote child health
- aid recovery and welfare in children
- promote overall development
- prevent deformity
- ameliorate handicap and distress
- provide support to children and families.

A unified team approach is required if services to the whole child and the family are not to be fragmented — the whole is greater than the parts (Fig. 24.1).

The shared identification of problems and their ascertainment in disease, disability or handicap should enable realistic team goal-setting for targeting of objectives and agreement to priorities and methods of management and resource use. This should ensure personal and professional accountabilities to client/s and funding agencies (Audit Commission 1988) (Fig. 24.2).

A medical diagnosis alone does not afford a sufficiently broad spectrum on which to base case management.

An accurate picture of a child and the presenting problems is only obtained from a careful, holistic assessment of that child (Table 24.1). This will normally require coordination of carefully planned inputs from many disciplines. Each individual disciplinary team member will concentrate upon aspects particular to his own disciplinary skills and each will contribute differing supplementary and complementary evidence, as summarised in Table 24.1.

WHAT IS A TEAM?

Many people may state they work in a multidis-

ciplinary team without understanding what this can truly mean.

A team is often described as a number of people associated in some joint venture and is applied to a group of people drawing together to achieve objectives through concerted effort. Strengths in one member of a team can balance weaknesses in another. Commitment is required of all team members to share in consultation, deliberation, decision-making and shared action.

Multidisciplinary and multiprofessional teams

Multidisciplinary and multiprofessional teams are composed of many professionals of several disciplines or agencies sharing common perspectives who work and act together with a common client or in a common client group as in a child development centre or mental handicap community service team or joint care planning team.

Team work of this philosophy and practice enhances understanding of each other's role and tends, gradually, to avoid role conflict and overlap. It should also lead to:

- agreements on curriculum planning
- skill sharing

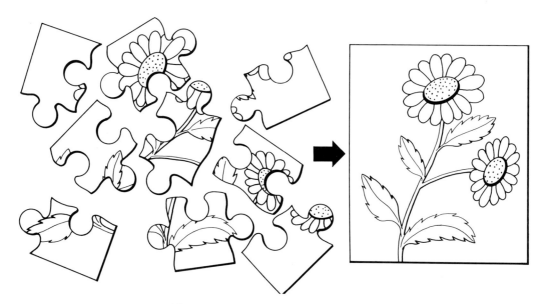

Fig. 24.1   The whole is greater than the parts.

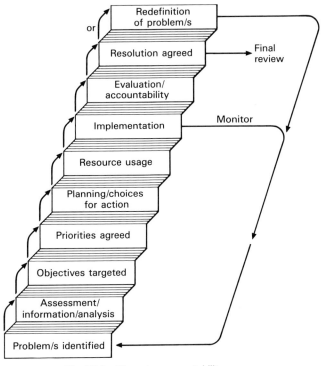

Fig. 24.2 Steps to accountability.

- the careful husbanding of scarce resources
- actions which are specific to child needs as opposed to professional abilities and variances.

There should be uniformity of attitudes as well as actions amongst a well coordinated and motivated team.

Interdisciplinary teams

Interdisciplinary team-working entails individual activities between, amongst or amidst others in a coordinated and cooperative fashion as in a hospital orthopaedic ward team.

Table 24.1 Factors affecting the health, welfare and development of a child

Personal/clinical	Organisational	Environmental
Motor (musculoskeletal)	Rules/schedules	Physical space
Postural, (ambulation),	Curriculum	Culture
Sensory, (perceptual),	Traditions	Socio-economic
Nutritional, (urological),	Beliefs	Geography
Neurological,	Expectations	Lifestyle
Pain/sleep/awakeness,	Attitudes	Transport
Emotional, (fear),	Family relationships	
Mental state/ability,	Peer pressures	
Exercise tolerance,	Models — medical	
Medication/drugs,	social	
	vocational	
	educational	

Example 1

In order to establish case management and care for people with problems in mental illness and mental handicap, multiprofessional team meetings are held.

Prior to discharge from a psychiatric ward a case conference would be called by the responsible Medical Officer.

Those taking part in the discussions and decisions would be the child's consultant psychiatrist and paediatrician, the appropriate hospital primary care nurse/sister, the specialist social worker, the general practitioner, a community psychiatric nurse, the child client and parent/surrogate.

With agreement from the client, other health, social or educational professionals and/or member of a voluntary agency would be invited to attend if they already are, or are soon to be, involved in care of that child.

Considerations for care would include:

• The views and wishes of the child and parent/carer.
• The need for agreement with the appropriate professionals and agencies for future action required to meet identified or special needs (e.g. housing adaptations, school transport, etc.).
• The possible involvement of other agencies for such as charity provision of equipment or voluntary body peer support groups.

Intradisciplinary teams

Intradisciplinary team-working is acting within one discipline or profession, as in peer consultation, or calling a senior colleague to demonstrate or help with a client and in peer clinical audit activities within a single discipline.

PROFESSIONAL RESPONSIBILITIES

Irrespective of any individual discipline, all professionals need to familiarise themselves with the various available statutory and voluntary provisions together with support services and available resources. In addition they must be aware of the paramount importance of effective liaison and interagency communication (APCP 1990).

Example 2

Another team example may be seen in the coordinated multidisciplinary work amongst the key worker, staff and therapists with a school child with special needs.

This group of professionals from health, education and social services will have knowledge of an individual child, having been involved in or received reports of assessments and statements of need for that child.

Taking into consideration identified needs of the child, ordinary classroom activities and demands, timetables, staff, skill and equipment resources available, they should plan together and agree with the parent and child a contract for a personal curriculum for that child and determine upon the best way this might be delivered.

A senior physiotherapist need not treat or physically handle a child all day and every day. A classroom care worker or general assistant may be designated to carry out the daily classroom therapeutic management schedule, i.e.:

• standing frame
• prone-lying on a prone board
• walking in an orthosis
• postural drainage positioning, etc.

As with parents of a preschool child, skilled professionals must educate the class teacher and carer into the rationale and techniques of such physical management and monitor the performance of delegated care workers. They must ensure that equipment used is safe and well-maintained and that they are also available for advice and trouble-shooting whenever this is needed by parent, carer or school staff.

The team leader will set up the statutory and needful intermittent reviews for identification of current performance, progress evaluation, problem identification and the resetting of objectives for the planning of education and therapeutic schedules and curricula.

Example 3

A child waiting for surgery on an orthopaedic ward may be visited by several people from different disciplines, after which a case conference, led by the orthopaedic surgeon, will be held. Each participant would bring their own perspectives to agree on common goals to meet individual client needs (Fig. 24.3). Subsequent decisions regarding the course of action would be made.

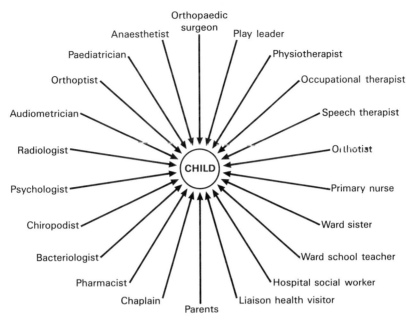

Fig. 24.3 Interdisciplinary team: orthopaedic ward.

Paediatric physiotherapists are reminded that, at all times, they are responsible for ensuring compliance with statutory, professional, managerial and local policies and procedures. They must know their local and their own professional policies (Chartered Society of Physiotherapy 1990).

Each person needs knowledge of local policies and procedures to follow for each service, site or team where they work (e.g. record-keeping, reporting, quality control mechanisms, etc.). Service and team managers have a responsibility to define this information at service induction and upon introduction of staff to new sites and teams.

TEAM WORKING FOR SUCCESS

Working in a multiprofessional or multidisciplinary team requires personal and professional qualities of trust, tolerance, wide vision, willingness to listen, knowledge of an individual's contributions of self and of others, accountability, sense of achievement, self and peer appraisal, awareness of authority and a personal sense of value in a group.

Working separately whilst simultaneously communicating clearly one's own findings to another or to a group of individual professionals can be a method of working across disciplines. Findings and reports may be collated by a lead professional, often a hospital consultant, general practitioner or assigned case manager. Such information may be disseminated amongst agency and professional team members but each professional would continue to interact directly with the client. Each member of the team should be aware that individual expertise and input might overlap and replication may result. This can become confusing and intrusive to the family, as well as exhausting to the child, when many different agents make domiciliary visits. Lack of cohesion may lead to duplication of effort and, as a consequence, service gaps may not be discovered or professional conflict may ensue.

To be a team, people have to work together. It is not a true team when each member is engrossed with his or her own issues and jealously guards professional boundaries. Confusion, conflict and consternation in a child abound unless therapeutic interventions, modalities and agents are kept to a minimum and individual personal perceptions in therapies are avoided.

Professional personnel and their skill inputs to a team may change from time to time and the child, and usually the family, are the only constants. Each client (child and family) requires inclusion in a team which has a coordinated, cooperative and integrated approach towards addressing needs. They require an advocate or 'named' constant — a key worker — to ensure team action decisions are followed through and minor difficulties are spotted before they become major problems.

Full team composition, the team leader or key workers may also change according to circumstances, choice, manpower, skills available and need, as shown in the examples in Table 24.2.

Team leadership

Drawing together the various strands linking team members requires good communication networks and accurate and shared records kept by all, with regular contact amongst team members. There should be constant review of these issues, together with monitoring of performance results by the team leader, who will require a knowledge of other disciplines combined with skills of communication and negotiation.

For the benefit of individual client families and other team members, the leader must arrange regular case consultation and discussion for a clear definition of the case management, tasks to be done and the results and standards expected or unmet. These definitions will include:

- how to meet agreed action objectives
- the timescale for achievement
- quality and consistency of input
- the allocated resources
- whom the team should involve in meeting objectives
- when the team will meet again.

The purposeful involvement of many agencies and professionals in the life of a child requires careful management and good team leadership. Coordination, direction and control in order to avoid overload on the child/family, the development or detection of duplication, or conflict or gaps in service and resource use is essential.

The Team Leader is responsible for drawing together the pieces to complete the jigsaw of the child and his problems and to ensure that all aim towards a diagnosis and action plan, be they social, educational, vocational, emotional, physical or medical in nature. He or she will also have a duty to ensure that things happen:

Table 24.2 Possibilities in health care team leadership

Forum	Team/committee	Possible team leader
Domiciliary — acute illness	Primary care team	General practitioner
Inpatient — trauma/surgery	Surgical team	Consultant surgeon
Orthopaedic/rehabilitation	Outpatient or continuation hospital team	Paediatric physiotherapist
Severe learning difficulties	Community mental handicap team	Clinical psychologist
Mental illness hospital — discharge	Mental health aftercare team	Community psychiatric nurse
Delayed child development	Child development unit team	Paediatric occupational therapist
Child handicap	District handicap team (Court 1976)	Community consultant Paediatrician
Physical disability	Joint care team physical disability	Social worker
Service planning/coordination	Joint client care planning team/s	Chairman: Unit General Manager
Joint service/s collaboration	Joint consultative committee	Chairman: District General Manager/Chief Executive

- that meeting places and times are prearranged
- that problems are raised and discussed
- that reports are presented and disseminated
- that answers and action plans are drawn up to meet needs whichever have been determined together.

Not all skilled professional practitioners have the qualities of team leadership. No one discipline has a monopoly of this role or responsibility to lead. Some teams elect a chair/leader, whereas others, for example, child development unit and community mental handicap service team members, assume the leadership role in rotation (see Table 24.2).

How should a team work?

1. Through cooperative coordination towards well-thought-out action plans with clear and controlled organisational procedures.
2. By being concerned with the long-term goals of the team and the quality of its service, as well as immediate and longer term fulfilment of client needs.
3. By balancing personal and professional advancement with the fulfilment of child-centred contracts.
4. By reaching wider team- and client-group-related goals.

This all takes effort and vision. It calls for strong motivation, commitment to quality and effective leadership.

Interdisciplinary cooperation and coordination is needed for many people from differing agencies to succeed on a client's behalf. Shared case presentation, audit and joint training activities are essential team building tools (Bauer 1989b). No single discipline can give all diagnostic, therapeutic, or educational inputs to meet the developmental, clinical, social, educational and vocational needs of a child. Neither should all children always have to receive inputs from every disciplinary member of a team!

Members of each discipline need to identify to each other the statutory obligations, duties, tasks and skills pertinent to their respective disciplines and then decide together what skill sharing and actions might take place following their own input to assessment and diagnosis (see Table 24.3).

Team objectives

In order to achieve an effective performance, the team needs to look at itself and ask:

- what are the team aims and objectives?
- how is the performance to be measured?
- how will the performance be reviewed against targets and comparisons?
- what changes and priority issues have been identified? (Audit Commission 1988).

These questions can relate to the team and its working, as well as to the way individual cases are managed amongst the team by its members.

All those persons from education, health or social services inputting to service provision must be accountable for decisions and action (and non-action) and subject themselves to the checks and balances of peer audit.

In sharing together the individual subjective and objective findings about the child, a comprehensive clinical, intellectual, social and emotional picture is built up. From joint

Table 24.3 Team questions

Work	People	Resources
What results are needed?	What is best use of time/abilities?	What resources/skills are available?
By when?	What motivates them?	How should they be used?
What quality is needed?	How can they be best be coordinated?	Is the budget adequate?
Met by what methods?		Can duplication or waste be avoided?

comparisons of these initial and individual data bases, hypotheses can be deduced and a framework designed and agreed for strategic action (or even inaction!) and evaluation.

The team, including child and parent/carer, will be enabled to identify true problems, to jointly set realistic child-oriented objectives, to plan goals, to choose targets, to develop strategies to reach these, to test out the results and to continue or to change direction.

Key worker

To act as the key worker is a role which may be held at differing times by different team members accommodating to developmental changes and needs of the child/family. The focus of need dictates the direction of effort.

The team should agree as to who amongst them is the key person to the child and family at that time. That key person is to ensure fulfilment of the plan for action and be the contact person for the family and other professionals.

The key worker is not to be seen as care team leader. That is a consistent and true management role ensuring that policy, procedures and team member practices are properly conducted. Nor is the team leader the special needs named person, although that person may well be the best key worker for an individual child.

Key working requires the ability to establish a rapport with a child, family and other team members. The worker needs knowledge of the problems presenting, the availability of resources, persistence, a sense of fairness, counselling skills and an ability or determination to get things done!

Team review

Planning together is most important for a team. When members are involved in putting their observations, findings, hypotheses, and projections together into the therapeutic management plan and educational curriculum, there is more motivation to win, to fulfil and succeed in those plans.

Integration and understanding of each others' services follow, with clearly defined time and action goals ensuring or questioning systematically the outcomes of intervention and negotiation of goal change if plans are unfulfilled. The key worker uses skills in diplomacy and problem solving to keep the 'finger on the pulse' on behalf of the child and family and will ensure action on their behalf.

SUMMARY

Paediatric physiotherapists need to be aware that services for children are not the prerogative of any one discipline or professional. They need to become proficient team members.

Team working necessitates use of management techniques such as problem-solving and decision-making. This leads to rationalisation of actions proposed, systematic evaluation of outcomes and optimal use of resources.

Team work encompasses knowledge of resource availability, scarcity, estimates of success, affordable risks and value to the child/family/carer/peers.

To be a team member needs interpersonal skills of written, verbal and non-verbal communication, negotiation, teaching, generosity and humour.

The APCP in 1990 (Dunn et al) stated: 'The paediatric physiotherapist must be able to communicate with three main groups of people; the child or young adult patient, the parent/carer and other involved professionals of the same and different disciplines' and that:

1. The development of effective and appropriate communication skills are requisite.
2. Communication should be clear, unambiguous and clearly understood.
3. The teaching of practical skills depends on the ability to communicate proficiently.
4. Appropriate terminology should be used in written reports.

The communication network and understanding from working closely together and using jargon-free language and records common to all builds up interdisciplinary trust, rapport and understanding to the benefit of child, family and all concerned. James Hogg, in 1984, called this 'complementary approaches to coactive behaviour and behavioural techniques' (Hogg 1984).

REFERENCES

Audit Commission 1988 Performance review. Planning, performance review in local government, action guide. HMSO, London

Bauer Doreen 1989a Introduction. Management model for rehabilitation programmes and service. Foundations of physical rehabilitation. A management approach. Churchill Livingstone, Edinburgh, p 7

Bauer Doreen 1989b Staffing, service leadership Foundations of physical rehabilitation. A management approach. Churchill Livingstone, Edinburgh ch 9, p 140

Chartered Society of Physiotherapy 1990 Standards of physiotherapy practice. Chartered Society of Physiotherapy, London

Court, S D M 1976 Handicap, Vol 1, Fit for the future. Report of the Committee on Child Health Services, CMND 6684. HMSO, London, ch 14, p 381

Dunn C, Williams V, Young C 1990 Communication and teamwork. APCP paediatric physiotherapy guidelines for good practice. APCP/CSP, London, ch 6

Hogg J 1984 Motor competence in children with mental handicap. In: Coupe J, Porter J (eds) The education of children with severe learning difficulties. Croom Helm, London

25

Legal aspects in paediatric physiotherapy

P. Eckersley

INTRODUCTION

Physiotherapists working with children operate within a complex framework which includes child and educational legislation as well as those issues encompassed by good practice and individual rights. In this chapter those Acts of Parliament relating to work with children are described and the legal responsibilities of clinical practice are discussed.

THE 1981 EDUCATION ACT

The 1981 Education Act is one of the landmarks in education legislation and is concerned specifically with children with special needs. It reflects the consensus view on special educational needs which emerged over the preceding two decades and owes much to the work of the Warnock Committee, which reported in 1978. In recent years much of what has been written about special education has encouraged:

1. Increased parental involvement and rights to information.
2. An emphasis on integrated educational provision.
3. A desire to identify children's needs and not merely categorise handicaps.
4. Moves towards continuous assessment procedures which are based on classroom

activities and children's experiences in school (Solity & Raybould 1988).

The Act came into force in April 1983 and established a new and comprehensive legal framework covering identification, assessment, advice, and the documentation of the provision required to meet a child's special educational needs. The procedural sections of the Act are detailed in Table 25.1.

STATUTORY ASSESSMENT PROCEDURES

Statutory assessment procedures are initiated under Section 5 of the Act (Table 25.1). In order to identify and make provision for children with learning difficulties it is necessary to gather advice from everyone who has relevant information about the child. All decisions about educational provision, including school placement and support services are made on the basis of this

Table 25.1 Sections of the 1981 Education Act

Section	Subject	Topics
1	Definitions	Special educational needs Learning difficulty Special educational provision
2	Provision	Conditions for integrated education Duties of governors Nominated member of staff
3	Provision	Other than in school
4	Duty of LEA	Determination of provision
5	Statutory Assessment	Procedures Advice givers
6	Assessment	Children under 2 years of age
7	Statement	Preparation
8	Appeals	Procedures Amended statements
9	Assessment	Parental requests
10	Health Authority	Duty to notify LEA of possible educational needs
11–14	Schools	Approval of special schools
15–16	Attendance	School attendance orders (see Children Act, p. 480)
17–21	Miscellaneous	Parental duties Powers of the Secretary of State

information. The procedures which form the statutory assessment are underpinned by a number of concepts and requirements:

- definition of special educational needs
- conditions of integration
- process of assessment
- format of statement
- maintenance of statement
- appeals procedures.

Definition of special educational needs

For the purposes of the 1981 Education Act a child has special educational needs if he has a learning difficulty which calls for special educational provision to be made for him. A child is considered to have a learning difficulty if:

1. He has a significantly greater difficulty in learning than the majority of children of his age.
2. He has a disability which either prevents or hinders him from making use of educational facilities of a kind generally provided within the area of the local authority concerned, for children of his age.
3. He is under the age of five years and is, or could be if special educational provision were not made for him, likely to fall within the above categories when over that age (Education Act (1981), Chapter 60: 1(2)).

The concept of special educational needs was introduced in the Warnock Report (Department of Education and Science 1978) and represents an abrupt departure from the practice of categorising children by type of handicap or primary disability: physical, mental, or sensory handicap.

Identification of special educational needs

The Act places a duty on each Local Education Authority (LEA) to identify those children for whom they are responsible who have special educational needs and to determine the provision

which will meet those needs. The formal processes of the 1981 Education Act are part of a
continuum of identification which may be initiated by a classroom teacher in a mainstream
school working individually with a pupil, by
parents who have concerns about the progress
their child is making, or by a health authority
nominee who informs the Education Authority
through a Section 10 referral that a child may
have special educational needs.

The Warnock Report suggested that as many
as 20% of children may experience learning difficulties at some stage in their school careers. For
the majority of these children their needs are
short-term and can be met by in-school learning
support and advice, consultation with parents
and individually established homework activities.
However, for a small number of children (approximately 2%) the nature, level and/or
complexity of their needs may indicate that it is
necessary to initiate formal assessment procedures to establish more clearly their particular
educational needs.

Process of assessment

The formal, statutory assessment procedures are
set out in Section 5 of the 1981 Education Act.
These include the time-scale and the format of
the assessment (Fig. 25.1).

The assessment of special educational needs is
not an end in itself; it is the first step towards a
better understanding of a child's learning difficulties for the practical purpose of providing
guidance both on the education needed and on
establishing a basis upon which to monitor the
child's progress (Department of Education and
Science 1989). It is suggested that where possible
assessments should take place in surroundings
which are familiar to the child, either at home or
at school.

Advice must be sought from the following:

1. Educational advice from the headteachers
   of all the schools the child has attended in
   the preceding 18 months.
2. Psychological advice from an educational
   psychologist nominated by the LEA.
3. Medical and health advice from a medical

officer nominated by the District Health
Authority (DHA).
4. Parental representations from the parent or
   through evidence submitted by a person
   acting on the parents' behalf.

All the advice must be relevant and usable in
an educational context and should focus on the
particular area of expertise of the advice giver. It
should not be influenced by consideration of
eventual school placements and should be written
in such a way as to enable teachers to develop
the information into a detailed programme of
education for the pupil. It is hoped that by bringing together the skills, perceptions and insights
of professionals in different disciplines, as well as
those of the parents, it should be possible to ar-
rive at a more complete understanding of a
child's special educational needs (Department of
Education and Science 1989). All information
from professionals must be made available to
parents.

Maintaining the statement

Each LEA is responsible for organising the col-
lection and collation of advice according to local
circumstances. Once collated the advice will be
drawn together into a draft statement which
analyses a child's difficulties and strengths;
specifies the approaches, facilities and resources
needed; and determines the provision required to
meet those needs (Eckersley 1987). The
Secretary of State has now indicated that the
time-scale from serving the Notice of Intention
to Assess to the compilation of draft statement
should be no more than 6 months.

The draft statement should be sent to all advice
givers for comment, and must be sent to parents
for their comments and agreement. It should be
noted that both the formal summative document
drawn up by the LEA and the separate sets of
professional advice which form the appendices
constitute the actual Statement. There must be
seven appendices:

- Appendix A — parental representation
- Appendix B — parental evidence
- Appendix C — educational advice
- Appendix D — medical advice

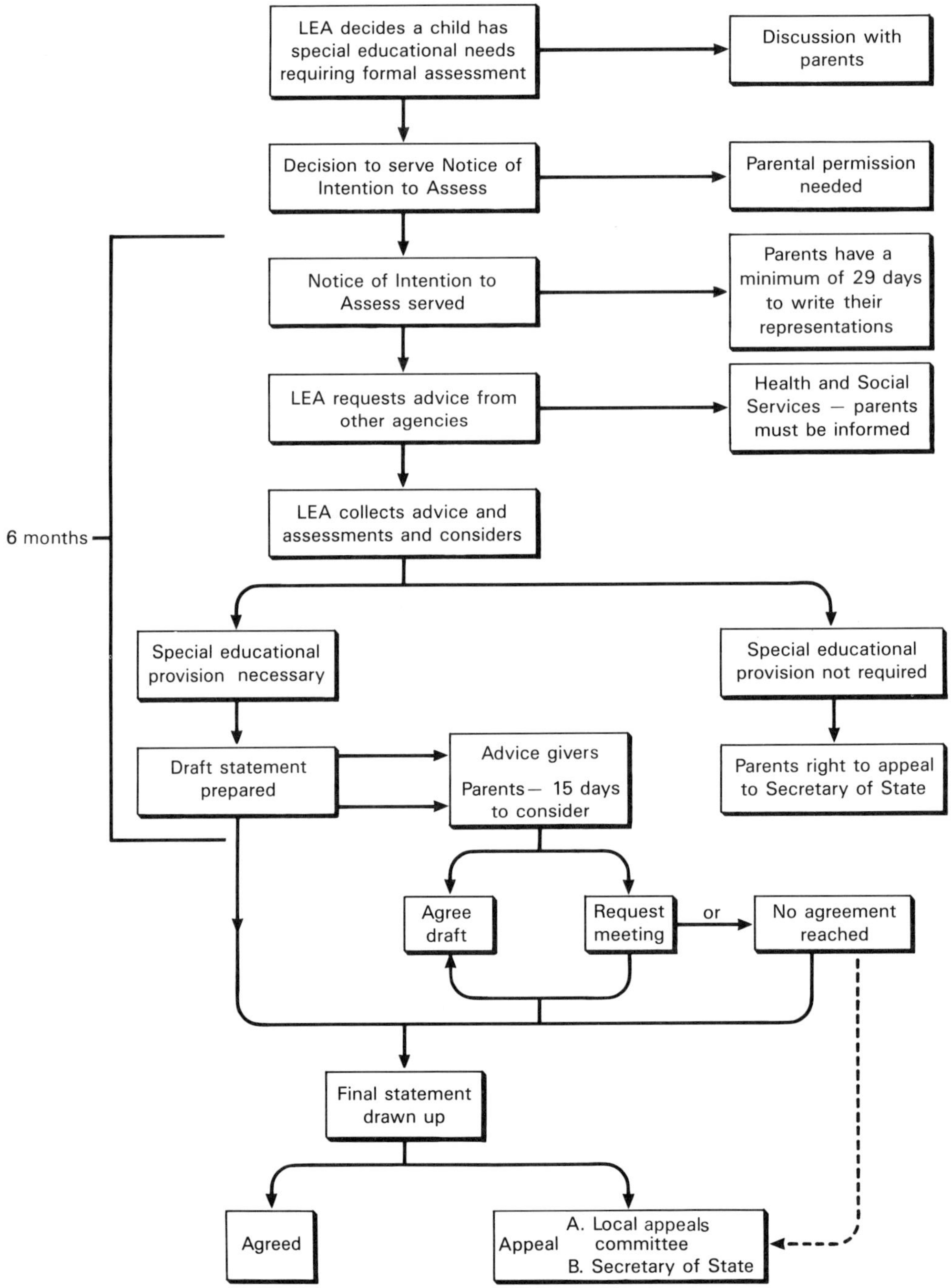

Footnote Parents can <u>only</u> appeal against a final statement

Fig. 25.1   Statutory Assessment Procedures: 1981 Education Act.

- Appendix E — psychological advice
- Appendix F — other education authority advice
- Appendix G — information from DHA or social services.

It should be noted that advice about non-medical support services such as physiotherapy should be sought through the medical officer, but that it should be collected and passed in full to the LEA to be attached at Appendix G to the statement (Department of Education and Science 1989).

Appeal procedures

On receipt of the draft statement a parent has 15 days to make representations and to request a meeting with the LEA nominated officer or an advice giver. Parents have a right to appeal against the content of the statement where it has not been possible to agree it in negotiation. The first stage is an appeal to a local panel which acts independently of the LEA but whose decision is not binding. Thereafter there is a further right of appeal to the Secretary of State, whose decision is binding.

Reviews and reassessment

Reviews must be held annually in order to update the statement and give an opportunity for everyone concerned with meeting a child's needs to come together to plan future objectives. Statements can now be amended under Section 9 of the Act as a result of reviews, but parents must consent to this. A statutory reassessment must be initiated when a child reaches the age of $13\frac{1}{2}$ in order to plan for the move towards independence and adulthood (see p. 476, 1986 Disabled Persons Act).

CONCEPT OF INTEGRATION

For many people, the most exciting and significant duties in the Act are those which promote the education of children with special needs in ordinary schools alongside children without such needs, rather than in separate and segregated schools and units (Advisory Centre for Education 1990). The Act stresses that where possible LEAs should ensure that children are educated in mainstream schools. School governors must also use their best endeavours to ensure that any pupil in their school secures the special educational provision he requires.

A number of qualifications are placed on the requirement to educate a child in a mainstream school. The provision and arrangements must be compatible with:

1. The child's receiving the special educational provision that he requires.
2. The provision of efficient education for the children with whom he will be educated.
3. The efficient use of resources (Education Act (1981) Chapter 60: 2(3)).

A select committee of the House of Commons (House of Commons 1987) suggested that placing the emphasis on interaction between children with special educational needs and other children is important in preparing such children for the social demands to be placed on them after leaving school. It emphasised that integration is a process in which children mix with their contemporaries in a regular and planned way whatever the school placement. The committee also concluded that the lack of specific resources has restricted implementation of the Act.

PARENTAL RIGHTS

The Warnock Report (Department of Education and Science 1978) recognised the invaluable experiences and skills which parents and carers brought to the process of assessment and decision making. This was reflected in the statutory rights given to parents to initiate and contribute to many of the procedures of the 1981 Education Act. The intention is not only to give parents a greater role in the education of their children but also to underpin this in statute. Those parental rights enshrined in the Act include the right to:

- initiate an assessment
- agree to the assessment process as a requirement before it can commence
- be informed who the advice givers will be

- write a parental report
- nominate their own representative
- be present during all assessments
- discuss the outcome of assessment with advice givers and LEA officers
- see all written reports specifically provided as part of the assessment
- appeal against the final decisions as they see fit.

These statutory rights are seen as ones which enable parents to act as equal partners with professional agencies and to be genuinely involved in and informed about meeting the needs of their own child. Many parents now have an expectation that they will be involved but in practice a number of barriers still remain:

1. Many parents feel they have inadequate information about assessment procedures and range of provision.
2. There may be insufficient help for parents in completing their parental contribution.
3. Some parents feel a lack of weight is given to their views.
4. There is a lack of choice in the range of forms of provision (House of Commons 1987).

ROLE OF THE PHYSIOTHERAPIST

The physiotherapist has an essential role to play in the assessment of the child with special educational needs with whom he is involved. The advice which is provided can have a direct impact on decisions about a child's future education and it is therefore essential that it is written from the perspective of a sound knowledge of child development, of paediatric therapy and a knowledge of school-based systems. It should also be remembered that a Statement of Special Educational Needs is primarily a document for parents and that advice should be written in a way which enables parents to develop a clear understanding of their child's needs and abilities.

The moves towards integration, the emphasis on liaison and coordination with school-based services and the requirement to consult parents have all increased the time needed to support individual children. It has also been suggested

that (House of Commons 1987) that steps should be taken to ensure that health authorities give increased priority to providing local education authorities with the necessary therapy inputs identified in statements. Despite recent cases which have gone to the Appeal Court the balance between the duty of Health Authorities to provide reasonable levels of services and the right of LEAs to employ their own therapists remains unclear.

Content of physiotherapy advice

The physiotherapy assessment should give a clear picture of the physical strengths and difficulties of the child. It should also indicate the level of provision which will be needed and on what basis this could be provided:

- as face-to-face contact
- on an advisory basis
- in an educational establishment
- on an out-patient basis.

The classroom teacher has the major responsibility for a pupil during the school day. The physiotherapy assessment should therefore address those issues which will assist the teacher in planning appropriate activities. It should also provide an opportunity to explore the potential to combine therapy activities within educational and learning experiences. Advice might include:

- are motor skills age-appropriate?
- will aids be needed for mobility and access?
- are there perceptual or fine motor problems?
- is special equipment needed for hand use?
- how does the child respond to individual and group work?
- can the child solve problems and ask questions?
- is advice needed on lifting?
- is a wheelchair needed on outdoor visits?
- can the child balance in a crowded playground?
- will the child tire easily during games?
- how much physical activity is safe?
- can he/she cope alone at mealtimes?
- can he/she carry his/her own books?
- can he/she get up from the floor alone?

- is it all right to let another pupil push the wheelchair?

It can also be helpful to indicate skills. The inclusion of 'regional champion wheelchair slalom' or 'enthusiastic basketball team member' can give a more positive impression of levels of independence than a list of itemised sub-skills.

Interagency collaboration

Involvement in the processes of assessment underpins the collaborative work of the physiotherapist with parents, statutory and voluntary agencies. Where a resulting Statement of Special Educational Needs is drawn up it should provide a baseline against which a child's progress can be monitored. This process involves:

- ascertaining relevant past and present levels of functioning, emotional states and interests
- assessing rate of development
- analysis of consequent learning difficulties
- specification of goals for change in the child and the environment
- specification of the child's requirements for differing approaches, facilities, resources or modification of the National Curriculum (see p. 476)
- perceptions and wishes of the parent and child
- special educational provision and services.

THE NATIONAL CURRICULUM

This chapter would be incomplete without introducing the reader to the structure of the National Curriculum as defined by the Education Reform Act (1988).

The National Curriculum consists of:

- three core subjects
  - English
  - mathematics
  - science
- Seven foundation subjects
  - technology
  - history
  - geography
  - music
  - art
  - physical education
  - modern foreign language.

Each subject is divided into a number of attainment targets which are in turn divided into ten levels of attainment. These levels define the age-appropriate stages in learning that children pass through as they grow and progress with their learning.

These stages in learning span the period of compulsory education, which is divided into four key stages (Fig. 25.2). From this figure it can be seen that pupils within any age band will be working towards different levels of attainment, i.e. a pupil aged 14 may be working at any level between 3 and 7, and for some attainment targets may be working at a similar level to a pupil aged 7. It is intended that the National Curriculum should give the flexibility for pupils to work at their own pace and have targets set for them which meet their own individually assessed needs.

At the end of each key stage standard assessment tasks (SATs) will be used to ascertain pupil progress and form a basis for recording pupil needs. The result of these tests must be reported to parents, governors and the LEA, and must be published.

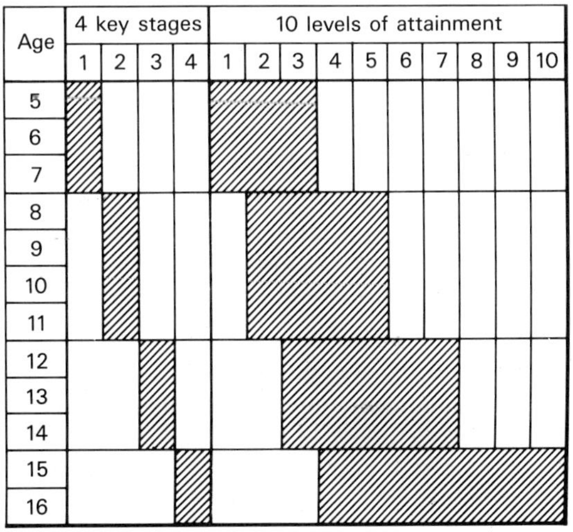

Fig. 25.2 Levels of attainment and key stages for science (14 attainment targets).

Exceptional arrangements

The National Curriculum is intended for all pupils. The Department of Education and Science (DES) and the National Curriculum Council (NCC) make it clear that all pupils share the same statutory entitlement to a broad and balanced curriculum, including the national curriculum. The NCC has. emphasised that exceptional arrangements should be made only rarely and that, for the majority of pupils, the national curriculum and its assessment arrangements will apply (Advisory Centre for Education 1990).

It is accepted that for a small number of pupils with Statements of Special Educational Needs some of the requirements of the National Curriculum may need to be modified or disapplied. However, this should not be taken as implying that the entitlement to follow the National Curriculum has been withdrawn.

Modification may include:

1. Use of a typewriter rather than writing.
2. Using a cassette recorder so that teacher instructions can be recorded.
3. Assistance to be given during practical subjects for physically disabled pupils.

Disapplication may include:

1. Taking part in SATs according to learning ability rather than chronological age.
2. Not being part of the published school results.
3. Exemption from a curriculum subject.

Any such modification or disapplication should only take place following a full formal assessment which includes the views of parents (Education Reform Act (1988) Section 18). All such exceptional arrangements must be detailed in the Statement.

However, it is also possible for headteachers to direct that a temporary exception should come into force for any individual pupil without the process of the 1981 Education Act being initiated. In this situation this direction is limited to 6 months, but can be extended for a further 6 months. The LEA and parents must be in-formed and parents have the right to appeal to the school governing body and, if dissatisfied, to the LEA and Secretary of State.

Parental involvement

An important aim of the introduction of the National Curriculum is to give parents the maximum information about the programmes their children are following, and regular reports on their progress (Maclure 1989). The information given to parents should include:

- admission procedures
- school organisation and policy
- complaints procedures
- curriculum policy
- disciplinary and exclusion procedures
- results of testing on their own child
- results of general school testing
- procedures for seeing their child's educational records.

DISABLED PERSONS ACT (1986)

The Disabled Persons Act (1986) received the Royal Assent in July 1986. It provides for the improvement of the effectiveness of, and the co-ordination of resources in, the provision of services for people with mental or physical handicap and for people with mental illness (Department of Health and Social Services 1986). The Act does not significantly change existing legislation but rather strengthens the rights of disabled persons and their carers in relation to services provided under the legislation (Radar 1988). It identifies a range of procedures to implement:

- effective provision of services
- assessment of consumers' need for services
- consultation with individuals and organisations on service provision
- the rights of disabled people and carers.

The Act is subdivided into 11 sections (Table 25.2).

Table 25.2 Sections of the 1986 Disabled Persons Act

Section	Subject	Topics
1	Authorised representatives	Procedures for appointment and termination. Rights of parents and disabled person over 16 to appoint
2	Authorised representatives	Function and rights Access to information
3	Assessment by Local Authorities of disabled persons	Requesting assessment Representations
4	Duty to consider needs of disabled people	Definitions Referrals
5	Children with Statements of Special Educational Needs	Procedures on leaving full-time education
6	Pupils with Statements leaving education	Review of dates
7	Patients discharged from inpatient treatment for mental illness	Assessment for provision Planning provision
8	Ability of carer	Local authority duty to consider
9	Information Services	Local authority duty to include information on relevant organisation providing services
10	Committees	Consultation with and representation by disabled people.
11	Reports to Parliament	Statistics Any information requested.

SECTIONS 5 AND 6

Sections 5 and 6 of the Act refer to children with statements of Special Educational Needs under the 1981 Education Act (see p. 469). The purpose of these sections is to ensure a smooth transition for a disabled child between full-time education and adult life (Department of Education and Science 1988). This is to be achieved by close cooperation between LEA and SSD as the child approaches the end of compulsory education through:

1. A review of procedures for speedy reliable transfer of information within and between the two departments.
2. The identification of appropriate contact points.

Section 5

Section 5 of the Disabled Persons Act (1986) requires the Local Education Department to inform the Social Services Department (SSD) of those pupils with Statements of Special Educational Need who will be reaching their 14th birthday. The LEA is then required to:

1. Seek the opinion from the SSD on whether a child who is the subject of a Statement is in its opinion a disabled person.
2. Receive an opinion from the SSD at the first annual review after the child's 14th birthday.
3. Notify the SSD when any such identified child will cease full-time education.

The first annual review after the child's 14th birthday may take place as a result of:

1. A mandatory 13+ assessment.
2. An annual review in the 15th year
3. Where a child over 14 has needs which change or who is assessed for the first time.

Notification from the LEA to SSD that a pupil will be leaving full-time education is to be given:

- not later than 8 months in advance.
- not more than 12 months in advance.

Where a pupil transfers from school to a part-time placement in college, this information must be given not later than 8 months in advance.

The Education (Special Education Needs) (Amendment) Regulations (1988) allow disclosure of a child's statement of Special Educational Needs to enable Social Services officers to identify those pupils who in their opinion are disabled and to undertake the assessment of a young person's needs in accordance with the terms of the 1986 Act. It seems probable that the SSD may decide to interview the young person and/or parents to reach an opinion as to whether a young person is a disabled person.

This assessment by the SSD is carried out following notification from the LEA of the date when a pupil will be leaving full-time education.

Where the LEA seeks an opinion from the SSD on whether a child is disabled the Act suggests that the LEA may wish to inform the parent, guardian or child (if over 16) that this is being done and explain the reasons.

It is regrettable that this process of informing parents is not included as a statutory right, the more so given the long-term implications of the decisions reached.

Where a parent/guardian of a child under 16 or a young person (over 16) requests that an assessment should not be carried out, then the officer of the SSD should comply with that request.

Section 6

Section 6 of the Disabled Persons Act (1986) requires LEAs to keep under review the leaving dates of young people in full-time education at school and those pupils in Further Education establishments who are under the age of 19 and have been identified as disabled.

The SSD is required to assess such young people within 5 months of receiving notification that a young person identified as disabled will be leaving school. The LEA is not statutorily required to notify the SSD if a pupil is over the age of 19.

The Act accepts that LEAs may not be able to state the precise date on which a child is expected to leave full-time education. It allows for the procedures to be varied where:

- Notification has been given to SSD but the leaving date is postponed or advanced.
- A child is to leave full-time education within 8 months.

In these circumstance, the SSD must be notified in writing as soon as reasonably practicable.

THE CHILDREN ACT (1989)

The Children Act received Royal Assent in November 1989 and was implemented as a whole in October 1991. It integrates the law relating to private individuals with the responsibilities of public authorities, in particular local authority social services departments, towards children (Table 25.3). In so doing the Act strikes a new balance between family autonomy and the protection of children (Department of Health 1989a and b).

In this section the two major themes of the Act are described:

- a child and family charter
- local authority responsibilities.

Table 25.3 Outline of the Children Act (1989)

Part	Title	Sections
I	Introductory	Welfare of the child Parental responsibility Appointment of guardians
II	Family proceedings	Residence orders Contact orders Family assistance
III	Local authority support	Children in need Day care Accommodation Advice and assistance to children
IV	Care and supervision	Application for orders Parental contact Education supervision orders Guardians *ad litem*
V	Protection of children	Child assessment orders Emergency protection orders
VI	Community homes	
VII	Voluntary homes and voluntary organisations	
VIII	Registered children's homes	
IX	Private fostering	
X	Child minding and day care	Registration Inspection
XI	Functions of Secretary of State	Inspection Research and returns
XII	General	Notification from Health and Education authorities Adoption Criminal care and supervision Jurisdiction of courts

CHILD AND FAMILY CHARTER

The Act is underpinned by the belief that children are generally best looked after within the family with both parents fully involved. It also stresses that, where possible, this should be achieved without resort to legal proceedings.

Rights of the child

The first principle of the Act is that the child's welfare must be the paramount consideration (National Children's Bureau 1989). Throughout the Act the importance of the child's own views and wishes is stressed. In the checklist for procedures recommended in the Act the first four items relate to:

1. The ascertainable wishes and feelings of the child.
2. The child's physical, emotional and educational needs.
3. The likely effect on the child of any change in his circumstances.
4. The child's age, sex, background and any other characteristics (Children Act (1989) Section 1(3)).

The express views of the child must be sought in all situations including:

1. *Section 43(8)*. The child may refuse an assessment or examination under child protection procedures provided he is of sufficient understanding to make an informed decision.
2. *Section 43(11)*. Reasonably practicable steps must be taken to ensure that prior notice is given to the child as well as his parents that an assessment order has been applied for.
3. *Section 46(3)*. The child must be informed of the steps which have been taken to protect him, especially where he is removed to a place of safety.
4. *Schedule 3*. Under education supervision orders the child's wishes must be taken into account when deciding where he/she should be educated.

The checklist given above (Section 1 (3)) is intended to remedy the situation where it was thought that the courts sometimes paid insufficient regard to the child's perspective. It is the duty of all those involved to take account of the child's views in all family proceedings including those of adoption and of place of residence following divorce. Where it is considered that the burden of resolving family problems might fall on the child, his views can be represented through a guardian *ad litem*. The child will also be entitled to separate legal representation which is instructed directly by him/her.

Parental responsibilities

The Act introduces and emphasises the concept of parental responsibility and hence of obligation towards a child rather than parental rights (National Children's Bureau 1989). The exercise of parental responsibility is left largely to the discretion of the adults concerned, even in divorce cases, and the law will intervene only as a last resort. After divorce or separation both parents retain their parental responsibility. Prior to October 1991, although joint custody could be given the court always directed care and residence to one parent. Under the Children Act this is no longer the situation and parents will be expected to resolve the issue unless the court feels that a residence order is necessary for the safety of the child.

Parental responsibility empowers a person (not necessarily a parent) to take most decisions in a child's life and can be acquired by:

1. Parents who were married or who have been married to each other after the time of the child's conception.
2. A single mother.
3. An unmarried father making a parental responsibility agreement with the mother.
4. An unmarried father applying to the court.
5. Private appointment of a guardian.
6. Court order to local authority for care, residence, emergency protection or guardianship.

Where more than one person has parental responsibility at the same time either may act independently of the other unless this is incompatible with a court order. Even when the child is under a care order the Act provides for parents to retain parental responsibility and to be involved in local authority decision-making.

Whilst the primary responsibility for the upbringing of children is described as resting with parents, it is considered that:

- The state should offer help where doing so lessens the risk of family breakdown.
- Transfer of parents' legal powers to local authorities should only be carried out following full court hearings.
- Parents and children should be full parties in court proceedings.
- All services should be arranged in voluntary partnership with parents.
- Support to families from other family members (grandparents, aunts, uncles) should be considered and, if offered, accepted before recourse to local authority care proceedings.

Family proceedings

The Children Act (1989) creates a single code for court orders concerning the welfare of children. It is expected that all court proceedings except those relating to emergency protection and child assessment will in future be heard in Family Proceedings Courts. The remit of these courts will be in connection with:

1. Divorce and separation.
2. Financial relief between spouses.
3. Domestic violence and occupation of matrimonial home.
4. Adoption.
5. High Court jurisdiction in relation to children.
6. Contact orders allowing a child to visit or stay with a person named in the order.
7. Residence order detailing arrangements of where the child will live.
8. Prohibited steps order limits the actions of a person with parental responsibility.
9. Care and supervision orders made on the application of the local authority.

Education supervision orders

Education supervision orders may be made on the application of a local education authority where a child who is of compulsory school age is not being properly educated. This situation would apply if a child failed to attend regularly the school at which he or she was registered or where a school attendance order is not being complied with.

As a result of the order a supervisor is allocated to advise, assist and befriend the child and his parents in a way which will ensure that the child is properly educated. The child's parents are required to follow the supervisor's directions. A supervision order lasts for 1 year and extensions of up to 3 years can be applied for.

Parental duty to comply with the education supervision order supersedes the parental duties to secure regular school attendance under the Education Act (1944).

Guardians *ad litem*

Each local authority must establish a panel of guardians *ad litem* from which individual appointments can be made. The guardian *ad litem*'s duty is to safeguard the interests of the child during emergency protection orders, child assessment orders, care and supervision orders, and contact orders.

In order to fulfil their functions they have the right to examine and take copies of any records held by the local authority and are also empowered to take an active role in all proceedings.

Care and supervision orders

These are the two main public law orders, which under the Children Act (1989) may only be granted on the application of a local authority or an authorised person (NSPCC and Secretary of State). In order to make a care or supervision order the following conditions must be satisfied. These are:

1. That the child concerned is suffering, or is likely to suffer, significant harm.
2. That the harm, or likelihood of harm, is attributable to:

— the care given to the child, or likely to be given to him if the order were not made, not being what it would be reasonable to expect a parent to give him

— the child's being beyond parental control (Section 31(2) The Children Act).

In these situations 'harm' includes both ill-treatment (physical, sexual and emotional abuse) and impairment of health. The harm suffered must be attributable to the absence of a reasonable standard of parental care. The transfer to the local authority of parents' legal powers and status can now only be achieved through a court hearing. Otherwise services to the family must be arranged on the basis of a voluntary partnership (Russell 1990). An emergency protection order lasts for 8 days, and is extendable to 15, and entitles the applicant to remove a child from a situation of immediate and apprehended danger.

LOCAL AUTHORITY RESPONSIBILITIES

The Children Act (1989) draws together the functions and responsibilities of the local authority in respect of children. The general duty of every local authority is to provide a range and level of services to safeguard and promote the welfare of children who are in need and to promote the upbringing of children by their families. In order to ensure this their duties include:

1. The identification of children in need.
2. Maintenance of a register of disabled children.
3. Publishing information about services provided and ensuring those who might benefit receive relevant information.
4. Assessing children's needs alongside the processes of the Education Act (1981) and the Disabled Persons Act (1986).
5. Providing day care for children in need who are aged 5 or under and not yet attending school.
6. Providing after-school care and supervised activities for children in need outside school hours and during school holidays.
7. Providing services to prevent children suffering abuse.
8. Providing family centres.
9. Providing services to enable disabled children to live as normal a life as possible.
10. Advising and assisting young people under 21 who cease to be looked after by the local authority.
11. Taking steps to prevent the need to bring care proceedings.

Central to these duties is the concept of 'children in need'.

Children in need

This concept is based on the belief that children's needs can usually best be catered for within their own families. The definition of need is intended to ensure that children whose parents can provide a reasonable upbringing within the family home *with* some assistance are enabled to do so (Department of Health 1990). The definition of need emphasises the role of preventative support and services to families.

A child is considered to be in need if:

1. He is unlikely to achieve or maintain, or to have the opportunity of achieving or maintaining, a reasonable standard of health or development without the provision for him of services by a local authority.
2. His health or development is likely to be significantly impaired, or further impaired, without the provision for him of such services.
3. He is disabled (Children Act (1989) Section A).

Under the Children Act (1989) services for children with disabilities are to be integrated with those provided for other children in need. The Act places a clear, positive and separate duty on local authorities to minimise the effect of their disabilities on children within their area and to give such children the opportunity to lead lives which are as normal as possible (Children Act (1989) Schedule 2).

To ensure appropriate services for children local authorities have the power to arrange for any assessment of a child. It is considered that health authorities will have a key role to play. Where the Local Authority makes a request to Education, Health or Housing Departments or to another Local Authority for help in fulfilling its duty under the Act then the other agency is duty bound to assess provided:

1. It is part of its statutory function.
2. Complying would not unduly prejudice its statutory function.

The thrust of the Act is to encourage genuine cooperation between agencies in order to meet the needs of children.

Additional duties

The Act also includes provision for the protection of children who are looked after away from home other than by local authorities (Department of Health 1989a and b). These arrangements include:

1. Ensuring the welfare of children in Health Service provision for more than 3 months through inspection.
2. Maintaining a register of persons who act as child minders on domestic premises or who provide day care on non-domestic premises for children under 8 for a period which exceeds 2 hours.
3. Responsibility to ensure appropriate private fostering and registered children's home arrangements.
4. Right to visit independent schools to ensure and safeguard a child's welfare.

SUMMARY

The Children Act is a comprehensive and far reaching reform of child law; its scope is unprecedented. It encompasses private disputes between parents about the future of their children, public child care law dealing with services to prevent family breakdown and with child protection and it includes those children with disabilities currently provided for by health and welfare legislation (National Children's Bureau 1989).

RESPONSIBILITIES IN WORKING PRACTICE

Physiotherapists working in all sectors have both a duty of care towards their patients and certain rights as employees to a safe working environment. Physiotherapists working in the community have the additional impact of working away from their base and from their colleagues. This section of the chapter concentrates on those duties and rights covered by:

- health and safety at work
- rights of children and families
- recording systems.

HEALTH AND SAFETY AT WORK
Health and Safety at Work Act (1974)

The Health and Safety at Work Act (HASAWA) came into force in April 1975. The aim of the Act is to protect both the employee at work and any member of the general public who may be affected by that work. Regulations implemented in 1978 gave trade unions the right to appoint safety representatives and to represent employees in safety matters. These legislative procedures meant that employees in education and medicine were protected for the first time.

In the NHS the employer is considered to be the District Health Authority or Health Trust and final responsibility in HASAWA issues rests with the District Management Team's named person. Day-to-day responsibility is delegated to the departmental superintendent.

In order to create an awareness of the need to achieve high standards of safety and to promote health and safety matters for all staff a number of issues must be addressed by any Superintendent Physiotherapist.

District policy

There should be a policy statement available to and followed by all employees. This policy will include:

1. Reporting of defective machinery and hazardous situations.
2. Cardiac arrest routines.
3. Queries on uncertain diagnosis and insufficient information.
4. Supervision of untrained persons.
5. Duties to patients and visitors.

Departmental policy

It is very important that Paediatric Physiotherapy Departmental Safety policies reflect the nature of the work which is being carried out. The list in Table 25.4 is intended as an initial guideline only.

The policy should also include:

- training on fire fighting and fire precautions
- first aid information

Table 25.4 Health and Safety at Work Act (1974): paediatric departmental policy (extracts)

Source of hazard	Nature	Precautions
Electrical equipment	Vibration therapy	Use of circuit breaker
	Intermittent positive pressure therapy (IPPT)	Regular maintenance
	Nebulisers	*No* child left unattended
General equipment	Plasterzote	Mask and goggles Position of child Size of room Temperature checks
	Toys and games*	Check eyes and limb attachment of soft toys Examine construction, sharp edges, splinters, etc. Regular cleaning
	Wheelchairs	Check brakes and tyres 'Parking' procedures 'Driving' regulations
Hydrotherapy pool	Drowning	Qualified staff for life-saving
	Allergies	Regular chemical level tests
	Infection	Toileting procedures Routine queries re ear infections, pressure sores

* This is particularly important where toys and games are given as gifts.

- staff illness
- infection control procedures
- registering and maintaining loaned equipment.

Student placement

Physiotherapy students are present for training and work experience in many departments. Legally they are not considered to be employees but have the same rights as any member of the general public in the department. Individual student timetables should be drawn up and made known to all staff. Students must know at all times which member or members of staff should be consulted on any issue. Great care must taken by all staff to ensure that students are competent to carry out any delegated tasks. Serious consideration should be given to ensuring knowledge through observation and closely supervised practice, with planned discussion and tutorial sessions prior to individual work.

Community work

A written safety policy should be drawn up for staff who work in the community.

Patients and home

Working in the patient's own home is a situation where the community physiotherapist faces a disadvantage to her physiotherapy counterparts who are working in hospitals, health clinics or local authority homes (Chartered Society of Physiotherapists 1988). The Health Authority is not liable for any negligent injury to the physiotherapist because it is not their property and the patient is not the employee of the Authority (Chartered Society of Physiotherapists 1988).

Where a paediatric community physiotherapist considers that working circumstances are unsafe as a result of environmental issues, attitude of family, unsafe house conditions or pets, defined working practice should be established. This practice should include:

1. The right *not* to visit a house but to offer physiotherapy elsewhere.

2. The duty to inform colleagues (i.e. health visitors) who may be affected by unsafe conditions.
3. Procedures for reporting such concerns to a departmental named person for necessary action.
4. Availability of joint visiting arrangements with colleagues (i.e. community preschool teacher, health visitor).
5. Timetabling systems which ensure that information is held on first and last visits of the day.
6. Ringing back to base systems for reporting in.
7. Consideration of personal alarms and car telephone systems.
8. Opportunities for training in the management and prevention of violent incidents.
9. Opportunities to discuss personal injury insurance.
10. Information on car insurance policy requirements.

Alternative work premises

Many community paediatric physiotherapists work in social services and education premises. In these circumstances the physiotherapist will need information on:

1. Reporting-in procedures to ensure:
   — those people on the premises have a right to be there
   — fire evacuation procedures can be followed.
2. Health and safety policy of the establishment.
3. A named contact person for liaison and coordination of work-related issues.

RIGHTS OF CHILDREN AND FAMILIES

The legislation already discussed in this chapter is based on the two concepts of partnership with parents and consideration of the views of the child.

Informed consent

The physiotherapist working with children must remember the professional duty to respect the rights and dignity of all people. In the context of paediatric physiotherapy informed consent has two elements:

1. The need to inform parents and carers of the nature of any physiotherapy intervention and to consider their views and wishes in carrying out treatment.
2. The need to involve children in the procedures of their own treatment.

Discussions and information-sharing sessions with parents and children are not always easy and it can be difficult to plan appropriate time into a busy schedule. However, Faulder (1985) believes that many of the objections health professionals put up against seeking informed consent are due to their shortcomings as communicators rather than their patients' inability to comprehend. It should also be recognised that in some cases, such as that of very young children, proxy consent from parents will be required.

Children

Informed consent for children should be seen as a continuum which ranges from discussion as to why it hurts to cough after surgery, to giving a favourite teddy bear passive movements, to choosing an appropriate range of exercises and activities to promote arm strength. Great care should be taken to ensure that there is an opportunity for the child to express any uncertainty and anxiety, and any misgivings or signs of reluctance to proceed with treatment must be attended to (Sim 1986).

Informed consent is particularly important in cases of non-accidental injury (NAI). The consequences of NAI may be head injury, chest infection or fractures. Physiotherapy intervention in these situations through chest percussion, exercise and passive movements may be seen by the child as a continuation of the abuse, or even as a punishment. Great sensitivity, ample time, comfortable surroundings and an opportunity to consult with colleagues will be essential.

Parents and carers

Discussions with parents are ineffectual if the information conveyed is not understood, and the therapist is duty-bound to ensure that understanding takes place (Sim 1986). All parents should be given the opportunity to discuss therapy programmes, to question and to give their own views. Their express consent to physiotherapy intervention should not be assumed and physiotherapists should:

1. Ensure that ward admission procedures explicitly inform parents of physiotherapy activity and its likely nature.
2. Resist requests from school and clinic staff to 'have a look' at a child without obtaining written parental permission.
3. Remember that they have no right of entry to a patient's own home.
4. Promote opportunities for parents to be present whilst their child is being treated.
5. Carry identity cards to reassure parents during home visits that the request to enter their home is a valid one.

Confidentiality

When working with children and families, and as a consequence of establishing a relationship based on trust and support, the paediatric physiotherapist frequently comes to hold information which is highly personal. This information must be treated no less confidentially than information related to the patient's social or medical condition; that is, it cannot and must not be discussed with others (Professional Practice Rule 6). Where case conferences and meetings are held to discuss children's progress it may be necessary to include only those people directly involved with the care of the child.

In some instances the fact of receiving physiotherapy may in itself be considered confidential and in these circumstances all staff should consider whether uniforms are appropriate for community work.

There may be situations where the physiotherapist becomes aware of situations relating to child abuse, criminal activity or to environmental hazards. In these situations confidentiality would be inappropriate and departmental and district guidelines should already be available to cover these instances. Immediate and urgent discussions with the departmental head should follow.

Disclosure of criminal background

All employing authorities are required to check with the police the possible criminal background of any person who applies to work in a post with access to children, whether as a paid employee or as a volunteer.

Negligence

Negligence within the law may be defined as the failure by an individual to exercise the degree of care which would be expected from a reasonable average person in the same circumstances (Hayne 1978).

Negligence follows when:

1. There is a duty of care owed to the patient.
2. The standard of care appropriate to that duty has been broken.
3. The breach caused the loss complained about.
4. The loss is of a type recognised by the court.
5. The loss must have been reasonably foreseeable (Carson 1988).

Appropriate standards of care are those which are drawn up and established by the Chartered Society of Physiotherapists and relate to the range of treatments and interventions in which therapists have been trained and are competent to practise. Physiotherapists working with children should consider carefully the concept of the duty of care owed to a patient/child as it relates both to the paediatric training they have received and to the HASAWA concept of insufficient information (see p. 482).

Particular consideration should be given to:

- Supervision of children during PE and games.
- Use of equipment and apparatus.

- Leaving children unattended during treatment, i.e. postural drainage, in standing frames, during intermittent positive pressure therapy.
- Decisions such as
  — walking unaided
  — standing unsupported } for the
  — getting from wheelchair } first time.
  'to floor alone'
- Moving from classroom to treatment area unattended.
- Delegating tasks to parents and carers.

RECORDING SYSTEMS

The rights and duties of paediatric physiotherapists as they relate both to health and safety and the duty of care can be effectively progressed and monitored through appropriate recording systems based on sound documented departmental procedures. These recording systems should include:

1. All accidents and near misses.
2. Progress of treatment including:
   — aims and objectives
   — changes in:
     • place of treatment (outdoors)
     • type of intervention
     • independent activity
   — reasons for changes
   — choice of equipment
   — parental knowledge of progress.
3. Discussions with parents and parental views.
4. Liaison with colleagues.
5. Delegation of tasks:
   — parents
   — support workers
   — students.
6. Training for and supervision of delegated tasks.
7. Information given to carers on safe lifting and carrying procedures.
8. Any significant event.

The paediatric physiotherapist is a member of a health team which has the responsibility for the effective care and treatment of children. In the course of work each physiotherapist is responsible and accountable for the quality and nature of his or her intervention. Specific and detailed records are not only appropriate for effective delivery of physiotherapy intervention but may also be needed in order to provide information should the nature of that intervention be called into question.

CONCLUSION

All physiotherapists working with children must have a sound knowledge of relevant legislation and effective departmental structures, and ensure that this knowledge is reflected in daily working practice. Legislative trends in all walks of life point towards enhanced rights for the consumer. Paediatric physiotherapists will wish to follow the trend as well as the letter of the law by:

1. Consulting parents, carers and children about their own priorities and wishes.
2. Ensuring information is available for parents, together with the time to discuss it.
3. Establishing joint working practices and liaison with other agencies.
4. Supporting activities which progress the involvement of children in their own local community.

REFERENCES

Advisory Centre for Education 1990 Special educational needs and the national curriculum, ACE Handbook. Advisory Centre for Education, London
Carson D 1988 Medical action litigation. Health Service Journal 21: January (Supplement)
Chartered Society of Physiotherapists 1988 Your job, your safety. Chartered Society of Physiotherapists. London
Department of Education and Science 1988 Disabled Persons Act — implementation of sections 5 and 6. Circular 2(88). Department of Education and Science, London
Department of Education and Science 1989 Circular 22(89): Assessments and statements of special educational needs. Procedures within the education, health and social services. Department of Education and Science, London

Department of Health 1989a An introduction to the Children Act 1989. HMSO, London

Department of Health 1989b Children Act 1989. HMSO, London

Department of Health 1990 Consultation paper number 3, Local Authority provision of service for families with children in need. Department of Health, London Department of Education and Science 1978 Warnock Report: Special Educational Needs. HMSO, London

Department of Health and Social Services 1986 Disabled Persons (Services, Consultation and Representation) Act 1986. HMSO, London, ch 33

Eckersley P 1987 The 1981 Education Act. Physiotherapy 73(9): 460–462

Faulder C 1985 Whose body is it? The troubling issue of informed consent. Virago, London

Hayne C R 1978 Safe . . . sure? Physiotherapy 64(1) 10–13

House of Commons 1987 Third report from education, science and arts committee: special educational needs: implementation of Education Act (1981). HMSO, London

Maclure S 1989 Education re-formed. Hodder and Stoughton, London

National Children's Bureau 1989 Information sheet no. 91 Highlight: the Children Act (1989). Barnardo's/National Children's Bureau, London

Radar (Royal Association for Disability and Rehabilitation) 1988 Act now: steering committee for the implementation of the Disabled Persons Act 1986. Radar, London

Russell P 1990 Introducing the Children Act. British Journal of Special Education 17(1): 35–37

Sim J 1986 Informed consent: ethical implications for physiotherapy. Physiotherapy 72(12): 584–587

Solity J, Raybould E 1988 A teacher's guide to special needs. Open University Press, Milton Keynes

Appendix

VOLUNTARY AND STATUTORY RESOURCES

Access Committee for England
35 Great Smith Street
London SW1P 3BJ
071 222–7980

ACE — Advisory Centre for Education
18 Victoria Park Square
London E2 9PB
081 980 4596

Action Against Allergy
43 The Downs
London SW20
081 947 5082

Arthrogryposis Group
The Oaks
Common Head Lane
Gillingham
Dorset SP8 4SW

Association for All Speech Impaired Children (AFASIC)
347 Central Markets
Smithfield
London EC1A 9NH
071 236 3632

Association of Parents of Vaccine-Damaged Children
2 Church Street
Shipston-on-Stour
Warwickshire
0608 61595

Association for Spina Bifida and Hydrocephalus
Tavistock House North
Tavistock Square
London WC1H 9HJ
071 388 1382

Association of Workers for Maladjusted Children
New Barns School
Church Lane
Toddington
Glos GL54 5DH
0236 689467

Asthma Society and Friends of the Asthma Research Council
300 Upper Street
London N1 2XX
071 928 3099

Barnardo's
Tanners Lane
Barkingside
Ilford
Essex IG6 1QG
081 550 8822

British Agencies for Adoption and Fostering
11 Southwark Street
London SE1 1RQ
071 407 8800

British Association of Music Therapy
Harperbury Hospital
Harper Lane
Shirley Radlett
Herts

British Association of Occupational Therapists
20 Rede Place
London W2 4TU

British Council for Rehabilitation of the Disabled
Tavistock House (South)
Tavistock Square
London WC1H 9LB
071 387 4037/8

British Diabetic Association
10 Queen Anne Street
London W1M 0BD
071 323 1531

British Dyslexia Association
98 London Road
Reading
Berkshire RG1 5AU
0734 668271

British Epilepsy Association
40 Hanover Square
Leeds
West Yorkshire LS3 1BE
0532 439393

British Institute of Mental Handicap
Wolverhampton Road
Kidderminster
Worcestershire DY10 3PP
0562 850251

British Rheumatism and Arthritis Association
6 Grosvenor Crescent
London SW1X 7ER
071 235 0902

British Sports Association for the Disabled
Hayward House
Barnard Crescent
Aylesbury
Bucks HP21 9PP
0296 27889

Brittle Bone Society
Unit 4
Block 20
Carlunie Rd
Dunsinane Estate
Dundee DD2 3QT
0382 67603

Chartered Society of Physiotherapy
14 Bedford Row
London WC1R 4ED
071 242 1941

Child Growth Foundation
2 Mayfield Avenue
Chiswick
London W4 1PW
081 994 7625

Children's Legal Centre
20 Compton Terrace
London N1 2UN
071 359 6251

Cleft Lip and Palate Association
1 Eastwood Gardens
Kenton
Newcastle-upon Tyne
NE3 3DQ
091 285 9396

College of Speech Therapists
Harold Poster House
6 Lechmere Rd
London NW2 5BU
081 459 8521

Contact-a-Family
16 Strutton Ground
London SW1
071 222 2211

Cystic Fibrosis Research Trust
Alexandra House
5 Blyth Road Bromley
Kent BR1 3RS
081 464 7211

DES Publications Despatch Centre
Honeypot Lane
Canons Park
Stanmore HA7 4PT
081 952 2366

Diabetes Foundation
177a Tennison Road
London SE25 5NF
081 656 5467

Disabled Living Foundation
346 Kensington High Street
London W14 8NS
071 289 6111

Down's Children's Association
4 Oxford Street
London W1N 9FC
071 580 0511

Down's Syndrome Association
12/13 Clapham Common
Southside
London SW4 7AA
071 720 0008

Dyslexia Institute
Head Office
133 Gresham Road
Staines
Middlesex TW18 8AJ
0784 59498

Education Otherwise
25 Common Lane
Hemingford Abbots
Cambridgeshire PE18 9AN

Enuresis Resource and Information Centre
65 St Michael's Hill
Bristol BS2 8DZ
0272 264920

Family Fund
PO Box 50
York YO1 1UY
0904 21115

Family Welfare Association
501–505 Kingsland Rd
Dalston
London E8 4AU
071 254 6251

Foresight — The Association for the Promotion of Preconceptual Care
The Old Vicarage
Church Lane
Witley
Godalming
Surrey GU8 5PN
0428 684500

Foundation for the Study of Infant Deaths
35 Belgrave Square
London SW1X 8QB
071 235 0965

Haemophilia Society
123 Westminster Bridge Rd
London SE1 7HR
071 928 2020

Handicapped Adventure Playground Association
Fulham Palace
Bishop's Avenue
London SW6 6EA
071 731 1435

Headway, National Head Injuries Association
200 Mansfield Road
Nottingham NG1 3HX
0602 622782

Health Education Council
78 New Oxford Street
London WC1A 1AH
071 631 0930

Hester Adrian Research Centre
The University of Manchester
Manchester M13 9P4

HMSO
PO Box 276
London SW8 5DT
071 211 5656

Hyperactive Children's Support Group
71 Whyke Lane
Chichester
Sussex PO19 2LD
0903 725182

Independent Panel of Special Education Experts
12 Marsh Road
Tillingham
Essex CM0 7SZ
0621 87781

Infantile Hypercalcaemia Foundation
Mulberry Cottage
37 Mulberry Green
Old Harlow
Essex CM17 0EY
0279 27214

King's Fund Centre
(Part of King Edward's Hospital Fund)
126 Albert Street
London NW1 7NF
071 267 6111

Leukaemia Care Society
PO Box 82
Exeter EX2 5DP
0392 64848

Mencap: Royal Society For Mentally Handicapped Children and Adults
Mencap National Centre
123 Golden Lane
London EC1Y 0RT
071 454 0454

Muscular Dystrophy Group of Great Britain and N. Ireland
Nattrass House
35 Macaulay Road
London SW4 0QP
071 720 8055

National Association for Deaf-Blind and Rubella Handicapped
311 Gray's Inn Road
London WC1X 8PT
071 278 1000

National Association for Gifted Children
Park Campus
Broughton Green Road
Northampton NN2 7AL
0604 792300

National Association for the Welfare of Children in Hospital
Argyle House
29–31 Euston Road
London NW1 25D
071 883 2041

National Autistic Society
276 Willesden Lane
London NW2 5RB
081 451 3844

National Bureau for Students with Disabilities (Skill) — Formerly National Bureau for Handicapped Students
336 Brixton Road
London SW9 7AA
071 274 0565

National Children's Bureau
8 Wakley Street
London EC1V 7QE
071 278 9441

National Council for Special Education
1 Wood Street
Stratford upon Avon CV37 6JE
0789 205332

National Deaf, Blind, and Rubella Association — Sense
311 Gray's Inn Road
London WC1X 8PT
071 278 1005

National Deaf Children's Society
45 Hereford Road
London W2 5AH
071 229 9272

National Eczema Society
Tavistock House East
Tavistock Square
London WC1H 9SR
071 388 4097

National Elfrida Rathbone Society
1st Floor
Princess House
105/107 Princess Street
Manchester M1 6DD
061 236 5358

National Society for Autistic Children
276 Willesden Lane
London NW2 5RB
081 451 1114

National Society for Phenylketonuria and Allied Disorders
26 Towngate Grove
Mirfield
West Yorkshire

National Society for the Prevention of Cruelty to Children
67 Saffron Hill
London EC1N 8RS
071 242 1626

Play Matters — National Toy Libraries Association
68 Churchway
London NW1 1LT
071 387 9592

PHAB
Tavistock House North
Tavistock Square
London WC1H 9HX
071 388 1963

Royal National Institute for the Blind (RNIB)
224 Great Portland Street
London W1N 6AA
071 388 1266

Royal National Institute for the Deaf
105 Gower Street
London WC1E 6AH
071 387 8033

Royal Society for the Prevention of Accidents (RSPA)
Cannon House
The Priory
Queensway
Birmingham B4 6BS
021 233 2461

Save the Children Fund
Mary Datchelor House
17 Grove Lane
Camberwell
London SE5 8RD
071 703 5400

Scoliosis Association (UK)
380–384 Harrow Road
London W9 2HU
071 289 5652

Sequal — Special Equipment and Aids for Living
27 Thames House
140 Battersea Park Road
London SW11

Spastics Society
12 Park Crescent
London W1N 4EQ
071 636 5020

Stillbirth and Neonatal Death Society
28 Portland Place
London W1N 4DE
071 436 5881

Toy Libraries Association
Seabrook House
Wyllyotts Manor
Darkes Lane
Potters Bar
Herts EN6 2HL
0707 44571

Tuberous Sclerosis Association of Great Britain
Little Barnsley Farm
Catshill
Bromsgrove
Worcs B61 0NQ
0527 71898

Twins and Multiple Birth Association
59 Sunnyside
Worksop
Notts S81 7LN
0909 479250

Voluntary Council for Handicapped Children
8 Wakley Street
London EC1V 7QE
071 278 9441

FURTHER READING

Disability Rights Handbook — published each April by The Disability Alliance, 25 Denmark St, London WC2H 8NS

Directory for Disabled People (1987) RADAR, Woodhead Faulkner, Cambridge, UK

Glossaries

PHYSIOTHERAPY TERMS

Acidosis — a disturbance of acid-base balance leading to a fall in blood pH.

Agnosia — inability to recognise the nature and significance of objects, sounds or images.

Amniocentesis — sampling the amniotic fluid surrounding the developing fetus to determine the presence or absence of abnormalities.

Antepartum — before birth.

Anticonvulsant — medication taken to control seizures.

Apgar score — scoring system used to evaluate a baby's physical condition. Used one and five minutes after birth.

Aphasia – loss of the ability to use expressive or to understand receptive language.

Apnoea — an episode of arrested breathing.

Apraxia — inability to plan and perform purposeful movements which are coordinated and understood.

Associated movement — a normal balancing or coordinating movement of one part of the body to compensate for or adjust to movement of another part.

Associated reaction — increased tone in an affected limb or limbs of a child with cerebral palsy following effort, the performance or the anticipation of movement.

Autosomes — the first 22 pairs of chromosomes.

Babbling — the different randomly repeated speech sounds made by babies from approximately 4 months onwards.

Backward chaining — the sequence of steps required to complete a particular task, i.e. drinking from a cup, learned from a reverse order. In this way the first skill learned is the one which completes the task.

Bone dysplasia — abnormally formed bone.

Bradycardia — a slow heart rate, usually considered to be below 60 beats per minute.

Case conference — a meeting of the people involved in working with a disabled child to discuss the current situation and to share and plan for future treatment and education.

Centile chart — reference charts used to establish appropriate rates of increase in height, weight and head circumference.

Cephalocaudal — neurological development proceeding from head to tail.

Chelator — a substance that binds and inactivates metals.

Clonus — rapid alternating muscle contraction and relaxation.

Cofactors — another chemical, often a vitamin, which helps enzymes in biochemical pathways work at maximum efficiency.

Compliance — the elasticity of the respiratory system.

Concept formation — an understanding of meaningful categories and groupings, i.e. shape, colour, size, function.

Congenital — present at or before birth.

Cyanosis — a blue tinge to the skin, lips and extremities due to a lack of oxygenated blood.

Delayed development — development in any or all areas which is significantly below the norm for the child's chronological age.

Disability — the limitation of a person's functional ability to carry out the everyday activities of daily living. See Handicap, Impairment.

Dysmorphic — unusual or striking facial features.

Dyspraxia — a partial loss of the ability to coordinate movement.

Echolalia — the automatic repetition of words or phrases, frequently parrot fashion, without fully understanding their meaning.

Epidemiology — a study of the pattern of frequency and distribution of disease.

FEV — Forced expiratory volume.

Functional assessment — an evaluation of the ability to carry out the tasks of daily living.

FVC — Forced vital capacity.

Grand mal — a form of seizure characterised by sudden loss of consciousness followed by a general convulsion.

Grunting — a sound made when an infant in respiratory distress breathes out against a partially closed glottis. (A self-administered and expiratory pressure which probably helps to keep airways patent.)

Handicap — a general term used to describe the effects of intellectual, emotional, social or physical disabilities which prevent an individual from leading an ordinary life. Also used when these factors affect a child's learning in a mainstream environment. See Disability, and Impairment.

Hepatomegaly — liver enlargement.

Hydrocephalus — an enlargement of the head due to the accumulation of cerebrospinal fluid in the ventricles of the brain.

Hyperactivity — constant movement from place to place; inability to attend to anything for longer than a few seconds.

Hyperammonaemia — an increased level of ammonia in the blood, above 50 µmol/l.

Hypertonia — increased muscle tone.

Hypoglycaemia — a low blood sugar, less than 2.8 µmol/l, after the first month of life.

Hypotonia — decreased muscle tone.

Idiopathic — a condition for which no cause can be found.

Impairment — any injury, damage or defect which prevents normal physical or mental functioning. See Disability, Handicap.

Incidence — the relative frequency of an event.

Interdisciplinary team — a group of people from various disciplines or sectors working jointly towards a common negotiated and agreed goal for a child or for a service. See Key worker.

Kernicterus — damage, usually in the newborn child, caused by jaundice resulting from incompatibility between the blood of the mother and the child.

Key worker — a team member nominated by the team and parents to act as coordinator and link person in the planning of services to an individual family. See Interdisciplinary team.

Kinaesthetic awareness — an awareness of the position of the body and the range, direction and extent of movement being performed, obtained through muscles, tendons and joints.

Laterality — an awareness of the right and left sides of the body. Frequently used to indicate a preference in usage.

Meconium — the dark green mucus present in the intestines of the fetus. Forms the first stool after birth.

Modelling — learning behaviour by observing and copying someone else.

Myoglobinuria — the presence in the urine of a special form of haemoglobin usually found in muscle due to muscle breakdown.

Neonate — infant aged from 0–1 month.

Norm — an acknowledged average or typical score used as a basis against which individual scores can be compared.

Objective — a precise statement which details what a child is expected to do, the way in which it will be observed and the means by which it will be carried out.

Object permanence — an awareness that objects still exist when they are out of sight, hidden, or have moved away.

Orthosis — an orthopaedic aid to improve movement function and to support and correct body alignment.

PEFR — Peak expiratory flow rate.

Preterm — born before 37 completed weeks of gestation.

Proprioception — knowledge and understanding of the position of joints in space during active or passive movement.

Pulmonary hypoplasia — incomplete development of the lungs.

Recession — indrawing of chest wall in child with respiratory distress.

Stereognosis — ability to recognise shape, size, texture and weight of objects placed in the hand by touch alone.

Stridor — harsh, high-pitched respiratory sound mainly caused by laryngeal oedema or narrowing.

Task analysis — breaking down a particular defined task into its component sub-skills.

Teratogenic — an agent that causes malformations in a developing embryo.

Visual discrimination — ability to differentiate visually between different shapes; essential for reading development.

Visual perception — ability to give meaning to what is seen.

SYNDROMES AND GENETIC DISORDERS

Achondroplasia — characterised by disproportionately short limbs, low nasal bridge, prominent forehead and lumbar lordosis. Mild hypotonia may be present but intelligence is usually normal.

Angleman syndrome — children present with developmental delay during the first year of life. Progressive, diffuse brain atrophy results in epilepsy, severe learning difficulties, an ataxic gait and jerky limb movements. Facial features are characterised by a prominent jaw and wide mouth.

Arthrogryposis multiplex congenita — joints fixed in flexion or extension at birth due to multiple joint contractures. Muscle wasting present.

Coffin–Lowry syndrome — a pattern of coarse facial features with prominent forehead, large hands with tapering fingers and moderate growth deficiency. Severe mental retardation present.

Cri-du-Chat syndrome — small-for-dates babies with growth retardation and microcephaly. Congenital heart defects. Characterised by mewing cry. Severe mental retardation present.

Cystic fibrosis — recurrent lung infections, combined with malabsorption problems and failure to thrive. Normal intelligence.

Down's syndrome — characterised by short stature, hypotonia, short fingers, small nose and upward slant to the eyes. Cardiac disease occurs in approximately 40% of cases. Severe mental retardation present.

Duchenne muscular dystrophy — a progressive muscle wasting with enlarged calf muscles, respiratory difficulty and heart failure. There may be some mental retardation.

Edwards syndrome or **Trisomy 18** — small-for-dates babies with hand deformities and congenital heart defects. Mental retardation present. Survival beyond 1 year of age in only 10% of cases.

Fetal rubella syndrome — effects range from deafness to severe learning difficulties with cataracts and heart defects.

Hunter syndrome — onset at approximately 2 to 4 years of age. Coarsening of facial features, joint contractures, progressive deafness. Variable mental retardation, the more severe the younger the onset.

Hurler's syndrome — characterised by severely retarded progress between the ages of 6 and 18 months, short stature, progressive mental retardation. Corneal clouding, spinal and limb abnormalities, and liver and spleen enlargement also present.

Klinefelter syndrome — growth characterised by long limbs and thin appearance. Moderate learning difficulties with late onset of speech. Tendency towards behavioural problems.

Marfan syndrome — characterised by tall stature and thin limbs, dislocation of the lens of the eye, myopia, aortic aneurysms. Intelligence not usually affected.

Neurofibromatosis syndrome — characterised by *cafe au lait* spots over the body with nerve tumours on the body and in eyes and ears. Intelligence usually normal.

Osteogenesis imperfecta — an increased susceptibility to fractures that results in bony deformities. Skin often appears translucent. Deafness often present.

Phenylketonuria — enzyme deficiency resulting in hyperactivity and profound mental retardation. Children usually have blond hair and blue eyes.

Pierre Robin syndrome — an early anomaly in the development of the mandible, combined with a cleft palate and posterior displacement of the tongue. Results in respiratory obstruction and failure to thrive.

Prader–Willi syndrome — onset of progressive obesity from infancy to 6 years. Small hands, feet and genitalia with severe hypotonia in early infancy. Severe mental retardation.

Retinitis Pigmentosa — a group of conditions resulting in retinal degeneration and progressive blindness.

Rubinstein–Taybi syndrome — characterised by short stature with large thumbs and toes and large beaked nose. Microcephaly and mental retardation present.

Tay–Sachs' disease — a degenerative disorder of the nervous system with profound mental retardation, deafness, blindness and epilepsy.

Tuberous sclerosis — calcium deposits in the brain result in mental retardation and infantile spasms. *Cafe au lait* spots appear on the skin together with fibromatous plaques and nodules.

Turner syndrome — a faulty chromosome distribution resulting in females of short stature. A webbed neck of ovarian disgenesis also present. Cardiac defects and hearing impairment may occur. Usually normal intelligence.

Werdnig–Hoffmann disease — infantile form of spinal muscular atrophy. An early onset progresses to death within a year or so; progression of the disease is slower with a later onset.

FURTHER READING

Smith D W (1982) Recognisable patterns of human malformation, W B Saunders, Philadelphia, USA

Index